THIRD EDITION

NUTRITION IN PUBLIC HEALTH

A Handbook for Developing Programs and Services

Edited by

Sari Edelstein, PhD, RD

Associate Professor
Department of Nutrition
School of Health Sciences
Simmons College
Boston, Massachusetts

JONES & BARTLETT
LEARNING

World Headquarters
Jones & Bartlett Learning
40 Tall Pine Drive
Sudbury, MA 01776
978-443-5000
info@jblearning.com
www.jblearning.com

Jones & Bartlett Learning Canada
6339 Ormindale Way
Mississauga, Ontario L5V 1J2
Canada

Jones & Bartlett Learning International
Barb House, Barb Mews
London W6 7PA
United Kingdom

Jones & Bartlett Learning books and products are available through most bookstores and online booksellers. To contact Jones & Bartlett Learning directly, call 800-832-0034, fax 978-443-8000, or visit our website, www.jblearning.com.

Substantial discounts on bulk quantities of Jones & Bartlett Learning publications are available to corporations, professional associations, and other qualified organizations. For details and specific discount information, contact the special sales department at Jones & Bartlett Learning via the above contact information or send an email to specialsales@jblearning.com.

This publication is designed to provide accurate and authoritative information in regard to the Subject Matter covered. It is sold with the understanding that the publisher is not engaged in rendering legal, accounting, or other professional service. If legal advice or other expert assistance is required, the service of a competent professional person should be sought.

Production Credits
Publisher, Higher Education: Cathleen Sether
Senior Acquisitions Editor: Shoshanna Goldberg
Senior Associate Editor: Amy L. Bloom
Senior Editorial Assistant: Kyle Hoover
Associate Marketing Manager: Jody Sullivan
Production Director: Amy Rose
Senior Production Editor: Renée Sekerak
Production Assistant: Sean Coombs
V.P., Manufacturing and Inventory Control: Therese Connell
Assistant Photo Researcher: Rebecca Ritter
Cover Design: Kristin E. Parker
Cover Image: © Peter Cox/ShutterStock, Inc.
Composition: Auburn Associates, Inc.
Printing and Binding: Courier Stoughton
Cover Printing: Courier Stoughton

Library of Congress Cataloging-in-Publication Data
Nutrition in public health : a handbook for developing programs and services
/ [edited by] Sari Edelstein.—3rd ed.
        p. ; cm.
    Includes bibliographical references and index.
    ISBN-13: 978-0-7637-7791-3 (pbk.)
    ISBN-10: 0-7637-7791-9 (pbk.)
    1. Nutrition—United States—Handbooks, manuals, etc. 2. Public
health—United States—Handbooks, manuals, etc. 3. Nutrition policy—United
States—Handbooks, manuals, etc. I. Edelstein, Sari.
    [DNLM: 1. Nutritional Physiological Phenomena—United States. 2. Needs
Assessment—United States. 3. Nutrition Policy—United States. 4. Public
Health Practice—United States. 5. Risk Factors—United States. QU 145
N9752 2011]
    RA601.N84 2011
    362.17′6—dc22
                                    2010024630

6048

Printed in the United States of America
14 13 12 11 10   10 9 8 7 6 5 4 3 2 1

Dedication

To all our wonderful students,
who will make a positive change worldwide for generations to come.

Contents

Foreword

The beginning of the 21st century is a time of contrasts. On one hand, our food supply continues to be reliable, abundant, and relatively cheap when compared with other countries. On the other hand, we are faced with a rapidly expanding epidemic of obesity in adults and children. Unfortunately, this problem is also emerging in many developing countries with increasing industrialization and adoption of industrialized lifestyle. Because of this, we will be facing a global problem of diseases related to obesity, such as type-2 diabetes and cardiovascular disease. In addition, we also face new challenges to safeguard our food supply from emerging infectious organisms to contamination.

At the same time, a tremendous amount of data is available on how nutrients and other dietary factors can enhance wellness and prevent diseases. This, together with sophisticated technology, provides us with the tools to turn around the nation's nutrition-related health problems, and move toward the goals of *Healthy People 2020*. Although our society is filled with constant messages for consumption (hence the risk of over-consumption), many governmental and nonprofit organizations have also launched efforts to curb over-consumption. This is the state of nutritional issues for the United States—a combination of problems and resources, and competing forces to influence the nation's consumption patterns.

In light of these issues, healthy eating and good nutrition need to be promoted on two fronts: personal knowledge of nutrition, skills, and responsibility to eat healthy, as well as a society that makes it easy to practice good nutrition for people at different stages in their lives. Both fronts are subjects of public health nutrition. The former should be taught in schools and other settings, while the latter in- volves policymaking in various institutions and at the government level and the need to seek cooperation from the food industry.

The knowledge of good health is not a secret, and the public health nutritionist plays a crucial role in steering a nation toward better health. Even for those who are not directly or primarily involved in this field, there is a little bit of public health nutritionist in all of us. We all can contribute to public health nutrition through civic involvement, such as working with public schools to improve school meals, and by making our voices heard to influence public policy. *Nutrition in Public Health* empowers professionals involved in public health nutrition to perform their jobs better, and to make an important impact on people's health. But it is also useful to all those in health professions.

Dr. Sari Edelstein has been involved in various aspects of nutrition for many years. She is an experienced dietitian, educator, and leader. Her experience in this area, plus the expertise of the contributing authors, represents an enormous wealth of knowledge. The subjects discussed in this book are timely and significant, and make this text a must-have for both students and practitioners of public health nutrition.

Teresa T. Fung, ScD, RD
Associate Professor in Nutrition
Simmons College
Boston, MA
Adjunct Assistant Professor in Nutrition
Harvard School of Public Health
Cambridge, MA

Preface

What Is Public Health Nutrition?
Sari Edelstein, PhD, RD

■ PUBLIC HEALTH NUTRITION

Public health nutrition is a complex, multifaceted set of programs that is dedicated to improving the health of the population through improved nutrition. In more detail, public health nutrition primarily exists to[1]:

- Improve the health of the whole population and teach high-risk subgroups within the population improved nutrition;
- Emphasize health promotion and disease prevention through improved nutrition; and
- Provide integrated community efforts for improved nutrition with leadership demonstrated by government offices.

In order to accomplish these three primary elements of public health nutrition, the U.S. Public Health Service has delineated 10 Essential Public Health Service Functions, as listed below.[2] Each of these 10 elements will assist the reader in understanding the steps that must be taken by public health professionals to bring about definitive qualitative and quantitative results.

1. Monitor health status to identify and solve community health problems
2. Identify and investigate the causes of health problems and health hazards in the community
3. Mobilize community partnerships and action to identify and solve health problems
4. Develop policies and plans that support individual and community health
5. Enforce laws and regulations that protect health and ensure safety
6. Link people to needed personal health services and assure the provision of health care when otherwise unavailable
7. Inform, educate, and empower people about health issues
8. Evaluate effectiveness, accessibility, and quality of personal and population-based health services
9. Assure a competent public health and personal healthcare workforce
10. Research for new insights and innovative solutions to health problems

When these 10 elements are expanded to full explanations for the reader, we create a compendium of information that mirrors the table of contents in this book. In this section, we recreate for the reader the organization of *Nutrition in Public Health, Third Edition* that embraces the Essential Public Health Service Functions.

■ PART I APPLYING NUTRITION TO PUBLIC HEALTH

Chapter 1 Nutritional Epidemiology: An Introduction

Chapter 2 Applying Nutrition Science to the Public's Health

In Part I, the reader is introduced to the role of nutritional epidemiology in public health.

In Chapter 2, we experience the various studies that have brought public health nutrition to the standards we enjoy today. The authors of Chapter 2 bring the reader through every hallmark of nutritional science, explain how these standards were attained, and translate what these standards mean for the public health recipients of today.

■ PART II ASSESSING AND INTERVENING IN THE COMMUNITY'S NUTRITION NEEDS

Chapter 3 Community Needs Assessment

Chapter 4 Reaching Out to Those at Highest Nutritional Risk

Chapter 5 Addressing Overweight in Children: A Public Health Perspective

Chapter 6 Intervening to Change the Public's Eating Behavior

In Part II, the reader is introduced to how public health nutritionists target care for those at highest risk. In order to find those at highest risk, a needs assessment of the community must be performed. Chapter 3 describes the concepts and issues involved in needs assessment of the public health arena. It is through proper needs assessment that the public health nutritionist can serve those who need help in ways that are most useful. In Chapter 4, we see the results of more than a century of needs assessments, with the designation of the young and the old as being those groups we must serve. In addition, those with illness and disability must be supported by public health nutrition services. Perhaps reaching those in need has been one of public health nutrition's most difficult challenges. In the 21st century, public health nutrition needs assessments have determined that America's indulgent eating habits have brought us to nutritional catastrophe. The epidemics of child (Chapter 5) and adult obesity (Chapter 6) are two additional areas in which public health nutrition must find a way to intervene and provide solutions.

■ PART III SHAPING THE POLICIES THAT AFFECT THE PUBLIC'S HEALTH

Chapter 7 Creating Public Policy

Chapter 8 Advocating and Influencing Health and Nutrition Policies

Chapter 9 Role of the United States Department of Agriculture in Public Health Nutrition

In Part III, we shift gears to investigate how science and needs assessment translate into public policy. It is through governmental policy that public health nutritionists are directed to educate and serve the public. Chapters 7 and 8 describe how nutrition policy is created, advocated, and influenced by the public, health practitioners, lobbyists, and legislators. What should be imparted to the reader in these chapters is the need for dietitians and nutritionists to get involved in advocating and influencing the passing of important nutrition policy. Chapter 9 demonstrates to the reader how the USDA acts on nutrition policy once it is made and illustrates the complexity of that role in fulfilling the challenges of public health nutrition.

■ PART IV PROMOTING THE PUBLIC'S NUTRITIONAL HEALTH

Chapter 10 Growing a Healthier Nation: Maternal, Infant, Child, and Adolescent Nutrition

Chapter 11 Importance of Public Health Nutrition Programs in Preventing Disease and Promoting Adult Health

Chapter 12 Assuring Nutrition for Older Adults

Chapter 13 Providing Nutrition Services in Public Health Primary Care

Chapter 14 The Baby Boomers: Identification of Wellness Needs

Chapter 15 Maintaining Nutrition and Food Service Standards in Group Care

Part IV includes those chapters that illustrate the programs and services public health nutrition provides for the differing groups of Americans. Through needs assessment, scientific study, and policy, many groups have been identified as recipients of public health nutrition. In Chapter 10, the programs and services, along with the challenges of serving children, adolescents, and women are discussed. In Chapters 11 through 15, the reader is educated about the public health nutrition programs that affect adults, a special subset of adults such as the baby boomers and the elderly. Each group differs in needs and challenges, but all will need to be provided for by public health nutrition now and in the future.

■ PART V PROTECTING THE PUBLIC'S NUTRITIONAL HEALTH

Chapter 16 Safeguarding the Food Supply

Chapter 17 Food Security and Adequate Food Access for the Public

Chapter 18 Security of the Food Supply and Bioterrorism Preparedness

Chapters 17 and 18 in Part V bring us to a whole new frontier of public health nutrition. That new frontier is securing adequate food for those who still live in poverty, as discussed in Chapter 17, and the fact that we must be protected from potential bioterrorism plots directed at our food supply, as discussed in Chapter 18. Despite the present outreach of public health nutrition, a hefty percentage of Americans still live without adequate food and/or live in a constant state of fear of being without food, thus showing that we have far to go in reaching those at highest risk. Yet we still face the stinging realization that food, too, must be kept secure because it can be a potent avenue for terrorism. Public health nutrition will now have to meet the challenge of keeping food safe from many forms of invasion.

■ PART VI MANAGING THE SYSTEM

Chapter 19 Planning and Evaluating Nutrition Services for the Community

Chapter 20 Managing Data

Chapter 21 Managing Money

Part VI provides the reader with fundamental information for how public health nutrition is funded. Chapter 19 details how nutrition services are planned and evaluated, such that targeted funds can be delineated to effective programs. In order to evaluate the effectiveness and cost of a program, data must be collected and managed appropriately, as discussed in Chapter 20. Lastly, a discussion on how money is managed will help the reader take public health nutrition from funding to appropriations is shown in Chapter 21.

■ PART VII MOBILIZING PERSONNEL

Chapter 22 Staffing Public Health Nutrition Programs and Services

Chapter 23 Managing Public Health Nutrition Personnel

Chapter 24 Leveraging Nutrition Education Through the Public Health Team

Chapter 22 in Part VII reviews the core functions of the professionals that comprise the public health nutrition team and designates the number needed to carry out the programs and services. In addition, Chapter 23 educates the reader on effective management skills that enable the public health nutrition professional to work through the ranks and perform those necessary services. Nutrition education services, as discussed in Chapter 24, are the final result of all the program planning, scientific data collection, nutrition policy, money appropriation, and safeguarding and distributing of the American public's food.

■ PART VIII SURVIVING IN A COMPETITIVE WORLD

Chapter 25 Networking for Nutrition

Chapter 26 Marketing Nutrition Programs and Services

Chapter 27 Earning Administrative Support

Chapter 28 Striving for Excellence and Envisioning the Future

Part VIII imparts important features to any program: networking, marketing, striving for excellence, and envisioning the future. For any program to be successful, these elements must be present and remain as one of public health nutrition's most daunting challenges. In order for programs to work and meet the needs of those targeted to receive help, networking and marketing must be carefully planned. Chapters 25 and 26 give the reader insight into these tools. Chapter 27 instills in the reader the need to market nutri-

tion programs within the organization of public health to assure survival. And, Chapter 28 reminds the reader that public health nutrition is a dynamic process and changes constantly. We must be able to anticipate needs and follow with provision of those needs to be successful.

■ BOOK FEATURES

Nutrition in Public Health, Third Edition has maintained the cutting edge relevance of the *Second Edition*, while adding several enhancement features.

- More in-depth information: Each chapter from the *Second Edition* has been updated and enhanced to give the reader a vast supply of background information and a full understanding of public health nutrition. In addition, new topics have been added to the *Third Edition* to reflect current public health issues. These include:
  - Obesity in America
  - Programs for the aged
  - Demands of the baby boomers
  - Food insecurity
  - Food bioterrorism
  - The role of the USDA in public health nutrition

- Section transitions: The text is divided into eight sections that pull the reader into the world of public health nutrition in a very organized fashion.

- Text Boxes: Interesting web sites, relevant information, and word definitions have been included in text boxes for easy reader viewing.

- Relevant appendices.
  - Appendix A: Helpful Nutrition Web Sites
  - Appendix B: State Health Department Web Sites
  - Appendix C: Learning Activities

- Instructor resources, including PowerPoint Presentations and an Instructor's Manual, are available as free instructor downloads from your sales representative.

References

1. *Division of Epidemiology*. School of Public Health, University of Minnesota. The LET Program, 1999.

2. *U.S. Public Health Service Essential Public Health Services*. Work Group of the Core Public Health Function Steering Committee, 1994.

Acknowledgments

The editor and contributing authors of *Nutrition in Public Health: A Handbook for Developing Programs and Services, Third Edition* would like to recognize the editor of the *First Edition*, Mildred Kaufman, MS, RD. Mildred is an alumnus of Simmons College, where the majority of contributing authors call home, and a past Department Head of University of North Carolina Chapel Hill's School of Public Health. It is Mildred's pioneering spirit and fine efforts on the *First Edition* of this book that have made the subsequent editions possible. We are grateful to Mildred for this and her contribution to the field of nutrition, dietetics, and public health.

Contributors

Deepa Arora, PhD
Middle Georgia College

Thelma B. Baker, PhD, RD, LD
Howard University

Elizabeth Barden, PhD
Northwestern University

Cynthia Taft Bayerl, MS, RD, LDN
Massachusetts Department of Public Health

Jeannette M. Beasley, PhD, MPH, RD
Group Health Cooperative

Margaret L. Bogle, PhD, RD, LD
United States Department of Agriculture

Lisa S. Brown, PhD, RD
Simmons College

Barbara Bruemmer, PhD, RD, CD
University of Washington

Katherine Cairns, MPH, MBA, RD
Summit Health Group

Joseph M. Carlin, MS, RD, LDN, FADA
Administration on Aging

Shirley Chao, MS, RD, LDN
Office of Elder Affairs, Boston

Stacey Chappa, RD
WIC, Kalamazoo, MI

Rachel Colchamiro, MPH, RD, LDN
Massachusetts Department of Public Health

Pamella Darby, MS, MPH, RD
New York University

Teresa T. Fung, ScD, RD
Simmons College
Harvard University

Stefanie Giampa, BA
Simmons College

Edna Harris-Davis, MS, MPH, RD, LD
Georgia Department of Public Health

Nancie Herbold, EdD, RD
Simmons College

David H. Holben, PhD, RD, LD
Ohio University

Jan Kallio, MS, RD, LDN
Altarum Institute

Patti S. Landers, PhD, RD, LD
University of Oklahoma

Beth Leonberg, MS, RD, CSP, FADA, LDN
Nutrition Outcomes, LLC

Beverly J. McCabe-Sellers, PhD, RD
United States Department of Agriculture

Shortie McKinney, PhD, RD, LDN, FADA
Marshall University

Elizabeth Metallinos-Katsaras, PhD, RD
Simmons College

Yeemay Su Miller, MS, RD
Simmons College

Julie M. Moreschi, MS, RD, LDN
Benedictine University

Theresa A. Nicklas, DrPH
Baylor College of Medicine

Esther Okeiyi, PhD, RD, LDN
North Carolina Central University

Carol E. O'Neil, PhD, MPH, LDN, RD
Louisiana State University

Bruce Rengers, PhD, RD
Metropolitan State College of Denver

Judith Sharlin, PhD, RD
Palm Beach State College

Arlene Spark, EdD, RD, FADA, FACN
Hunter College

Bonnie Spear, PhD, RD
University of Alabama at Birmingham

Inger Stallmann-Jorgensen, MS, RD, LD
Georgia Prevention Institute, Medical College of Georgia

Paul N. Taylor, PhD
Simmons College

Marcia Thomas, MS, MPH, RD
New York University

Dolores M. Wolongevicz, PhD, MS, RD, LDN
Boston University

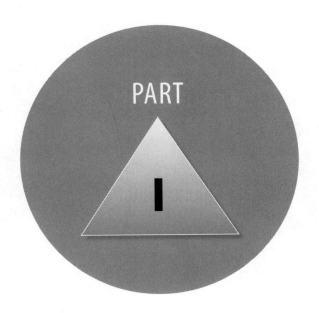

PART

I

Applying Nutrition to
Public Health

CHAPTER 1

Nutritional Epidemiology: An Introduction

LISA S. BROWN, PhD, RD
DOLORES M. WOLONGEVICZ, PhD, MS, RD, LDN
STEFANIE GIAMPA, BA

CHAPTER 2

Applying Nutrition Science to the Public's Health

CAROL E. O'NEIL, PhD, MPH, LDN, RD
THERESA A. NICKLAS, DrPH

Chapter 1 reviews public health nutrition epidemiology. *Epidemiology* is the study of disease distribution within a population and the factors, both protective and promoting, that influence the occurrence of disease. Epidemiology utilizes both observational and experimental techniques to discover patterns related to disease development. Chapter 2 describes the various studies that brought about the public health nutrition standards we enjoy today.

Nutritional Epidemiology: An Introduction

Lisa S. Brown, PhD, RD

Dolores M. Wolongevicz, PhD, MS, RD, LDN

Stefanie Giampa, BA

READER OBJECTIVES   After studying this chapter and reflecting on the contents, you should be able to:

1. Define nutritional epidemiology and understand its role in health and disease.
2. Identify the various types of study designs commonly used in nutritional epidemiologic research.
   a. Discuss the strengths and weaknesses of each study design.
3. Describe the commonly used dietary assessment methods in nutritional epidemiologic research.
   a. Discuss the strengths and weaknesses of each dietary assessment method.
4. Discuss important methodological issues in dietary data collection and analyses in nutritional epidemiologic research.

■ OVERVIEW OF EPIDEMIOLOGY

Epidemiology is the study of disease distribution within a population and the factors, both protective and promoting, that influence the occurrence of disease. Epidemiology utilizes both observational and experimental techniques to discover patterns related to disease development. One of the first epidemiologic studies of the modern era occurred in 1854 when John Snow discovered that a water pump on Broad Street in the Soho district of London was the source of a cholera outbreak within the city. His systematic technique of counting the number of cases in each area of London led him to Soho and eventually to the pump on Broad Street.[1] Once he identified the water as the suspected cause he could then test his theory to be sure that it was the source of the outbreak using experimental techniques. Based on Snow's work the pump was closed and the outbreak ended.

Although this is a very clear demonstration of a disease that could be traced to a single source, the same basic principles are used today to connect disease with potential causes. First the cases are tracked to identify potential causes. Causes may be as simple as a water source or a complex interaction between several factors such as exercise and diet. Next, hypotheses are created and tested using observational techniques and, finally, if possible, using experimental designs (to be expanded in a later section). It is precisely this set of steps that has led to many health-related discoveries allowing for the development of interventions to decrease the spread of disease within a population. **Figure 1–1** illustrates this process. For example, the discovery that exposure to tobacco smoke causes cancer led to labeling and education campaigns, taxation on cigarettes, and finally limitations in many places regarding where smoking is permitted.[2]

■ OVERVIEW OF NUTRITIONAL EPIDEMIOLOGY

In nutritional epidemiology, researchers apply epidemiologic methods to specifically study the connection between dietary factors and health outcomes. As with the broader field of epidemiology, the purpose is to identify targets for intervention that could reduce the burden of disease within a population. For example, nutritional epidemiologists have spent decades examining the connection between dietary fat intake and development of cardiovascular disease. The result of these investigations has led to expert guidelines recommending limited total and saturated fat intake, while

1. Suspect that a factor (exposure/independent variable/X) influenced disease (outcome/dependent variable/Y) occurrence.

   ■ Descriptive epidemiology

   –Examining disease patterns

   –Descriptive studies (ecological and cross sectional studies)

   ↓

2. Form specific hypotheses regarding the exposure-disease association.

   ↓

3. Conduct epidemiologic study to determine relationship between exposure and disease ("analytic epidemiology")

   ↓

4. Judge whether association may be causal. <u>Need to consider:</u>

   –Chance, bias, confounding

   –Strengths and weaknesses of study design

   –Context of study in other epidemiologic research

5. Create intervention strategies to reduce the burden of disease

FIGURE 1–1 Common Pathway for Epidemiologic Research of Nutrition

endorsing the benefits of more liberal consumption of mono- and polyunsaturated fat.[3-5]

Early observations of the role of diet in disease prevention and health promotion are evident in the writings of Hippocrates, who is considered the Father of Medicine. Hippocrates wrote over two thousand years ago: "A low diet of food and drink is on the whole a surer way to health than violent changes from one diet to another."[6] It was not until the 18th century, however, that one of the first controlled clinical trials into the relationship between food, nutrition, and disease risk was conducted.

In 1747, James Lind divided 12 sailors with scurvy into pairs and assigned five of the pairs to receive a different treatment currently accepted as a remedy for the condition.[7] The sixth pair received lemons and oranges, considered an experimental treatment at the time. The only sailors to recover from scurvy were those who received the citrus fruits. Not long after this experiment the English Navy became the dominant force of the seas, all because they could stay out longer without getting sick. English sailors became known as "Limys" because of their new association with citrus fruit. It can be said that nutrition conquered the sea! While Lind could not identify the exact compound responsible for the effect, he was among the first to demonstrate that scurvy was the result of a dietary deficiency. As we now know, the vitamin in question is vitamin C, which was not isolated until 1928.[8]

Early experiments like Lind's showed that there was something within certain foods that had an essential role in human functioning, but recognition of the actual vitamins and minerals necessary for human health did not occur until the late 19th and the 20th centuries.[9,10] Early nutritional investigations focused on identifying deficiency diseases associated with specific vitamins and minerals. As new vitamins were discovered and applied to populations deficient in them, certain diseases almost miraculously disappeared including beriberi, scurvy, and pellegra.

While the single nutrient model remains important today (e.g., the fortification of folic acid in the American food supply in 1998 has greatly reduced the occurrence of neural tube defects in newborns), this model has many limitations as well. Specifically, it does not seem to fit well when applied to complex diseases including obesity, diabetes, and cardiovascular disease. In more recent years, the field of nutritional epidemiology has moved beyond the single nutrient/deficiency disease model to include multifaceted investigations of the nutritional determinants of disease related to excess nutrient consumption.[10,11] The connections between excess nutrition and chronic disease development are generally much more complicated than the single nutrient model and can only be studied by observing free living populations on a larger scale over long periods of time. The complex model has become the face of modern nutritional epidemiology moving forward investigation into the determinants of diseases of overnutrition including obesity, type 2 diabetes, certain cancers, and cardiovascular disease, and has taken shape in the study of dietary patterns, nutrition indices, and nutrient risk scores.

One of the first large-scale studies of the modern era of nutritional epidemiology is the Framingham Heart Study (FHS) initiated in 1948 to identify factors contributing to cardiovascular disease (CVD) development.[12] Cardiovascular disease had become the leading cause of death in the United States by the mid-twentieth century, although it barely made the top 10 causes in 1900.[13,14] In response, the United States government held a contest to find a "typical" American town that would be followed medically over many years to determine potential causes of cardiovascular disease. Framingham, Massachusetts was selected as the representative American town and two-thirds of the residents agreed to participate. Early findings included the discovery of a link between blood cholesterol levels and development of heart disease. While early single-nutrient–driven investigations found no connection between nutrition and cardiovascular disease development, later research used a more complex model of looking for dietary patterns and stratified participants by age, gender, and other pertinent factors such as smoking status. These studies have greatly contributed to our knowledge of the connections between diet and several chronic diseases.[15-22]

The Nurses' Health Study (NHS)[23] initiated in 1976 has also been an extremely valuable source of information in nutritional epidemiology. The NHS originally included approximately 122,000 female nurses and has been instrumental in advancing our understanding of the effect of diet and lifestyle factors on health. One of the unique features of both the NHS and its male counterpart, the Health Professionals Follow-Up Study (HPFS),[24] is that population was defined by professional status instead of physical location. While that may have caused relative homogeneity within the population in terms of socioeconomic and education status, it also allowed for much greater diversity in terms of environmental and cultural exposures. Unlike Framingham, which was a geographically homogenous population, the NHS included women from all around the United States. By redefining population, these studies were able to look at many new factors related to chronic disease development that were not possible in a geographically and culturally similar population. Another major strength of having a broader definition of population was the ability to recruit large numbers of subjects. With such a large-scale study, investigations into less common diseases including many cancers is made possible, and both the NHS and the HPFS have been invaluable in their contributions to the field of nutritional epidemiology.

Like the Framingham and the Nurses' Health studies described above, many other community-based cohorts have been recruited and followed to help illuminate the complex connections between lifestyle behaviors and health outcomes. Some like Bogalusa[25] focus on a younger population and others such as The Strong Heart Study[26] focus on a minority population, but, combined, we are able to observe patterns that help put together the pieces of the multipart puzzle that connects lifestyle and disease.

■ TYPES OF STUDY DESIGNS USED IN NUTRITIONAL EPIDEMIOLOGY

Once a hypothesis is created, the first thing to be decided is how best to test if there is a possible link. The main tool used by the epidemiologist to determine potential connections is study design. A variety of study designs or methodologies are utilized to conduct nutritional epidemiologic investigations. The type of study design that is selected depends on the research question to be investigated, the type of data available to answer the question, time frame (past, present, or future) of data collection, feasibility (cost, time allotted for data collection, staff and technical resources to carry out the study, etc.), and ethical considerations.

The most common research designs used in nutritional epidemiology are descriptive studies, such as ecological and cross-sectional investigations and analytic studies, including case-control, cohort, and experimental investigations. Descriptive studies are considered less scientifically rigorous than analytic designs. However, it is important to emphasize that all study designs have a place in the hierarchy of research methodologies (Figure 1–1). For example, descriptive research often provides valuable information for generating hypotheses (research questions) that can then be tested using analytic research techniques.

Descriptive studies also tell us about the current status of a problem. For example, a cross-sectional study could be done to identify what percentage of the population is anemic, vitamin D–deficient, smoking, exercising regularly, etc. This process measures the prevalence of a disease. The term *prevalence* in epidemiology refers to the percentage of the population that has a disease at any given point; for example, the percentage of the population living with diabetes in the United States on a given date. Prevalence numbers can be compared over time to create an ongoing picture of progress toward a public health goal or simply indicate the severity of a problem at any given time point.

Analytic study designs are considered better for determining whether certain factors may be a potential cause or protective factor for a certain disease. With the exception of the case-control study, analytic studies follow populations over time, which is considered a key factor in determining a potential causal link between the exposure and outcome. Using a time element, incidence can be calculated. *Incidence* is another important concept in epidemiology. It refers to the occurrence of new cases of disease in a specific population within a certain time frame, for example, how many people develop diabetes in the United States within a given year. Incidence and prevalence are discussed in depth later in this chapter.

An understanding of the characteristics, strengths, and limitations of each study design is necessary to determine the most appropriate method to address a particular nutritional concern. **Table 1–1** describes each of the study designs in more detail and gives examples of some of the landmark studies that represent that study design. Nutritional epidemiologic investigations take a common path (Figure 1–1).

Choice of study design is largely driven by the exact nature of the study question, type of data available to answer the question, and financial resources available. Other issues such as the ethics of answering that question with certain experimental techniques is also an issue that every researcher must confront. It would be unethical to expose someone to a factor that you are reasonably sure would do them harm. An example is purposely exposing a group to cigarette smoke after it was suspected to cause cancer. On the other side of the ethical question, it is not considered ethical to withhold a treatment that appears significantly protective.

For these important ethical considerations, there are many protections that have been developed for human and animal subjects, including the use of Institutional Review Boards (IRBs) to approve studies and study review panels to assess results for experimental trials during the course of the investigation.

TABLE 1–1	**Descriptive Study Designs**

Ecological/Correlational

Examines relationships between a risk factor and a disease outcome at the population level

Strengths:

- Relatively quick and inexpensive
- Utilizes available data
- Takes advantage of large differences in exposure to a given risk factor between different populations
- Good for hypothesis generation
- Random error is relatively small

Weaknesses:

- Only shows potential association, NOT causation
- Cannot be applied directly to individuals
- Assumes exposure to the risk factor is equal across the entire population
- Assumes other factors are the same between the two populations being compared

Examples:

- Keys, A.—Coronary Heart Disease in Seven Countries[27,28]

Cross-Sectional/Prevalence

Creates a "snapshot" of an existing disease and factors that may be associated

- Data on exposure, disease, and confounders are all collected at the same time

Strengths:

- Relatively quick and inexpensive
- Utilizes available data
- Good for hypothesis generation
- Good for diseases with long latency
- Provides information about a causal relationship when:
  —Exposure is immutable or unlikely to change (sex, blood type, etc.)
- Measures prevalence
  —Good for assessing burden of disease, targeting the need for intervention programs
  —Comparison of several surveys can indicate the trend of a variable

Weaknesses:

- Lack of temporality between exposure and disease (gathering information about exposure and disease at the same time)
- Difficult to use to assess causation (outcome may have affected "exposure")
- Number of prevalent cases may be affected by incidence and duration

Examples:

- National Health and Nutrition Examination Survey[29,30]
- Behavioral Risk Factor Surveillance System (BRFSS)[31]

Analytic Study Designs

Case-Control

Used to determine potential exposures in relation to a disease outcome. A group with the disease is recruited and compared to an equivalent group without disease. Information on the disease and possible exposures are collected at the same time and the two groups are compared for differences in exposure history.

- People with disease are defined as *cases* and those without are *controls*.
- Often is used for rare diseases or diseases that take a long time to develop.

Strengths:

- Same method of obtaining exposure history from all respondents
- Efficient for diseases that take a long time to develop
- Efficient for rare diseases
- Good for diseases where little is known about etiology (can evaluate multiple exposures in relation to disease)
- Good for dynamic populations
- Less cost and time than prospective cohort studies (because no f/u and smaller sample)

Examples:

- Wu et al.—Green tea and breast cancer[32]
- Shaw et al.—Periconceptual vitamin and folate use and neural tube defects[33]
- Doll, R.—Smoking and lung cancer[2,34]
- Wu et al., Hercberg, S.—Plasma carotene and cancer[35,36]

| TABLE 1–1 | *(Continued)* |

Weaknesses:

- Recall bias: Information about previous diet is collected from those with and without the disease. Cases may recall exposures differently than controls because they are more motivated to discover what caused their disease.

- Interviewer bias: If interviewers know status of cases and controls, and also know the hypothesis, they may ask questions differently to cases and controls. They may probe cases for more information on exposures.

- Temporality between exposure and disease sometimes uncertain

- Inefficient for rare exposures

- Control group selection may be difficult

- Cannot estimate relative risk directly must use odds ratio

- Only show association NOT causation

Cohort

Examines relationships between an exposure and a disease outcome at the population level, subjects are followed over time and information on exposures is collected prior to the development of disease

Prospective Cohort

Subjects are grouped according to exposure and then followed to see who develops the disease

Strengths:

- Estimate risk directly using incidence

- Good for assessing causal relationships

- Good for minimizing selection bias and confounding.

- Good for studying rare exposures

- Collect exposure data (i.e., current diet) without being biased by already having the disease

Examples:

- Nurses' Health Study (NHS)[23,24,37,38]

- Framingham Heart Study (FHS)[12,16,39]

- Strong Heart Study[26,40]

- Health Professionals Follow-up Study[24]

- Honolulu Heart Program[41]

Weaknesses:

- Difficult with rare outcomes because even very large cohorts will not accumulate a sufficient number of cases within a reasonable amount of time

- Difficult for long latency because too long to follow

- Best for studying a particular exposure

- Costs

- Potential problem with subjects lost to follow-up

Retrospective Cohort

Investigator evaluates association between exposure and incidence of disease in a sample where exposure and disease have already occurred.

Strengths:

- Estimate risk directly using incidence

- Excellent for diseases with long latency periods

- Good for studying rare exposures

- Less expensive than prospective studies

Weaknesses:

- Difficult with rare outcomes

- Heavy reliance on data from memory, preexisting records, and quality of record keeping

- Problem with subjects lost to follow-up

- Many inherent problems with internal validity

continues

TABLE 1–1	*(Continued)*

Clinical/Controlled Trial

Applies a controlled intervention to test the effect in prevention or treatment of disease, investigators assign who receives treatment, and what treatment is given.

- Subjects are randomized into either a treatment or control group.
- Ideally neither the subject nor the investigator knows whether the subject receives the treatment or the placebo

Strengths:

- High validity
- Can distinguish small and modest effects
- Randomization should ensure that both known and unknown associated risk factors are evenly distributed between the treatment and control groups.

Weaknesses:

- Expense
- May be unethical if the "treatment" is potentially harmful; potential benefit must outweigh potential harm
- Subject compliance with treatment may not be good, especially if the treatment is complicated or difficult

Examples:

- The Dietary Approaches to Stop Hypertension (DASH)[42,43]
- Women's Health Initiative (WHI)[44,45]
- Dean Ornish—The Lifestyle Heart Trial[46]
- Child & Adolescent Trial for Cardiovascular Health (CATCH)[47,48]
- OMNI-Heart[49]
- Pathways Project[50]

Criteria for Causality

One important goal of epidemiologic investigations is to prove that factor x causes outcome y and subsequently design an intervention to alter that relationship. Some study designs are well-suited to prove causality, with the randomized controlled trial (RCT) considered the gold standard.[51] **Figure 1–2** shows the "hierarchy of study design." *Hierarchy* in this context refers to the ability of these study designs to determine causality. Observational techniques are considered less convincing than experimental design, but there are several elements that can raise the validity of the results.

In 1965 Austin Bradford Hill proposed criteria for assessing causation. The guidelines he created are referred to as the *Bradford-Hill criteria*, and are still used extensively to help researchers determine if there is indeed a causal link between an exposure and an outcome.[52]

1. **Strength**: The larger the effect or strength of association, the more likely it is causal. Caveat: A small association does not mean that there is not a causal effect. The effect may be weak or the sample size small.
2. **Consistency**: Consistent findings observed by different persons in different places with different samples strengthens the likelihood of an effect. For this reason, studies must be replicated multiple times to confirm results.
3. **Specificity**: Causation is likely when a specific population at a specific site shows incidence of a specific disease with no other explanation. The more specific an association between a factor and an effect is, the bigger the probability of a causal relationship.
4. **Temporality**: The effect has to occur after the cause (and if there is an expected delay between the cause and expected effect, then the effect must occur after that delay).
5. **Biological gradient**: Greater exposure should generally lead to greater incidence of the effect. However, in some cases, the mere presence of the factor can trigger the effect. In other cases, an inverse proportion is observed: greater exposure leads to lower incidence.

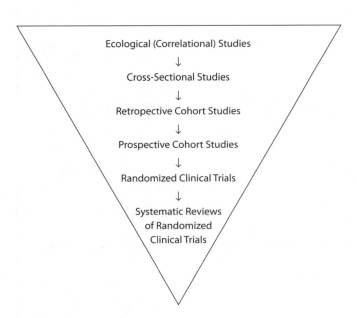

Ecological (Correlational) Studies
↓
Cross-Sectional Studies
↓
Retropective Cohort Studies
↓
Prospective Cohort Studies
↓
Randomized Clinical Trials
↓
Systematic Reviews of Randomized Clinical Trials

FIGURE 1–2 Hierarchy of Study Designs

6. **Plausibility**: A plausible mechanism between cause and effect is helpful although it should be kept in mind that knowledge of the mechanism is limited by current knowledge.

7. **Coherence**: Coherence between epidemiological and laboratory findings increases the likelihood of an effect. However, Hill noted that "... lack of such [laboratory] evidence cannot nullify the epidemiological effect on associations."[52]

8. **Experiment**: "Occasionally it is possible to appeal to experimental evidence."[52]

9. **Analogy**: The effect of similar factors may be considered.

This is not to say that if a hypothesis passes all the tests the relationship is indisputably causal, it is simply a good way to rule out those that are likely not. Hill himself said, "None of my nine viewpoints can bring indisputable evidence for or against the cause-and-effect hypothesis and none can be required *sine qua non*."[52]

Incidence and Prevalence

Incidence and prevalence are the two main numbers used to measure disease frequency within a population. They allow us to compare groups or to monitor progress.

Incidence measures the development of new cases of disease in a population during a given time period while prevalence measures the proportion of the population that has the disease at a given time. One of the best ways to visualize these concepts is to imagine a faucet dripping water into a sink. Incidence would be measured by the number of drops of water that fall from the faucet in a given time frame such as an hour. *Prevalence* would be the total amount of water in the sink at any given time.

Some diseases have a relatively low incidence but a high prevalence. This would occur when a disease is common within a population and people tend to live for a long time after diagnosis. For example, heart disease and diabetes are both very common in the American population and, although they are two of the leading causes of death in the United States, numerous people live many years with them. Other diseases may have an incidence that is relatively high compared to a low prevalence. This would happen if people who are diagnosed with the disease are either quickly cured or die. For example, the common cold occurs frequently within a population over a given time span, but a relatively small percentage of the population has it at any one time.

Measuring Dietary Exposure: Dietary Assessment Methods

At the core of nutritional epidemiologic investigations is the ability to define nutritional/dietary exposures, including the estimation of population and individual food and nutrient intake and characterization of long-term, habitual dietary intake patterns. Several dietary assessment methods are available to measure diet in nutrition research. These include 24-hour recalls, food records or diaries, and food frequency questionnaires.[53,54] Each method is briefly discussed in the following sections. Detailed descriptions of each method can be found elsewhere.[55] All of them rely on self-reported data and each has its own set of strengths and weaknesses[56] that are also discussed below. Like study designs, it is important to be able to distinguish between the characteristics of each technique to determine which dietary assessment tool would be the most appropriate to use for the nutrition question and population under investigation.

Dietary Recalls

The 24-hour recall requires the respondent to retrospectively recall everything he/she ate and drank during the previous 24-hour period. In standard application, a trained interviewer asks the subject what they consumed and records it. Newer techniques include multiple "passes" and strategic prompting to help the subject recall any drinks, condiments, snacks, etc. that otherwise may be forgotten. Respondents are asked to report portion size usually based on standard sizes (i.e., a cup of milk) and/or using food models to improve accuracy of portion size estimation. A 24-hour recall can be quickly done during a clinic visit; it is then coded and matched to foods in the corresponding nutrient analysis database, and analyzed for nutrient content.

A single 24-hour recall is generally thought to be effective at quantifying mean group intake over a large population but an inaccurate method for estimation of usual intake for an individual.[56,57] Alternatively, multiple 24-hour recalls may be used to estimate usual intake on the individual level. The primary limitation generally cited for the 24-hour recall is that they are dependent on the ability of the subject to comprehensively remember what they consumed and accurately report portion sizes.[58–61] Although this is generally assumed to be true when recall data are interpreted, it has been shown that subjects may not accurately remember and report their intake. Karvetti and Knuts,[59] in a group of 140 subjects who provided recalls one day after their food intake was directly observed and measured, found that the subjects only accurately remembered 58%–74% of what they had eaten. Inaccuracy of this type is referred to as *recall bias* and would clearly lead to some level of error when correlating the reported dietary intake with disease outcomes.

Food Records

Food records attempt to avoid recall bias by requiring the respondent to immediately record what they eat and drink during a given period of time. A minimum of three days of records are collected to estimate usual intake for an individual and/or population, with one weekend day and two weekdays as a standard protocol, but some studies may collect as many as seven to ten days.[11,55,56] Dietary intake is recorded by the respondent in real time and is turned in to the research team that manually codes and inputs the information into a nutrient analysis database to create a nutrient profile.

Food records are considered to be better estimates of an individual's intake compared with recalls and are equally good or better estimates of group intake compared with recalls.[56–58] The primary limitations cited for the dietary record method include a high respondent burden leading to failure of subjects to comply and fill out the records or fill them out incompletely. Food records are often also criticized for suspected respondent failure to fill them out in real time, making them, in effect, subject to the same limitations of the recall. Methods to address portion size are similar to that of the 24-hour recall.

As with the food recall, it has been found that the assumptions upon which the accuracy of the food record are based are not always met. A major limitation of food records is reporting bias in which a subject may not wish to disclose everything he/she consumed, may limit what he/she eat and drink on the days the record is kept, or may selectively report only "healthier" foods. One common form of reporting bias is underreporting of true intake either intentionally or due to poor estimation of portion size. Underreporting is thought to be widespread and has been demonstrated to be a problem. Several studies have quantified underreporting by comparing the food record with a biological marker.[62–64]

Food Frequency Questionnaires

Food frequency questionnaires (FFQs) became popular in the 1980s to facilitate collection of dietary data in large cohort studies. The respondent is asked to estimate frequency of consumption of foods listed on a predetermined food list. The majority of FFQs are designed to be *self-administered*, meaning that the subject fills out the form him/herself, with a trained professional assigned to review the form for completeness.[11,55,56]

Unless directed by a specific research question, food items are usually listed using generic names; cooking methods are often not specified, for example, French fries that are baked in the oven versus fried in a fryolator. FFQs generally include several similar foods on the same line (e.g., "potato chips, pretzels, and tortilla chips"), and groups may vary between different FFQs depending on the decisions made by the investigators. A food frequency questionnaire may contain as many as 200 or more line items or as few as 30 to 40 lines, with longer questionnaires demonstrating a higher validity compared with shorter.[65,66] Portion size may be specified for every item on the FFQ (known as *quantitative*), specified for some items but not others (known as *semiquantitative*), or may be left unspecified. Controversy remains regarding the value of including portion size.[67,68] A nutrient analysis

database specific to each FFQ is created to analyze nutrient content; forms are generally created to be either scanned directly by the computer or input by hand by a data entry specialist. No literature exists in the public domain documenting the process of creating the FFQ database and there is currently no standard procedure established.

Food frequency questionnaires are generally acknowledged as the least precise method of estimating nutrient intake, and as such are often validated against other diet assessment methods when biomarkers are not available.[11,55–58,69–71] Error implicit in the FFQ includes the generic nature of the foods listed and the corresponding generic nature of the nutrient values assigned in the database. FFQs may not accurately represent the usual diet if foods commonly consumed by an individual are not listed on the form. Respondents may not understand how to fill out the form correctly and may not accurately account for things such as eating a double portion of a food at the same meal or on the same day. As with recalls, FFQs are not filled out in real time, so recall bias may be a problem. Likewise, respondents may not wish to report less healthy foods that they consume making reporting bias a concern, similar to diet records.

Currently, FFQs are widely used despite their limitations; they are well known to be the most cost-effective method of collecting dietary data within a large cohort and *reasonably* valid when compared with biomarkers and other dietary collection methods including multiple 24-hour recalls and 3-day food records. It is generally recommended that nutrient profiles derived from FFQs should not be used to characterize an individual's absolute nutrient intake given the generic nature of the assessment, but instead are used for relative ranking of individuals within a cohort.[56–58,72]

Validity of Dietary Data

Several potential sources of error have been identified in the collection and analysis of usual dietary intake, and these may contribute to the attenuation between estimated diet and risk of disease development.[55–58] As discussed above, bias related to the dietary assessment tool is an area of concern when interpreting correlations. Confounding is also a concern to be considered when determining if a relationship truly exists between a dietary variable and disease outcome.

A *confounder* is a variable that is associated with both the outcome and the exposure. Confounding occurs when the effect attributed to the variable of interest is possibly due to another highly correlated, potentially unmeasured factor. Theoretically, statistical modeling will account for such effects, but as Fraser highlights in his commentary, "dietary analyses are peculiarly predisposed to confounding simply because of the complexity of this variable."[73] He goes on to discuss that an investigator may believe she or he is studying the effect of a particular nutrient of interest, but in reality may be studying the effect of another nutrient or food-based chemical that is highly correlated, but is not measured or defined poorly.

■ GENERAL CONSIDERATIONS IN NUTRITIONAL EPIDEMIOLOGIC STUDIES

Epidemiologic study techniques can be invaluable tools to identify underlying causes of disease within a population, allowing for intervention to moderate or eliminate disease. There are several limitations of epidemiologic research, however, and a good understanding of these limitations is important to designing and interpreting studies.

One of the biggest obstacles to drawing connections between diet and disease outcomes is that measuring diet is a difficult process. As discussed above, a self-reported diet usually includes several forms of bias that create error in measurement of dietary variables. Even if diet could be measured without any source of error, there are other challenges, not the least of which is the fact that diet is a complex set of exposures that are strongly inter-correlated. For example, an individual who eats a diet high in saturated fat also may eat a diet high in cholesterol, sodium, and trans fat, making it hard to tease out the effects of each variable. To make matters worse, people who have these sorts of diets also may get less exercise, be more obese, and engage in several other behaviors that make it very hard to isolate the effects of one specific factor.

Another major challenge for the nutritional epidemiologist is that it is almost impossible to compare a truly unexposed group to an exposed group. Unlike with behaviors such as smoking, all individuals are exposed to dietary factors to some degree. For example, it is impossible to completely avoid consumption of saturated fat. The best we can do is compare those who appear to be less exposed to those who have relatively higher exposure. When the range of intake of a certain nutrient is narrow, it is very difficult to see the impact of that nutrient on health outcomes. For example, it is likely that early investigations into whether saturated fat and cholesterol are linked to heart disease failed to find a connection because the American public had a very high intake across the population.

To further complicate the problem, eating patterns evolve over time. It is possible that dietary habits in childhood are a major determinant of future health. Unfortunately, current study techniques either poorly reflect or completely fail to capture dietary habits practiced over a lifetime.

Another obstacle to determining the influence of diet on health is that individuals are biologically different from each other and may process nutrients differently. There are some individuals who may tolerate a high fat or high carbohydrate diet well, while others develop disease on the exact same diet.

Finally, there is the problem that food is not a constant thing. Vitamin content can vary by the soil where the food is grown, how it is stored, and how it is prepared. Farming techniques also change our food supply on the most basic level. A cow fed a corn-based diet is not nutritionally the same as a cow that grazes on grass. We may think we are comparing the proverbial apples to apples, but in reality often those apples have very different nutrient contents that make our results incomprehensible.

This is not to say that there is no point to trying to study the connections between diet and disease; it simply explains why it is a much more difficult process than the public expects. Only through the refining of our study techniques and continuing to perform well-designed studies across a variety of populations in a variety of circumstances can we ever answer the great questions of nutritional epidemiology and effectively intervene to help people live longer, healthier lives.

■ SUMMARY

Epidemiology has evolved over the past few centuries to help researchers connect disease with their underlying causes. Although this is not always a straightforward process, it is very valuable in helping direct intervention efforts to minimize the impact of disease. Traditional epidemiologic techniques have been extremely effective in eliminating certain nutrition-related diseases that can be linked to a single cause, such as a vitamin deficiency. More recent applications of epidemiology have become more complex as diseases with multiple causes are studied.

Issues for Discussion

1. Discuss how nutrient recommendations have been affected by epidemiological studies.

2. Describe the different factors that can be measured for nutritional epidemiological studies.

3. List and discuss the techniques used to gather information for nutritional epidemiological studies.

References

1. Summers J. *Soho—A History of London's Most Colourful Neighborhood.* London, UK: Bloomsbury; 1989:113–117.

2. Doll R, Peto R, Boreham J, Sutherland I. Mortality in relation to smoking: 50 years' observations on male British doctors. *BMJ.* 2004;328:1519–1528.

3. U.S. Department of Health and Human Services and U.S. Department of Agriculture. *Dietary Guidelines for Americans,* 6th ed. Washington, DC: U.S. Government Printing Office; 2005, 2010.

4. American Heart Association Nutrition Committee, Lichtenstein AH, Appel LJ, et al. Diet and lifestyle recommendations revision 2006: a scientific statement from the American Heart Association Nutrition Committee. *Circulation.* 2006;114:82–96.

5. National Cholesterol Education Program (NCEP) Expert Panel on Detection, Evaluation, and Treatment of High Blood Cholesterol in Adults (Adult Treatment Panel III). Third Report of the National Cholesterol Education Program (NCEP) Expert Panel on Detection, Evaluation, and Treatment of High Blood Cholesterol in Adults (Adult Treatment Panel III) final report. *Circulation.* 2002;106: 3143–3421.

6. Hippocrates. *Hippocratic Writings.* London, UK: Penguin Books; 1983:193.

7. Lind J. *A Treatise on the Scurvy in Three Parts.* London, UK: Millar; 1753.

8. Svirbely J, Szent-Gyorgyi A. The chemical nature of vitamin C. *Biochem J.* 1932;26:865–870.

9. Langseth L. *Nutritional Epidemiology: Possibilities and Limitations.* Washington, DC: International Life Sciences Institute; 2000.

10. Caballero B. Fortification, Supplementation, and Nutrient Balance. *Eur J Clin Nutr.* 2003;57(suppl 1):S76–S78.

11. Willett W. *Nutritional Epidemiology,* 2nd ed. New York: Oxford University Press; 1998.

12. Feinleib M, Kannel WB, Garrison RJ, McNamara PM, Castelli WP. The Framingham Offspring Study. Design and Preliminary Data. *Prev Med.* 1975;4:518–525.

13. Hinman A. 1889 to 1989: a century of health and disease. *Public Health Rep.* 1990;105:374–380.

14. Greenlund KJ, Giles WH, Keenan NL, et al. Heart disease and stroke mortality in the 20th century. In: Ward J, Warren C, eds. *Silent Victories: The History and Practice of Public Health in Twentieth Century America.* Oxford, UK: Oxford University Press; 2006.

15. Millen BE, Quatromoni PA, Gagnon DR, Cupples LA, Franz MM, D'Agostino RB. Dietary patterns of men and women suggest targets for health promotion: the Framingham Nutrition Studies. *Am J Health Promot.* 1996;11:42–52.

16. Millen BE, Quatromoni PA, Copenhafer DL, Demissie S, O'Horo CE, D'Agostino RB. Validation of a dietary pattern approach for evaluating nutritional risk: the Framingham Nutrition Studies. *J Am Diet Assoc.* 2001;101:187–194.

17. Millen BE, Quatromoni PA, Pencina M, et al. Unique dietary patterns and chronic disease risk profiles of adult men: the Framingham Nutrition Studies. *J Am Diet Assoc.* 2005;105: 1723–1734.

18. Millen BE, Pencina MJ, Kimokoti RW, et al. Nutritional risk and the metabolic syndrome in women: opportunities for preventive intervention from the Framingham Nutrition Study. *Am J Clin Nutr.* 2006;84:434–441.

19. Quatromoni PA, Copenhafer DL, D'Agostino RB, Millen BE. Dietary patterns predict the development of overweight in women: the Framingham Nutrition Studies. *J Am Diet Assoc.* 2002;102:1239–1246.

20. Quatromoni PA, Pencina M, Cobain MR, Jacques PF, D'Agostino RB. Dietary quality predicts adult weight gain: findings from the Framingham Offspring Study. *Obesity.* 2006;14:1383–1391.

21. Fogli-Cawley JJ, Dwyer JT, Saltzman E, McCullough ML, Troy LM, Jacques PF. The 2005 Dietary Guidelines for Americans Adherence Index: development and application. *J Nutr.* 2006; 136:2908–2915.

22. Fogli-Cawley JJ, Dwyer JT, Saltzman E, et al. The 2005 Dietary Guidelines for Americans and risk of the metabolic syndrome. *Am J Clin Nutr.* 2007;86:1193–1201.

23. Belanger CF, Hennekens CH, Rosner B, Speizer FE. The Nurses' Health Study. *Am J Nurs.* 1978;78:1039–1040.

24. Hu FB, Willett WC. Diet and coronary heart disease: findings from the Nurses' Health Study and Health Professionals Follow-up Study. *J Nutr Health Aging.* 2001;5:132–140.

25. Mohindra NA, Nicklas TA, O'Neil CE, Yang SJ, Berenson GS. Eating patterns and overweight status in young adults: the Bogalusa Heart Study. *Int J Food Sci Nutr.* 2009;3:14–25.

26. Lee ET, Welty TK, Fabsitz R, et al. The Strong Heart Study. A study of cardiovascular disease in American Indians: design and methods. *Am J Epidemiol.* 1990;132:1141–1155.

27. Keys AC. *Seven Countries: A Multivariate Analysis of Death and Coronary Heart Disease.* Boston: Harvard University Press; 1980:362–371.

28. Kromhout D, Menotti A, Blackburn H. *Prevention of Coronary Heart Disease: Diet, Lifestyle, and Risk Factors in the Seven Countries Study.* Norwell, MA: Kluwer Academic Publishers; 2002.

29. Center for Disease Control and Prevention. *National Health and Nutrition Examination Survey.* Available at http://www.cdc.gov/nchs/nhanes/about_nhanes.htm. Accessed January13, 2010.

30. Alexander C, Landsman P, Teutsch S, Haffner S. NCEP-Defined Metabolic Syndrome, Diabetes, and Prevalence of Coronary Heart Disease Among NHANES III Participants Age 50 Years and Older. *J Am Diabet Assoc.* 2003;52:1210–1214.

31. Remington PL, Smith MY, Williamson DF, Anda RF, Gentry EM, Hogelin GC. Design, characteristics, and usefulness of state-based behavioral risk factor surveillance: 1981–87. *Public Health Rep.* 1988;103:366–375.

32. Wu AH, Yu MC, Tseng CC, Hankin J, Pike MC. Green tea and risk of breast cancer in Asian Americans. *Int J Cancer.* 2003;106:574–579.

33. Shaw GM, Schaffer D, Velie EM, Morland K, Harris JA. Periconceptional vitamin use, dietary folate, and the occurrence of neural tube defects. *Epidemiology.* 1995;6:219–226.

34. Doll R. How it really happened. *Am J Respir Crit Care Med.* 2000; 162;4.

35. Wu AH, Henderson BE, Pike MC, Yu MC. Smoking and other risk factors for lung cancer in women. *J Natl Cancer Inst.* 1985;74: 747–751.

36. Hercberg S. The history of ß-carotene and cancers: from observational to intervention studies. What lessons can be drawn for future research on polyphenols? *Am J Clin Nutr.* 2005; 81:218S–222S.

37. Grodstein F, Manson J, Stampfer M. Postmenopausal hormone use and secondary prevention of coronary events in the Nurses' Health Study: a prospective, observational study. *Ann Intern Med.* 2001;135:1–8.

38. Hung H-C, Joshipura KJ, Jiang R, et al. Fruit and vegetable intake and risk of major chronic disease. *JNCI.* 2004;96:1577–1584.

39. Splansky GL, Corey D, Yang Q, et al. The third generation cohort of the National Heart, Lung, and Blood Institute's Framingham Heart Study: design, recruitment, and initial examination. *Am J Epidemiol.* 2007;165:1328–1335.

40. North KE, Howard BV, Welty TK, et al. Genetic and environmental contributions to cardiovascular disease risk in American Indians. *Am J Epidemiol.* 2003;157:303–314.

41. Goldberg RJ, Burchfiel CM, Benfante R, Chiu D, Reed DM, Yano K. Lifestyle and biologic factors associated with atherosclerotic disease in middle-aged men. 20-year findings from the Honolulu Heart Program. *Arch Intern Med.* 1995;155:686–694.

42. Obarzanek E, Sacks FM, Vollmer WM, et al. Effects on blood lipids of a blood pressure–lowering diet: the Dietary Approaches to Stop Hypertension (DASH) Trial. *Am J Clin Nutr.* 2001;74:80–89.

43. Appel LJ, Moore TJ, Obarzanek E, et al. A clinical trial of the effects of dietary patterns on blood pressure. DASH Collaborative Research Group. *N Engl J Med.* 1997;336:1117–1124.

44. Writing Group for the Women's Health Initiative Investigators. Design of the Women's Health Initiative clinical trial and observational study. The Women's Health Initiative Study Group. *Control Clin Trials.* 1998;19:61–109.

45. Kooperberg C, Cushman M, Hsia J, et al. Can biomarkers identify women at increased stroke risk? The Women's Health Initiative Hormone Trials. *PLoS Clin Trials.* 2007;2:e28.

46. Ornish D, Brown SE, Scherwitz LW, et al. Can lifestyle changes reverse coronary heart disease? The Lifestyle Heart Trial. *Lancet.* 1990;336:129–133.

47. Lytle LA, Eszery MK, Nicklas T, et al. Nutrient intakes of third graders: results from the Child and Adolescent Trial for Cardiovascular Health (CATCH) Baseline Survey. *J Nutr Educ.* 1996;28:338–347.

48. Perry CL, Stone EJ, Parcel GS, et al. School-based cardiovascular health promotion: the child and adolescent trial for cardiovascular health (CATCH). *J Sch Health.* 1990;60:406–413.

49. Carey VJ, Bishop L, Charleston J, et al. Rationale and design of the Optimal Macro-Nutrient Intake Heart Trial to Prevent Heart Disease (OMNI-Heart). *Clin Trials.* 2005;2:529–537.

50. Caballero B, Clay T, Davis SM, et al. Pathways: a school-based, randomized controlled trial for the prevention of obesity in American Indian schoolchildren. *Am J Clin Nutr.* 2003;78: 1030–1038.

51. Jadad A. *Randomized Controlled Trials; a User's Guide.* London, England. BMJ Books. 1998.

52. Hill AB. The environment and disease: association or causation? *Proc Royal Soc Med.* 1965;58:295–300.

53. Thompson FE, Byers T. Dietary assessment resource manual. *J Nutr.* 1994;124(suppl):2245S–2317S.

54. Johnson RK. Dietary intake–how do we measure what people are really eating? *Obes Res.* 2002;10(suppl):63S–68S.

55. Friedenreich CM, Slimani N, Riboli E. Measurement of past diet: review of previous and proposed methods. *Epidemiol Rev.* 1992;14:177–196.

56. Bingham SA. The dietary assessment of individuals: methods, accuracy, new techniques and recommendations. *Nutr Abstr Rev.* 1987;57:705–742.

57. Anderson SA. Guidelines for use of dietary intake data. *J Am Diet Assoc.* 1988;88:1258–1260.

58. Sempos CT, Flegal KM, Johnson CL, Loria CM, Woteki CE, Briefel RR. Issues in the long-term evaluation of diet in longitudinal studies. *J Nutr.* 1993;123(2 Suppl):406–412. Review.

59. Karvetti RL, Knuts LR. Validity of the 24-hour dietary recall. *J Am Diet Assoc.* 1985;85:1437–1442.

60. Carter RL, Sharbaugh CO, Stapell CA. Reliability and validity of the 24-hour recall. *J Am Diet Assoc.* 1981;79:542–547.

61. Kahn HA, Whelton PK, Appel LJ, et al. Validity of 24-hour dietary recall interviews conducted among volunteers in an adult working community. *Ann Epidemiol.* 1995;5:484–489.

62. Hill RJ, Davies PS. The validity of self-reported energy intake as determined using the doubly labelled water technique. *Br J Nutr.* 2001;85:415–430. Review.

63. Cook A, Pryer J, Shetty P. The problem of accuracy in dietary surveys. Analysis of the over 65 UK National Diet and Nutrition Survey. *J Epidemiol Community Health.* 2000;54:611–616.

64. Martin LJ, Su W, Jones PJ, Lockwood GA, Tritchler DL, Boyd NF. Comparison of energy intakes determined by food records and doubly labeled water in women participating in a dietary-intervention trial. *Am J Clin Nutr.* 1996;63:483–490.

65. Subar AF, Ziegler RG, Thompson FE, et al. Prostate, Lung, Colorectal, and Ovarian Cancer Screening Trial Investigators. Is shorter always better? Relative importance of questionnaire length and cognitive ease on response rates and data quality for two dietary questionnaires. *Am J Epidemiol.* 2001;153:404–409.

66. Molag ML, de Vries JH, Ocké MC, et al. Design characteristics of food frequency questionnaires in relation to their validity. *Am J Epidemiol.* 2007;166:1468–1478.

67. Noethlings U, Hoffmann K, Bergmann MM, Boeing H. European Investigation into Cancer and Nutrition. Portion size adds limited information on variance in food intake of participants in the EPIC-Potsdam study. *J Nutr.* 2003;133:510–515.

68. Thompson FE, Subar AF, Brown CC, et al. Cognitive research enhances accuracy of food frequency questionnaire reports: results of an experimental validation study. *J Am Diet Assoc.* 2002;102:212–225.

69. Porrini M, Gentile MG, Fidanza F. Biochemical validation of a self-administered semi-quantitative food-frequency questionnaire. *Br J Nutr.* 1995;74:323–333.

70. Briefel RR, Flegal KM, Winn DM, Loria CM, Johnson CL, Sempos CT. Assessing the nation's diet: limitations of the food frequency questionnaire. *J Am Diet Assoc.* 1992;92:959–962.

71. Kushi LH. Gaps in epidemiologic research methods: design considerations for studies that use food-frequency questionnaires. *Am J Clin Nutr.* 1994;59(1 suppl):180S–184S.

72. Carroll RJ, Freedman LS, Hartman AM. Use of semiquantitative food frequency questionnaires to estimate the distribution of usual intake. *Am J Epidemiol.* 1996;143:392–404.

73. Fraser GE. A search for truth in dietary epidemiology. *Am J Clin Nutr.* 2003;78(3 suppl):521S–525S.

CHAPTER 2

Applying Nutrition Science to the Public's Health

CAROL E. O'NEIL, PhD, MPH, LDN, RD

THERESA A. NICKLAS, DrPH

If we could give every individual the right amount of nourishment and exercise, not too little and not too much, we would have found the safest way to health.

—Hippocrates 460–377 BCE

READER OBJECTIVES

After studying this chapter and reflecting on the contents, you should be able to:

1. Explain how and why nutrition policies, programs, and practice must be evidence-based.

2. Evaluate the peer-reviewed literature and assess bodies of evidence used to form nutrition policies and recommendations.

3. Compare and contrast different types of research studies and explain how they are used to form policies, programs, and consumer information.

4. Explain how and why nutrition policies, recommendations, and programs are changed at regular intervals.

5. Defend U.S. nutrition policies and recommendations.

6. Use the same resources as public health nutritionists to keep pace with current research or available programs that are grounded in research.

■ INTRODUCTION

Hippocrates was right, but for the rest of us, appreciation of this relationship was a long time in coming. Prior to the 1970s, public health nutrition was focused primarily on feeding programs and preventing nutrient deficiency diseases. Early in the 20th century, there was a general lack of understanding of the relationship between diet and disease, and diseases such as pellagra and rickets were common. As food availability improved and the prevalence of deficiency diseases decreased, there was a growing awareness that dietary excess and imbalance increased the risk of developing chronic disease, such as coronary heart disease (CHD), hypertension, type 2 diabetes mellitus, and cancer.[1]

In 1977, the U.S. Senate Select Committee on Nutrition and Human Needs, under the leadership of Senator George McGovern, issued *Dietary Goals for the U.S.*[2] The goals engendered controversy among health professionals and the food industry because of the way they were conceived and presented. At that time, there was also a lack of consensus on the impact of food/nutrients on chronic disease risk. In retrospect, the authors of these dietary goals were remarkably perspicuous. The statement by Dr. C. Edith Weir, Assistant Director of the Human Nutrition Research Division,

U.S. Department of Agriculture (USDA), that "Most all of the health problems underlying the leading causes of death in the U.S. could be modified by improvements in diet"[2] remains the cornerstone of public health nutrition and nutrition policy in the United States.

Today, the preponderance of epidemiologic, clinical, and laboratory data have clearly linked both diet and physical inactivity with chronic disease. Four of the leading causes of death—heart disease, cancer, cerebrovascular disease, and diabetes mellitus—are related directly to poor diet, physical inactivity, and other lifestyle factors.[3] The cost of these diseases to society is staggering; for example, in 2007 chronic cardiovascular disease (CVD) cost approximately $149 billion annually.[4] On an individual level, after controlling for covariates, subjects with diabetes had approximately 239% of the healthcare costs of those without diabetes.[5]

Not included among the four major causes of death, but a major contributor to these and other health problems, is obesity. Obesity has reached epidemic proportions. National Health and Nutrition Examination Survey (NHANES) data from 2005–2006[6] showed that among adults, 33.3% of males and 35.3% of females (more than 72 million people) were obese.

An animated map showing obesity trends in the United States between 1985 and 2008 can be found at http://www.cdc.gov/obesity/data/trends.html

These statistics were not significantly higher than the prevalence of obesity in 2003–2004.[7] Among children and adolescents 2–19 years of age ($n = 8,165$) participating in the NHANES in 2003–2004 and 2005–2006, 31.9% were overweight and 16.3% were obese. There was no difference in the prevalence of overweight or obesity between 2003–2004 and 2005–2006 and no significant trend between 1999 and 2006.[8] In the United States, obesity was responsible for approximately $40 billion of increased medical spending through 2006, with $7 billion in Medicare prescription drug costs. It was projected that medical costs associated with obesity could rise to $147 billion per year by 2008.[9] These statistics do not include the nearly $66 billion dollars in indirect costs, such as absenteeism from work, disability, and worker's compensation.[10] Obesity has surpassed tobacco, alcohol, and poverty as a public health risk.[11,12] Thus, it is crucial to work toward reducing disease risk and promoting healthy behaviors in all individuals.

These health problems are not unique to the United States. Globally, largely preventable chronic diseases account for 60% of all deaths (35 million people), 80% of whom live in low- or middle-income countries.[13] Over the next decade, it is estimated that more than 75% of deaths worldwide will result from these diseases, with 60% occurring in developing countries that are experiencing rapid health transitions. The World Health Organization (WHO)[13] has compared the spread of chronic diseases to that of communicable diseases; however, chronic diseases appear to be "spread" by the Westernization of diets and the decline in physical activity associated with increasing industrialization, rather than by infectious or parasitic agents. The WHO finalized a global strategy to improve diet and increase physical activity for 2008–2013 to reduce the risk of chronic non-communicable diseases while continuing to carry forward the long-term WHO goals on other nutrition-related areas, including undernutrition.

Relatively few modifiable risk factors—for example, a lack of fruit and vegetables in the diet, obesity, smoking, inappropriate use of alcohol, and physical inactivity—cause the majority of the chronic disease burden. Changes in diet and physical activity patterns can significantly reduce disease risk, often in a surprisingly short time period. It has been estimated that a 1% reduction in intake of fat and saturated fatty acids and a 0.1% reduction in intake of cholesterol would, over 20 years, prevent over 56,000 cases of CHD[14] and more than 18,000 deaths; these changes would also save more than 117,000 life-years. Improved dietary patterns could save more than $43 billion in medical care costs and lost productivity resulting from CHD, cancer,

stroke, and diabetes and prevent over 119,900 premature deaths among individuals 55 to 74 years of age. As the average life expectancy in the United States continues to rise, and if current dietary and physical activity patterns remain unchanged, the incidence and prevalence of chronic diseases will continue to increase.

PUBLIC HEALTH NUTRITION AND PUBLIC HEALTH NUTRITIONISTS

The Institute of Medicine's (IOM) *The Future of the Public's Health in the 21st Century* states that the mission of public health is "to assure conditions where people can be healthy."[15] This report extends the *Future of Public Health* report, which asserted that public health is "what we as a society do collectively to assure the conditions in which people can be healthy."[16] Public health nutritionists or registered dietitians working in public health settings can play decisive roles in improving our nation's health.[16,17] Challenges for health professionals in the 21st century include shifting demographics, changes in eating and physical activity patterns, disparities in health care, and global economic pressures.

Public health nutritionists need to be able to understand what drives food and physical activity choices by the public. Food choices are driven by: taste; convenience; accessibility, availability, and affordability of foods; ethnic or religious preferences; socioeconomic status; health and nutrition knowledge; shopping practices; and time.[18–22] The decision not to engage in regular physical activity may be driven by lack of knowledge and attitudes about physical activity recommendations, lack of a safe place to exercise or of social support, and lack of access to programs.[23–28]

Without this knowledge, it is difficult to understand why people eat what they do, why they do or do not engage in physical activity, or why they are or are not able to plan interventions and design policies and recommendations that change behavior that will lead to a healthier lifestyle.

Public health nutritionists also need to have a broad grasp of the sciences, including the pathophysiology of disease, genetics, biotechnology and its impact on sustainable agriculture, nutritional biochemistry and

The first detailed recommendations for physical activity were published in 2008 by the Department of Health and Human Services (available at http://www.health.gov/paguidelines/guidelines/default.aspx#toc).

Nutrigenomics: The study of the effects of food or food components on gene expression and how individual genetic differences can affect the way we respond to foods or nutrients. Need to know more? The CDC provides an online tutorial on Genomics for Public Health Practitioners: http://www.cdc.gov/genomics/training/GPHP/menu.html

molecular biology, nutrigenomics, informatics, biostatistics, epidemiology, and of course, nutritional sciences. Finally, public health nutritionists need to know what information and resources are available to them to help plan and assess programs at the national, state, local, or individual levels.

Today, for consumers and health professionals alike, there is a bewildering array of information available.[29–31] A 2009 survey of more than 1,000 adults conducted by the American Dietetic Association showed that nearly 80% were interested in finding nutrition information on the Internet, and 70% visited two or three Web sites when using the Internet to find food and nutrition information. Virtually all participants believed the information they found online was reliable and trustworthy.[32] For health professionals, information is also available on the Internet and through standard media channels; but it is through peer-reviewed journals that we must obtain the scientific information that allows us to evaluate or even generate information used in ethical practice.

In this chapter, we will look at examples of how to interpret and evaluate the professional literature to 1) make evidence-based practice decisions in public health; 2) learn the science behind nutrition recommendations, policy, and legislation; and 3) find ways for nutritional science to be translated into messages for consumers.

> Anybody can post anything on the Internet—and very little information is removed. To determine if the site you've chosen for information is accurate, reliable, and timely, get in the habit of evaluating Web sites and teaching your clients to evaluate them. Need help? Learn how to do it from a reliable source: http://www.library.cornell.edu/olinuris/ref/research/webeval.html.

■ PEER-REVIEWED LITERATURE AND EVIDENCE-BASED PRACTICE

Peer-reviewed literature is the *gold standard* for scientific information provided to the public as well as the information used for setting recommendations and policies, designing and evaluating nutrition programs, and conducting ethical evidence-based nutrition and dietetics practice. Unfortunately, the literature can be difficult to understand and the data often appear contradictory. Use of different study designs, populations, and/or methods—including statistical analyses—contribute to the confusion.

Assessing the science behind the policies, programs, practice, and consumer information begins with asking a question and

> Not familiar with PubMed? Work through the online tutorials to help with your literature searches or ask your university librarian to help you. http://www.nlm.nih.gov/bsd/disted/pubmed.html

finding, reading, and evaluating the articles needed to answer it. **PubMed** is the premiere database for articles on nutrition topics. This database is comprised of more than 19 million citations for biomedical articles from MEDLINE and life science journals. Many citations in PubMed include links to full-text articles from PubMed Central or publisher Web sites. Other important databases for nutrition-related research are shown in **Table 2–1**.

After asking a question and determining the appropriate database to use, the next stage is selecting the descriptors and conducting the search. The descriptors and the search limits depend on the question(s) you are asking. For example, if your question is, "What is the effect of 100% fruit juice consumption on weight in children?" your descriptors could be "fruit juice" OR "fruit" AND "weight" OR "BMI" AND "children" OR "adolescents." The search might be easier if your search limits are "All Children," then the last two descriptors could be eliminated.

Scanning the abstracts will allow you to determine which articles are appropriate for your question. Obtaining the full-text articles, either by downloading them or visiting the library, and assessing them are the next steps (**Table 2–2**). This is not a casual reading to prepare a summary but a critical evaluation of the published study. However, a single peer-reviewed article is not sufficient for making ethical evidence-based practice decisions; setting public health goals (e.g., Healthy People [HP] 2020); developing dietary recommendations, (e.g., Dietary Reference Intakes [DRI]); mandating nutrition policy (e.g., Dietary Guidelines for Americans [DGA]); or designing nutrition programs for health professionals and the public (e.g., the Centers for Disease Control and Prevention's [CDC] Fruits and Veggies More Matters™). To do this, the strength of a body of scientific studies must be assessed.[33–36]

The Agency for Healthcare Research and Quality (AHRQ), through its Evidence-Based Practice Centers, sponsors the development of evidence reports and technology assessments to assist public- and private-sector organizations in their efforts to improve the quality of health care in the United States.[37] The AHRQ identified three important domains that should be addressed to grade the strength of the evidence: 1) the quality of the studies—including the extent to which bias was minimized, 2) the quantity of the studies—including the magnitude of effect, the number of studies conducted, and the sample size or power of the study, and 3) the consistency of results—whether or not similar studies produce similar results.[37]

Another critical consideration when assessing the body of evidence is the study design: what type of study was used to produce the test results, and what was the relevance to the disease/condition/program under study? Some study designs are more powerful than others in providing evidence on a topic; this has given rise to the concept of a "hierarchy of evidence"[38] about the effectiveness of interventions,

| TABLE 2–1 | Databases Important for Nutritional Sciences |

Database	Purpose
AGRICOLA	Provides citations in agriculture and related fields.
AGRIS	International information system for the agricultural sciences and technology; created by the Food and Agriculture Organization of the United Nations (FAO).
BRFSS Behavioral Risk Factor Surveillance System: Survey Data	Includes eight databases on specific illnesses or aspects of chronic disease prevention and health promotion; designed to help public health professionals and educators locate program information.
CARIS Current Agricultural Research Information System	Created by FAO to identify and to facilitate the exchange of information about current agricultural research projects being carried out by or on behalf of developing countries.
The Cochrane Library	Contains reliable evidence from Cochrane and other systematic reviews, clinical trials, and more. Cochrane reviews bring you the combined results of the world's best medical research studies, and are recognized as the gold standard in evidence-based health care.
Directory of Open Access Journals	This database increases the visibility and ease of use of open access journals and promotes their increased usage and impact.
EMBASE	The most comprehensive course for answers on biomedical answers.
ERIC Educational Resources Information Center	Includes educational research and resources; early childhood education, junior colleges and higher education; reading and communications skills; languages and linguistics; education management; counseling and personnel services; library and information science; information resources.
Food Safety Research Database	The Food Safety Research Information Office is located at the National Agricultural Library. This office provides information on publicly funded, and to the extent possible, privately funded food safety research initiatives to prevent unintended duplication of food safety research and to assist the executive and legislative branches of the government and private research entities to assess food safety research needs and priorities.
FSTA Food Science and Technology Abstracts	The largest collection of food science, food technology, and food-related human nutrition abstracts. It contains over 580,000 records with approximately 2000 new records added every month. FSTA covers journal articles (~80%) plus patents, theses, standards, legislation, books, reviews, and conference proceedings.
Health Source: Nursing/Academic Edition	Provides ~600 scholarly full text journals, including nearly 450 peer-reviewed journals focusing on many medical disciplines. Also features abstracts and indexing for nearly 850 journals.
Index to Scientific and Technical Proceedings	Indexes the published literature of the most significant conferences, symposia, seminars, colloquia, workshops, and conventions in a wide range of disciplines in science and technology over the last five years.
LILACS Latin American and Caribbean of Health Sciences Information System	Includes bibliographic control and dissemination of health scientific-technique literature from Latin American and Caribbean countries, absent from other the international databases.
MEDLINE	Sponsored by the National Library of Medicine, contains citations and abstracts to international biomedical literature from over 3,700 journals on topics including research, clinical practice, administration, policy issues, and healthcare services.
Merck Index Online	A one-volume encyclopedia of chemicals, drugs, and biologicals that contains more than 10,000 monographs, 32 supplemental tables, and 450 Organic Name Reactions. Entries cover drugs and pharmaceuticals, describe common organic chemicals and laboratory reagents, cover naturally occurring substances and plants, the elements and on inorganic chemicals, and compounds of agricultural significance.
Nursing and Allied Health Source	Provides reliable healthcare information covering nursing, allied health, alternative and complementary medicine, and related topics.
Science Citation Index	This database covers the journal literature of the sciences.
Science Direct	A Web information source for scientific, technical, and medical research. It offers access to more than 1,100 journals in 16 fields of science, including the social sciences.
Scopus™	The largest abstract and citation base of the peer-reviewed literature.
Web of Science	Indexes more than 5,800 major journals across 164 scientific disciplines.

TABLE 2–2	**How to Assess an Article from the Peer-Reviewed Literature**

Title

1. Did the title reflect what was actually done in the study? The purpose, the populations used, the findings, and conclusions can be reflected in the title. A positive statement about the contents, rather than a title that is a question is preferred.

Abstract

1. Did the abstract clearly outline all aspects of the manuscript?
    a. The purpose of the study
    b. The methods
    c. The results
    d. The conclusions

2. Was enough information provided to understand what was done and what was found?

Introduction

1. Did the authors provide enough background information to understand why the study was done?

2. Did the authors provide enough background information to let you know what others have done on this topic and where there might be gaps in the literature?*

3. Were important studies omitted from the introduction? This might suggest bias.

4. Did the authors clearly state the purpose of the study? A hypothesis or research question should have been stated. Not all study designs are appropriate for testing hypotheses; for example, cross-sectional studies are hypothesis generating.

Materials and Methods (could be phrased Subjects and Methods)

1. Was the type of study clearly defined?

2. Did the experimental design allow the research question or hypotheses to be tested?

3. If appropriate, was a control group included? Was it comparable to the test group?

4. Was the population appropriate for the study?

5. Was the population suitable to generalize results?

6. Was the population well defined?
    a. Number/adequate sample size for appropriate statistical power
    b. Gender, age, race/ethnicity, income, etc.
    c. Inclusion/exclusion criteria for the study
    d. If the study population was a subset of a larger population, was it clear how the study population differed from the larger population? This could indicate bias.
    e. Was a convenience sample used or were the participants randomized?

7. Were there ethical concerns if human subjects or vertebrate animals were used? Was there a clear statement that the research has been approved by the appropriate committee?

8. Were the methods presented in enough detail so that the research could be repeated (or built upon) by another research team?

9. Were the methods used reliable and valid?

10. Statistical methods:
    a. Were they appropriate?
    b. Were outcome variables clearly defined?
    c. Did the authors control for potential confounding variables?
    d. Was a statistical probability level clearly stated?

11. Was it clearly stated how the data will be presented in the results (e.g., data are presented as mean ± standard error [SE])?

12. Were all terms defined?

Results

This section should present study results only. No methodology should be presented and unless it is a combined Results and Discussion section; there should be no interpretation of the information.

1. Were results organized in a logical sequence?
    a. Did the results follow the same order as the methods?

2. Were demographics presented?

3. Were the graphics appropriate?
    a. Were they needed? Should more/less be included?
    b. Was the information clearly presented in labeled tables and figures? Can the tables and figures stand alone?
    c. From a biological standpoint were the data reasonable?

Discussion

1. Were the study objectives met?

2. Did the authors adequately interpret their results?

3. Did the authors discuss their results and compare them with the current literature?

4. Was the discussion related directly to the results or was it overly speculative?

5. If non-standard methods were used, were they adequately discussed?

6. Were limitations of the study clearly stated?

7. Were conclusions drawn? Were they supported by the results?

References

1. Were appropriate citations listed? Were they accurate? Were they timely?

2. Were enough references presented so that a cogent whole presentation was in the manuscript?

Acknowledgments

1. Were the funding sources clearly identified?

2. Were there real or apparent conflicts of interest, which could suggest bias?

*This is difficult for those unfamiliar with the literature but becomes easier with practice and familiarity with the topic.

treatments, practice protocols, or policies (discussed in depth in Chapter 1). From bottom (least convincing) to top (best evidence) the hierarchy is generally presented as: expert opinion, case reports, case series, case-control studies; cross-sectional surveys; cohort studies (prospective or retrospective); randomized clinical trials (RCT); and systematic reviews of RCT with or without meta-analysis. It should be kept in mind; however, that this hierarchy assumes that all studies were well designed and executed. A poor RCT may not provide the same level of evidence as a very well designed cross-sectional survey.

To assess a body of evidence, many organizations, including the National Heart, Lung, and Blood Institute (NHLBI), the American Dietetic Association (ADA), and the American Diabetes Association, have grading scales. The NHLBI uses a four-point scale to grade the scientific evidence from different study types (**Table 2–3**). The Evidence Analysis Library (EAL) of the ADA uses a five-step process; the fourth of which is to summarize evidence and the last is to develop a conclusion statement and assign a grade.

Grades I and II are considered "Strong—where benefits clearly exceed harms, [with] excellent supporting evidence." Examples of evidence statements for a wide variety of nutrition-related topics are found on the EAL's Web site. A caveat that should be considered for all of these scales is that they are time-consuming and new studies are continually being

> American Dietetic Association (ADA) members have full online access to the Evidence Analysis Library (EAL) at http://www.adaevidencelibrary.com

published. Be sure the information you use in your practice is the most recently available.

■ NUTRITION MONITORING

Collecting nutrition and health-related information from a population is critical for designing and evaluating policies and programs that improve health status and decrease risk factors. Scientists analyze data from nutrition monitoring programs and use these analyses to contribute to the literature. To be useful, information must be collected in a timely manner and presented to scientists, policy makers, and the public in a readily understandable form. Without current monitoring, decisions may be made using insufficient information or incorrect assumptions. Nutrition and health-related information can be obtained using several methods, notably through nutrition screening, assessment, and surveillance; these are often collectively referred to as nutrition monitoring.

Nutrition screening is a systematic approach to identify quickly nutrition problems or individuals at nutritional risk that are in need of further assessment or an intervention. The Nutrition Screening Initiative's DETERMINE questionnaire and the mini-nutritional assessment, used in screening elderly populations[39] are two widely used screening instruments. Many other screening tools are available for

> Stay on top of nutritional monitoring and other events in public health by subscribing online to the *Morbidity and Mortality Weekly Report* at http://www.cdc.gov/mmwr/mmwrsubscribe.html

TABLE 2–3	National Heart, Lung, and Blood Institute's Evidence Categories	
Category	**Sources of Evidence**	**Definition**
Category A	Randomized controlled trials (rich body of data)	Well-designed, randomized clinical trials that provide a consistent pattern of findings in the population for which the recommendation is made. Category A requires substantial numbers of studies involving substantial numbers of participants.
Category B	Randomized controlled trials (limited body of data)	Limited randomized trials or interventions, post-hoc subgroup analyses, or meta-analyses of randomized clinical trials. These are used when there are a limited number of existing trials, study populations are small or provide inconsistent results, or when the trials were undertaken in a population that differs from the target population of recommendation.
Category C	Observational or non-randomized studies	Evidence is from outcomes of uncontrolled or non-randomized trials or from observational studies.
Category D	Panel Consensus Judgment	Expert judgment is based on the panel's synthesis of evidence from experimental research described in the literature or derived from the consensus of panel members based on clinical experience or knowledge that does not meet the above criteria. This category is used only where the provision of some guidance was deemed valuable but an adequately compelling clinical literature addressing the subject of the recommendation was deemed insufficient to place in one of the other categories.

Source: U.S. Department of Health and Human Services, *The Obesity Initiative.* Available at http://www.nhlbi.nih.gov/guidelines/obesity/ob_gdlns.pdf. Accessed February 25, 2010.

nutrition professionals, including, but not limited to those designed to determine malnutrition,[40] diabetes risk,[41] and food security.[42]

Nutrition assessment measures indicators of dietary status, using such methods as 24-hour diet recalls, food frequency questionnaires (FFQ) as discussed in Chapter 1, food diaries, or newer dietary assessment methods including digital photography[43–47] or use of mobile phones to keep food records.[48] Principal strengths of 24-hour diet recalls are that they provide detailed information about the types and amounts of food consumed on a given day,[49] have a low response burden, and are cost-effective.[50] The principal limitations are that they are memory-dependent, respondents may under- or over-report consumption, and 24-hour diet recalls should not be used to assess individual diets. Collection of group data from 24-hour diet recalls with mean reporting, for example, as used by the NHANES, is an appropriate use of 24-hour diet recalls[51]; however, it has long been recognized that 24-hour diet recalls may not be reflect usual intake.[52,53] In 2003, staff members of NHANES began collecting two recalls and the National Cancer Institute (NCI), coupled with the Center for Nutrition Policy and Promotion (CNPP), developed a statistical method to calculate usual intake using both recalls.[54–57] The multiple pass method for the 24-hour dietary recalls[58–60] should be used (**Table 2–4**). The standard for assessing intake is multiple 24-hour dietary recalls using the multiple pass method. Because intake may change on weekend days, it is important to include both weekday and weekend days in the recalls.

Food Frequency Questionnaires vary in the number of food items, food groups, and food portion assessments—all of which affect nutrient intake.[61,62] Similar to 24-hour diet

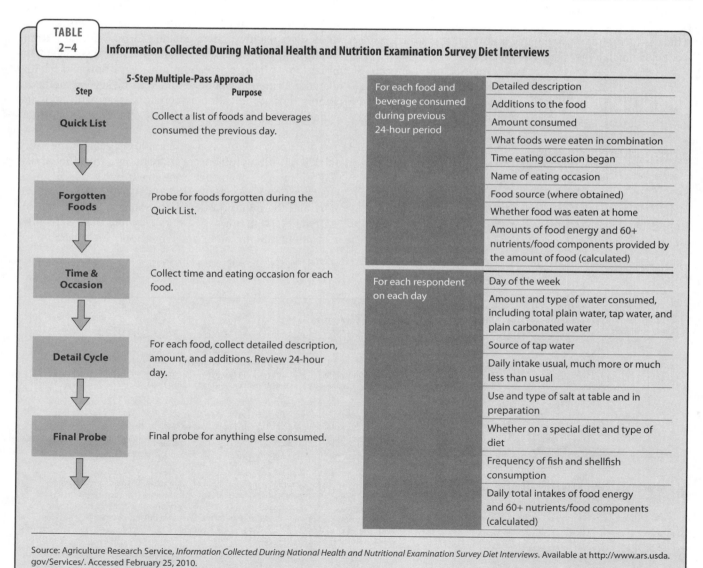

| **TABLE 2–4** | **Information Collected During National Health and Nutrition Examination Survey Diet Interviews** |

5-Step Multiple-Pass Approach

Step	Purpose
Quick List	Collect a list of foods and beverages consumed the previous day.
Forgotten Foods	Probe for foods forgotten during the Quick List.
Time & Occasion	Collect time and eating occasion for each food.
Detail Cycle	For each food, collect detailed description, amount, and additions. Review 24-hour day.
Final Probe	Final probe for anything else consumed.

For each food and beverage consumed during previous 24-hour period
Detailed description
Additions to the food
Amount consumed
What foods were eaten in combination
Time eating occasion began
Name of eating occasion
Food source (where obtained)
Whether food was eaten at home
Amounts of food energy and 60+ nutrients/food components provided by the amount of food (calculated)

For each respondent on each day
Day of the week
Amount and type of water consumed, including total plain water, tap water, and plain carbonated water
Source of tap water
Daily intake usual, much more or much less than usual
Use and type of salt at table and in preparation
Whether on a special diet and type of diet
Frequency of fish and shellfish consumption
Daily total intakes of food energy and 60+ nutrients/food components (calculated)

Source: Agriculture Research Service, *Information Collected During National Health and Nutritional Examination Survey Diet Interviews.* Available at http://www.ars.usda.gov/Services/. Accessed February 25, 2010.

recalls, FFQs often underestimate intake of total energy,[63,64] and energy adjustment can be used to reduce the effects of measurement error, that is, regression dilution.[65,66] It is also important that appropriate racial and ethnic foods consumed by the population of interest be included when designing FFQ. Although a wide variety of FFQs are in use, some have not been validated against 24-hour recalls or direct observation. Using meta-analyses, FFQs with longer food lists (200 items) were shown to have 0.01 to 0.17 higher correlation coefficients than FFQs with shorter food lists (≤ 100 items) for most nutrients.[67] An advantage of FFQs is that they can be self-administered and thus, are suitable for large epidemiologic studies.

Digital photography[44–47] and cell phones[48] to determine food intake are also used. They are appealing with their use of technology, but accuracy is dependent on training staff, study participants, or clients to take consistent photographs. Other methods used to determine intake include direct observation, plate waste, and food records with or without the weighing of foods.

Accurate determination of intake is critical. Intake of food groups can be determined from using instruments as conventional as the MyPyramid tracking system,[68] which is appropriate for the public, and the MyPyramid Equivalents Database,[69] which may be more appropriate for health professionals. Nutrient intake can be assessed using the Nutrient Data Laboratory of the Agricultural Research Service,[70] the Food and Nutrient Database for Dietary Studies,[71] and commercial diet analysis programs. Whenever possible, dietary intake should be confirmed using appropriate biomarkers.[72,73] Intake of nutrients or food groups can be compared with recommended values for specific populations and, in turn, with the prevalence or incidence of chronic disease.

Surveillance comes from the French verb *surveiller*, "to watch over." In 1968, the World Health Assembly described surveillance as "the systematic collection and use of epidemiologic information for planning, implementation, and assessment of disease control."[74] Surveillance, in contrast to surveys, is continuous, and data that are collected can be used to provide the framework for public health policies and rationale for intervention. Surveillance also provides a way to monitor the effectiveness of specific interventions. This completes the loop–surveillance studies that can be used to determine nutritional problems or nutritional needs, and after the intervention, they can be used to determine whether the problems remain or if the intervention was effective.

Most governments track the health and nutrition status of their population. For example, the U.S. government has tracked information on food and the food supply for more than 100 years, starting with the USDA's Food Supply Series in 1909. The first USDA Household Food Consumption Survey (known as the Nationwide Food Consumption Survey after 1965) was begun in the 1930s. In 1960, the National Health Examination Survey was initiated; however, it did not include information on nutrition and its link with diet. Federal officials thus could not provide information on diet and disease or undernutrition to Congress. The nation's first comprehensive nutrition survey was the Ten-State Nutrition Survey conducted between 1968 and 1970 in 10 states: California, Kentucky, Louisiana, Massachusetts, Michigan, New York, South Carolina, Texas, Washington, and West Virginia. The NHANES I and II and the Pediatric Nutrition Surveillance Systems were initiated in the 1970s.

In 1990, the National Nutrition Monitoring and Related Research Program (NNMRRP) (PL 101-445) established a comprehensive, coordinated program for nutrition monitoring and related research to improve health and nutrition assessment in U.S. populations. The NNMRRP required a program to coordinate federal nutrition monitoring efforts and assisted state and local governments in participating in a nutrition monitoring network; an interagency board to develop and implement the program; and a nine member advisory council to provide scientific and technical advice and to evaluate program effectiveness. The NNMRRP also required that dietary guidelines (Dietary Guidelines for Americans [DGA]) be issued every five years, and that any dietary guidance issued by the federal government for the general public be reviewed by the Secretaries of Agriculture and Health and Human Services (HHS).

The NNMRRP encompasses more than 50 surveillance activities that monitor and assesses health and nutritional status in the United States. Monitoring efforts are divided into five overarching areas: nutrition and related health measurements; food and nutrient consumption; knowledge, attitude, and behavior assessments; food composition and nutrient data bases; and food supply determinants. Important monitoring programs are summarized in **Table 2–5**. Most of the data sets generated through this program are available to the public. Some are restricted, due to confidentially or disclosure rules/regulations, and can be accessed by researchers through application to the Research Data Center (RDC) in the National Center for Health Statistics (NCHS) headquarters in Hyattsville, Maryland.

Goals of NHANES

- Estimate the number and percent of persons in the U.S. population, and designated subgroups, with selected diseases and risk factors
- Monitor trends in the prevalence, awareness, treatment, and control of selected diseases
- Monitor trends in risk behaviors and environmental exposures
- Analyze risk factors for selected diseases
- Study the relationship between diet, nutrition, and health
- Explore emerging public health issues and new technologies
- Establish a national probability sample of genetic material for future genetic research
- Establish and maintain a national probability sample of baseline information on health and nutritional status

TABLE 2–5 National Nutrition Related Health Assessments[a]

Survey Name	Date	Target	Data Collected	Dept/ Agency
Nutritional and Related Health Measurements				
NHANES[b]	1999–present	Civilian, non-institutionalized persons 2 months or older; oversampling of adolescents, African-Americans, Mexican-Americans, and adults ≥ 60 yrs	Survey elements are similar to NHANES III & NHIS.[c] This is a continuous monitoring system.	NCHS, CDC (HHS)
NHANES III	1988–1994	Civilian, non-institutionalized persons 2 months or older; oversampling of adolescents, non-Hispanic blacks, Mexican-Americans, children < 6 yrs and adults ≥ 60 yrs	Demographics, dietary intake (24-hour recall & food frequency), biochemical analysis of blood and urine, physical examination, anthropometry, blood pressure, bone densitometry, diet and health behaviors, health conditions	NCHS, CDC (HHS)
NHANES III Supplemental Nutrition Survey of Older Persons	1988–1994	Representative U.S. elderly population	See above	NCHS, NIH/NIA
HHANES	1982–1984	Civilian, non-institutionalized Mexican Americans in five southwestern states, Cuban Americans in Dade Co. FL, and Puerto Ricans in New York, New Jersey, and Connecticut, 6 months to 74 years	Demographics, dietary intake (24-hour recall & food frequency), biochemical analysis of blood and urine, physical exam, anthropometry, blood pressure, diet and health behaviors, health conditions	NCHS (HHS)
NHANES II	1976–1980	Civilian, non-institutionalized persons 6 months to 74 yrs	Demographics, dietary intake, biochemical analysis of blood & urine, physical exam, anthropometry	NCHS (HHS)
NHANES I	1971–1974	Civilian, non-institutionalized population of the conterminous states 1 to 74 yrs	Demographics, dietary information, biochemical analysis of blood & urine, physical exam, anthropometry	NCHS (HHS)
PedNSS	1973, continuous	Low-income, high-risk children, birth to 17 yrs, emphasis on birth to 5 yrs	Demographics, anthropometry, birth weight, hematology	NCCDPHP, CDC (HHS)
PNSS	1973, continuous	Convenience sample of low-income, high-risk pregnant women	Demographics, pregravid weight and maternal weight gain, anemia, behavioral risk factors, birth weight, and formula-feeding data	NCCDPHP, CDC (HHS)
Food and Nutrient Consumption				
CSFII[d]	1994–1996 1989–1991 1985–1986	Individuals of all ages with oversampling in low-income households	One and three day food intakes, times of eating events, sources of food eaten away from home	ARS, HNIS
TDS	1961, annual	Specific age and gender groups	Determines levels of nutrients and contaminants in the food supply—analyses are performed on foods that are "table-ready"	FDA (HHS)
Consumer Expenditure Survey	1980, continuous	Non-institutionalized population and a portion of the institutionalized population in the United States	Demographics, food stamp use, average annual food expenditures	U.S. Bureau of Labor Statistics
NFCS	1987 1977–1978	Households in the conterminous states—all income and low income	Households: quantity (pounds), money value (dollars), and nutritive value of food eaten. Individuals: food intake, times of eating events, and sources of foods eaten away from home	HNIS (USDA), ARS (USDA)
SNDA II	1998	Public schools in the 48 contiguous states and the District of Columbia that participate in the National School Lunch Program	School and food service characteristics, nutrients by food group and relationship to the RDA and DGA by meals, source of meals, and nutrient content of USDA meals	FNS/USDA
WIC Feeding Practices Study	1994–1995	Pre- and post-natal women and their children who participate in WIC	Demographics, rates of breast and formula feeding, factors associated with breast feeding.	FNS/USDA

TABLE 2–5 *(Continued)*

Survey Name	Date	Target	Data Collected	Dept/Agency
5-A-Day for Better Health Baseline Survey	1991	Adults 18 years and older	Demographics, fruit and vegetable intake, and knowledge, attitudes, and practices regarding intake	NCI (HHS)
Knowledge, Attitude, and Behavior Assessments				
YRBBS	Biennial	Civilian, non-institutionalized adolescents 12 to 18 yrs	Demographics, diet and weight; drug, alcohol & tobacco use; seat belt and bicycle helmet use; behaviors that contribute to violence; suicidal tendencies[e]	CDC (HHS)/ NCCDPHP
BRFSS	1984, continuous	Adults 18 yrs and older in households with telephones located in participating states	Demographics, questions that assess risk factors associated with leading causes of death: alcohol and tobacco use, weight, seat belt and helmet use; use of preventative medical care[f]	CDC (HHS)/ NCCDPHP
DHKS	1994–1996	Adults 20 yrs and older who participated in CSFII 1994–1996	Demographics, self-perceptions of relative intake, awareness of diet and health relationships, food label use, perceived importance of following diet and health recommendations, beliefs about food safety, and knowledge of sources of nutrients; data can be linked with intake through CSFII data	ARS/USDA
Infant Feeding Practices Survey	1993–1994	New mothers and healthy infants to 1 year of age	Demographics, prior infant feeding practices, baby's social situation, characteristics associated with breast feeding, development of allergies	FDA
Consumer Food Handling Practices	1998 1992–1993	Civilian, non-institutionalized over 18 yrs with telephones	Demographics, prevalence of unsafe food handling practices, knowledge of food safety principles, use of sources of information about safe food handling, incidence of food borne illnesses	FDA
Food Composition and Nutrient Data Bases				
National Nutrient Data Bank	–	–	This is the repository for values of approximately 7,100 foods and up to 80 components. Essentially all food composition databases are derived from this data bank	ARS (USDA)
Food Label and Package Survey	1977–1996, biennially	All brands of processed foods regulated by the FDA	Prevalence of nutrition labeling, declaration of select nutrients, prevalence of label claims and other descriptors	FDA (HHS)
Food Supply Determinations				
AC Nielsen SCANTRACK	1985, monthly	~ 3,000 U.S. Supermarkets	Sales and physical volume of specific market items, selling price, percent of stores selling the product	ERS/USDA
U.S. Food and Nutrient Supply Series	1909, annually	U.S. Population	ERS = Amount of food commodities that disappear into the food distribution system; CNPP = nutrient levels of food supply. Results are totaled for each nutrient and converted to per day basis.	ERS/CNPP/ USDA

[a] A complete guide to nutrition monitoring in the United States can be found at: http://www.cdc.gov/nchs/data/misc/nutri98.pdf

[b] Abbreviations: ARS = Agricultural Research Service; BRFSS = Behavioral Risk Factor Surveillance System; CDC = Centers for Disease Control and Prevention; CNPP = Center for Nutrition Policy and Promotion; CSFII = Continuing Survey of Food Intakes by Individuals; DHKS = Diet and Health Knowledge Survey; ERS = Economic Research Service FDA = Food and Drug Administration; HHANES = Hispanic Health and Nutrition Examination Survey; HHS = Health and Human Services; HNIS = Human Nutrition Information Service; NFCS = Nationwide Food Consumption Survey; NCCDPHP = National Center for Chronic Disease Prevention and Health Promotion; NCHS = National Center for Health Statistics; NCI = National Cancer Institute; NHANES = National Health and Nutrition Examination Survey; NHIS = National Health Interview Survey; NIA = National Institute on Aging; NIH= National Institutes of Health; PedNSS = Pediatric Nutrition Surveillance System; PNSS = Pregnancy Nutrition Surveillance System; SNDA = School Nutrition Dietary Assessment Study; TDS = Total Diet Study; USDA = United States Department of Agriculture; WIC = Women, Infants, and Children; YRBSS = Youth Risk Behavioral Surveillance System.

[c] http://www.cdc.gov/nchs/nhanes.htm complete survey content of NHANES 1999–2004

[d] CSFII and NHANES have now been combined into a single survey

[e] http://www.cdc.gov/mmwr/PDF/SS/SS302.pdf = YBRSS report 2004; *MMWR* summary reports available through CDC Web site

[f] http://www.cdc.gov/brfss/#about_BRFSS = Behavioral Risk Factor Surveillance System full information

In 2002, the Department of HHS and the USDA integrated NHANES and the Continuing Survey of Food Intakes by Individuals (CSFII), the two major diet and health surveys, into a continuous data collection system. Diet and nutrition information thus can be linked directly to health status information. The integrated dietary component of the NHANES is entitled, *"What We Eat in America."*[75]

The NHANES is a program of studies designed to assess the health and nutritional status of the U.S. population. The survey combines health interviews and physical examinations with dietary information (**Table 2–6**).

Beginning in 1999, the NHANES survey became a continuous surveillance program with data released to the public biannually. Rather than using a random sample, the

---

TABLE 2–6	**Data Available Through NHANES**

Health Exam Tests

Health Measurements by Participant Age and Gender

- Physician's exam – all ages
- Blood pressure – ages ≥ 8 years
- Bone density – ages ≥ 8 years
- Condition of teeth – ages ≥ 5 years
- Vision test – ages ≥ 12 years
- Hearing test – ages 12–19 years and ≥ 70 years
- Height, weight, and other body measures – all ages
- Ophthalmology exam for eye diseases – ages ≥ 40 years
- Breathing tests – ages 6–79 years

Lab Tests on Urine: (≥ 6 years)

- Kidney function tests – ages ≥ 6 years
- Sexually transmitted disease (STD)
  —Chlamydia and gonorrhea – ages 14–39 years
- Exposure to environmental chemicals – selected persons ages ≥ 6 years
- Pregnancy test – girls and women ages ≥ 12 years and girls ages 8–11 years who have periods

Lab Tests on Blood: (≥ 1 year and older)

- Anemia – all ages
- Total cholesterol and high density lipoprotein (HDL) – ages ≥ 6 years
- Glucose measures – ages ≥ 12 years
- Infectious diseases – ages ≥ 2 years
- Kidney function tests – ages ≥ 12 years
- Lead – ages ≥ 1 years
- Cadmium – ages ≥ 1 years
- Mercury – ages ≥1 years
- Liver function tests – ages ≥ 12 years
- Nutrition status – ages ≥ 1 years
- Thyroid function test – ages ≥ 12 years
- Prostate specific antigen (PSA) – men ages ≥ 40 years
- Sexually transmitted diseases (STD)
  —Genital herpes – ages 14–49 years
  —Human immunodeficiency virus (HIV) – ages 18–49 years
  —Human papillomavirus (HPV) antibody – ages 14–59 years
- Exposure to environmental chemicals – selected persons ages ≥ 6 years

Lab Tests on Water

- Environmental chemicals – ages ≥ 12 years in half of households

Other Lab Tests

- Vaginal swabs (self-administered) – girls and women ages 14–59 years
- Human papillomavirus (HPV) – ages 14–59 years

Private Health Interviews

- Health status – ages ≥ 12 and older
- Questions about drug and alcohol use – ages ≥ 12 years (no drug testing will be done)
- Reproductive health – girls and women ages ≥ 12 years
- Questions about sexual experience – ages 14–69 years
- Tobacco use – ages ≥ 12 years

Anthropometry from the Mobile Examination Center

- Body mass index (BMI); for children ages 2–19 years; BMI z-score is also determined
- Waist circumference
- Skinfold measurements and body fat measures through DXA

Dietary Information from the Mobile Examination Center

- 24-hour dietary recalls; parents or guardians report for children 0–5 years of age; children 6–11 years are assisted by an adult; children ≥ 12 years self-report
- Food frequency questionnaire

After the Visit to the NHANES Examination Center

- Persons asked about the foods they eat will receive a phone call 3–10 days after their exam for a similar interview, all ages.
- Then participants, or an adult for participants 1–15 years old, are asked about food shopping habits.
- Persons who test positive for hepatitis C will be asked to participate in a brief telephone interview 6 months after the exam. Parents will respond for children.

NHANES uses a complex, multistage, probability sampling design to select participants representative of the civilian, non-institutionalized U.S. population. Oversampling of population subgroups at different times (e.g., Hispanic Americans) increases the reliability and precision of health status indicator estimates for these subgroups. Data collection by the NHANES occurs at three levels: a brief household screener interview, an in-depth household survey interview, and a medical examination. Because detailed interviews, clinical, laboratory, radiological examinations are conducted, the response burden to participants is significant. Interviews and medical examinations take place in a mobile examination center. Because of this sampling design, using appropriate statistical analyses of NHANES data are critical. To assure that NHANES analyses reflect a nationally representative sample, it is important to use the described weighting system and specialty software (e.g., SUDAAN).

Take a guided tour of the mobile examination center at http://www.cdc.gov/nchs/nhanes/about_nhanes.htm

It is difficult to quantify the tremendous impact that NHANES and related programs have had on health policy and health research in the United States.[76] One way is to look at this is the number of publications generated using NHANES data. A PubMed search in January 2010 using the term "NHANES" produced 16,621 publications on topics as diverse as national trends in self-reported physical activity/sedentary behavior in pregnant women; trends in cardiovascular risk; prevalence and treatment of mental disorders in U.S. children and television viewing, computer use; body mass index in children and adolescents; and the association of consumption of 100% fruit juice and nutrient intake in children. NHANES has also shown that there are ethnic and racial differences in dietary intake[77,78]; food sources for different nutrients are different in different ethnic groups[79]; cardiovascular risk factors cluster according to socioeconomic status[80]; and hypertension varies according to geographical region.[81] These findings have important implications for intervention strategies.

■ EPIDEMIOLOGIC STUDIES

In addition to the NCHS data, a number of long-term, primarily government funded, epidemiologic studies on adults and children/adolescents have provided critical information used to guide the nation's health policies and federal programs. The Bogalusa Heart Study (BHS), the Framingham Heart Study (FHS), and

To learn more about working with NHANES data, complete the online tutorial at http://www.cdc.gov/nchs/tutorials/nhanes/index_current.htm

the Coronary Artery Risk Development in Young Adults (CARDIA) are leading examples. Other important U.S. epidemiologic studies that have contributed to our knowledge of risk reduction and disease prevention are The Nurses' Health Study (NHS; $N = 170,000$ women registered nurses between the ages of 30 and 55 years at the beginning of the study) and the Nurses' Health Study II (NHS II established in 1989, $N = \sim 117,000$ women nurses aged between 25 and 42 years); and the all-men Health Professional Follow-up Study (initiated in 1986 with 2-year scheduled follow-ups), which was designed to complement the NHS, relating nutritional factors to the incidence of serious illnesses, such as cancer, heart disease, and other vascular diseases in 51,529 male health professionals. Also of import is the Iowa Women's Health Study with a cohort of 41,837 post-menopausal women who have been followed since 1985. These studies combined have produced more than 2000 scientific publications and have helped shape medical care, risk reduction and health promotion, and public policy.

The Bogalusa Heart Study

The (BHS)[82–84] was designed initially to examine the early natural history of coronary heart disease and essential hypertension in a biracial (black/white) pediatric population. The BHS population consists of approximately 5,000 individuals who have been studied at various growth phases and have been followed for as long as 15 years. The mixed epidemiologic design of the study has included cross-sectional and longitudinal surveys to provide information on three questions: 1) what are the distribution and prevalence of CVD risk factors in a defined pediatric population and how are abnormal serum lipid levels, blood pressure, and other risk factors are defined in children; 2) do cardiovascular risk factors track and change over time; and 3) what is the interrelationship among these risk factors? Other questions, notably what is the interaction of genetics and the environment, were also posed.

Data from the BHS have contributed significantly to our knowledge and understanding of cardiovascular risk factors in children as well as the history of CVD in early life. For example, information on children, adolescents, and young adults from birth to 31 years of age has provided the framework to establish desirable cholesterol levels in children, and has led investigators to recommend screening of cardiovascular risk factors for all children, not only those with a parental history of heart disease or dyslipidemia, beginning at elementary school age.

Data have also suggested that risk factors for cardiovascular disease "track," that is, they remain in a rank

The Bogalusa Heart Study (BHS) was extended and many findings were duplicated in another population through the Young Finns Study. To learn more about the Young Finns Study, go to http://vanha.med.utu.fi/cardio/youngfinnsstudy

relative to peers over time. For example, children with elevated serum total cholesterol or low density lipoprotein cholesterol (LDL-C) levels are likely to become adults with dyslipidemia. Bogalusa Heart Study data have been used to characterize diets of children and secular trends in children's diets for more than 30 years.[85] BHS data were used as the rationale by the American Academy of Pediatrics for their recommendation that the DGA could apply to healthy children 2 years of age and older, and to develop the ADA's position paper on dietary guidance for healthy children 2 to 11 years of age.[86]

One of the major accomplishments of the BHS did not come from epidemiologic data per se, but from autopsy studies of participants,[87] usually those killed in accidents. BHS data confirmed and extended earlier studies[88] that showed fatty streaks in the aorta were evident in the first decade of life and that the extensiveness of these lesions was highly associated with serum total cholesterol and LDL-C levels.

Framingham Heart Study

The FHS has been described as "one of the most impressive medical works in the 20th century."[89] The Framingham Study has provided information critical to the recognition and management of atherosclerosis, and its causes and complications. Initiated under the auspices of the National Heart Institute (now the NHLBI) in 1948, 1,980 men and 2,421 women were enrolled originally in a three-year observational study in Framingham, Massachusetts, which at the time was a novel idea. Published in 1961, the first report entitled, "Factors of risk in the development of coronary heart disease—six-year follow-up experience; the Framingham Study," identified high blood pressure, smoking, and high cholesterol levels as major factors in heart disease and conceptualized them as risk factors. Continued study of the population has provided health professionals with multifactorial risk profiles for cardiovascular disease that have assisted in identifying individuals at high risk as well as providing the basis for preventative measures. During its more than 50 year history, the FHS has introduced the concept of biologic, environmental, and behavioral risk factors; identified major risk factors associated with heart disease, stroke, and other diseases; revolutionized preventive medicine; and changed how the medical community and general population regard disease pathogenesis. The National Cholesterol Education Program (NCEP)[14] uses the Framingham risk scoring system to determine the 10-year risk of CHD in adults. The Framingham study has also supplied valuable information to the Seventh Report of the Joint National Committee on the Prevention, Detection, Evaluation, and Treatment of High Blood Pressure.[90]

In 1971, the Framingham Heart Offspring Study began, consisting of 5,124 men and women, ages 5 to 70 years, who were offspring and spouses of the offspring of the original Framingham cohort. The objectives of this study were to determine the incidence and prevalence of CVD and its risk factors, trends in CVD incidence and its risk factors over time, and family patterns of CVD and risk factors. The Offspring Study provided the opportunity to evaluate a second generation of participants, assess new or emerging risk factors and outcomes, and provide a resource for future genetic analyses.

The quality of data from surveys and epidemiologic studies depends on the training of personnel and adherence to rigid protocols. It also depends on the validity and reliability of the test instruments used as well as on the responses of the subjects. Instruments may need to be modified for specific populations. For example, in the BHS the 24-hour diet recall method had to be adapted for use in children.[91,92] To improve the reliability and validity of the 24-hour diet recall, quality controls included the use of a standardized protocol that specified exact techniques for interviewing, recording, and calculating results; standardized graduated food models to quantify foods and beverages consumed; a product identification notebook for probing of snack consumption, and foods and beverages most commonly forgotten; school lunch assessment to identify all school lunch recipes, preparation methods, and average portion sizes of menu items reflected in each 24-hour diet recall; follow-up telephone calls to parents to obtain information on brand names, recipes, and preparation methods of meals served at home; products researched in the field to obtain updated information on ingredients and preparation, and their weights (primarily snack foods and fast foods).[93] All interviewers participated in rigorous training sessions and pilot studies before the field surveys to minimize interviewer effects. One 24-hour diet recall was collected on each study participant, and duplicate recalls were collected from a 10% random subsample to assess interviewer variability.[94]

■ METABOLIC DIET STUDIES

Metabolic diet studies are conducted in clinical research centers where study participants are randomized into test or control groups and are fed an experimental diet or "regular" diet, respectively. Different designs are available for metabolic diet studies,[95] but the one that provides the most valid results is a double-blind, placebo-controlled study. In these studies, neither the investigator nor the participant knows whether the test or control diet is offered. Because it is difficult and expensive to do these studies, they are usually short term and have a small sample size; compliance and drop-out rates are problems.

The Dietary Approaches to Stop Hypertension (DASH)[96] and DASH sodium[97] trials are examples of metabolic diet studies. Epidemiologic, clinical trials, and studies using experimental animals showed that consumption of nutrients, notably low levels of sodium, and high levels of potassium, and calcium lowered blood pressure; however, people eat food—not isolated nutrients. To test the impact that combination diets incorporating foods high in these nutrients had on blood pressure, the DASH study was conducted. DASH was a randomized controlled trial conducted at four academic medical centers with 459 adult participants. Inclusion criteria were untreated systolic blood pressure less than 160 mm Hg and diastolic blood pressure 80 to 95 mm Hg. For three weeks, participants ate a control diet. They were then randomized to eight weeks of a control diet; a diet rich in fruits and vegetables; or a combination diet rich in fruits, vegetables, and low-fat dairy foods, and low in saturated fatty acids, total fat, and cholesterol. Salt intake and weight were held constant, and diets were isoenergic. All food was prepared in a metabolic kitchen and was provided to participants. The combination diet (or "DASH diet") was shown to quickly (within 2 weeks) and substantially lower blood pressure. In DASH sodium, a subsequent study, 412 participants were assigned to a control diet or a DASH diet; within the assigned diet, participants ate meals with high (3,450 mg/2100 kcals), intermediate (2,300 mg/2,100 kcals) and low (1,150 mg/2,100 kcals) levels of sodium for 30 consecutive days each, in random order. Reduction of sodium intake to levels below the current recommendation of 100 mmol/day and the DASH diet substantially lowered blood pressure, with the most significant effect seen in lowering blood pressure with the lowest sodium concentration coupled with the DASH diet. The DASH diet has been widely embraced for the treatment of hypertension and nutrition education materials are readily available. As elegant and persuasive as the DASH studies were, one drawback to feeding studies is that participants receive all foods. The studies thus cannot assess how compliant people are after the study ends.[95] The PREMIER study[98] demonstrated that free-living individuals were able to make the lifestyle changes associated with decreased blood pressure.

CLINICAL TRIALS

Clinical trials are commonly used to determine the efficacy of drugs or other pharmacologic agents; however, they can also be used to assess diet or dietary interventions. They have many of the same advantages and disadvantages of metabolic studies. Because clinical trials of diet may involve pharmacologic intervention, they carry a risk that is not usually seen with metabolic diet studies. The classical example of this was seen in the Alpha-Tocopherol, Beta-Carotene Cancer Prevention Study (ATBC Study)[99] and the Beta-Carotene and Retinol Efficacy Trial (CARET).[100] Based on epidemiologic data that showed a relationship between dietary intake of fruits and vegetables[101,102] or, specifically, of beta carotene[103] and a reduced risk of developing lung cancer, especially in smokers,[103] the ATBC and CARET studies used high dose beta-carotene in major cancer chemopreventive trials.[104] Investigators expected to see reductions in

lung cancer by as much as 49% in some high-risk groups.[100] In actuality, the opposite was seen and beta-carotene increased the risk of lung cancer, forcing the CARET study to be stopped early.[105] These studies clearly point to the necessity of additional research, and have important public health implications.[106]

ANIMAL STUDIES

Animal studies are important in nutrition research for many reasons. Laboratory animals that are genetically identical and exposed to the same environmental conditions can be fed carefully characterized diets with different combinations of nutrients; thus, the number of variables studied are limited. Special treatments, such as ovariectomies to mimic the physiologic state of postmenopausal women,[107] can be performed on animals. Because the lifespan of most laboratory animals is short, the effects of dietary manipulation can be followed over several generations. Animals can be sacrificed at the end of the experiment and the effect of the treatment can be examined closely at the organ, tissue, or cellular level. Animal studies can explore molecular mechanisms behind a given observation in humans. For example, ferrets were used to determine that high doses of beta-carotene caused keratinized squamous metaplasia in lung tissues that was exacerbated by exposure to cigarette smoke.[108] This explains the paradoxical relationship between beta-carotene and smoking seen in the clinical trials above. It points out another use of animal studies: that the metabolism of natural products should be investigated using animal models *before* beginning intervention trials, particularly if nutrient doses exceed recommended levels.[109]

Animals most commonly used in nutrition research are rats, mice, rabbits, guinea pigs, dogs, sheep, and monkeys. The species selected for a given experiment should be that which is the most similar to human metabolism for a particular nutrient. The importance of this is illustrated in the classic studies of vitamin C metabolism. Guinea pigs are the only laboratory animal that, like humans, have an obligatory requirement for this nutrient; thus, a review of the literature shows only guinea pigs were used for vitamin C research.

Many of the elements that make animal studies so appealing in nutrition research are also drawbacks. With the exception of monozygotic twins, humans are not genetically identical; thus, no matter how carefully a human experiment is controlled, responses to dietary manipulations may be different due to individual genetic backgrounds. Interactions between genetics and the environment are easy to study in animals, but results are difficult to translate to humans.

HEALTHY PEOPLE 2010/2020

Individual health is closely linked to community health—the health of the community and environment in which individuals live, work, and play. Community health, in turn, is profoundly affected by the collective beliefs, attitudes, and behaviors of everyone who lives in that community. *Healthy People 2010 (HP)*, published by the Department of Health and Human Services (DHHS),[110] is the comprehensive health promotion and disease prevention agenda for the nation; the goals for HP 2010 will remain in place until superseded by HP 2020. The HP program grew out of health initiatives pursued over the last 25 years. In 1979, *Healthy People: The Surgeon General's Report on Health Promotion and Disease Prevention*[111] provided nutritional goals for reducing premature deaths and preserving independence for older adults. In 1980, *Promoting Health/Preventing Disease: Objectives for the Nation*, targeted 226 health objectives for the nation to achieve over the next 10-year period.[112] These were followed by HP 2000, HP 2010, and, now 2020 goals.

The NCHS is responsible for coordinating efforts to monitor progress toward the HP objectives. National data are gathered from more than 190 different data sources, from more than seven federal government departments (DHHS as well as the Departments of Commerce, Education, Justice, Labor, Transportation, and the Environmental Protection Agency), and from voluntary and private nongovernmental organizations. As appropriate, data for the objectives are provided for subgroups defined by relevant dimensions (e.g., sociodemographic subgroups of the population, health status, or geographic classifications) through DATA 2010,[113] an interactive database system and the CDC Wonder System.[114] Quarterly reports are made available to the public.[115]

Many states have developed their own HP plans.[116] Development of state-specific plans allows states to prioritize health problems, address needs of specific racial or ethnic groups, and develop solutions that are economically feasible for state budgets. Other specific interest groups have developed similar plans—for example, Healthy Workforce 2010[117] provides a resource for large and small employers and Rural *Healthy People 2010*, a companion document for rural areas,[118] focuses on health problems and solutions of rural Americans. The NHLBI's HP 2010 Cardiovascular Gateway[119] illustrates how this agency links goals from HP 2010, the DGA, and the NCEP to provide information and ideas to the public and health professionals. Improving Health/Changing Lives: Communities Taking Action illustrates effective health campaigns in America. Programs of excellence funded by the NHLBI; these include the Healthy Heart Project in rural West Virginia and Helping Educators Attack Cardiovascular Risk Factors Together programs. To support the HP initiative, the NHLBI also has nutrition education material available as well as access to conferences, meetings, exhibits, and distance learning opportunities.

At this time, the Secretary of HHS is overseeing the update of the HP objectives. The process for reformulating the nation's public health goals is ongoing and transparent.[1]

The proposed overarching goals for HP 2020 are more ambitious than for HP 2010:

- Eliminate preventable disease, disability, injury, and premature death.
- Achieve health equity, eliminate disparities, and improve the health of all groups.
- Create social and physical environments that promote good health for all.
- Promote healthy development and healthy behaviors across every stage of life.

A feedback loop of intervention, assessment, and dissemination of evidence and best practices would enable achievement of HP 2020 goals. The Action Model to Achieve HP Goals (**Figure 2–1**) represents the impact of interventions (i.e., policies, programs, and information) on determinants of health at multiple levels (e.g., individual; social, family, and community; living and working conditions; and broad social, economic, cultural, health, and environmental conditions) to improve outcomes. Results of these interventions can be demonstrated through assessment, monitoring, and evaluation. Through dissemination of evidence-based practices and best practices, these findings would feed back to intervention planning to enable the identification of effective prevention strategies in the future.

The objectives related to Nutrition and Weight Status for HP 2020 is presented in Table 2–7. Objectives 1 to 4 were retained directly from HP 2010; objectives 5 to 14 were retained but modified from HP 2010; objectives 15 to 20 are new to HP 2020; and 3 objectives were archived from HP 2010. It is important to note that the data sources used to generate the objectives are included in HP 2020; often NHANES data were used. Why were these changes made? Objectives were retained because they remain important or were not met in HP 2010. For example, the first objective is to "Increase the proportion of adults who are at a healthy weight." This objective was not met—in fact, 50% moved away from the target (**Figure 2–2**). It's noteworthy that when public comments were examined, many asked the question, "what is a healthy weight?" Without this knowledge, it is unlikely that the public can meet the HP goals.

■ NUTRIENT REQUIREMENTS

The first Recommended Daily Allowances (RDAs) were published in 1941 "as a guide for advising on nutrition problems in connection with national defense."[120] The first edition included recommendations for only nine nutrients: protein, thiamine, riboflavin, niacin, ascorbic acid, vitamins A and D, calcium, and iron. In the seventh edition (1968), additional nutrients were included: folate, vitamins B_6 and B_{12}; vitamin E, phosphorous, magnesium, and iodine. The last edition of the RDAs (1989) added vitamin K, zinc, and selenium. The RDAs should be geared to groups of healthy

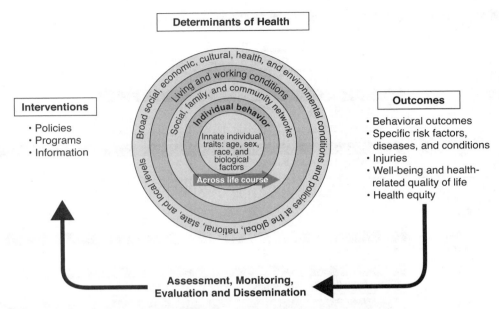

FIGURE 2–1 Action Model to Achieve *Healthy People 2020* Overarching Goals

Source: U.S. Department of Health and Human Services, *Secretary's Advisory Committee on National Health Promotion & Disease Prevention Objectives for 2020.* Available at http://www.healthypeople.gov/hp2020/advisory. Accessed February 24, 2010.

people, such as the military or school feeding programs, rather than to individuals. The RDAs are, however, often used to assess the adequacy of an individual's diet.

In 1993, the question of whether the RDAs should be changed was posed by the Institute of Medicine's (IOM) Food and Nutrition Board (FNB). Support for change included that: 1) sufficient new scientific information had accumulated to substantiate reassessment of these recommendations; 2) sufficient data for efficacy and safety existed; reduction in the risk of chronic diet-related diseases needed to be considered—previously, the RDA had focused on preventing deficiency diseases; 3) upper levels of intake should be established where there were data concerning risk of adverse effects; and 4) components of food that gave possible health benefits. Components of food, not meeting the traditional concept of a nutrient—such as phytochemicals, should be reviewed, and if adequate data existed, reference intakes should be established.

Between 1994 and 2004, the IOM's FNB DRI extended and replaced the former RDAs and the Canadian Recommended Nutrient Intakes.[121] The DRIs are available on the IOM Web site or the Web site of the Food and Nutrition Information Center of the National Agricultural Library.[122] The DRIs are specified on age, gender, and lifestage (e.g., pregnancy or lactation),

> Phytochemicals are chemicals found in plants that may have non-nutritive health benefits. Examples are antioxidants (e.g., carotenoids) or antibacterials (e.g., garlic).

and cover more than 40 nutrient substances. Conceptually, the DRIs are the same as the RDAs in that their formulation relies on the best scientific evidence available at the time of issuance,[123] are designed for healthy individuals over time, and can vary depending on life cycle stage or gender. The reference values for heights and weights of adults and children used in the DRIs are from NHANES III. The DRIs differ from the original RDAs in that they incorporate the concepts of disease prevention, upper levels of intake and potential toxicity, and non-traditional nutrients. The latter establishes a precedent; as scientists learn more about the relationship of phytochemicals, herbals, or botanicals and health, these too can be incorporated into the recommendations. Where scientific evidence is available, the DRIs are a set of at least four nutrient-based reference values. Briefly, the four reference values are the estimated average requirement (EAR), RDA, tolerable upper intake level (UL), and adequate intake (AI). The EAR is the median usual intake value estimated to meet the requirements of half the healthy individuals; it is based on specific criteria of adequacy and is based on careful review of the scientific evidence. Not all nutrients have an EAR since there may not be an acceptable science base upon which to define one. The EAR is used to calculate the RDA (RDA = EAR + 2 standard deviation [SD] of the requirement), which is the average daily dietary intake level sufficient to meet the nutrient requirement of approximately 98% of individuals. If there is no EAR for a nutrient, there can be no RDA. If this is the case, an AI for the nutrient is provided. This value is deemed by experts and is intended to meet or to exceed the needs of a healthy population. The

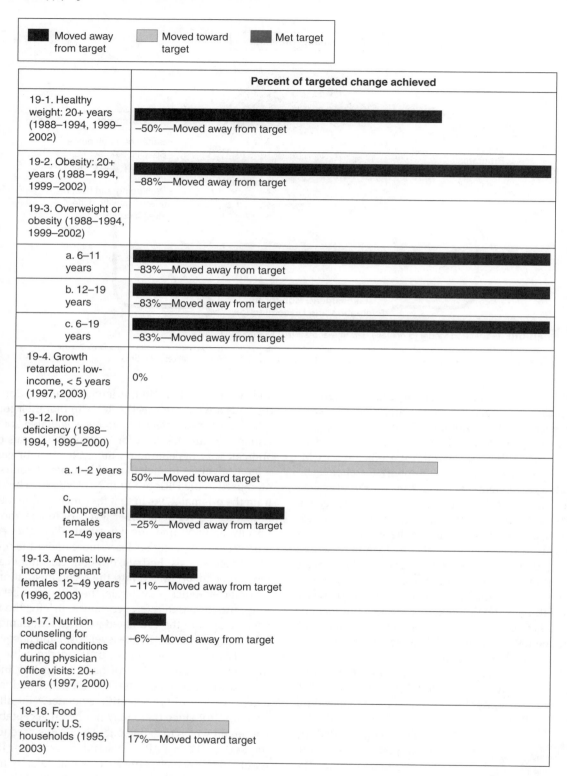

| Moved away from target | Moved toward target | Met target |

	Percent of targeted change achieved
19-1. Healthy weight: 20+ years (1988–1994, 1999–2002)	–50%—Moved away from target
19-2. Obesity: 20+ years (1988–1994, 1999–2002)	–88%—Moved away from target
19-3. Overweight or obesity (1988–1994, 1999–2002)	
a. 6–11 years	–83%—Moved away from target
b. 12–19 years	–83%—Moved away from target
c. 6–19 years	–83%—Moved away from target
19-4. Growth retardation: low-income, < 5 years (1997, 2003)	0%
19-12. Iron deficiency (1988–1994, 1999–2000)	
a. 1–2 years	50%—Moved toward target
c. Nonpregnant females 12–49 years	–25%—Moved away from target
19-13. Anemia: low-income pregnant females 12–49 years (1996, 2003)	–11%—Moved away from target
19-17. Nutrition counseling for medical conditions during physician office visits: 20+ years (1997, 2000)	–6%—Moved away from target
19-18. Food security: U.S. households (1995, 2003)	17%—Moved toward target

FIGURE 2–2   Progress Quotient Chart for Focus Area 19: Nutrition and Overweight. Data shown are selected data.

Source: U.S. Department of Health and Human Services, *Healthy People 2010 Midcourse Review*. Available at http://www.healthypeople.gov/Data/midcourse/html/tables/pq/PQ-19.htm. Accessed February 24, 2010.

TABLE 2–7	Proposed *Healthy People 2020* Objectives Related to Nutrition and Weight Status (NWS)*

Number	Objective
NWS HP2020–1:	Increase the proportion of adults who are at a healthy weight.
NWS HP2020–2:	Reduce the proportion of adults who are obese.
NWS HP2020–3:	Reduce iron deficiency among young children and females of childbearing age.
NWS HP2020–4:	Reduce iron deficiency among pregnant females.
Objectives Retained but Modified from Healthy People 2010	
NWS HP2020–5:	Reduce the proportion of children and adolescents who are overweight or obese.
NWS HP2020–6:	Increase the contribution of fruits to the diets of the population aged 2 years and older.
NWS HP2020–7:	Increase the variety and contribution of vegetables to the diets of the population aged 2 years and older.
NWS HP2020–8:	Increase the contribution of whole grains to the diets of the population aged 2 years and older.
NWS HP2020–9:	Reduce consumption of saturated fat in the population aged 2 years and older.
NWS HP2020–10:	Reduce consumption of sodium in the population aged 2 years and older.
NWS HP2020–11:	Increase consumption of calcium in the population aged 2 years and older.
NWS HP2020–12:	(Developmental) Increase the proportion of worksites that offer nutrition or weight management classes or counseling.
NWS HP2020–13:	Increase the proportion of physician offices visits that include counseling or education related to nutrition or weight.
NWS HP2020–14:	Eliminate very low food security among children in U.S. households.
Objectives New to Healthy People 2020	
NWS HP2020–15:	(Developmental): Prevent inappropriate weight gain in youth and adults.
NWS HP2020–16:	Increase the proportion of primary care physicians who regularly measure the body mass index of their patients.
NWS HP2020–17:	Reduce consumption of calories from solid fats and added sugars in the population aged 2 years and older.
NWS HP2020–18:	Increase the number of States that have State-level policies that incentivize food retail outlets to provide foods that are encouraged by the Dietary Guidelines.
NWS HP2020–19:	Increase the number of States with nutrition standards for foods and beverages provided to preschool-aged children in childcare.
NWS HP2020–20:	Increase the percentage of schools that offer nutritious foods and beverages outside of school meals.
Objectives Archived from Healthy People 2010[†]	
HP2010 19-4:	Reduce growth retardation among low-income children under age 5 years.
HP2010 19-9:	Increase the proportion of persons aged 2 years and older who consume no more than 30 percent of calories from total fat.
HP2010 19-13:	Reduce anemia among low-income pregnant females in their third trimester.

*http://www.healthypeople.gov/hp2020/objectives/TopicArea.aspx?id=35&TopicArea=Nutrition+and+Weight+Status. On the original Web page, students can click on the hyperlinks and read the public comments on individual objectives.

[†]Archived objectives are *Healthy People 2010* objectives that are not included in the proposed set of *Healthy People 2020* objectives for data, target, or policy reasons.

Source: U.S. Department of Health and Human Services, *Nutrition and Weight Status*. Available at http://www.healthypeople.gov/data/midcourse/. Accessed February 25, 2010.

The National Agricultural Library has a new interactive DRI for Health Professionals at http://fnic.nal.usda.gov/interactiveDRI.

DRI tables are available at http://iom.edu/en/Global/News%20Announcements/~/media/Files/Activity%20Files/Nutrition/DRIs/DRISummaryListing2.ashx

AI can be used as a guide for intake, but cannot be used for all the applications for which the EAR can; it is also an indication that additional research is required for a nutrient. The assumption is that when this research is completed and evaluated, the AI can be replaced by an EAR and RDA. The UL is the highest level of continued daily nutrient intake that is unlikely to pose an adverse health effect. It is important to note that the word "tolerable" was chosen to avoid implying a possible beneficial effect.

The IOM has published DRIs and related information for: electrolytes and water[123]; energy, carbohydrate, fiber, fat, fatty acids, cholesterol, protein, and amino acids; vitamin A,

The National Agricultural Library has a new interactive DRI for Health Professionals at http://fnic.nal.usda.gov/interactiveDRI.

DRI tables are available at http://iom.edu/en/Global/News%20Announcements/~/media/Files/Activity%20Files/Nutrition/DRIs/DRISummaryListing2.ashx vitamin K, arsenic, boron, chromium, copper, iodine, iron, manganese, molybdenum, nickel, silicon, vanadium, and zinc[124]; dietary antioxidants and other related compounds[125]; folate and other B vitamins[126]; and calcium, phosphorus, magnesium, vitamin D, and fluoride.[127] A complete set of the DRI books is available online or can be ordered in book form or read online.

Important uses of the DRIs include individual diet planning, dietary guidance, institutional food planning, military food and meal planning, planning for food assistance programs, food labeling and fortification, developing new or modified food products, and guaranteeing food safety. In planning menus/diets for individuals or groups, it is important to meet the RDA or AI without exceeding the UL. The IOM has incorporated the DRIs and other data into a series of reports, including School Meals: Building Blocks for Healthy Children,[128] Local Government Actions to Prevent Childhood Obesity,[121,129] the Public Effects of Food Deserts[130] (Workshop Summary), Nutrition Standards and Meal Requirements for National School Lunch and Breakfast Programs: Phase I. Proposed Approach for Recommending Revisions,[131] and the Use of Dietary Supplements by Military Personnel.[132] Summaries of the development of the DRI[133] as well as the uses of the DRI in dietary assessment[134,135] and to plan menus[136] can be found in the literature.

■ THE CENTER FOR NUTRITION POLICY AND PROMOTION

The Center for Nutrition Policy and Promotion (CNPP), created in December 1994, is an office of the USDA's Food, Nutrition, and Consumer Services. Its mission is "to improve the health of Americans by developing and promoting dietary guidance that links scientific research to the nutrition needs of consumers."[137] The CNPP carries out its mission to improve the health of Americans by: 1) advancing and promoting food and nutrition guidance for all Americans; 2) assessing diet quality; and 3) advancing consumer, nutrition, and food economic knowledge. Major projects administered by CNPP are shown in **Figure 2–3.**

The three major divisions of the CNPP are:

- The Nutrition Marketing and Communication Division (NMCD) established and maintains communication and outreach programs and consumer materials, in coordination with The Nutrition Guidance and Analysis Division. A principal function of the NMCD is to design, implement, and magnify the reach of the MyPyramid Food Guidance System.
- The Nutrition Guidance and Analysis Division (NGAD) administers the process for setting the DGA. It also establishes USDA diet, health, and wellness policies, and applies the information from EALD and

other sources to conduct research and develop the content of nutrition education and outreach programs in these areas. The NGAD also designs, leads, and reports on projects that inform policy related to the USDA Healthy Eating Index (HEI), USDA Food Plans, U.S. Food Supply Series, and Expenditures on Children by Families Project.
- The Evidence Analysis Library Division (EALD) leads scientific review projects that inform and support nutrition policy and guidance and serve as the basis for nutrition promotion and education activities. The EALD supports the DGA process and the Dietary Guidelines Advisory Committee (DGAC).

■ DIETARY GUIDELINES FOR AMERICANS

The Dietary Guidelines for Americans (DGA) are the foundation of federal nutrition policy, nutrition education programs, and information activities. The DGA provide nutrition and dietary advice designed to promote health and reduce the risk of chronic disease for healthy Americans age 2 years and older. By law (PL 101-445), the DGA are developed and published jointly by the Departments HHS and Agriculture every five years. The seventh edition (2010) was released in April 2010 (earlier editions were published in 1980, 1985, 1990, 1995, 2000, and 2005).[138] The 2010 DGA will remain in effect until the 2015 DGA are released. Changes in the DGA must reflect current scientific and medical knowledge available at the time of publication.[139] Two important documents demonstrate the necessity of relying on a science base: The 1988 *Surgeon General's Report on Nutrition and Health*[140] and 1989 *National Research Council's Report, Diet and Health: Implications for Reducing Chronic Disease Risk* (**Table 2–8**, footnote).

The DGA dictates U.S. federal nutrition policies, which directly affect nearly 32.6 million Americans receiving electronic benefits from the Supplemental Nutrition Assistance Program (SNAP); 30.5 million children participating in USDA Child Nutrition Programs; approximately 8.7 million women, infants, and children receiving benefits under the Women, Infants, and Children (WIC) program; and more than 3 million adults over 60 years of age through the Elderly Nutrition Program. The DGA also affects information policy, as evidenced in MyPyramid, food labels, and federal nutrition education programs, such as the SNAP-education program. These pivotal uses of the DGA assure that nutrition information promulgated by the government is consistent. Although not mandated, the DGA also provide the foundation for nutrition recommendations and programs from non-federal agencies such as the American Heart Association and the American Cancer Society.

The DGA appear most frequently as succinct statements of nutrition recommendations for the public (Table 2–8). The

MyPyramid replaced the Food Guide Pyramid in 2005 (En Español)

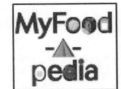 MyFoodapedia provides quick access to food groups, calories, & comparisons

 The Dietary Guidelines for Americans give the basics for healthy eating

 The MyPyramid Menu Planner helps you reach your personal goals

 Get a MyPyramid Plan for Kids (6-11yrs) and Preschoolers (2-5yrs) today

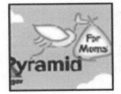 Start out right as a new mom or mom-to-be with MyPyramid for Moms

 Get feedback on your food & physical activity with MyPyramid Tracker

 Know Your Farmer, Know Your Food: Nutrition from farm to table

 Expenditures on Children reports estimate the cost of raising children

 Try out the Cost of Raising a Child Calculator

 USDA Food Plans represent a nutritious diet at 3 different cost levels

 Listen to one of many audio podcasts with MyPyramid tips and advice

FIGURE 2–3   Projects of the Center for Nutrition Promotion and Policy

Source: U.S. Department of Agriculture, *Center for Nutrition Policy and Promotion.* Available at http://www.cnpp.usda.gov. Accessed February 24, 2010.

DGA have three central points: 1) make smart choices from every food group; 2) find your balance between food and physical activity; and 3) get the most nutrition out of calories. As the DGA have evolved more specific information is given—including key recommendations to special populations—such as pregnant women or people with hypertension.

Information that encourages the use of the DGA is available to consumers and to nutrition educators. The full 40-page bulletin, consumer pamphlets, and the report from the DGAC are available online or through the Government Printing Office; a downloadable Power Point presentation for nutrition educators is also available online.

TABLE 2–8	The 2010 Dietary Guidelines for Americans*

Adequate Nutrients within Calorie Needs: Key Recommendations

- Consume a variety of nutrient-dense foods and beverages within and among the basic food groups while choosing foods that limit the intake of saturated and *trans* fats, cholesterol, added sugars, salt, and alcohol.
  - Meet recommended intakes within energy needs by adopting a balanced eating pattern, such as the USDA Food Guide or the DASH Eating Plan.

- **Weight Management**
  - To maintain body weight in a healthy range, balance calories from foods and beverages with calories expended.
  - To prevent gradual weight gain over time, make small decreases in food and beverage calories and increase physical activity.

- **Physical Activity**
  - Engage in regular physical activity and reduce sedentary activities to promote health, psychological well-being, and a healthy body weight.
  - To reduce the risk of chronic disease in adulthood: Engage in at least 30 minutes of moderate-intensity physical activity, above usual activity, at work or home on most days of the week.
  - For most people, greater health benefits can be obtained by engaging in physical activity of more vigorous intensity or longer duration.
  - To help manage body weight and prevent gradual, unhealthy body weight gain in adulthood: Engage in approximately 60 minutes of moderate-to-vigorous–intensity activity on most days of the week while not exceeding caloric intake requirements.
  - To sustain weight loss in adulthood: Participate in at least 60 to 90 minutes of daily moderate-intensity physical activity while not exceeding caloric intake requirements. Some people may need to consult with a healthcare provider before participating in this level of activity.
  - Achieve physical fitness by including cardiovascular conditioning, stretching exercises for flexibility, and resistance exercises or calisthenics for muscle strength and endurance.

- **Food Groups to Encourage**
  - Consume a sufficient amount of fruits and vegetables while staying within energy needs. Two cups of fruit and 2-½ cups of vegetables per day are recommended for a reference 2,000-calorie intake, with higher or lower amounts depending on the calorie level.
  - Choose a variety of fruits and vegetables each day. In particular, select from all five vegetable subgroups (dark green, orange, legumes, starchy vegetables, and other vegetables) several times a week.
  - Consume 3 or more ounce-equivalents of whole-grain products per day, with the rest of the recommended grains coming from enriched or whole-grain products. In general, at least half the grains should come from whole grains.
  - Consume 3 cups per day of fat-free or low-fat milk or equivalent milk products.

- **Fats**
  - Consume less than 10 percent of calories from saturated fatty acids and less than 300 mg/day of cholesterol, and keep *trans* fatty acid consumption as low as possible.
  - Keep total fat intake between 20 to 35 percent of calories, with most fats coming from sources of polyunsaturated and monounsaturated fatty acids, such as fish, nuts, and vegetable oils.
  - When selecting and preparing meat, poultry, dry beans, and milk or milk products, make choices that are lean, low-fat, or fat-free.
  - Limit intake of fats and oils high in saturated and/or *trans* fatty acids, and choose products low in such fats and oils.

- **Carbohydrates**
  - Choose fiber-rich fruits, vegetables, and whole grains often.
  - Choose and prepare foods and beverages with little added sugars or caloric sweeteners, such as amounts suggested by the USDA Food Guide and the DASH Eating Plan.
  - Reduce the incidence of dental caries by practicing good oral hygiene and consuming sugar- and starch-containing foods and beverages less frequently.

- **Sodium and Potassium**
  - Consume less than 2,300 mg (approximately 1 tsp of salt) of sodium per day.
  - Choose and prepare foods with little salt. At the same time, consume potassium-rich foods, such as fruits and vegetables.

- **Alcoholic Beverages**
  - Those who choose to drink alcoholic beverages should do so sensibly and in moderation—defined as the consumption of up to one drink per day for women and up to two drinks per day for men.
  - Alcoholic beverages should not be consumed by some individuals, including those who cannot restrict their alcohol intake, women of childbearing age who may become pregnant, pregnant and lactating women, children and adolescents, individuals taking medications that can interact with alcohol, and those with specific medical conditions.
  - Alcoholic beverages should be avoided by individuals engaging in activities that require attention, skill, or coordination, such as driving or operating machinery.

- **Food Safety**
  - To avoid microbial foodborne illness:
    - Clean hands, food contact surfaces, and fruits and vegetables. Meat and poultry should not be washed or rinsed.
    - Separate raw, cooked, and ready-to-eat foods while shopping, preparing, or storing foods.
    - Cook foods to a safe temperature to kill microorganisms.
    - Chill (refrigerate) perishable food promptly and defrost foods properly.
    - Avoid raw (unpasteurized) milk or any products made from unpasteurized milk, raw or partially cooked eggs or foods containing raw eggs, raw or undercooked meat and poultry, unpasteurized juices, and raw sprouts.

*Key recommendations for special groups were omitted from this table, but are available on the Internet.
Source: U.S. Department of Agriculture, *Dietary Guidelines for Americans* 2005. Available at http://www.health.gov/dietaryguidelines/dga2005/document/html/executivesummary.htm. Accessed February 24 , 2010.

■ FOOD GROUP PLANS

In the United States, food group plans have provided dietary guidance based on current scientific knowledge for almost 100 years.[141] The USDA published its first recommendations in 1916. Between 1916 and the 1940s, plans had between 5 and 16 separate food groups and were published by various government agencies. In 1943, as part of the wartime effort, the USDA published the *National Wartime Nutrition Guide*. *The Basic Seven Food Guide*, derived from the *Wartime Guide*, was issued and was used until 1955 when the Department of Nutrition at the Harvard School of Public Health recommended collapsing the groups to four. This format was accepted by the USDA in 1956 and in 1979 a fifth group—fats, sweets, and alcohol—was added. These plans had two things in common: they were designed to meet nutrient requirements and to prevent nutritional deficiencies. With the recognition of the relationship between diet and chronic disease risk and the development of the DGA, it was important to develop a food guidance system that included recommendations to prevent the excesses or poor food choices associated with chronic disease.[142] These efforts culminated with the Food Guide Pyramid (FGP) released in 1992.[141,143] Like the DGA, it emphasized overall health, was based on current scientific research, addressed the total diet, and was built on successful elements of previous food plans.[144] The food patterns of the original FGP were designed to help Americans make food choices adequate in meeting nutrition standards but moderate in energy, total and saturated fatty acids, sugar, and salt. The patterns were assessed by comparing them to the 1980 RDAs and the 1980 DGA.[142] Later, they were assessed to the 1989 RDAs and the 1985 and 1990 DGA.[143] The FGP supported the 2000 DGA; however, it was more specific and allowed consumers to understand food choice more fully. Consumer testing prior to its original release showed a pyramid to be the most effective graphic because that shape helped to convey key dietary concepts of variety, proportionality, and moderation.[145] The foundation of the FGP was comprised of: grains and cereals; fruits and vegetables constituted the next tier; these were followed by milk and dairy products, and meat and meat alternates; fats, oil, and sweets constituted the tip of the pyramid (**Figure 2–4a**). Serving sizes were based on common household measures, and provided the basis for serving size recommendations for the DGA and dietary guidelines from other agencies.[141] The number of servings recommended from each food group from the pyramid is based on the number of calories an individual needs.

Advantages of the FGP included that it provided a clear graphic of familiar food groups, offered a flexible eating plan, promulgated choosing a variety of foods, and focused on sugars and fats. Disadvantages included that no distinction was made among types of fats and oils, simply looking at the FGP provided ambiguous information on serving

sizes and consumption of fruit and vegetables, some graphics were not clear, and no specific recommendations for physical activity were made.

With the revision of the DGA in 2005, and with the recognized ambiguities of the FGP, the Food Guidance System was changed to My-Pyramid. This is now the most recognized nutrition education tool in the United States (**Figure 2–4b**). MyPyramid translates the 2005 DGA into a total diet that meets nutrient needs from food sources and engenders concepts of *variety*, *proportionality*, *moderation*, and *activity*. Variety is symbolized by the six colored bands that represent the five food groups (grains, vegetables, fruit, meat, and dairy) and oils. Proportionality is portrayed by food group band thickness and that the food

> Challenge yourself by completing the Continuing Professional Education credits program for MyPyramid http://www.cnpp.usda.gov/CPEcredits.htm

a

Key

● Fat (naturally occurring and added)
▼ Sugars (added)

These symbols show fats, oils and added sugars in foods.

FATS, OILS & SWEETS
Use sparingly

MILK, YOGURT & CHEESE GROUP
2-3 servings

MEAT, POULTRY, FISH, DRY BEANS, EGGS & NUTS GROUP
2-3 servings

VEGETABLE GROUP
3-5 servings

FRUIT GROUP
2-4 servings

BREAD, CEREAL, RICE & PASTA GROUP
6-11 servings

b

MyPyramid.gov
STEPS TO A HEALTHIER YOU

FIGURE 2–4   (a) The Food Guide Pyramid. (b) MyPyramid.
Source: Courtesy of U.S. Department of Agriculture/U.S. Department of Health and Human Services. Available at http://www.mypyramid.gov. Accessed February 25, 2010.

group band narrows at the top, suggesting moderation. The steps at the side along with the person climbing them represent engaging in regular physical activity. *Personalization* is suggested by the name "MyPyramid" and by the human figure climbing the steps. Finally, *gradual improvement* is shown by the slogan—Steps to a Healthier You—which suggests that changes in diet and physical activity can be made in steps.

MyPyramid provides food recommendations in common household measures, such as cups and ounces, rather than the more ambiguous "servings" of the FGP. All food recommendations are made in the lowest fat and no added sugar forms. Fats and sugars (and alcohol) exceeding this recommendation or added at the table are called discretionary calories.

Learn more about the development of MyPyramid by going to the MyPyramid Web site for Professional Use: Development of MyPyramid at http://www.mypyramid. gov/professionals/MyPyramid Development/MyPyramid Development.html.

Interactive tools at My Pyramid.gov provide consumers and health professionals alike with a wide array of information, including: the ability to personalize and track diets, plan menus, and learn about food groups; there are also podcasts, nutrition education materials, and continuing education opportunities available. Special sections on MyPyramid are for children and MyPyramid can be followed using Twitter.

The United States is not the only country to have a food group plan.[146] Many other countries have them, but not all are in a pyramid form. Various cultural food pyramids and pyramids for different age groups are available also. For any food guidance system, recommendations and plans should be appropriate for each nation, based on their national food supply, food consumption pattern, nutrition status, and nutritional standards.

■ HEALTHY EATING INDEX

The Healthy Eating Index (HEI) was developed to provide a single summary method of assessing adherence to dietary recommendations. It was originally developed in 1995 using 1989–1990 CSFII data,[147] and was updated using 1994–1996 data and 1999–2000 NHANES data[148,149] to assess and monitor the dietary status and dietary changes of Americans.[150]

The revision of the DGA in 2005 called for a new HEI (HEI-2005) to accommodate the changes in recommen-

Encouraging children to consume a healthy diet is especially important. Have a classroom discussion to determine the reasons. Turn your discussion to the current diets of children. Then conclude with ways to improve their diets.

dations for whole grains, variety in vegetables, whole fruits, saturated fatty acids, and discretionary calories. The HEI-2005[151,152] measures diet quality in terms of conformity with MyPyramid[153] and the standards use a density approach and they are expressed as a percent of calories or per 1,000 calories (**Figure 2–5**).

The HEI-2005 has been used in several ways. The CNPP has examined the quality of diets from children and adolescents from 2 to 17 years of age and found that their diets needed improvement. Overall, these children and adolescents needed to increase their consumption of whole fruit, whole grains, dark green and orange vegetables, and legumes. In these children, solid fat, alcohol, and added sugar (SoFAAS) calories should be reduced.

Others have looked at whether the HEI-2005 score was associated with improved end points for chronic disease.[154] Results showed that adherence to the DGA was associated with only a small reduction in major chronic disease risk in a population of over 100,000 U.S. adult men and women. A limitation of this study was that few people adhered to the DGA.

■ THE FOOD LABEL

The Nutrition Labeling and Education Act (NLEA) of 1990 (Public Law 101-535) amended the Federal Food, Drug, and Cosmetic Act to provide, among other things, that certain nutrients and food components be included on the label. The regulatory authority for the food label rests with the Food and Drug Administration (FDA) and the Federal Trade Commission. The Secretary of HHS (and by delegation, the FDA) can add or delete nutrients included in the food label or labeling if this action is necessary to assist consumers in maintaining healthy dietary practices. In response to these provisions, in the Federal Register of November 27, 1991 (**Figure 2–6**), the FDA published a proposed rule entitled "Food Labeling; Reference Daily Intakes and Daily Reference Values; Mandatory Status of Nutrition Labeling and Nutrient Content Revision." In that document, the agency proposed to require that foods bear nutrition labeling listing certain nutrients and the amount of those nutrients in a serving of the food.

Under the NLEA, some foods are exempt from the food labeling laws: food served for immediate consumption (i.e., that served in hospital cafeterias and airplanes, and sold by food service vendors, e.g., mall cookie counters, sidewalk vendors, and vending machines); ready-to-eat food that is not for immediate consumption but is prepared primarily on site (e.g., bakery, deli, and candy store items); food shipped in bulk as long as it is not for sale in that form to consumers; medical foods (i.e., those used to address the nutritional needs of patients with certain diseases); plain coffee and tea, some spices; and other foods with no significant amounts of any nutrients.

Healthy Eating Index-2005 Components and Standards for Scoring[a]

Component	Maximum points	Standard for maximum score	Standard for minimum score of zero
Total fruit (includes 100% juice)	5	≥0.8 cup equiv. per 1,000 kcal	No fruit
Whole fruit (not juice)	5	≥0.4 cup equiv. per 1,000 kcal	No whole fruit
Total vegatables	5	≥1.1 cup equiv. per 1,000 kcal	No vegatables
Dark green and orange vegatables and legumes[b]	5	≥0.4 cup equiv. per 1,000 kcal	No dark green or orange vegetables or legumes
Total grains	5	≥3.0 oz. equiv. per 1,000 kcal	No grains
Whole grains	5	≥1.5 oz. equiv. per 1,000 kcal	No whole grains
Milk[c]	10	≥1.3 cup equiv. per 1,000 kcal	No milk
Meat and beans	10	≥2.5 oz. equiv. per 1,000 kcal	No meat or beans
Oils[d]	10	≥12 grams per 1,000 kcal	No oil
Saturated fat	10	≤7% of energy[e]	≥15% of energy
Sodium	10	≤0.7 grams per 1,000 kcal[e]	≥2.0 grams per 1,000 kcal
Calories from solid fats, alcoholic beverages, and added sugars (SoFAAS)	20	≤20% of energy	≥50% of energy

[a]Intakes between the minimum and maximum levels are scored proportionately, except for saturated fat and sodium (see note 5).
[b]Legumes count as vegetables only after meat and beans standard is met.
[c]Includes all milk products, such as fluid milk, yogurt, and cheese, and soy beverages.
[d]Includes nonhydrogenated vegetable oils and oils in fish, nuts, and seeds.
[e]Saturated fat and sodium get a score of 8 for the intake levels that reflect the 2005 Dietary Guidelines, < 10% of calories from saturated fat and 1.1 grams of sodium/1,000 kcal, respectively.

FIGURE 2-5 Components of the 2005 Healthy Eating Index
Source: Center for Nutrition Policy and Promotion, *Healthy Eating Index-2005*. Available at http://www.cnpp.usda.gov/Publications/HEI/healthyeatingindex2005factsheet.pdf. Accessed February 25, 2010.

60856   Federal Register / Vol. 56, No. 229 / Wednesday, November 27, 1991 / Proposed Rules

[FR Doc. 91-27168 Filed 11-26-91; 8:45 am]
BILLING CODE 4160-01-M

21 CFR Parts 5, 20, 100, 101, 105, and 130

[Docket No. 91N-0219]

RIN 0905-AD08

Regulatory Impact Analysis of the Proposed Rules to Amend the Food Labeling Regulations

AGENCY: Food and Drug Administration, HHS.

ACTION: Regulatory impact analysis statement.

SUMMARY: The Food and Drug Administration (FDA) is publishing herein the regulatory impact analysis (RIA) that it has prepared under Executive Order 12291 and the Regulatory Flexibility Act (Pub. L. 96-354) on the costs and benefits of the food labeling regulations that FDA is currently proposing to amend. FDA is issuing these proposals (published

prepared by the Economics Section of the Office of Compliance in FDA's Center for Food Safety and Applied Nutrition (CFSAN).

The food labeling reform initiative, taken as a whole, will have associated costs in excess of the $100 million threshold that defines a major rule. Therefore, in accordance with Executive Order 12291 and the Regulatory Flexibility Act (Pub. L. 96-354), FDA has developed one comprehensive RIA that presents the costs and benefits of all of the food labeling proposals taken together. FDA requests comments on the RIA.

I. Introduction

The 1990 amendments amend the Federal Food, Drug, and Cosmetic Act (the act) to expand the coverage of nutrition labeling to all food products (except meat and poultry), produce more ingredient labeling, regulate health claims, and standardize nutrient content claim definitions and serving sizes. The 1990 amendments require that the nutrition information on both the food label and on eating establishment

inventory, and reformulation. Administrative costs are management costs which are often high because of the prominence of the food label as an advertising tool for packaged foods. Analytical costs are costs of testing products for nutrient composition to comply with labeling provisions. Printing costs are the costs of printing new labels which may be either glue-on labels or the food package itself. These costs may include redesign costs where extensive labeling changes are undertaken. In the model, estimates of printing costs take into account normal firm relabeling.

Inventory costs are the costs of disposal of existing labels where firms have inventories that outlast the compliance period, i.e., the period of time between issuance of a final rule and its effective date. Inventories of labels, both glue-on labels and packages, range from only a few months to well over 10 years in the food industry. The last cost category reformulation includes the costs of reformulating products and introducing new ones in response to labeling

FIGURE 2-6 Comments on Food Labeling Regulations Published in the *Federal Register*
Source: Food and Drug Administration/HHS, *Federal Register*. 1991; 56: 60689-60726.

Placement of information on the label, type size, manufacturer name and contact information, and other information related to content are also mandated. To accommodate foods sold in small packages, there are special requirements. Further, the USDA regulates poultry in accordance with the Poultry Products Inspection Act and meat under the Federal Meat Inspection Act. Daily values (DV) are one of the key elements of the food label; these are the daily dietary intake standards used for nutrition labeling. The first daily intake standards, referred to as the U.S. Recommended Daily Allowances, for the nutrition label were established in 1973 and were based on the RDAs.[155,156]

Helping clients understand food labels—including 1) how to use them to make careful food selections, which may reduce or even prevent chronic disease, 2) how the information is especially important to individuals in certain disease states, and 3) how the food in question integrates into a total food plan—is clearly within your purview as a nutrition professional. Information on how to read the food label and consumer information is available online.[157]

As mandated by the NLEA of 1990, the FDA issued the final food labeling rules for health claims. Updated in 2008, information on the FDA Web site qualifies and explains claims that can be made for convention food and dietary supplements. The claims fall into four categories[158]: 1) Nutrient Content Claims; 2) Health Claims; 3) Qualified Health Claims (QHC); and 4) Structure Function Claims. Nutrient Content Claims are fairly straightforward (e.g., "contains 100 calories"). In addition, disclosure statements should be made; this is a statement that calls the consumer's attention to one or more nutrients in the food that may increase the risk of a disease or health-related condition that is diet-related. The disclosure statement is required when a nutrient in a food exceeds certain prescribed levels. For example, if a low fat food is high in sodium, this must be noted on the label. Other claims may be made on the label; for example, claims that a food is a "good source" of a nutrient may be made when a food contains 10% to 19% of the RDI (declared on the label as the DV) or claims that a food is a "high" source of a nutrient may be made when a food contains at least 20% of the RDI.

Health claims on foods and dietary supplements, can be made after such statements have been reviewed and authorized by FDA. Before industry can place such a claim on a label, stringent requirements must be met[159]; there are also specific criteria that all foods allowed to bear such health claims must fulfill. The FDA has provided industry guidance on the *evidence-based review system* that FDA uses to evaluate the publicly available scientific evidence for significant scientific agreement (SSA) health claims or qualified health claims on the relationship between a substance and a disease or health-related condition.[159] **Table 2–9** shows the health claims and qualified health claims allowed on food labels.[160,161]

Through the Consumer Health Information for Better Nutrition Initiative,[162] the FDA acknowledged that consumers benefit from more information on food labels about diet and health. The FDA thus established interim procedures whereby QHCs can be made for conventional foods and for dietary supplements. Past court decisions have clarified the need to provide for health claims based on less scientific evidence rather than just on the standard of SSA as long as the claims do not mislead the consumers. The FDA began considering QHCs under its interim procedures on September 1, 2003.

One example of a Qualified Health Claim (QHC) is that scientific evidence suggests but does not prove that eating 1.5 ounces per day of most [tree] nuts as part of a diet low in saturated fat and cholesterol may reduce the risk of heart disease. (See nutrition information for fat content.)

Finally, structure/function claims are allowed on labels. These differ from health claims in that structure/function claims describe the role of a substance intended to maintain the structure or function of the body. Structure/function claims do not require preapproval by FDA. Products with structure/function claims must include this disclaimer: "This statement has not been evaluated by the Food and Drug Administration. This product is not intended to diagnose, treat, cure, or prevent any disease." Examples are "calcium builds strong bones" and "antioxidants maintain cell integrity."

As seen above, food label criteria continue to change to meet current scientific research and public demand. Another example is the Food Allergen Labeling and Consumer Protection Act of 2004 (Public Law 108-282, Title II), which mandated that as of January 1, 2006, foods containing or potentially containing any of the eight most common food allergens—milk, eggs, fish, Crustacean shellfish, tree nuts, peanuts, wheat, and soybeans—include the food name on the label in "plain English" (e.g., this product contains EGGS). These foods account for 90% of food allergic reactions in children and adults. The FDA also provides guidance for industry from a standpoint of allergens and potential allergens in the food.

■ COMMUNICATING NUTRITION RECOMMENDATIONS TO THE PUBLIC

A number of programs exist with a scientific base that are designed to improve the health of the nation. The Centers for Disease Control and Prevention's (CDC) Fruits and Veggies More Matters™ [163] (**Figure 2–7**) serves as a model program. This program has an impressive partnership whose members include the NCI, CNPP, The American Cancer Society, the FDA, and the National Council of Fruit and Vegetable Nutrition Coordinators.[164] This exten-

---

TABLE 2–9 **Health Claims and Qualified Health Claims Subject to FDA Enforcement Discretion**

Table 9a. Health Claims Subject to Enforcement Discretion

- Calcium and Osteoporosis and Calcium, Vitamin D, and Osteoporosis
- Dietary Lipids and Cancer
- Saturated fat, Trans-fat, and Cholesterol and the Risk of Coronary Heart Disease
- Dietary Non-Cariogenic Carbohydrate Sweeteners and Dental Caries
- Fiber-containing Grain Products, Fruits and Vegetables and Cancer
- Folic Acid and Neural Tube Defects
- Fruits and Vegetables and Cancer
- Fruits, Vegetables and Grain Products that contain Fiber, particularly Soluble fiber, and the risk of Coronary Heart Disease
- Sodium and Hypertension
- Soluble Fiber from Certain Foods and Risk of Coronary Heart Disease
- Soy Protein and Risk of Coronary Heart Disease
- Stanols/Sterols and Risk of Coronary Heart Disease

Table 9b. Qualified Health Claims Subject to Enforcement Discretion

Qualified Claims about Cancer Risk
- Tomatoes and/or Tomato Sauce and Prostate, Ovarian, Gastric, and Pancreatic Cancers
- Calcium and Colon/Rectal Cancer and Recurrent Colon/Rectal Polyps
- Green Tea and Cancer
- Selenium and Cancer
- Antioxidant Vitamins and Cancer

Qualified Claims about Cardiovascular Disease Risk
- Nuts and Heart Disease
- Walnuts and Heart Disease
- Omega-3 Fatty Acids and Coronary Heart Disease
- B Vitamins and Vascular Disease
- Monounsaturated Fatty Acids from Olive Oil and Coronary Heart Disease
- Unsaturated Fatty Acids from Canola Oil and Coronary Heart Disease
- Corn Oil and Heart Disease

Qualified Claims about Cognitive Function
- Phosphatidylserine and Cognitive Dysfunction and Dementia

Qualified Claims about Diabetes
- Chromium Picolinate and Diabetes

Qualified Claims about Hypertension
- Calcium and Hypertension, Pregnancy-Induced Hypertension, and Preeclampsia
- Qualified Claims about Neural Tube Birth Defects
- 0.8 mg Folic Acid and Neural Tube Birth Defects

---

sive partnership reinforces the importance of this health message.

Like the MyPyramid Web site, the Fruits and Veggies More Matters™ on the Internet is geared to both health professionals and consumers. For health professionals, information on the surveillance of fruit and vegetable intake, research to practice information, the research behind the program, and state indicator reports are available. Surveillance data are from the Behavioral Risk Factor Surveillance System (BRFSS),[165] which is the world's largest, ongoing telephone health survey system, tracking health conditions and risk behaviors in the United States yearly since

1984. Data are also collected from the Youth Risk Behavior Surveillance System (YRBSS),[166] which monitors priority health-risk behaviors and the prevalence of obesity and asthma among youth and young adults. These surveillance systems clearly show that individuals are not consuming the recommended amounts of fruit and vegetables daily. For example, in 2007, the last year for which compiled survey data are available, only 21.4% of students had eaten fruits and vegetables five or more times per day during the seven days before the survey.[167] This finding has been supported repeatedly in the literature and clearly shows that there is a need to increase consumption across all age and ethnic

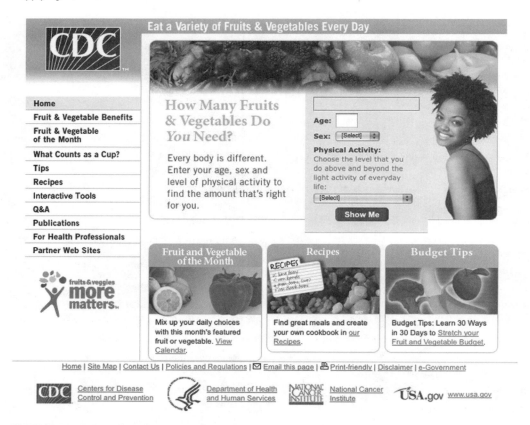

FIGURE 2–7 Fruits and Veggies More Matters

Source: Center for Disease Control and Prevention, *Fruits and Veggies More Matters*. Available at http://www.fruitsandveggiesmatter. gov. Accessed February 25, 2010.

groups. To help consumers meet the recommendations, a wide array of resources for professional presentations and consumer brochures are also available on this site.

The science behind the program is clear. The inverse relationship between eating fruit and vegetables and reducing the risk of some types of cancer is one of the best established tenets of nutritional epidemiology.[168–188] It's important to understand, however, that the studies supporting this finding are not consistent for all types of cancer.[173,186,187] Other studies have shown that consuming fruit,[176] but not vegetables, reduced the risk of some types of cancer whereas others showed the effect was linked with vegetable intake only.[175] Some studies have shown no association or only a weak one.

Intake of fruit and vegetables also has been reported to reduce the risk of other chronic diseases, notably hypertension.[188] The importance of including fruit and vegetables in the diet is underscored by their prominent recommendations in HP 2020, DGA, and MyPyramid. Every major diet and health organization recommends a diet rich in fruits and vegetables for prevention of chronic disease. Therapeutic diet regimens, including the DASH Diet[96,97,189] and the National Cholesterol Education Program's Adult Treatment Plan III diet,[14] recommend diets rich in fruit and vegetables.

Is this program effective in helping Americans to meet program and national recommendations? It's unclear at this time. The Fruits and Veggies More Matters™ program is relatively new and is an extension of the 5-a-Day marketing campaign. For the 5-a-Day campaign, some studies did show that the program was successful[190–193] and others did not.[194] Studies have indicated, however, that it is important to consider characteristics of the specific target population—including barriers to consumption and stages of change—and to deliver positive messages.[195–197] Despite the success of some intervention studies, a recent report suggested that nationally, there has been no change in consumption of fruit and vegetables in adults during the period from 1994 to 2005.[198] This clearly indicates that more work needs to be done to encourage individuals to consume fruit and vegetables and to provide them with the resources to do so.

■ **SUMMARY**

Often there are complaints that nutrition recommendations are conflicting and confusing; these actually are remarkably similar across agencies (**Table 2–10**). Why? Because this is what the science behind the programs dictates. The

TABLE 2–10	Weight, Diet, and Physical Activity Recommendations for Health Promotion and Disease Prevention[h]				
	2005 DGA/MyPyramid	**ATP III**	**DASH[i] for Hypertension**	**AHA**	**NCI**
Weight	Maintain in healthy range/lose weight if needed	Maintain desirable weight/lose weight if needed	Maintain a healthy weight	Use up as many calories as you take in	Avoid obesity
Grains	6 ounce equivalents with half whole grains	≥ 6 servings	6–8 servings	6–8 servings with half as whole grains	
Fruit	2 cups	2–4 servings	2–2.5 cups	4–5 servings	Women 7 servings Men/Teenage Boys 9 servings
Vegetables	2-½ cups	3–5 servings	2–2.5 cups	4–5 servings	
Dairy	3 cups low-fat or fat-free	2–3 servings low-fat or fat-free	2–3 cups low-fat or fat-free	2–3 servings low-fat or fat-free	
Meat/Alternates	5.5 ounce equivalents lean, low-fat, or fat-free	< 5 ounces	≥ 6 ounces	< 6 ounces low fat eat fish at least 2×/ week	
Fat Total SFA *Trans* MUFA PUFA	20%–35% energy < 10% energy	25%–35% energy < 7% energy ≤ 20% of energy ≤ 10% of energy	DASH had 27% of energy from fat; no other recommendations	< 7% of energy < 1% of energy	
Nuts, Seeds, Legumes	Legumes 3 cups/ week	Encouraged, but no specific recommendation	4–5 servings/week	4–5 servings/week	
Cholesterol	< 300 mg	< 200 mg	150 mg	< 300 mg	
Sodium	< 2,300 mg[j]	< 2,400 mg	< 2,300 mg–then lower to 1,500 mg	< 2,300 mg	Minimize salt-cured, salt-pickled, or smoked foods
Fiber	14 g/1,000 kcals	20–30 g	30 g	25 g	20–30 g with upper limit of 35 g
Added Sugar	No recommendation	No recommendation	~ 2 teaspoons	Women 100 kcals Men 150 kcals	
Alcohol	Men ≤ 2 Women ≤ 1 if at all	Men ≤ 2 Women ≤ 1 if at all	Men ≤ 2 Women ≤ 1 if at all	Men ≤ 2 Women ≤ 1 if at all	Men ≤ 2 Women ≤ 1 if at all
Physical Activity	30 minutes most days of the week	Follow Surgeon General's recommendations	30 minutes of brisk exercise on most days for persons with hypertension	30–60 minutes on most days of the week at 50%–80% capacity	Moderate intensity at least 30 minutes a day for most days

[h]For the Dietary Guidelines for Americans and American Heart Association, amounts presented are for a 2,000 kcal reference diet.
  Abbreviations: ATP III = Third Report of the Expert Panel on Detection, Evaluation, and Treatment of High Blood Cholesterol in Adults; DASH = Dietary Approaches to Stop Hypertension; AHA = American Heart Association; NCI = National Cancer Institute. Unless otherwise stated, recommendations are per day. The Centers for Disease Control and Prevention recommends that individuals follow either MyPyramid or the DASH diet.
[i]The Seventh Report of the Joint National Committee on the Prevention, Detection, Evaluation, and Treatment of High Blood Pressure recommends that people follow a DASH diet plan to help reduce blood pressure.
[j]Individuals with hypertension, blacks, and older Americans should limit intake to 1,500 mg/day.

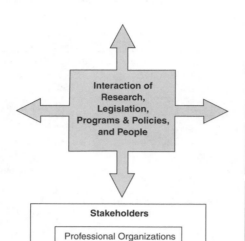

FIGURE 2–8   Relationships Among Nutrition Research, Legislation, Stakeholders, and Nutrition Programs and Policies. Abbreviations: BRFSS = Behavioral Risk Factor Surveillance System; CDC = Centers for Disease Control and Prevention; CNPP = Center for Nutrition Policy and Promotion; DASH = Dietary Approaches to Stop Hypertension; EFNEP = Expanded Food and Nutrition Education Program; HEI = Healthy Eating Index; NHANES = National Health and Nutrition Examination Survey; SNAP = Supplemental Nutrition Assistance Program; YRBSS = Youth Risk Behavior Surveillance System.

Source: U.S. Department of Health and Human Services, *Secretary's Advisory Committee on National Health Promotion & Disease Prevention Objectives for 2020.* Available at http://www.healthypeople.gov/hp2020/advisory. Accessed February 24, 2010.

challenge for all nutritionist professionals is to evaluate critically the scientific evidence before it is translated into public health practice. Nutrition professionals need to use this information to design, execute, and evaluate programs and policies so that positive recommendations are communicated to the public in a unified way. Doing so assures that consumers are getting the most accurate and comprehensive information available, which allows them to make positive lifestyle changes. This chapter reviewed the science behind public health policies, programs, nutrition education materials, and legislation. **Figure 2–8** shows the interrelationship among these elements to summarize this chapter.

Issues for Discussion

1. Dietary recommendations for the public change as scientific studies discover new information. How can these changes be brought to the public in a way that doesn't confuse them or make them feel resentful?

2. What ethical responsibility, if any, does industry or the media have in assuring the public's health?

3. The Dietary Guidelines for Americans and MyPyramid promulgate prudent diets, but Americans clearly have

difficulty following these recommendations. Why? If people can't follow them, should we continue to make these recommendations?

References

1. National Academy of Sciences, National Research Council, Food and Nutrition Board. *Diet and Health: Implications for Reducing Chronic Disease Risk.* Washington, DC: National Academy Press; 1989.

2. U.S. Senate Select Committee on Nutrition and Human Needs. *Dietary Goals for the United States*, 2nd ed. Washington, DC, U.S. Government Printing Office; 1977.

3. Centers for Disease Control and Prevention. *FastStats*. Available at http://www.cdc.gov/nchs/FASTATS/lcod.htm. Accessed January 17, 2010.

4. Trogdon JG, Finkelstein EA, Nwaise IA, Tangka FK, Orenstein D. The economic burden of chronic cardiovascular disease for major insurers. *Health Promot Pract*. 2007;8:234–242.

5. Trogdon JG, Hylands T. Nationally representative medical costs of diabetes by time since diagnosis. *Diabetes Care*. 2008;31:2307–2311.

6. Ogden CL, Carroll MD, McDowell MA, Flegal KM. Obesity among adults in the United States—no statistically significant chance since 2003–2004. *NCHS Data Brief*. 2007;1:1–8.

7. Ogden CL, Carroll MD, Curtin LR, McDowell MA, Tabak CJ, Flegal KM. Prevalence of overweight and obesity in the United States, 1999-2004. *JAMA*. 2006;295:1549–1555.

8. Ogden CL, Carroll MD, Flegal KM. High body mass index for age among US children and adolescents, 2003-2006. *JAMA*. 2008;299:2401–2405.

9. Finkelstein EA, Trogdon JG, Cohen JW, Dietz W. Annual medical spending attributable to obesity: payer- and service-specific estimates. *Health Aff (Millwood)*. 2009;28:w822–831. Epub 2009 Jul 27.

10. Trogdon JG, Finkelstein EA, Hylands T, Dellea PS, Kamal-Bahl SJ. Indirect costs of obesity: a review of the current literature. *Obes Rev.* 2008;9:489–500.

11. Sturm R. The effects of obesity, smoking, and problem drinking on chronic medical problems and health care costs. *Health Affairs.* 2002;21:245–253.

12. Sturm R, Wells KB. Does obesity contribute as much to morbidity as poverty or smoking? *Public Health.* 2001;115: 229–295.

13. World Health Organization. *2008-2013 Action Plan for the Global Strategy for the Prevention and Control of Noncommunicable Diseases.* Available at http://www.who.int/nmh/publications/ncd_action_plan_en.pdf. Accessed January 5, 2010.

14. *Third Report of the Expert Panel on Detection, Evaluation, and Treatment of High Blood Cholesterol in Adults (Adult Treatment Panel III).* National Institutes of Health; National Heart, Lung, and Blood Institute. Final Report, 2002. Available at http://www.nhlbi.nih.gov/guidelines/cholesterol/atp3full.pdf. Accessed March 16, 2010.

15. *The Future of the Public's Health in the 21st Century.* Institute of Medicine. Board on Health Promotion and Disease Prevention. Washington DC: The National Academies Press; 2003.

16. Institute of Medicine. *The Future of Public Health.* Washington DC, The National Academy Press; 1989.

17. Stitzel KF. The roles of registered dietitians and dietetic technicians, registered in health promotion and disease prevention. *J Am Diet Assoc.* 2006;106:1875–1884.

18. Cassady D, Jetter KM, Culp J. Is price a barrier to eating more fruits and vegetables for low-income families? *J Am Diet Assoc.* 2007;107:1909–1915.

19. Glanz K, Basil M, Maibach E, Goldberg J, Snyder D. Why Americans eat what they do: taste, nutrition, cost, convenience, and weight control concerns as influences on food consumption. *J Am Diet Assoc.* 1998;98:1118–1126.

20. Jetter KM, Cassady DL. The availability and cost of healthier food alternatives. *Am J Prev Med.* 2006;30:38–44.

21. French SA. Pricing effects on food choices. *J Nutr.* 2003;133: 841S–843S.

22. Furst T, Connors M, Bisogni CA, Sobal J, Falk LW. Food choice: a conceptual model of the process. *Appetite.* 1996;26:247–265.

23. Casagrande SS, Whitt-Glover MC, Lancaster KJ, Odoms-Young AM, Gary TL. Built environment and health behaviors among African Americans: a systematic review. *Am J Prev Med.* 2009; 36(2):174–181.

24. Yap TL, Davis LS. Process of behavioral change as it relates to intentional physical activity. *AAOHN J.* 2007;55:372–378; quiz 379–380.

25. Gordon-Larsen P, Griffiths P, Bentley ME, Ward DS, Kelsey K, Shields K. Barriers to physical activity: qualitative data on caregiver-daughter perceptions and practices. *Am J Prev Med.* 2004;27:218–223.

26. Irwin JD, He M, Bouck LM, Tucker P, Pollett GL. Preschoolers' physical activity behaviours: parents' perspectives. *Can J Public Health.* 2005;96:299–303.

27. Thompson JL, Davis SM, Gittelsohn J. Patterns of physical activity among American Indian children: an assessment of barriers and support. *J Community Health.* 2001;26:423–445.

28. Weir LA, Etelson D, Brand DA. Parents' perceptions of neighborhood safety and children's physical activity. *Prev Med.* 2006;43:212–217.

29. Borra ST, Earl R, Hogan EH. Paucity of nutrition and food safety 'news you can use' reveals opportunity for dietetics practitioners. *J Am Diet Assoc.* 1998;98:190–193.

30. Keenan DP, AbuSabha R, Robinson NG. Content analysis of media coverage of the *1995 Dietary Guidelines for Americans. J Extension.* 2001;39. Available at http://www.joe.org/joe/2001october/rb5.html. Accessed March 16, 2010.

31. Shine A, O'Reilly S, O'Sullivan K. Consumer attitudes to nutrition labeling. *Br Food J.* 1997;99:283–289.

32. American Dietetic Association. Survey says consumers hungry for accurate nutrition information. Available at http://www.eatright.org/Media/content.aspx?id=4294967816. Accessed March 16, 2010.

33. Cooper MJ, Zlotkin SH. An evidence-based approach to the development of national dietary guidelines. *J Am Diet Assoc.* 2003;103(Suppl 2):S28–33.

34. Dourson ML, Andersen ME, Erdreich LS, MacGregor JA. Using human data to protect the public's health. *Regul Toxicol Pharmacol.* 2001;33:234–256.

35. Kroke A, Boeing H, Rossnagel K, Willich SN. History of the concept of 'levels of evidence' and their current status in relation to primary prevention through lifestyle interventions. *Public Health Nutr.* 2004;7:279–284.

36. Myers EF. ADA Evidence Analysis Library. *J Am Diet Assoc.* 2005;105(5 Suppl 1):S79.

37. West S, King V, Carey TS, et al. *Systems to Rate the Strength of Scientific Evidence.* Evidence Report/Technology Assessment No. 47 (Prepared by the Research Triangle Institute-University of North Carolina Evidence-based Practice Center under Contract No. 290-97-0011). AHRQ Publication No. 02-E016. Rockville, MD: Agency for Healthcare Research and Quality; April 2002.

38. Akobeng AK. Understanding randomized controlled trials. *Arch Dis Child.* 2005;90:840–844.

39. American Society on Aging. *Live Well, Live Long. Health Promotion and Disease Prevention for Older Adults.* Available at http://www.asaging.org/cdc/module8/phase5/phase5_2a3.cfm. Assessed March 16, 2010.

40. Isenring EA, Bauer JD, Banks M, Gaskill D. The Malnutrition Screening Tool is a useful tool for identifying malnutrition risk in residential aged care. *J Hum Nutr Diet.* 2009;22:545–550.

41. Bang H, Edwards AM, Bomback AS, et al. Development and validation of a patient self-assessment score for diabetes risk. *Ann Intern Med.* 2009;151:775–783.

42. United States Department of Agriculture, Economic Research Service. *Food Security in the United States.* Available at http://www.ers.usda.gov/Briefing/FoodSecurity/surveytools.htm#household. Accessed March 16, 2010.

43. Jonnalagadda SS, Mitchell DC, Smiciklas-Wright H, et al. Accuracy of energy intake estimated by a multiple pass, 24-hour dietary recall technique. *J Am Diet Assoc* 2000;100:303–308.

44. Subar AF, Crafts J, Zimmerman TP, et al. Assessment of the accuracy of portion size reports using computer-based food photographs aids in the development of an automated self-administered 24-hour recall. *J Am Diet Assoc.* 2010;110:55–64.

45. Martin CK, Newton RL Jr, Anton SD, et al. Measurement of children's food intake with digital photography and the effects of second servings upon food intake. *Eating Behaviors.* 2007;8:148–156.

46. Martin CK, Han H, Coulon SM, Allen R, Champagne CM, Anton SD. A novel method to remotely measure food intake of free-living individuals in real time: the remote food photography method. *Br J Nutr.* 2009;101:446–456.

47. Williamson DA, Allen HR, Martin PD, Alfonso AJ, Gerald B, Hunt A. Comparison of digital photography to weighed and visual estimation of portion sizes. *J Am Diet Assoc.* 2003;103:1139–1145.

48. Six BL, Schap TRE, Zhu FM, et al. Evidence-based development of a mobile telephone food record. *J Am Diet Assoc.* 2010;110: 74–79.

49. Dodd KW, Guenther PM, Freedman LS, et al. Statistical methods for estimating usual intake of nutrients and foods: a review of the theory. *J Am Diet Assoc.* 2006;106:1640–1650.

50. Johnson RK, Driscoll P, Goran MI. Comparison of multiple-pass 24-hour recall estimates of energy intake with total energy expenditure determined by the doubly labeled water method in young children. *J Am Diet Assoc.* 1996;96:1140–1144.

51. Hennekens CH, Buring J. *Epidemiology in Medicine.* Baltimore, MD. Lippincott, Williams, & Wilkins; 1987:400.

52. Garn SM, Larkin FA, Cole PE. The real problem with 1-day diet records. *Am J Clin Nutr.* 1978;31:1114–1116.

53. Hegsted DM. Problems in the use and interpretation of the Recommended Dietary Allowances. *Ecol Food Nutr.* 1972; 1:255–265.

54. Subar AF, Dodd KW, Guenther PM, et al. The food propensity questionnaire: concept, development, and validation for use as a covariate in a model to estimate usual food intake. *J Am Diet Assoc.* 2006;106:1556–1563.

55. Tooze JA, Midthune D, Dodd KW, et al. A new statistical method for estimating the usual intake of episodically consumed foods with application to their distribution. *J Am Diet Assoc.* 2006;106:1575–1587.

56. Dodd KW, Guenther PM, Freedman LS, et al. Statistical methods for estimating usual intake of nutrients and foods: a review of the theory. *J Am Diet Assoc.* 2006;106:1640–1650.

57. *Usual Dietary Intakes: The NCI method.* The National Cancer Institute. Available at http://riskfactor.cancer.gov/diet/ usualintakes/method.html. Accessed January 17, 2010.

58. Bliss RM. Researchers produce innovation in dietary recall. *Agric Res* 2004; 52:10–12.

59. Raper N, Perloff B, Ingwersen L, Steinfeldt L, Anand J. An overview of USDA's Dietary Intake Data System. *J Food Compos Anal.* 2004;17:545–555.

60. McBride J. Was it a slab, a slice, or a sliver? High tech innovations take survey to new level. *Agric Res.* 2001;49:4–7.

61. Jain M, McLaughlin J. Validity of nutrient estimates by food frequency questionnaires based either on exact frequencies or categories. *Ann Epidemiol.* 2000;10:354–360.

62. Kuskowska-Wolk A, Holte S, Ohlander EM, et al. Effects of different designs and extension of a food frequency questionnaire on response rate, completeness of data and food frequency responses. *Int J Epidemiol.* 1992;21:1144–1150.

63. Kroke A, Klipstein-Grobusch K, Voss S, Möseneder J, Thielecke F, Noack R, Boeing H. Validation of a self-administered food-frequency questionnaire administered in the European Prospective Investigation into Cancer and Nutrition (EPIC) Study: comparison of energy, protein, and macronutrient intakes estimated with the doubly labeled water, urinary nitrogen, and repeated 24-h dietary recall methods. *Am J Clin Nutr.* 1999;70:439–447.

64. Andersen LF, Tomten H, Haggarty P, Løvø A, Hustvedt BE. Validation of energy intake estimated from a food frequency questionnaire: a doubly labelled water study. *Eur J Clin Nutr.* 2003;57:279–284.

65. Day NE, Ferrari P. Some methodological issues in nutritional epidemiology. In: Riboli E, Lambert R. *Nutrition and Lifestyle: Opportunities for Cancer Prevention.* IARC Scientific Publications No. 156;2002:5–10.

66. Willett WC. Dietary diaries versus food frequency questionnaires—a case of undigestible data. *Int J Epidemiol.* 2001;30:317–319.

67. Molag ML, de Vries JH, Ocké MC, et al. Design characteristics of food frequency questionnaires in relation to their validity. *Am J Epidemiol.* 2007;166:1468–1478.

68. *MyPyramid Tracker.* United States Department of Agriculture. Available at http://www.mypyramidtracker.gov. Accessed January 17, 2010.

69. *MyPyramid Equivalents Database.* United States Department of Agriculture. Available at http://www.ars.usda.gov/Services/ docs.htm?docid=17558. Accessed January 17, 2010.

70. United States Department of Agriculture. National Nutrient Database for Standard Reference. Nutrient Database Laboratory. Available at http://www.nal.usda.gov/fnic/foodcomp/search. Accessed January 17, 2010.

71. United States Department of Agriculture. Food and nutrient database for dietary studies. Available at http://www.ars. usda.gov/Services/docs.htm?docid=12089. Accessed January 17, 2010.

72. Bingham SA. Biomarkers in nutritional epidemiology. *Public Health Nutr.* 2002;5:821–827.

73. Kaaks RJ. Biochemical markers as additional measurements in studies of the accuracy of dietary questionnaire measurements: conceptual issues. *Am J Clin Nutr.* 1997;65 (4 Suppl):1232S–1239S.

74. World Health Organization. *Report of the technical discussions at the twenty first World Health Assembly on "national and global surveillance of communicable diseases."* A2.1. 18-5-1968. Geneva, Switzerland.

75. United States Department of Agriculture. *What we eat in America.* Available at http://www.ars.usda.gov/Services/docs. htm?docid=15044. Accessed January 17, 2010.

76. Woteki CE. Integrated NHANES: uses in national policy. *J Nutr.* 2003;133:582S–584S.

77. Arab L, Carriquiry A, Steck-Scott S, Gaudet MM. Ethnic differences in the nutrient intake adequacy of premenopausal US women: results from the Third National Health Examination Survey. *J Am Diet Assoc.* 2003;103:1008–1014.

78. Ford ES, Ballew C. Dietary folate intake in US adults: findings from the third National Health and Nutrition Examination Survey. *Ethn Dis.* 1998;8:299–305.

79. Looker AC, Loria CM, Carroll MD, et al. Calcium intakes of Mexican Americans, Cubans, Puerto Ricans, non-Hispanic whites, and non-Hispanic blacks in the United States. *J Am Diet Assoc.* 1993;93:1274–1279.

80. Sharma S, Malarcher AM, Giles WH, Myers G. Racial, ethnic and socioeconomic disparities in the clustering of cardiovascular disease risk factors. *Ethn Dis.* 2004;14:43–48.

81. Hicks LS, Fairchild DG, Cook EF, Ayanian JZ. Association of region of residence and immigrant status with hypertension, renal failure, cardiovascular disease, and stroke, among African-American participants in the third National Health and Nutrition Examination Survey (NHANES III). *Ethn Dis.* 2003;13:316–323.

82. Berenson GS (ed). *Causation of Cardiovascular Risk Factors in Childhood: Perspectives on Cardiovascular Risk in Early Life.* New York: Raven Press; 1986:408.

83. Berenson GS, McMahan CA, Voors AW, et al. *Cardiovascular Risk Factors in Children–The Early Natural History of Atherosclerosis and Essential Hypertension.* New York: Oxford University Press; 1980:450.

84. Berenson GS, Wattigney WA, Bao W, et al. Rationale to study the early natural history of heart disease: The Bogalusa Heart Study. *Am J Med Sci.* 1995;310(suppl 1):S22–S28.

85. Nicklas TA, Demory-Luce D, Yang SJ, et al. Children's food consumption patterns have changed over two decades (1973–1994): The Bogalusa Heart Study. *J Am Diet Assoc.* 2004;104:1127–1140.

86. Nicklas TA, Hayes D. Position of the American Dietetic Association: nutrition guidance for healthy children ages 2 to 11 years. *J Am Diet Assoc.* 2008;108:1038–1044, 1046–1047.

87. Berenson GS, Wattigney WA, Tracy RE, et al. Atherosclerosis of the aorta and coronary arteries and cardiovascular risk factors in persons aged 6 to 30 years and studied at necropsy (The Bogalusa Heart Study). *Am J Cardiol.* 1992;70:851–858.

88. Strong JP, McGill HC Jr. The natural history of coronary atherosclerosis. *Am J Pathol* 1962;40:37–49.

89. Metha NV, Khan AI. Cardiology's 10 greatest discoveries of the 20th century. *Tex Heart Inst J.* 2002;29:164–171.

90. The Seventh Report of the Joint National Committee on Prevention, Detection, Evaluation, and Treatment of High Blood Pressure (JNC 7). Available at http://www.nhlbi.nih.gov/guidelines/hypertension. Accessed March 16, 2010.

91. Framingham Heart Study. Offspring Cohort. Available at http://www.framinghamheartstudy.org/participants/offspring.html. Accessed January 17, 2010.

92. Farris RP, Nicklas TA. Characterizing children's eating behavior. In: *Textbook of Pediatric Nutrition.* Suskind RM, Suskind LL, eds. New York: Raven Press; 1993:505–516.

93. Nicklas TA, Forcier JE, Webber LS, Berenson GS. School lunch assessment as part of a 24-hour dietary recall for children. *J Am Diet Assoc.* 1991;91:711–713.

94. Frank GC, Hollatz AT, Webber LS, Berenson GS. Effect of interviewer recording practices on nutrient intake—Bogalusa Heart Study. *J Am Diet Assoc.* 1984;84:1432–1436.

95. Most MM, Ershow AG, Clevidence BA. An overview of methodologies, proficiencies, and training resources for controlled feeding studies. *J Am Diet Assoc.* 2003;103:729–735.

96. Appel LJ, Moore TJ, Obarzanek E, et al. A clinical trial of the effects of dietary patterns on blood pressure. DASH Collaborative Research Group. *N Engl J Med.* 1997;336:1117–1124.

97. Sacks FM, Svetkey LP, Vollmer WM, et al. Effects on blood pressure of reduced dietary sodium and the Dietary Approaches to Stop Hypertension (DASH) diet. DASH-Sodium Collaborative Research Group. *N Engl J Med.* 2001;344:3–10.

98. Funk KL, Elmer PJ, Stevens VJ, et al. PREMIER—a trial of lifestyle interventions for blood pressure control: intervention design and rationale. *Health Promot Pract.* 2008;9:271–280.

99. Albanes D, Heinonen OP, Taylor PR, et al. Alpha-tocopherol and beta-carotene supplements and lung cancer incidence in the alpha-tocopherol, beta-carotene cancer prevention study: effects of base-line characteristics and study compliance. *J Natl Cancer Inst.* 1996;88:1560–1570.

100. Omenn GS, Goodman G, Thornquist M, et al. The beta-carotene and retinol efficacy trial (CARET) for chemoprevention of lung cancer in high risk populations: smokers and asbestos-exposed workers. *Cancer Res.* 1994;54(7 suppl):2038s–2043s.

101. Block G, Patterson B, Subar A. Fruit, vegetables, and cancer prevention: a review of the epidemiological evidence. *Nutr Cancer.* 1992;18:1–29.

102. Steinmetz KA, Potter JD. Vegetables, fruit, and cancer. I. Epidemiology. *Cancer Causes Control.* 1991;2:325–357.

103. Le Marchand L, Hankin JH, Kolonel LN, et al. Intake of specific carotenoids and lung cancer risk. *Cancer Epidemiol Biomarkers Prev.* 1993;2:183–187.

104. Steinmetz KA, Potter JD, Folsom AR. Vegetables, fruit, and lung cancer in the Iowa Women's Health Study. *Cancer Res.* 1993;53:536–543.

105. Smigel K. Beta carotene fails to prevent cancer in two major studies; CARET intervention stopped. *J Natl Cancer Inst.* 1996; 88:145.

106. Pryor WA, Stahl W, Rock CL. Beta carotene: from biochemistry to clinical trials. *Nutr Rev.* 2000;58(2 Pt 1):39–53.

107. Roy HJ, Keenan MJ, Zablah-Pimentel E, et al. Adult female rats defend "appropriate" energy intake after adaptation to dietary energy. *Obes Res.* 2003;11:1214–1222.

108. Wolf G. The effect of low and high doses of beta-carotene and exposure to cigarette smoke on the lungs of ferrets. *Nutr Rev.* 2002;60:88–90.

109. Russell RM. The enigma of beta-carotene in carcinogenesis: what can be learned from animal studies. *J Nutr.* 2004;134: 262S–268S.

110. *Healthy People 2010.* Available at http://www.healthypeople.gov. Accessed January 17, 2010.

111. US Department of Health and Human Services. *Healthy People: The Surgeon General's Report on Health Promotion and Disease Prevention.* Washington, DC: Government Printing Office; 1979: section 25.

112. Perspectives in Disease Prevention and Health Promotion Implementing the 1990 Prevention Objectives: Summary of CDC's Seminar. *Morbid Mortal Wkly Rpt.* 1983;32:21–24.

113. Centers for Disease Control and Prevention. *CDC Wonder. Data 2010: the Healthy People Database.* Available at http://wonder.cdc.gov/data2010. Accessed March 17, 2010.

114. Centers for Disease Control and Prevention. *CDC Wonder.* Available at http://wonder.cdc.gov. Accessed March 17, 2010.

115. Centers for Disease Control and Prevention, National Center for Health Statistics. *Healthy People.* Available at http://www.cdc.gov/nchs/hphome.htm. Accessed March 17, 2010.

116. *Healthy People 2010. State Healthy People Plans.* Available at http://www.healthypeople.gov/implementation/stateplans.htm. Accessed March 17, 2010.

117. Partnership for Prevention. Available at http://www.prevent.org.

118. Southwest Rural Health Research Center. *Rural Healthy People 2010.* Available at http://srph.tamhsc.edu/centers/rhp2010. Accessed March 17, 2010.

119. National Institutes of Health, National Heart Lung and Blood Institute (NHLBI). *HP 2010 Cardiovascular Gateway.* Available at http://hp2010.nhlbihin.net/cvd_frameset.htm. Accessed March 17, 2010.

120. *Food and Nutrition Board. Recommended Dietary Allowances,* 10th ed. Washington DC: National Academy Press; 1989.

121. Yates AA. National nutrition and public health policies: issues related to bioavailability of nutrients when developing dietary reference intakes. *J Nutr.* 2001;131:1331S–1334S.

122. Food and Nutritional Information Center. National Agricultural Library. *Dietary Reference Intakes.* Available at http://fnic.nal.usda.gov/nal_display/index.php?info_center=4&tax_level=3&tax_subject=256&topic_id=1342&level3_id=5141. Accessed March 17, 2010.

123. Institute of Medicine (U.S.). Panel on Dietary Reference Intakes for Electrolytes and Water. *DRI, Dietary Reference Intakes for Water, Potassium, Sodium, Chloride, and Sulfate.* Washington, DC: National Academies Press; 2005.

124. Institute of Medicine (U.S.). *Dietary Reference Intakes for Energy, Carbohydrate, Fiber, Fat, Fatty Acids, Cholesterol, Protein, and Amino Acids (Macronutrients).* National Academy of Sciences, Institute of Medicine, Food and Nutrition Board. Washington, DC: National Academies Press; 2005.

125. Institute of Medicine (U.S.). *Dietary Reference Intakes: Proposed Definition and Plan for Review of Dietary Antioxidants and Related Compounds.* National Academy of Sciences. Institute of Medicine. Food and Nutrition Board. Washington, DC: National Academies Press; 1998.

126. Institute of Medicine (U.S.). *Dietary Reference Intakes for Thiamin, Riboflavin, Niacin, Vitamin B6, Folate, Vitamin B12, Pantothenic Acid, Biotin, and Choline.* National Academy of Sciences. Institute of Medicine. Food and Nutrition Board. Washington, DC: National Academies Press; 1998.

127. Institute of Medicine (U.S.). Standing Committee on the Scientific Evaluation of Dietary Reference Intakes. *Dietary Reference Intakes: For Calcium, Phosphorus, Magnesium, Vitamin D, and Fluoride.* Washington, DC: National Academies Press; 1997.

128. Institute of Medicine. *School Meals: Building Blocks for Healthy Children.* Washington, DC: National Academies Press; 2009. Available at http://books.nap.edu/openbook.php?record_id=12751. Accessed January 17, 2010.

129. Institute of Medicine. *Local Government Actions to Prevent Childhood Obesity*. 2009. Available at http://www.iom.edu/ Reports/2009/ChildhoodObesityPreventionLocalGovernments. aspx. Accessed March 17, 2010.

130. Institute of Medicine. *The Public Health Effects of Food Deserts. Workshop Summary*. Washington, DC: National Academies Press. Available at http://www.iom.edu/Reports/2009/ FoodDeserts.aspx. 2009. Accessed March 17, 2010.

131. Institute of Medicine. *Nutrition Standards and Meal Requirements for National School Lunch and Breakfast Programs: Phase I. Proposed Approach for Recommending Revisions*. Washington, DC: National Academies Press; 2008. Available at http://www.nap.edu/catalog.php?record_ id = 12512. Accessed March 17, 2010.

132. Institute of Medicine. *The Use of Dietary Supplements by Military Personnel*. Washington, DC: National Academies Press; 2008. Available at http://books.nap.edu/openbook.php?record_ id = 12095. Accessed March 17, 2010.

133. Yates AA. Process and development of dietary reference intakes: basis, need, and application of recommended dietary allowances. *Nutr Rev*. 1998 Apr;56(4 Pt 2):S5–S9.

134. Murphy SP, Poos MI. Dietary Reference Intakes: summary of applications in dietary assessment. *Public Health Nutr*. 2002; 5:843–849.

135. Murphy SP, Barr SI, Poos MI. Using the new dietary reference intakes to assess diets: a map to the maze. *Nutr Rev*. 2002; 60:267–275.

136. Barr SI, Murphy SP, Agurs-Collins TD, Poos MI. Planning diets for individuals using the dietary reference intakes. *Nutr Rev*. 2003;61:352–360.

137. United States Department of Agriculture. Center for Nutrition Policy and Promotion. *Improving the nutrition and well-being of Americans*. Available at http://www.cnpp.usda.gov. Accessed March 17, 2010.

138. United States Department of Agriculture, National Agriculture Library. Available at http://www.cnpp.usda.gov/ dietaryguidelines.htm. Accessed March 18, 2010.

139. Dwyer JT. Nutrition guidelines and education of the public. *J Nutr*. 2001;131(11 suppl):3074S–3077S.

140. U.S. Department of Health and Human Services, Public Health Service. *The Surgeon General's report on nutrition and health*. DHHS (PHS) Publication No. 88-50215; 1988.

141. Welsh S, Davis C, Shaw A. A brief history of food guides in the United States. *Nutr Today* 1992;November/December:6–11.

142. Cronin FJ, Shaw AM, Krebs-Smith SM, et al. Developing a food guidance system to implement the dietary guidelines. *J Nutr Ed*. 1987;19:281–302.

143. Welsh S, Davis C, Shaw A. *USDA's Food Guide: Background and Development*. Washington, DC: U.S. Department of Agriculture, Human Nutrition Information Service; 1993. Misc. Publication 1514.

144. Davis CA, Britten P, Myers EF. Related articles, past, present, and future of the Food Guide Pyramid. *J Am Diet Assoc*. 2001;101:881–885.

145. Goldberg JP, Belury MA, Elam P, et al. The obesity crisis: don't blame it on the pyramid. *J Am Diet Assoc*. 2004;104:1141–1147.

146. Painter J, Rah JH, Lee YK. Comparison of international food guide pictorial representations. *J Am Diet Assoc*. 2002;102(4):483–489.

147. Kennedy ET, Ohls J, Carlson S, Fleming K. The Healthy Eating Index: Design and applications. *J Am Diet Assoc*. 1995;95:1103–1108.

148. Bowman SA, Lino M, Gerrior SA, Basiotis PP. *The Healthy Eating Index: 1994-96*. U.S. Department of Agriculture, Center for Nutrition Policy and Promotion. Washington, DC: CNPP-5; 1998.

149. Basiotis PP, Carlson A, Gerrior SA, Juan WY, Lino M. *The Healthy Eating Index: 1999–2000*. U.S. Department of Agriculture, Center for Nutrition Policy and Promotion. Washington, DC: CNPP-12; 2002.

150. Kennedy ET, Ohls J, Carlson S, Fleming K. The Healthy Eating Index: design and applications. *J Am Diet Assoc*. 1995;95:1103–1108.

151. Guenther PM, Krebs-Smith SM, Reedy J, et al. USDA Center for Nutrition Policy and Promotion Fact Sheet No. 1, 2008. Available at http://www.cnpp.usda.gov/Publications/HEI/ healthyeatingindex2005factsheet.pdf. Accessed March 17, 2010.

152. Guenther PM, Reedy J, Krebs-Smith SM. Development of the Healthy Eating Index-2005. *J Am Diet Assoc*. 2008;108:1896–1901.

153. Britten P, Marcoe K, Yamini S, Davis C. Development of food intake patterns for the MyPyramid Food Guidance System. *J Nutr Educ Behav*. 2006;38(6 Suppl):S78–S92.

154. Willett WC, McCullough ML. Dietary pattern analysis for the evaluation of dietary guidelines. *Asia Pac J Clin Nutr*. 2008;17(suppl 1):75–78.

155. Pennington JA, Hubbard VS. Derivation of daily values used for nutrition labeling. *J Am Diet Assoc*. 1997;97:1407–1412.

156. Origin and framework of the development of dietary reference intakes. *Nutr Rev*. 1997;55:332–334.

157. U.S. Department of Health and Human Services, U.S. Department of Agriculture. Eating Healthier and Feeling Better Using the Nutrition Facts Label. Available at http://www.fda. gov/downloads/Food/LabelingNutrition/ConsumerInformation/ ucm120909.pdf. Assessed March 17, 2010.

158. U.S. Department of Health and Human Services, U.S. Food and Drug Administration. *Food. VIII. Claims*. Available at http://www.fda.gov/Food/GuidanceComplianceRegulatory Information/GuidanceDocuments/FoodLabelingNutrition/ FoodLabelingGuide/ucm064908.htm. Accessed March 17, 2010.

159. U.S. Department of Health and Human Services, U.S. Food and Drug Administration. *Guidance for Industry: Evidence-Based Review System for the Scientific Evaluation of Health Claims*—Final. January 2009. Available at http://www.fda. gov/Food/GuidanceComplianceRegulatoryInformation/ GuidanceDocuments/FoodLabelingNutrition/ucm073332.htm. Accessed March 17, 2010.

160. U.S. Department of Health and Human Services, U.S. Food and Drug Administration. *Health Claims Meeting Significant Scientific Agreement (SSA)*. Available at http:// www.fda.gov/Food/LabelingNutrition/LabelClaims/ HealthClaimsMeetingSignificantScientificAgreementSSA/default. htm. Accessed March 17, 2010.

161. U.S. Department of Health and Human Services, U.S. Food and Drug Administration. Summary of Qualified Health Claims Subject to Enforcement Discretion. Available at http://www.fda.gov/Food/LabelingNutrition/LabelClaims/ QualifiedHealthClaims/ucm073992.htm. Accessed March 17, 2010.

162. U.S. Department of Health and Human Services, U.S. Food and Drug Administration. *Consumer Health Information for Better Nutrition Initiative*. Available at http://www.fda.gov/ Food/LabelingNutrition/LabelClaims/QualifiedHealthClaims/ QualifiedHealthClaimsPetitions/ucm096010.htm. Accessed March 17, 2010.

163. Centers for Disease Control and Prevention. Eat a Variety of Fruits & Veggies Every Day. Available at http://www. fruitsandveggiesmatter.gov. Accessed March 17, 2010.

164. Association of State and Territorial Public Health Nutrition Directors. *Fruit and Vegetable Nutrition Council*. Available at http://www.astphnd.org/chapter_contents. php3?sid = fbf4ae&chapter_id = 5&member_id = . Accessed March 17, 2010.

165. Centers for Disease Control and Prevention. *Behavioral Risk Factor Surveillance System*. Available at http://www.cdc.gov/ brfss. Accessed March 17, 2010.

166. Centers for Disease Control and Prevention. YRBSS: Youth Risk Behavior Surveillance System. Available at http://www.cdc. gov/healthyyouth/yrbs. Accessed March 17, 2010.

167. Centers for Disease Control and Prevention. *2007 National Youth Risk Behavior Survey Overview*. Available at http://www.cdc.gov/healthyyouth/yrbs/pdf/yrbs07_us_overview.pdf. Accessed March 18, 2010.

168. Block G, Patterson B, Subar A. Fruit, vegetables, and cancer prevention: a review of the epidemiological evidence. *Nutr Cancer*. 1992;18:1–29.

169. Steinmetz KA, Potter JD. Vegetables, fruit, and cancer. I. Epidemiology. *Cancer Causes Control*. 1991;2:325–357.

170. Le Marchand L, Hankin JH, Kolonel LN, et al. Intake of specific carotenoids and lung cancer risk. *Cancer Epidemiol Biomarkers Prev*. 1993;2:183–187.

171. Key TJ, Schatzkin A, Willett WC, et al. Diet, nutrition, and the prevention of cancer. *Public Health Nutr*. 2004;7:187–200.

172. Chainani-Wu N. Diet and oral, pharyngeal, and esophageal cancer. *Nutr Cancer*. 2002;44:104–126.

173. Key TJ, Schatzkin A, Willett WC, et al. Diet, nutrition and the prevention of cancer. *Public Health Nutr*. 2004;7(1A):187–200.

174. Steinmetz KA, Potter JD. Vegetables, fruit, and cancer prevention: a review. *J Am Diet Assoc*. 1996;96:1027–1039.

175. Riboli E, Norat T. Epidemiologic evidence of the protective effect of fruit and vegetables on cancer risk. *Am J Clin Nutr*. 2003;78(3 suppl):559S–569S.

176. Kampman E, Arts IC, Hollman PC. Plant foods versus compounds in carcinogenesis; observational versus experimental human studies. *Int J Vitam Nutr Res*. 2003;73:70–78.

177. Temple NJ, Gladwin KK. Fruit, vegetables, and the prevention of cancer: research challenges. *Nutrition*. 2003;19:467–470.

178. Smith-Warner SA, Spiegelman D, Yaun SS, et al. Intake of fruits and vegetables and risk of breast cancer: a pooled analysis of cohort studies. *JAMA*. 2001;285:769–776.

179. Kim DJ, Holowaty EJ. Brief, validated survey instruments for the measurement of fruit and vegetable intakes in adults: a review. *Prev Med*. 2003;36:440–447.

180. Ziegler RG. Vegetables, fruits, and carotenoids and the risk of cancer. *Am J Clin Nutr*. 1991;53(1 suppl):251S–259S.

181. Duthie GG, Gardner PT, Kyle JA. Plant polyphenols: are they the new magic bullet? *Proc Nutr Soc*. 2003;62:599–603.

182. La Vecchia C, Altieri A, Tavani A. Vegetables, fruit, antioxidants and cancer: a review of Italian studies. *Eur J Nutr*. 2001;40:261–267.

183. Reddy L, Odhav B, Bhoola KD. Natural products for cancer prevention: a global perspective. *Pharmacol Ther*. 2003;99:1–13.

184. Van Duyn MA, Pivonka E. Overview of the health benefits of fruit and vegetable consumption for the dietetics professional: selected literature. *J Am Diet Assoc*. 2000;100:1511–1521.

185. van't Veer P, Jansen MC, Klerk M, Kok FJ. Fruits and vegetables in the prevention of cancer and cardiovascular disease. *Public Health Nutr*. 2000;3:103–107.

186. Bazzano LA, Serdula MK, Liu S. Dietary intake of fruits and vegetables and risk of cardiovascular disease. *Curr Atheroscler Rep*. 2003;5:492–499.

187. Hu FB. Plant-based foods and prevention of cardiovascular disease: an overview. *Am J Clin Nutr*. 2003;78(3 suppl):544S–551S.

188. Dauchet L, Amouyel P, Dallongeville J. Fruits, vegetables and coronary heart disease. *Nat Rev Cardiol*. 2009;6:599–608.

189. National Heart Lung and Blood Institute. *Your Guide to Lowering Your Blood Pressure with DASH*. Available at http://www.nhlbi.nih.gov/health/public/heart/hbp/dash/new_dash.pdf. Accessed March 18, 2010.

190. Anderson JV, Bybee DI, Brown RM, et al. 5-a-Day fruit and vegetable intervention improves consumption in a low-income population. *J Am Diet Assoc*. 2001;101:195–202.

191. Havas S, Anliker J, Damron D, et al. Final results of the Maryland WIC 5-A-Day Promotion Program. *Am J Public Health*. 1998;88:1161–1167.

192. Sorensen G, Stoddard A, Peterson K, et al. Increasing fruit and vegetable consumption through worksites and families in the treatwell 5-a-day study. *Am J Public Health*. 1999;89:54–60.

193. Beresford SA, Thompson B, Feng Z, et al. Seattle 5 a Day worksite program to increase fruit and vegetable consumption. *Prev Med*. 2001;32:230–238.

194. Stables GJ, Subar AF, Patterson BH, et al. Changes in vegetable and fruit consumption and awareness among US adults: results of the 1991 and 1997 5 A Day for Better Health Program surveys. *J Am Diet Assoc*. 2002;102:809–817.

195. Havas S, Treiman K, Langenberg P, et al. Factors associated with fruit and vegetable consumption among women participating in WIC. *J Am Diet Assoc*. 1998;98:1141–1148.

196. Langenberg P, Ballesteros M, Feldman R, et al. Psychosocial factors and intervention-associated changes in those factors as correlates of change in fruit and vegetable consumption in the Maryland WIC 5 A Day Promotion Program. *Ann Behav Med*. 2000;22:307–315.

197. Campbell MK, Reynolds KD, Havas S, et al. Stages of change for increasing fruit and vegetable consumption among adults and young adults participating in the national 5-a-Day for Better Health community studies. *Health Educ Behav*. 1999;26:513–534.

198. Blanck HM, Gillespie C, Kimmons JE, Seymour JD, Serdula MK. Trends in fruit and vegetable consumption among U.S. men and women, 1994-2005. *Prev Chronic Dis*. 2008;5:A35.

PART

II

Assessing and Intervening in the
Community's Nutrition Needs

Part II introduces how public health nutritionists target care for those at highest risk. Chapter 3 explains the role of needs assessment in public health and how it helps Americans. Proper needs assessment allows the public health nutritionist to serve most usefully those who need help. In Chapter 4, we see the results of more than a century of needs assessment, with the designation of the young and the old as well as people coping with illness and disability as those who must be supported by public health nutrition services. Reaching those in need has been one of public health nutrition's most difficult challenges.

In the 21st century, public health nutrition needs assessments have determined that the indulgent eating habits of Americans in the United States has brought about a nutritional catastrophe. The epidemics of overweight in children (Chapter 5) and adult obesity (Chapter 6) are two additional areas in which public health nutrition must find a way to intervene and provide solutions.

CHAPTER

3

Community Needs Assessment

ELIZABETH METALLINOS-KATSARAS, PhD, RD

READER OBJECTIVES

After studying this chapter and reflecting on its contents, you should be able to:

1. Define community in the context of public health nutrition.
2. Explain the rationale for community needs assessment.
3. Define the terms used in community needs assessment.
4. Describe the steps to follow when conducting a community needs assessment.
5. Describe the types of data that can be collected about a community and how these data can be obtained.
6. Identify existing sources of data that can be used.
7. Describe the types of data that can be used to assess the nutritional status of the target population.
8. Compare assessed needs with the capacity of existing services to meet these needs and identify unmet needs.

■ INTRODUCTION

The commissioner of public health in your town has come to you with the following question: "What are the major nutritional problems of our community that are currently not being addressed effectively?" Embedded within this question are several additional queries, including "Who is most affected by the nutritional problems? What are some of the barriers to their improvement? What is the healthcare system doing about them?" The overarching goal of the task you have been handed is to develop new programs or to identify ways in which existing public health nutrition programs can address the most pressing nutritional needs of a community. Such a request from a high-ranking official may sound a bit far-fetched; however, in an era in which the obesity epidemic is at the forefront of not only scientific inquiry but also the media, there is a renewed interest in prevention. Prevention is, after all, the hallmark of public health nutrition.

How would you go about responding to this inquiry? What would you do first? What information or data would

you need and where would you get it? This chapter describes the process you can use to determine the unmet nutrition-related needs of a community. Both hypothetical and actual needs assessment examples are used to exemplify both nutritional status and community resource data.

■ COMMUNITY NEEDS ASSESSMENT: DEFINITION AND OVERVIEW

An integral step in the public health process is determining the nutritional needs of the community and population with which you are working. Accurate and focused needs assessment is an essential step in the planning, implementation, and evaluation of public health programs for several reasons.

First, public health departments and agencies must know about the primary problems and unmet needs of the community prior to developing a new program, modifying existing programs, or distributing resources. Second, in order to allocate resources to program development and implementation, it is also essential to determine the most important and pressing needs. Although we as community and public health nutritionists are committed to improving all aspects of nutrition-related community health, resource allocation constrains most programmatic decisions. One thus needs to identify the most pressing nutrition-related problems, the underlying causes in the specific group in question, and which problems are not being met by existing resources in order to prioritize and distribute resources.

Equally important in the description of the nutrition problems is who will be affected in order to address their issues. A community can be defined broadly as a group of people with common characteristics. The individuals within the community—who are the focus of the needs assessment—comprise the target population. For example, Roxbury is a low-income, inner-city neighborhood of Boston, Massachusetts. In recognition of the importance of obesity prevention, you as the public health nutritionist would like to conduct a community needs assessment of school-age children living in Roxbury, Massachusetts. Therefore, the community is Roxbury, while the target population is school-age children.

> A community is a group of people with common characteristics. These can include a location or region; sociodemographic characteristics such as ethnicity, age, education, or occupation; a nutritional problem (e.g., obesity); or a common bond (e.g., members of an organization).[1]

Community needs assessment includes both an assessment of the community resources and an assessment of the nutritional status/concerns of the target population. The scope of the community needs assessment can be large (e.g., a nationwide maternal and child nutrition needs assessment) or small (e.g., determining the need for breast-feeding support among Laotian-American participants of a specific Special Supplemental Nutrition Program for Women, Infants and Children [WIC] program).

> A target population is the group that is the focus of an assessment, a study, an intervention[2] or a program.[1]

The types of data and methods of obtaining data vary greatly as well. The foundation of some needs assessments is the identification, compilation, and interpretation of existing (i.e., secondary) data, whereas others incorporate a primary data collection component. Which data collection route should be taken depends on the purpose of the needs assessment, but it is important to note that numerous existing data sources are publicly available to the public health nutritionist. **Table 3–1** lists some of these. Some public health nutritionists may embark on primary data collection prematurely, unknowingly ignoring existing data pertinent to their needs assessment. This can waste precious resources; therefore, we cannot overstate the importance of investigating existing data sources and research in the published literature that may be relevant to your specific needs assessment.

Who will conduct the community needs assessment? You might envision a lonely public health nutritionist setting out to complete all the phases of the assessment. In reality, in most cases a team is assembled to conduct the assessment. The desirability of this approach is underscored by the fact that numerous and varied skills are needed to effectively conduct a community needs assessment. The public health nutritionist is the nutrition expert but may not be a data or survey development expert. Nor can public health nutritionists alone represent the stakeholders. Others on the team thus will complement the public health nutritionist with their expertise in qualitative or quantitative research methods, data analysis, and interpretation.

> **Qualitative research:** Any method of data collecting that generates narrative data or words rather than numerical data or numbers. The words must reflect the study participant perspective.[3]
>
> **Quantitative research:** Hypothesis-testing research that gathers numerical data or data that can be quantified.

As some have noted,[4] needs are in the eye of the beholder, and many decisions can be based on value judgments about the problems that exist in a target population. For example, most consider obesity to be a serious public health problem, but there are some who disagree.[5] The fact that a public health nutritionist's perceived need may not be met with unanimous agreement by the public makes it important to engender community support for the methods and the findings of the needs assessment.[4] The needs assessment process thus includes not only a scientific and analytic component but also a political one. Therefore, it is important to include those individuals or groups in the needs assessment process who will be affected by the findings.[4] These stakeholders include:

- Consumers/program recipients
- Policymakers
- Target population
- Nutrition program providers
- Nutrition program funders

The individuals represented within each of these groups provide a unique perspective that informs not only the development of the needs assessment process but also how the nutrition problem in question should be addressed.

TABLE 3–1	Examples of Secondary Datasets that Could Be Sources for a Community Needs Assessment	
Dataset and Source	**Description**
2010 Census Datasets	Data warehouse for NCHS public use data files for: • National Health and Nutrition Examination Survey • National Health Care Survey • National Health Interview Survey • National Immunization Survey • Longitudinal studies on aging
Youth Risk Behavior Surveillance System	Monitors priority health risk behaviors that contribute markedly to the leading causes of death, disability, and social problems among youth and adults in the United States. Data files and documentation.
DataFerrett System	NCHS and the Bureau of the Census collaborated to provide NCHS datasets in the Census's DataFerrett system. This unique data mining and extraction tool allows you to select a data basket full of variables, recode those variables as needed, and then develop and customize tables and charts.
United States Department of Agriculture (Economic Research Service)	Food Security in the United States

Web sites

ftp://ftp2.census.gov/census_2000/datasets
http://www.cdc.gov/nchs/datawh/ftpserv/ftpdata/ftpdata.htm
http://www.cdc.gov/HealthyYouth/yrbs/about_yrbss.htm
http://www.cdc.gov/nchs/datawh/ferret/ferret.htm
http://www.ers.usda.gov/data/foodsecurity/ECLS

■ STEPS TO CONDUCT A COMMUNITY NEEDS ASSESSMENT

The community needs assessment includes a planning phase in which the public health nutritionist makes a case for the needs assessment, a methodology development phase, a data collection and analysis phase, and a utilization phase.[2,4] The following describes one set of steps to conduct a community needs assessment. Other valuable resources on conducting community needs assessment, program planning, and evaluation have been developed by the Association of State and Territorial Public Health Nutrition Directors (www.movingtothefuture.org; **Table 3–2**).

Phase 1: Needs Assessment Planning

In the first phase of the needs assessment, the public health nutritionist not only must make a case for the needs assessment in a specific community but also must lay out the organizational framework that will guide the process. The following sections describe the steps necessary to achieve this end.

Step 1: Identify the Community of Interest

At this initial stage of the needs assessment, you need to articulate which community is of concern. This community can include the group of people who are the focus of your needs assessment (i.e., the target population) or a specific region or neighborhood in which they live (e.g., Roxbury, MA), the nutritional problem of concern (e.g., obesity), or all of the above (e.g., overweight children living in Roxbury, MA). It is important to be as specific as possible in order to focus your needs assessment efforts.

Step 2: Describe the Problem, Research Its Underlying Causes, and State Why a Needs Assessment Is Necessary

In this step, you as the public health nutritionist prepare a brief, but compelling, statement of the problem.[2] It should include a description of the nutritional problem of concern, who is affected, the magnitude of the problem, what is known about its causes, and why there is justification for the needs assessment. An essential component of this step is to comprehensively review the research in the published literature in terms of both underlying causes and public health impact. Fortunately, resources such as PubMed on the Internet can be used to identify relevant research articles; in many cases, full text articles are available online. In order to minimize the possibility that you are missing important research in this area, you should utilize a reference librarian to guide you in your use of key words and finding the best databases for your topic. Public health nutritionists often are not in a position to conduct scientific research into the underlying causes of nutrition-related problems; however, the wealth of published research available precludes the need for them to do so.

To return to the former example regarding the nutrition-related problem of overweight children in Roxbury, one needs to examine the literature regarding:

- *Magnitude of the problem.* This includes determining the percentage of children who are overweight or at risk of becoming overweight, and identifying which specific groups of children are most at risk.
- *Importance of addressing this problem in children.* This includes the tracking of overweight people from childhood to adulthood; chronic disease consequences, both in childhood and adulthood; and cost to the healthcare system.
- *Define the known causes of children being overweight.* What is known about how overweight indices have increased among children in general? These include increases in sedentary behavior (e.g., TV watching), reductions in physical activity, and increased consumption of specific types of food (e.g., fast food, processed foods, soft drinks).
- *Gaps in the scope of influence.* This refers to those individuals living in a community in whom there are gaps in nutrition knowledge relevant to the identification and resolution of the nutritional problem in the target

population. In this case, these would include parents, teachers, school administrators, and other community members who can influence children's macro- or micro-environment

Step 3: Define the Target Population

At this point, you have research and data that identify which groups are most at risk for a specific nutritional problem or overall poor nutritional status, and the groups in which the nutritional problem has the greatest effect on public health. This knowledge will guide you to define more clearly the target population for your needs assessment. For example, in the case of overweight children in Roxbury, from your review of the published literature you may have found that the prevalence of obesity increases substantially during adolescence. This could provide the justification for choosing pre-teens living in Roxbury as the target population, if your needs assessment is for obesity prevention programs.

Prevalence, also called *prevalence proportion,* is the proportion of people in a population who have a disease.[6,p.41]

Step 4: Determine the Purpose, Goals, and Objectives of the Community Needs Assessment

The purpose is a general description of the intent of the needs assessment. A community needs assessment may be conducted for any of the following reasons[2]:

- To identify groups of people in the community who are at nutritional risk[2]
- To determine which factors are underlying contributors to the nutritional problem in the particular community in question[2]
- To discover the community's or target population's most critical unmet nutritional needs and prioritize them[2]
- To assess the degree to which existing programs and services meet the needs of the target population[2]
- To distribute resources either within a program (regionally) or between different types of programs based on nutrition needs in the community

It is important to note that the underlying contributors to the problem (second bullet above) must be distinguished from the research question, which is often epidemiological in nature regarding what causes a disease or condition. Although, for example, in the case of the community needs assessment, there is evidence that TV watching may contribute to the development of obesity in children, a nutrition needs assessment will ascertain: a) whether TV watching is high among children in that community, and b) the factors in the community that may contribute to this behavior. As part of the community needs assessment, factors such as unsafe neighborhoods, lack of parks, and lack of affordable after school and summer youth programs may all contribute to the high TV watching among children in this community and subsequent childhood obesity.

Goals and objectives lay the foundation for all activities subsequently conducted for the needs assessment, including data gathering, analysis, and utilization. Goals drive the type of data that will be needed and how it will be used. As McKenzie et al.[1] noted, goals will be the basis for all subsequent activities and is the "hoped for end result." There may be more than one goal for the needs assessment. Objectives, on the other hand, are statements that describe the specific result or outcome that will be achieved or activity accomplished (one result or activity per statement). According to Boyle and Holben,[2] strong verbs should be used in objective statements; examples of such verbs are increase, decrease, reduce, assess, and identify. What is described in each objective should be measurable in some way; thus, by collecting data you should be able to assess the degree to which you were successful at achieving each specific objective. There are usually two or more objectives per goal.

Step 5: Determine the Organizational Structure for the Needs Assessment

It is important that the organizational structure for the needs assessment be determined at the outset.[4] This includes identifying who will direct the needs assessment and all agency and non-agency members of the needs assessment team. What resources will be assigned to this activity, including dedicated staff? How will community members be involved? The composition of the team responsible for conducting the needs assessment depends on the goals and objectives of the needs assessment. Some important members of the needs assessment team include a nutrition professional, staff responsible for nutrition program service delivery and program administration, and someone with expertise in quantitative or qualitative data collection/management/analysis methods (depending on the data needed, expertise will vary). In order for the needs assessment to be conducted thoroughly and effectively, resources need to be allocated consistent with the scope of the needs assessment. This can be a challenge for public health agencies at times, and this is one of the underlying reasons for determining resource allocation at the outset. If adequate resources cannot be allocated, then the scope of the needs assessment may need to be narrowed.

Phase 2: Methodology Development

In this phase of the community needs assessment process, the team will lay out in detail which data will be needed to meet each objective of the needs assessment and how they will obtain these data. Although time-consuming, this type of planning in advance will facilitate all activities related to the needs assessment. As with the literature review, careful and systematic attention to completeness and detail will minimize surprises and ensure that all data that are needed can be obtained.

Step 6: Specify the Data Needed and Design a Plan for Acquiring the Data

The data that may be needed for a nutrition needs assessment likely will fall under one or more of the following four categories:

- Community data
  - Community organizational structure and authorities: Data related to how the community is organized politically and socially
  - Community services and usage: Data related to nutrition-related programs, services, and usage in the community
  - Community demographics and health: The overall health of the community
  - Community environment: Includes local, state, and national policies and systems as well as the specific community's physical environment that can affect the nutritional status of the target population

- Target population data
  - Data related to the nutritional status of the target population
  - Lifestyle factors affecting nutritional status
  - Sociodemographic factors; living and working conditions
  - Data related to attitudes, perceptions, and opinions of the target population

As noted by Peterson and Alexander,[4] the wealth of data potentially available can be both advantageous and disadvantageous. Having numerous indicators implies that the degree to which nutrition-related needs/status is measured is improved (as opposed to having only a few indicators available). Conversely, having too many indicators available can be overwhelming for data management, and tabulation can become unmanageable. Thus, is important to carefully choose the best indicators that relate to the objectives of your nutrition needs assessment. The following specific criteria can be used to assess the potential costs and benefits of choosing indicators[4]:

- *Simplicity:* An indicator needs to be conceptually straightforward, well defined, and a valid and reliable measure of what it purports to represent. Both the public and policy makers should be able to understand it.
- *Stability:* Estimates derived from these indicators should be based on large enough numbers so that they do not fluctuate dramatically due to small sample size.
- *Availability:* Ideally, the indicator is available at national, state, and local levels, so that even if your needs assessment is conducted on a local community, it is possible to examine relative health as compared to state and national status.
- *Broad representation:* An indicator should reflect the potential nutrition-related concerns of most of the target population as well as higher risk groups within the target population.
- *Political feasibility:* Although the public health impact of the nutrition-related problem is one of the most important considerations, one must also consider whether the political environment will facilitate or hinder an intervention to deal with this problem.

The types of data that will be obtained for the needs assessment fall under two general categories: qualitative data and quantitative data. In addition, there are two types of data acquisition: data already collected and in a database or report (i.e., *secondary data sources*) and data that must be collected directly from the community or target population as part of the needs assessment (i.e., *primary data collection*).

Plan to Obtain Community Data

1. Community data, including the organizational structure and authorities.   How the community's governmental agencies

and healthcare organizations are organized and who is in power can affect the healthcare as well as the preventative service delivery for the target population. Community leaders are also important to identify because not only will they be invaluable sources of information about the unmet needs in the community, but also they will be essential to any successful strategy to address the unmet need identified by the needs assessment. One method that can be used to identify such individuals is obtaining organizational charts of government offices and healthcare organizations, either through the Internet or through visiting the offices. In addition, reading the local newspapers and listening to local radio stations will provide information on both community and business leaders as well as influential media groups. Finally, those who have particular influence on, involvement with, or a vested interest in the well-being of the target population (i.e., *stakeholders*) should be identified and included.

American Heart Association is available at www.americanheart.org.

American Red Cross is available at www.redcross.org.

American Diabetes Association is available at www.diabetes.org.

United Way is available at http://www.liveunited.org/.

2. Community services and usage. Information on which nutrition-related services and programs are available in the community can be obtained from the Internet (i.e., government and nonprofit organizations' Web sites as well as online library sources), local health organizations, government agencies and civic groups, the Yellow Pages of the telephone directory, and voluntary health organizations such as the American Heart Association, the American Red Cross, the American Diabetes Association, and the United Way directories. Usage data includes the number of people using services as well as segments of the target population that are more or less likely to use specific services. This type of information can be obtained from the agencies and programs delivering the services; however, some of this information may not be available to the public. Involving key personnel who are involved in delivering programs relevant to the specific goals of the nutrition needs assessment thus facilitates access to such data.

3. Community demographics and health. Demographic data and health data can be obtained from a variety of sources (see Table 3–2). Some important demographic data include ethnicity, age distribution, gender, marital status, income, and poverty statistics. These all provide a description of who lives in the community. A variety of health statistics reflect overall health of the community, and these can point to segments of the population that are at risk for malnutrition. The following are some health statistics that are available at the national and state level available through the Centers for Disease Control and Prevention (www.cdc.gov/data/-statistics); some may be available for the local level as well:

- Age-adjusted mortality: These include overall rates of death, both in general and from specific diseases.
- Natality: These statistics include the percent of mothers with adequate prenatal care, the infant mortality rate, average birth weights, and the percent of unmarried mothers.
- Leading causes of death: This is a rank order list of those causes to which deaths are most frequently attributable.
- Morbidity: These statistics include rates of nutrition-related diseases such as obesity, hypertension, heart disease, arthritis, and diabetes (as well as complications from diabetes).
- Health risk behaviors: These include sedentary activities, smoking, serum cholesterol concentration, lead exposure, and iron deficiency anemia.

Some of these statistics are also stratified by demographic characteristics, which can then be more accurately compared to the target population demographics. This is particularly useful if local data on a particular health outcome is not available for the specific community.

4. Environmental conditions within the community. This includes availability of food, access to medical care, and access to preventative services, transportation, parks, walkways, and bicycle paths. All of these factors comprise the environment of the community that can affect the nutritional status of the target population. Availability of food, for example, is determined by variety, cost, and quality of the food that community grocery stores, supermarkets, co-ops, farmer's markets, restaurants, or fast food establishments in the area provide. For many community residents, food availability within the specific community determines what they can buy and have in their homes. How can we ascertain food availability? One of the best ways, if logistically possible, is to walk around the community and visit supermarkets and grocery stores, also

TABLE 3–2	Sources for Demographic and Health Statistics for the Community Needs Assessment
Source	**Description**
U.S. Census Bureau Census Data	The 2009 Statistical Abstract American Community Survey. Includes state and county data.
Health, United States	2008 National Health statistics produced in report format by the National Center for Health Statistics (NCHS). Comprehensive report drawing from a variety of data sources.
FastStatsAtoZ	Provides state and territorial-specific natality and mortality statistics as well as health and health risk behavior data.
National Health and Nutrition Examination Survey (NHANES)	Reports and study results.
Links to NCHS surveys related to health and health care	
National Vital Statistics	Annual reports present detailed vital statistics data, including natality, mortality, marriage, and divorce.
The Behavioral Risk Factor Surveillance System (BRFSS)	World's largest telephone survey; tracks health risks in the United States; includes national and state statistics as well as statistics on selected metropolitan areas.
Youth Risk Behavior Surveillance System (YRBSS)	Developed in 1990 to monitor priority health risk behaviors that contribute markedly to the leading causes of death, disability, and social problems among youth and adults in the United States.
The Pediatric Nutrition Surveillance System (PedNSS) and the Pregnancy Nutrition Surveillance System (PNSS)	Program-based surveillance systems that monitor the nutritional status of low-income infants, children, and women in federally funded maternal and child health programs.
Data Warehouse for NCHS data	Includes links to detailed statistical tables on a variety of health topics.
United States Department of Agriculture (USDA)	International food consumption patterns Economic Research Service Food Stamp Program statistics WIC Program statistics Food security in the United States links to a variety of data sources on food security.
Association of State and Territorial Public Health Nutrition Directors (ASTPHND)	Provides tools for planning nutrition and physical activity programs.

Web sites with links to statistical information

http://www.census.gov/compendia/statab/
http://www.census.gov/acs/www/
http://www.cdc.gov/nchs/hus.htm
http://www.cdc.gov/nchs/fastats/map_page.htm
http://www.cdc.gov/nchs/nhanes/nhanes_products.htm
http://www.cdc.gov/nchs
http://www.cdc.gov/nchs/products/vsus.htm
http://www.cdc.gov/brfss/
http://www.cdc.gov/HealthyYouth/yrbs
http://www.cdc.gov/pednss/
http://www.cdc.gov/nchs/datawh.htm
http://www.ers.usda.gov/data/InternationalFoodDemand/
http://www.ers.usda.gov
http://www.fns.usda.gov/pd/snapmain.htm
http://www.fns.usda.gov/fns/data.htm
http://www.ers.usda.gov/Data/foodsecurity/
http://www.movingtothefuture.org

noting types of restaurants and transportation availability. Visiting stores and noting food quality, availability, and cost provides valuable qualitative information on what the target population faces in their food procurement on a day-to-day basis. In addition, it also provides an opportunity for you to get a true feel of the community, the ethnic groups represented, and the physical surroundings that can affect opportunities for physical activity.

The National Nutrition Monitoring and Related Research Program (http://www.cdc.gov/nchs/about/otheract/nutrishn/nutrishn.htm) includes all data on the collection and analysis activities of the federal government related to measuring the health and nutritional status, food consumption, dietary knowledge, and attitudes about diet and health of the U.S. population, and measuring food consumption and quality of the food supply.

Plan to Obtain Data on the Target Population

Data on the nutritional status of the target population can be obtained through either secondary data sources or primary data collection. The former is desirable, if it is appropriate for the needs assessment, because it requires much fewer resources and can be obtained much more quickly. The National Nutrition Monitoring and Related Research Program publishes statistics at the national and state levels. In addition, you can obtain some of these datasets and conduct further analyses as part of the needs assessment. For example, it may be that your target population is Puerto Rican, but the statistics you identify are described for those of Hispanic descent as a whole. If the dataset is available, then the member of your team who is responsible for data management and analysis can analyze the data for Puerto Ricans, specifically.

Existing datasets, if they include the indicators pertinent to the nutrition needs assessment, thus can be used to describe the target population's health and nutritional status. These also can be used as a basis to compare the target population's nutritional status with national and state statistics.

Nutritional status indicators fall under one of the following four categories[7]:

- Dietary assessment
- Laboratory/biochemical assessment
- Anthropometric assessment
- Clinical assessment

Dietary Assessment

Dietary assessment methods are used to collect data on usual food and nutrient intake of individuals. Some frequently used dietary assessment methods are 24-hour recalls (single or repeated), estimated or weighed food records, dietary history, and food frequency questionnaires.[7]

All of the aforementioned methods have systematic errors.[7] The goal is to minimize these errors as much as possible. There is an extensive literature in the area of dietary assessment, and many research articles that describe improved methodology[8] and their validity and reliability in various populations. The following is simply a summary of the most important points to consider.

There are various challenges to obtaining dietary data that reflect usual diet, not the least of which is that among free-living individuals, dietary intake exhibits variation from day to day. This variation is superimposed on a consistent pattern.[9,p.33] What the researcher is attempting to ascertain is that consistent pattern. Depending on the dietary assessment method used, the accuracy of intake data often reflects a person's literacy and educational level (for all methods, but especially food records), memory (24-hour recall and food frequency questionnaire), and ability to accurately quantify foods (24-hour recall and food frequency questionnaire). Another source of error is that individuals often alter their dietary intake while undergoing the assessment, thus reducing the accuracy with which the foods reflect what is usually eaten.

If you are considering collecting dietary data, you need to review several factors. First, who is your population and what method is most appropriate? If your population is a well-educated one, then using food records[9] may be a good choice. On the other hand, if the population has limited literacy, then repeated 24-hour recalls may be a better choice.

Second, the number of days of dietary intake affects the validity with which the data reflects the individual's usual intake. A single day, whether it be a 24-hour recall or a food record, is not adequate to estimate a person's true usual intake for any macro- or micro-nutrient[9,p.41]; a single day, however, can provide an estimate of the average usual nutrient intake of a large population group if all the days of the week are represented.[7,p.50] The degree of day-to-day variability affects the number of days needed, and this also depends on the nutrient under examination. For example, it has been stated that in order to obtain an estimate of an individual's vitamin A intake, such that 95% of observed values are within 10% of the true mean, one needs 105 days of dietary intake data.[9,p.44] This may seem absurd, but this example illustrates that it is virtually impossible to estimate an individual's intake based on one 24-hour recall. However, by administering repeated 24-hour recalls, you can improve the validity with which they represent the individual's usual diet.

The third issue is how the data will be analyzed. For 24-hour recalls and food records, you need to use a nutrient analysis program to assess the macro- or micro-nutrient content of the diet. If using a validated Food Frequency Questionnaire, such as the Harvard Semiquantitative Food Frequency Questionnaire (FFQ), then often the nutrient analysis is provided for a fee by the institution that sponsors that FFQ.

The following are generally recommended methods based on the objective of the dietary assessment:

- Average usual intakes of a population group: Can use a single 24-hour recall or food record,[7] although repeated measures are always better.
- Proportion of the population "at risk" for a nutrient deficiency or excess: Repeated 24-hour recalls or food records.[7] The number of days depends on the nutrient(s) that are the focus of the needs assessment.[7,9]
- Usual nutrient intakes of individuals: Repeated 24-hour recalls or food records.[7] The number of days depends on the nutrient(s) that are the focus of the needs assessment.[7,9]
- Pattern of food use for a group or individual or ranking of individuals: Food frequency questionnaires.[7]

To summarize, if a dietary assessment is needed as a part of the needs assessment, you should choose the method that will produce the most valid and reliable data for the target population that will meet the objectives of the needs assessment in the most succinct manner. Ideally, someone on the needs assessment team should have expertise in the area of dietary assessment, and a review of the literature should be conducted prior to choosing a method.

Laboratory/Biochemical Assessment

This is an objective measure of subclinical nutrient deficiency; it involves measurement of nutrient level, a nutrient's metabolite, or functional tests that measure nutrient-dependent enzyme activity or concentrations.[7,pp.285-295] The aforementioned may be measured in blood, urine, hair, fingernails, or toenails. Many other functional tests exist as well but are likely beyond the scope of a public health nutrition needs assessment. One of the most common laboratory tests used in nutritional surveillance and in programs such as WIC is hemoglobin or hematocrit, which is used as an indicator of iron deficiency anemia. Note, however, that hemoglobin is a relatively insensitive indicator and nonspecific; this means that a significant proportion of people may truly have iron deficiency anemia but be classified as having normal hemoglobin (insensitivity), while others may be diagnosed with iron deficiency anemia based on their hemoglobin levels but are not truly anemic (nonspecific). Part of the problem is that hemoglobin (and hematocrit) is affected by many factors other than iron, including inflammation, infections, protein energy malnutrition, thalassemia minor,

vitamin B_{12}, or folate deficiencies, to name a few.[7,p.352] In order to more accurately identify those who have iron deficiency anemia, other indicators of iron status (e.g., transferrin saturation, serum ferritin) should also be collected. In addition, hemoglobin and hematocrits' predictive value (i.e., positive predictive value is the percent of those who are diagnosed with anemia based on either of these screening tools that are truly anemic) has declined because the prevalence of anemia in the U.S. population has been successfully reduced.[10]

Anthropometric Assessment

This type of nutritional assessment includes all measures of physical dimensions and body composition.[7] Two general objectives of anthropometric assessments are to assess growth and body composition.[7] The most commonly used indices of linear growth are recumbent length (in those under 2 years or older) and standing height (in those 2 years of age or older). Head circumference in children under 3 years of age is related to brain size. Weight along with height is used to calculate body mass index (BMI), which is used as an indirect measure of obesity.[7,p.178] Other anthropometric measurements used to assess body composition are skinfold (e.g., triceps skinfolds) and circumferences (waist and mid-arm).

> Body mass index (BMI) = weight (kg)/height (m)^2

Note that interpretation of these data requires a comparison to reference data and/or prediction equations to calculate body composition from the data. The Centers for Disease Control and Prevention has reference growth charts for infants and children (2000 CDC Growth Charts, see below) available and a module for using the BMI for age growth charts. In 2006, the World Health Organization also released growth standards for infants and children up to 71 months of age that were based on an international sample of well nourished children who have breast-fed and whose mothers have followed the WHO guidelines for breastfeeding support and infant feeding (http://www.who.int/childgrowth/standards/en/). Both CDC (http://www.cdc.gov/nccdphp/dnpa/growthcharts/resources/sas.htm) and WHO (http://www.who.int/childgrowth/software/en/) have software that can be used to convert raw weights, heights into percentiles, and z scores.

Whether you use secondary or primary data, it is essential for the needs assessment that you use standardized protocols to collect these data (usually height/length

> For a description of the semiquantitative food frequency questionnaire used in the Nurses Health Study at the Harvard School of Public Health, visit http://www.hsph.harvard.edu/Academics/nutr/department/Nurses%20Study.html.

or weight). If you use reference data to convert raw data into either percentiles or z-scores, these must be based on the CDC 2000 growth curves. The Health Resources and Services Administration (HRSA) has produced a training module, available on the Web, that describes how to accurately measure height and weight in children and adolescents.

Clinical Assessment

Clinical assessment occurs via a physical examination and medical history in order to detect physical signs and symptoms of under- or overnutrition.[7,p.577] This requires expertise and training on the part of the examiner in order to accurately associate these signs with a nutritional deficiency. These signs are generally nonspecific, so they should be used in conjunction with one or more of the other nutritional assessment methods.[7] Note that by the time clinical signs develop, there already will be a manifestation of an advanced stage of nutrient deficiency, because clinical signs occur when malnutrition is chronic in nature. An example of a clinical sign of vitamin C deficiency is swollen red gums[7,p.583]; however, swollen red gums also could be due to various non-nutritional problems (e.g., periodontal disease). Combined with other information (such as a dietary assessment showing a low intake of vitamin C–containing foods), the accurate attribution of this clinical sign to vitamin C deficiency may be made.

For a copy of the 2000 CDC Growth Charts, along with a comprehensive description, see: http://www.cdc.gov/growthcharts/

For a module on using the BMI-for-age growth charts for infants and children, see: http://www.cdc.gov/nccdphp/dnpa/growthcharts/training/modules/module1/text/intro.htm

For training on accurate measurement in children and adolescents, see the HRSA training module: http://depts.washington.edu/growth/module5/text/page7b.htm

Other Types of Data

There are many determinants of food and nutrient intake, nutritional status, and health. Many of these have been summarized in a conceptual framework elsewhere (Nutrition Monitoring in the United States) and Boyle and Holben[2] in more detail. Many of the following interact with one another to affect actual food intake, health beliefs and practices.

- Health risk behaviors: This includes tobacco or alcohol use and drug abuse.
- Availability and use of health care: health insurance, disease screening, annual physical exams, and frequency of visits to a healthcare professional.
- Lifestyle practices: These include time spent engaging in physical activity and sedentary behavior (leisure time and non-leisure time).

- Income: Income distribution and percentage of population living below the poverty level.
- Cultural factors: ethnic group and degree of acculturation.
- Religion and degree of adherence to religious beliefs.
- Educational level: Distribution and percentage attaining specific levels of education.
- Household composition and size: Who lives in the household (e.g., mother, father, grandmother, 3 children) and how many people live in the household.
- Occupation: Can refer to the occupation of any or all the adults living in the household.
- Working conditions: Hours of work, job benefits, and job stress.
- Living conditions: Potential health risks associated with the housing (e.g., lead paint).
- Primary social groups: Family, friends, and work groups.[2]

In addition, data on attitudes, perceptions, and opinions can be a critical component of the needs assessment data collection plan because it is often the lack of insight into the target population's attitudes and perceptions about a nutrition or health problem, the contributing factors, and workable solutions that hinder the successful implementation of an effective plan of action. This type of data can be qualitative in nature.

Methods for Obtaining Data on the Target Populations (Primary Data Collection)

Surveys can be used to obtain data about health risk behaviors, such as use of health care; physical activity and sedentary behaviors; socioeconomic factors; working and living conditions; and attitudes, perceptions, and opinions. Although many set out to develop their own surveys, this is not recommended unless there are survey development experts on the needs assessment team. Although it may seem simple enough, survey development is complicated and time-consuming, and if it is not done correctly, the derived data may be unusable. If you are going to use a survey to collect primary data for the needs assessment, it is recommended that you use the following series of steps that prioritize validated and extensively used surveys over survey development. Note that some resources include copies of existing health surveys.[11]

1. Identify surveys in the research literature or those used in the National Nutrition Monitoring and Related Research Program (NNMRRP) that address the question of interest.
2. Give preference to those surveys that have strong evidence of validity (i.e., construct and predictive validity) and reliability.
3. If there is no strong evidence of survey validity (i.e., no validation or only face or content validity assessed),

give preference to those existing surveys used in national nutrition surveillance or monitoring. Although formal validation may not have been done, the questions have been used on large population groups and the data have been analyzed and utilized; this implies that the data were usable for the purpose intended. In addition, this will enable comparison of your local or regional needs assessment data to national statistics.

4. If a set of survey questions comprise a scale (e.g., body image), it is important to use the entire set of questions that form that scale.

Detailed guidance for survey development is beyond the scope of this chapter; however, there are several excellent reference books that provide guidance in developing surveys.[11,12] Drafting questions for a survey seems deceptively simple but, in fact, writing questions that are straightforward, universally understood by all respondents, and truly answer the question the researcher sets out to answer is complicated. The final wording (and formatting) of the question and response categories evolve from a process of obtaining input from experts, pre-testing, and reliability and validity testing. For many, resource constraints preclude such survey development. Unfortunately, what results from hurried attempts at drafting questions are data of questionable quality that may not prove to have been worthwhile to collect using such a survey. **Exhibit 3–1** is a compilation of some important points to consider when drafting your own survey. In addition, if the instrument that you select has been used in samples that are sociodemographically or ethnically different from your target population, you need to test it with your target population prior to its use for the needs assessment.

Focus Groups

A focus group usually consists of 7 to 10 people who are relatively homogeneous and whose input or opinion is sought through broad open-ended questions about a research topic.[13] Focus group participants are selected because they are considered knowledgeable about the topic. Focus groups are often used to obtain qualitative data on perceptions, attitudes, or opinions about a specific issue or product. This can be an extremely important method in the needs assessment process because it can provide a method for eliciting opinions from the target population on their perceived needs, barriers to preventing disease, or even why certain programs are not working. For example, in the case of the nutrition problem of childhood obesity in Roxbury, a focus group of teenagers may provide insight as to why they choose what they do after school, why they don't use certain after school programs, and what kinds of activities they would participate in that would get them moving.

Key Informant Interviews

Key informant interviews consist of structured or unstructured interviews (phone or face-to-face) of individuals (i.e., key informants) who have been identified as having specific knowledge about the topic of interest. In this case it would be someone who has knowledge about the community, target populations, services, or other efforts (past or present) to address health- or nutrition-related problems, or stakeholders who may have important insights about the needs of the community or target population.

Phase 3: Data Collection and Analysis

By the time this phase is reached, all of the methods for the needs assessment, including indicators, existing datasets that will be used, or the methods for primary data analysis, will have been determined. This is the phase in which data will be collected, either directly from participants or from existing reports, or additional analysis will be completed from secondary data sets.

Step 7: Collect Data on the Community and the Target Population

Irrespective of the methods used for the needs assessment data collection, it is imperative that someone be responsible for overseeing the following:

- Data collection progress and troubleshooting
- Data entry and cleaning (if primary data collection)
- Data management in terms of how databases will be designed and what software will be used
- Quality or limitations of the data

Step 8: Analyze and Interpret Data

In this stage, the pertinent data will be summarized for the community and target population. As Boyle and Holben[2] note, the following steps must be undertaken in the analysis stage in order to "diagnose" the community; that is, to describe the unmet needs in the community:

- Interpret the health status of the target population that lives in the community.
- Interpret the pattern of health care, health services, and nutrition- or health-related programs that are designed to reach the target population.
- Assess the relationship between the health/nutrition needs of the target population and the pattern of services available in the community.

The results of the needs assessment should then be summarized in a report. This summary should include the needs assessment methods used, a description of the nutritional problems, their severity and prevalence, their distribution across the community and target population (e.g., is it worse in urban areas or in specific age or ethnic groups?), causes

Exhibit 3–1 Survey Checklist

This checklist is intended to be a guide for you in the development of your survey. However, following all of these recommendations cannot replace extensive pre-testing of your survey instrument to determine what is working and what isn't. In addition to wording and formatting, pre-testing can help you determine optimal question and response order. This list combines and summarizes Fowler's guidelines[12,14] for conducting survey research and improving survey questions along with the author's observations regarding common errors made when reviewing surveys that students as well as non-survey experts attempt to draft. It is not intended to be an exhaustive list, nor can it be used in lieu of the guidance of survey development experts and a good reference on survey development such as those noted herein. It also does not address other aspects such as mode of administration, training of interviewers, and other facets of collecting high-quality survey data. In addition, because many surveys are now computer assisted, the aforementioned reference books[12] also address newer issues of computer assisted administration.

Questions: Wording, Content, and Order

- Use full sentences.
- Ask all respondents the same questions.[12]
- To ensure consistent meaning for all respondents, define all words that people may interpret differently.[12]
- Be as specific as possible. For example, if asking about smoking, you need to specify the type, and what you are defining as a person who smokes.
- Language level should match respondent ability.
- Avoid hypothetical questions, avoid asking about causality, ask only one question at a time, and so on.[12]
- Include all the domains laid out in your conceptual framework in your survey.
- Avoid words like typical, usually, and on average. Use a specific time frame whenever possible.
- If using a self-administered survey, it is very important that you place the most critical information needed for your research near the beginning. This is also important in an interviewer-administered survey, but less so.
- Place sensitive questions appropriately. For an interviewer-administered survey, these need to be near the end. For a self-administered survey they can be closer to the beginning.
- Avoid derogatory or negative terms/words that may cause bias in response. If there is something threatening or negative in your survey, attempt to neutralize it by inserting an introductory sentence acknowledging that some people do this behavior or have this problem.

If you are asking about a list or want multiple responses, then specify in your question the number of points to be made.[12]

Response Categories

- List all possible responses, but only once. Possible responses should be listed after the question.[12]
- If you determine that a respondent can provide a relatively accurate quantitative response, then ask for the actual number instead of selecting categories. This is desirable as long as it doesn't make completing the survey more difficult for the respondent. For example, if you want to know how many siblings a person has, simply leave a space or two (depending on the range of sibling number in the population) and let them supply the actual number.
- Specify the response format (e.g., if you want years, include that in the response).
- If only one answer is required, make response categories mutually exclusive.
- Ensure that the number of response categories captures the full range of possible responses, including adequate variability (e.g., if most people are going to check the last category, then you need to break down that category further so that you can differentiate better among people).
- Make the order of responses consistent throughout the survey. For example, if numerical categories are listed, then they all need to be listed in the same order (lowest to highest is most common).
- Use specified frequencies whenever possible instead of vague words like "often, sometimes," and so on.
- Make sure there is a space for the respondent to respond. For example, if you say "check off one answer," then you need a space (__) or check-off box.

Introductions and Transition Statements and Instructions

- Provide an introduction to the survey itself. Here you generally describe the purpose of the survey, what you expect the respondent to do, and what she or he should do if they don't understand something or have questions. Also, this is where you should assure the respondent of confidentiality or anonymity (whichever applies in your case).
- If the survey is broken up into sections (which it should be if the survey is longer than a few pages), then number and label the sections with section headings, and have a brief introduction to each section.
- Although you may have instructed the respondent at the beginning of a section or at the beginning of the survey, you still need to provide instructions to tell the respondent exactly what to do for every question. The instructions should be in a different font than the question (they can be italicized, bolded, or capitalized). Be consistent throughout in terms of how you want the

person to respond (e.g., circle or check off responses). In the instructions, also include how many they can choose (i.e., all that apply or one).
- If you have an "other" option, then ask respondents to specify or describe what that is.

Survey Format and Layout
- General rule: Avoid crowding and maximize white space.
- There should be space between questions as well as between questions and response categories.
- Provide plenty of space for the responses (whether it be a number written in or room for them to check something off).
- If you have contingency questions (i.e., questions that depend on a response to another question) and it is a self-administered questionnaire, it is best to use arrows to actually lead the person to the next question. The arrow normally stems from the response. If it is an interviewer-administered survey, it is OK to say "Go

to question ___," but these instructions should also be adjacent to the response category.
- However you decide to lay out your response categories, be consistent (columnar or in rows).
- If you have a series of questions with the same response categories and decide to lay them out in a tabular format, shade every other row so that people won't lose their place.
- Make sure that the question and the response categories are on the same page.

General
- Number all pages.
- Each page should have a place for an ID number.
- At the end of each page note that there are more pages to the survey. You can say "Next page" with an arrow or something else that will tell the respondent that there is more to complete. On the next to the last page of the survey, note "only one more page left." This is essential for any survey that is more than two pages long.

specific to that target population and community, and the consequences in terms of morbidity and mortality.[2,p.430] In addition, you should prepare an executive summary, no longer than one to two pages, that highlights the key points of the needs assessment.

Phase 4: Using the Needs Assessment Results

Step 9: Share the Findings of the Assessment

The findings of the needs assessment must be shared not only with others in the agency that undertook the lead for the needs assessment and participating agencies and organizations, but also with the stakeholders who either provided advice and key information or work with the target population.

Step 10: Prioritize the Needs of the Community and Target Population

Many unmet needs may be identified as a result of the needs assessment; however, resource limitations often constrain the degree to which all unmet needs can be addressed. It thus is essential that needs be prioritized. Various methods of prioritization have been proposed[15,p.37–40]; two will be reviewed here.

In their seminal book, *Community Nutritional Assessment*, Jelliffe and Jelliffe[16] laid out five principles that can be used to set priorities. First, priority should be given to what the community identifies as its priorities, preferences, or concerns. Second, common problems should be given priority over rare ones. Third, serious problems should be

prioritized over less critical ones. Fourth, easily preventable problems should have higher priority than those for which prevention is more difficult. Finally, those health problems that have exhibited increases over time should be given preference over those whose frequencies are decreasing or have stabilized.

Another simple method of prioritization is to use members of the target population and program providers who may have been included on the needs assessment team to rank the top five needs. The series of rankings assigned to each need is reverse-scored (i.e., if a need is ranked as 1, it is given a score of 5); scores are then summed, and those with the highest numbers are given priority.[15,p.37–38]

Step 11: Develop a Plan of Action to Use the Needs Assessment Findings to Improve the Nutritional Status of the Target Population

Once the needs assessment is completed and unmet needs are identified and prioritized, a plan of action to address the priority needs must be developed. This may involve modifying an existing program or programs to better meet the need or developing new programs, or advocating for funding to address the unmet need, utilizing the needs assessment results as ammunition. The team needs to include stakeholders in the process of developing this plan of action.

Needs Assessment in Practice: Massachusetts WIC Needs Assessment

The Massachusetts WIC Needs Assessment (WIC NA) was developed in 1983 by the Massachusetts Department of

Public Health (MDPH) Advisory Committee in order to guide the allocation of caseload and resources (i.e., the statewide distribution of funds). Some of the methodology was derived from a broader needs assessment process whose goal was to distribute funds statewide for primary prenatal and pediatric care services.[17] In 1993, MDPH revised the WIC needs assessment in order to: 1) to compensate for the reported 2000 census undercount and to update economic indicators (e.g., poverty); 2) to compensate for economic changes that have occurred since the release of the 1990 poverty data; and, 3) to better account for variation in ethnicity distribution by communities.

The methodology is composed of what is referred to as both a qualitative score for ranking cities and towns, in terms of variables correlated with the need for WIC services (considered indicators of risk) and a quantitative estimate of the number of people eligible for WIC services at the local level.

Read more about the Special Supplemental Nutrition Program for Women, Infants and Children in Chapters 4 and 5.

The methodology takes into consideration the eligibility requirements of the WIC program. In Massachusetts, infants and children under five years of age, and pregnant, postpartum, and breastfeeding/lactating women whose household income is below 185% of the poverty line, are eligible to receive WIC services. This plan is the result of a well thought out and detailed methodology; its original framework continues to be in use (Stella Uzogara, personal communication, August 3, 2009). A person with strong quantitative, programming, and data skills is needed to conduct this needs assessment.

For the qualitative indicator of overall need for nutrition services, various health and socioeconomic indicators are used in a principal component analysis to produce composite z-scores, which reflect risk. Cities and towns are then ranked according to the magnitude of these scores. The following health and socioeconomic indicators comprise this score.

Health Indicators for the Five Most Recent Years

All the health indicators are taken from the birth file, which includes all birth data for the entire state. Because MDPH (Vital statistics division in the Bureau of Health Information, Statistics, Research and Evaluation [BHISRE]) is the agency responsible for the birth data, WIC does not have to wait for the public release of these data, and therefore has access to the most current data (i.e., the open surveillance file). The following up-to-date data were available:

- Neonatal mortality rate
- Proportion of adolescent pregnancies
- Percent low birth weight

The birth file data were chosen over the census data because these data are timelier and have been shown to be a better reflection of the true population of infants, children, and mothers.[18]

Socioeconomic Indicators

The following socioeconomic indicators are used:

- The annual unemployment rate for the previous year: This information is obtained from the Department of Education and Training (e.g., for 2009 WICNA, the 2008 annual unemployment rate for Massachusetts cities and towns was used).
- Percentage of the population under 5 years old who are living under 100% of the poverty line: This information (annual poverty rate) is obtained from the most current rate listed by the Current Population Survey or CPS of the U.S. Census Bureau (toll free 1-866-758-1060 or Web site: http://pubdb3.census.gov/macro/032008/pov/new46_100125_01.htm).
- Percentage of the population that is a minority (using race/ethnicity): This is based on the race/ethnic distribution of births as indicated by the city and town birth data.

The estimate of the number of WIC-eligible individuals is derived from the sum of eligible mothers (pregnant, postpartum and breastfeeding) and eligible children (children 0–5 years of age) who are living near poverty and below poverty. Children near poverty are those living between 100% and 200% of the poverty line. Children below poverty are those living below 100% of the poverty line. Birth certificate data is again used because it is considered to be a more accurate reflection of the population than the census data for reasons previously noted.

The following are used to estimate the total number of eligible people:

Total eligible number of infants and children. This is calculated using the 5-year birth totals multiplied by the percent below 100% of poverty. The percent of those under 5 years of age living at the poverty line could not be derived directly from the census data because only the percent of those living under 100% of poverty is available. Information about children 0 to 5 years old living between 100% and 200% of poverty are not available, so the percentage of the total population that lived between 100% and 200% of poverty had to be used instead. In addition the actual income cut-off of < 185% of the poverty threshold that determines WIC eligibility is not available in any of the datasets; thus the closest cut-off of < 200% of poverty is used.

The estimate of the number of 0- to 5-year-olds who were eligible for WIC thus was calculated by adding together the following two estimates:

1. Number of children living below poverty level = 5-year birth totals multiplied by the proportion of 0- to 5-year-olds < 100% of poverty

2. Number of children living at poverty or between 100% and 200% of poverty = 5-year birth totals multiplied by percent of population between 100% and 200% of poverty.

Total number of pregnant women. This was calculated using the total number of unborn and born eligible infants and women who knew that they were pregnant. It was assumed that a woman can begin to receive WIC services when she is 1-month pregnant, or alternatively for 8 months of her pregnancy (i.e., 66.7% of the year).

- Estimate of number of eligible pregnant women = eligible infants × 0.667
- Estimate of number of eligible postpartum non lactating women = eligible infants × 0.5
- Estimate of number of eligible postpartum breastfeeding women = eligible infants × 0.5

Total number of postpartum women. This was considered equal to the number of eligible infants.

In order to combine the socioeconomic and health risk factors with the size of the population who are in need of WIC services into a single indicator that would be used to guide caseload allocation decisions, the qualitative needs assessment z-score is combined with the quantitative measure of estimated eligible individuals; this combines to produce the "risk-adjusted" eligible population by city and town.

In summary, the WIC NA is the result of a well thought out, complex methodology developed by an advisory group for allocating caseload and resources for the WIC program statewide. It estimates the numbers of individuals eligible for WIC and adjusts for other health and socioeconomic risk factors, using a variety of internal (e.g., birth, death data) and external (e.g., census data, unemployment data) data sources, and has allocated appropriate staff to carry it out. It was developed and continues to be carried out through a collaborative effort between administrative, management, and other personnel with strong data and analytic skills. It exemplifies the best of public health needs assessment efforts.

■ CONCLUSIONS

This chapter provided an overview of community needs assessment, an integral component of the pubic health process in general, and public health nutrition in particular. This overview is intended to act as a starting point for those planning to undertake a community needs assessment. The aspiring public health nutritionist is encouraged to use the more detailed references noted in this chapter at the early stages of the needs assessment planning process in order to obtain more thorough information about the many steps involved in this process.

Unmet need should be at the forefront of public health consciousness, and designing the strategy and obtaining the tools to identify this need in a specific community and target population lay the foundation for its identification. The scope of a community needs assessment can be broad or limited in nature; its success doesn't lie in its breadth but rather in its ability to meet its objectives, identify unmet need within the scope defined, and design effective action plans that are inclusive of the public health program personnel, community, and stakeholders. After all, effective teamwork is both the challenge and reward of public health.

Issues for Discussion

1. Why would it be important to include program providers as part of your needs assessment team?

2. What is the rationale for examining the leading causes of death as a measure of the community's health? In relation to mortality, what else could you examine?

3. If the purpose of the Roxbury example provided in this chapter is to identify the causes of the high prevalence of obesity among children living in Roxbury, lay out one goal and at least two objectives for such a needs assessment.

References

1. McKenzie JF, Pinger RR, Kotecki JE. *An Introduction to Community Health*, 4th ed. Sudbury, MA: Jones & Bartlett; 2002:3, 123.

2. Boyle MA, Holben DH. *Community Nutrition in Action: An Entrepreneurial Approach*, 5th ed. Independence, KY: Brooks Cole; 2010:39–87.

3. Achterberg CL, Shepherd SK. The philosophy and role of qualitative inquiry in research. In: *Research Successful Approaches*, 2nd ed. Monsen E, Van Horn L, eds. Chicago: American Dietetic Association; 2003:120–128.

4. Peterson DJ, Alexander GR. *Needs Assessment in Public Health: A Practical Guide for Students and Professionals*. New York: Kluwer Academic/Plenum Publishers; 2001:15–37.

5. Campos P. *The Obesity Myth: Why America's Obsession with Weight Is Hazardous to Your Health*. New York: Gotham; 2004.

6. Rothman KJ. *Epidemiology: An Introduction*. Oxford, NY: Oxford University Press; 2002.

7. Gibson RS. *Principles of Nutritional Assessment*. Oxford, NY: Oxford University Press; 1990.

8. Jonnalagadda SS, Mitchell D, Smickilas-Wright H, et al. Accuracy of energy intake data estimated by a multi-pass, 24-hour recall technique. *J Am Dietetics Assoc.* 2000;100: 303–308, 311.

9. Willett W. *Nutritional Epidemiology*. Oxford, NY: Oxford University Press; 1998.

10. Monsen ER. *Research Successful Approaches*, 2nd ed. Chicago, IL: American Dietetic Association; 2003.

11. Aday LA, Cornelius LJ. *Designing and Conducting Health Surveys*, 3rd ed. San Francisco: Jossey-Bass, John Wiley & Sons; 2006.

12. Fowler FJ Jr. *Survey Research Methods*, 4th ed. Applied Social Research Methods Series, vol. 1. Bickman L, Rog DJ, eds. Newbury Park, CA: Sage; 2009.

13. Morse JM, Field PA. An overview of qualitative methods. In: *Qualitative Research Methods for Health Professionals*, 2nd ed. Chapman and Hall, Thousand Oaks, CA; 1995:31–32.

14. Fowler FJ Jr. *Improving Survey Questions, Design and Evaluation*. Applied Social Research Methods Series, vol. 38. Newbury Park, CA: Sage; 1995.

15. Gilmore GD, Campbell MD. *Needs Assessment Capacity Assessment Strategies for Health Education and Health Promotion*, 3rd ed. Sudbury, MA: Jones and Bartlett; 2005.

16. Jelliffe DB, Jelliffe EFP. *Community Nutritional Assessment: With Special Reference to Less Technically Developed Countries*. New York: Oxford Medical Publications; 1989:452–453.

17. Guyer B, Schor L, Messenger K, Prenney B, Evans F. Needs assessment under the Maternal and Child Health Services block grant: Massachusetts. *Am J Public Health*. 1984;74:1014–1019.

18. Massachusetts Public Health Department. March 2009. Internal memo.

CHAPTER 4

Reaching Out to Those at Highest Nutritional Risk

Rachel Colchamiro, MPH, RD, LDN

Jan Kallio, MS, RD, LDN

READER OBJECTIVES

After studying this chapter and reflecting on the contents, you should be able to:

1. List social and environmental factors that contribute to nutritional risk in communities, families, and individuals.

2. Describe the extent to which these factors affect various populations in the United States and how these factors impact nutritional status in families and individuals.

3. Describe information needed by nutritionists to assess and effectively respond to factors in communities, families, and individuals that increase nutritional risk.

4. Describe the community services available to provide food, nutrition education, financial assistance, and health insurance to at-risk populations in the United States.

■ DEFINING HIGH-RISK FACTORS

A high-risk factor is a biological, economic, environmental, or social insult that increases risk. Factors that place individuals, families, and communities at risk must be investigated and described in the community needs assessment. Social, economic, and environmental factors that contribute to nutritional risk include but are not limited to:

- Poverty
- Unemployment and underemployment
- Inadequate education and literacy
- Immigration and cultural background
- Substandard housing and homelessness
- Hunger and food insecurity
- Geographic or social isolation
- Limited or inadequate health care

These complex societal issues require the concerted attention of all those who are concerned about the nutritional health and well-being of community members. The immediate needs of families and individuals are a shared responsibility of the interdisciplinary teams and networks

that provide health and human services. Many clients and their families are known to multiple programs and agencies. Assessment and eligibility information should be shared among service providers, and services should be coordinated to ensure comprehensive, unduplicated efforts.

Poverty

Poverty income guidelines were first set in 1964, using the index developed by Mollie Orshansky of the Social Security Administration. Findings of the 1955 U.S. Department of Agriculture (USDA) National Food Consumption Study indicated that at that time the average American family spent approximately one-third of its net income for food. In the early 1960s, the USDA developed cost-specific, nutritionally balanced food plans and designated the Economy Food Plan as the least expensive food purchasing plan to meet a family's nutritional needs. Therefore, the poverty line was established at three times the cost of the Economy Food Plan for a family of four.

In 1975, the USDA replaced the Economy Food Plan with the similarly cost-defined Thrifty Food Plan, which became the national standard for a low-cost nutritious diet. Poverty

Portions of this chapter were reprinted or compiled with permission from the publisher of the *First Edition* of *Nutrition in Public Health* by M. Kaufman. New York: Aspen Publishers; 1990.

thresholds continue to be based on the 1963–1964 calculation of the Economy Food Plan for a specific household size multiplied by three, with adjustments for price changes only using the Consumer Price Index. These guidelines are used by federal agencies as criteria for eligibility for various federal assistance programs and as a basis for compiling data on poverty. **Table 4–1** shows the 2009 poverty income guidelines used by federal government agencies.[1]

Poverty guidelines are set annually by the U.S. government. Check http://www.nutrition.gov for current guidelines.

Unfortunately, the current poverty guidelines may no longer accurately measure poverty. Since the creation of the original poverty thresholds in the 1960s, the relative prices of the basic necessities of life for a family have changed considerably. Housing, transportation, childcare, and health care now comprise a larger proportion of a family's budget, while the relative cost of food has declined. It is estimated that today's families spend less than one-fifth of their incomes on food; therefore, a more appropriate poverty guideline would be more than five times the cost of the Thrifty Food Plan.[2]

In 2008, an estimated 13.2% of the U.S. population lived in poverty (39.8 million individuals), defined that year for a family of four, including two children under the age of 18, as having an annual income of less than $21,200. For African Americans, 24.7% lived in poverty, and 23.2% of Hispanic Americans lived in poverty. The poverty rate for Americans over the age of 65 was 9.7% (3.7 million individuals).[3]

A disproportionate number of children live in poverty. Children represent 25% of the total population but only 35% of the poor population. In 2006, 18% of all children lived in poor households (at or below 100% of the federal poverty level); 8% of all children lived in extreme poverty (at 50% of the federal poverty level). Child poverty rates are highest for African-American children (35%), American Indian and Alaskan-Native children (33%) and Hispanic-American children (27%). The most at-risk children are those living in single-parent–headed households. In 2007, 32% of single-parent– families with children had incomes below the poverty line, compared to 6% of married-couple families with children.[4]

Poverty is a clear predictor of health status. Premature death is more than twice as likely for middle-income Americans as for those at top of the income ladder, and more than three times as likely for those at the bottom than those at the top.[5]

Babies in households near or below the poverty line are at greater risk for infant mortality than babies born to more affluent families, and research shows that disparities in infant mortality based on household income have increased substantially since 1985.[6] Low-income children with chronic health conditions, such as asthma or diabetes, have worse overall health, spend more days in bed, and face more hospitalizations than do higher-income children with the same conditions.[7] One study reported that while only 2.6% of children of higher income were reported to have a fair or poor health status, 8.3% of low-income children were reported to have the same.[8]

The health disparities associated with poverty grow more apparent with age and persist through adulthood. More than 22% of individuals living under the poverty line report limitation of activity caused by chronic health conditions, whereas less than 9% of the non-poor (individuals at or greater than 200% of the poverty line) report the same.[9]

Assessing an individual's or family's income with the poverty guidelines can give initial critical information regarding the ability to meet immediate basic needs. Even if a family does not meet the definition of poverty, their housing and utility costs may use up the major portion of their income. Therefore, they are left with little or no money for food and other basic household essentials. To determine an individual's or family's ability to buy food, nutritionists must compare total net income with fixed costs for housing, utilities (heat, gas, electricity, water, telephone), medical care, transportation to and from work, and child care. This calculation will assist in identifying their needs for financial and food assistance, health care, and social service programs.

Unemployment and Underemployment

The economic downturn of the last few years has resulted in higher numbers of unemployed individuals, as well as

TABLE 4–1	2004 Poverty Guidelines for the 48 Contiguous States and the District of Columbia[a]
Size of Family Unit	**Poverty Guideline**
1	$ 9,310
2	$12,490
3	$15,670
4	$18,850
5	$22,030
6	$25,210
7	$28,390
8[b]	$31,570

[a]There are separate poverty guideline figures for Alaska and Hawaii that reflect the Office of Economic Opportunity administrative practice, which began in the 1966–1970 period.

[b]For family units with more than eight members, $3,180 is added for each additional member.

Source: Nord, M., Andrews, M., Carlson, S. *Household Food Security in the United States, 2002.* Washington, DC: Economic Research Service, U.S. Department of Agriculture; October 2003.

underemployed persons, who are working in jobs below their job training or work experience, part-time, or in low-paying jobs. The recession that began in December of 2007 has hit the labor market particularly hard. Increases in unemployment during 2008 were the largest fourth-quarter-to-fourth-quarter increase since 1982.[10]

The unemployment rate in the summer of 2009 was at 9.7%, accounting for 14.9 million Americans.[11] In 2006, 5.5 million children lived in households with no employed parent, a number that has surely grown since the beginning of the most recent recession.[12]

Although most policy and service planners focus on issues related to unemployment, underemployment is a hidden issue and rarely recognized. Individuals employed in low-paying jobs, particularly at minimum wage, do not earn a "living wage," which is sufficient earnings to provide for basic household needs. An individual earning the federal minimum wage of $7.25 per hour, working 40 hours a week, 52 weeks a year, will earn only $15,080 annually, about 68% of the 2009 poverty level for a family of four. In 2006, 56% of children in low-income families had at least one parent who worked full-time and year-round and 25% of children in low-income families had at least one parent who worked part-time, or full-time, part-year.[12]

With the rapid advances of technology in the United States, there are fewer blue-collar jobs (industrial or factory jobs with unskilled or skilled manual labor) than ever before. Recent years have experienced instability of high-tech jobs, resulting in workers who once thought they had secure jobs being laid off. Service jobs (maids, housecleaning, janitorial, maintenance, food service) continue to be low paying and very often inadequate to meet family household needs.

Assessment of the food intake of the unemployed and underemployed may show consistent inadequacy or an episode when the individual or family had little or no food and nutrient intake was poor. Surveys indicate that an initial consequence of unemployment is to cut back on the spending for food, as well as to postpone medical or dental treatment, as reported by half of survey respondents.[13]

It must be realized that the needs of the newly unemployed differ from the needs of those who have been unemployed for extended periods of time. For the newly unemployed, it is important to know if their income prior to unemployment was moderate, low, or below the poverty level; if their previous work had been continuous or sporadic; and if there is another wage earner in the household. First-time unemployed individuals and families working in low-paying jobs are less likely to know about available food and financial assistance programs and services, and may not be familiar with their eligibility and the application processes.

Inadequate Education and Literacy

According to 2008 U.S. Census data, 14% of adults in the United States have an 11th-grade education or less. This varies widely by ethnicity; 9% of Caucasians, 18% of African Americans, and 37% of Hispanic Americans have not graduated from high school.[14] Young people in the lowest quartile of income levels are more than five times as likely to drop out of school as their counterparts in the highest quartile of income.[15]

Twenty percent of American adults read at less than a fifth-grade level. It is estimated that nearly 50% of Americans do not have the literacy proficiency considered the minimum standard to be employable in today's labor market.[16] These adults generally have sufficient skills to cope with their usual daily activities but are not eligible for jobs that require reading and writing proficiency.

Most jobs require basic skills in reading, writing, and mathematics. Additionally, many require computer skills. As the educational requirements of jobs increase, people with less education do not qualify. In 2000, 31.4% of job applicants lacked the basic skills necessary to perform the jobs they sought.[17] Clearly, poor literacy is tightly linked to poverty. Among adults at the lowest level of literacy proficiency, 43% live in poverty. Among adults with strong literacy skills, only 4% live in poverty.[18]

For families in the cycle of inadequate education, unemployment, and poverty, improving the education of one or more family members can be the key to breaking the cycle.

Refugees and immigrants may have limited literacy in their own language, making learning to communicate in a new language even more difficult. They may learn to understand some English to meet basic needs for daily living before they learn to speak, read, and write this new language.

Low literacy affects the nutritional health of individuals and families by limiting access to the understanding of basic nutrition and health information, including food labels, medical or food preparation instructions (e.g., infant formula preparation), and dietary plans. Nutritionists should provide educational interventions and materials that consider the clients' ability to speak, read, write, and comprehend English. Many tools are available, including the SMOG Readability Formula and

The SMOG (Simplified Measure of Gobbledygoop Grading) Readability Formula is a method for determining the reading level of written materials. It is based on how many three-syllable words you use in your writing. See the Web site http://www.med.utah.edu/pated/authors/readability.html for more information.

the Fry Graph Reading Level Index, which can be utilized to evaluate written materials to determine the appropriateness of their reading level.

Programs presented to non-English-speaking populations must build on their cultural food preferences and customs. Written materials should use pictorial graphics to communicate nutrition messages. Pictures and text should be field tested with the target audience to assure that the materials are acceptable and easy to understand.

Data regarding educational attainment and language spoken is collected by many public health assistance programs. This information can be utilized to plan and to respond more effectively to the needs of the populations served.

In most cases, nutritionists will not be assessing an individual's literacy level. However, it should not be assumed that all clients are able to read either in English or in their native language. There are simple, informal methods to easily identify individuals with low literacy skills, without causing embarrassment to the client. Methods include asking open-ended questions about the materials received or handing written materials to clients upside down to observe if they turn it right side up to read. Nutritionists should also listen for comments commonly given to mask the inability to read, such as "I left my reading glasses at home" or "I'll read this later."

Cultural Barriers

During the past three decades, political, social, cultural, religious, and economic oppression in Central America, South America, the Caribbean Islands, Eastern Europe, Africa, and Southeast Asia has brought an influx of refugees into the United States. Nearly 1,170,000 individuals obtained legal resident status in the United States or entered the country as asylees or refugees in 2008.[19] It is estimated that almost 40% of those migrating to the United States between 2004 and 2005 entered the country illegally.[20] An estimated 11.5% of the U.S. population (approximately 32.5 million people) are now foreign-born.[21] New immigrants need guidance and support as they resettle in an adopted land.

Citizenship status affects family members' employability, income, and eligibility for tax-supported services. Immigrants and refugees—who are not naturalized citizens or legal residents—may have difficulty finding jobs with adequate pay or even finding work at all. They may hesitate to follow through on referrals to government assistance programs, because they fear deportation or future problems in obtaining citizenship.

Within each cultural group, patterns and practices of families and individuals differ according to their socioeconomic status, religion, education, and age when they immigrated to the United States. Immigrants face an unfamiliar choice of foods in large and impersonal supermarkets, more "high-tech" kitchen and other equipment, and high prices for their traditional foods. They frequently give up their

more nutrient-dense traditional foods in favor of U.S. snack foods and fast foods. Many choose to feed their babies formula instead of following traditions of breast-feeding.

Religion, tradition, beliefs, taboos, medical uses and philosophies, and the traditional roles of family members influence food habits. Nutritionists should be knowledgeable about common cultural food patterns and should complete an individual assessment to determine the core foods that are a regular part of a client's daily diet, considering the nutrient contributions and typical preparation of these foods. This knowledge should serve as the beginning point for nutrition education, suggesting more emphasis on familiar or similar foods before introducing new foods.

When working with undocumented clients, their fears and concerns must be respected. Professionals must know about program eligibility, make referrals on a case-by-case basis, and maintain the family's confidentiality.

Substandard Housing and Homelessness

The past few decades have brought dramatic rises in rents and housing costs, a decreased availability of newly built government-subsidized housing, and condominium conversion of sizeable amounts of rental property. The homeownership and mortgage crisis of 2008 forced many families into foreclosure, further burdening a system in which secure housing is either unavailable or unaffordable to families who must live on a fixed income, limited budget, or public assistance allowance.

The cost of renting a two-bedroom apartment rose 41% between 2000 and 2009. Roughly a third of American households live in rented housing; more than half of these do not earn enough to afford the average fair market rent for an appropriately sized home. On average, a renter earning the federal minimum wage must work 109 hours to afford a two-bedroom rental unit at the fair market rent.[22]

As housing costs rise beyond the means of low-income families and as affordable rental units are more difficult to obtain, many move in with friends and extended family. Families who are guests in someone else's household have little or no control over the kinds or quality of foods purchased or how foods are prepared.

Although they may have a roof over their heads, many low-income families live in substandard housing, lacking an adequate refrigerator, range, oven, or running water to prepare foods. Facilities to wash dishes, pots, and pans may be inadequate. There may be improper food storage or trash and garbage disposal, with rampant rodent and insect infestation. Older housing may have lead-containing paint that is peeling, cracked, or chipped. Lead poisoning can result in impaired growth, learning disabilities, and even mental retardation for infants and children if the peeling paint is ingested.

For some families the housing crisis has resulted in homelessness, which is a growing problem among women, children, and young families. Approximately 664,000 individuals in the United States are homeless on any given night; two-fifths of these individuals are part of a homeless family. Half of all the children in these families are age five or younger.[23] Recent estimates suggest that 1 in 50 children are homeless at some point during the course of a year.[24] Homeless children are 2.5 times more likely to have a health problem than housed children and more than 6 times as likely to have multiple health problems versus a single health problem.[25]

Many homeless families are housed temporarily in hotels, motels, or shelters, while some find themselves on the street. Often, mothers who live in shelters or on the streets feel guilty when they are not able to prepare adequate and nutritious meals for their children. Some shelters for the homeless serve meals or provide refrigerators and possibly hot plates. However, many of the hotels and motels do not provide refrigerators, hot plates, group kitchens, or any place to store food, and they may even prohibit the use of small appliances to cook food in the rooms. These hotel and shelter residents may need to choose between spending their few dollars on high-priced restaurants or ready-to-eat foods and not eating.

Nutritionists should assess the housing issues in their community and identify potential problems experienced by families or individuals that relate to food access. Nutritionists should be aware of the food storage and food preparation resources available to individuals and families living in hotels, motels, or shelters. Nutritionists must identify individuals potentially at-risk for nutrition deficiencies in the homeless population. They must advocate and assist in improving the availability of nutritious food for homeless individuals and families and those living in substandard housing. Nutrition education and food assistance should be responsive to the needs and resources of the individual or family.

Hunger and Food Insecurity

Food insecurity and hunger are persistent problems in our society. Food security is defined as the assured access at all times to enough food for an active, healthy life, as well as access to enough food that is safe, nutritious, and acquired in socially acceptable ways.[26] Hunger is an outcome of limited or uncertain access to food.

A 2007 survey by the United States Department of Agriculture found that more than 11% of participating households were food insecure at least some time during the year.

About one-third of food-insecure households had very low food security. This means that, at times during the year, the food intake of one or more adults in the household was reduced and their eating patterns were disrupted because of a lack of money and other resources for food. In 2007, food-secure households typically spent 35% more on food than food-insecure households of the same size and household composition. Just over half of all food-insecure households participated in one or more of the three largest Federal food and nutrition assistance programs during the month prior to the survey.[27]

A recent study found that food insecurity is linked to the ability of a family to pay for their household energy needs. Children and families who struggle to maintain heating and cooling costs were more likely to report food insecurity during those months with highest household energy needs.[28] Nutritionists can help families to achieve food security by assuring that all eligible families utilize the federally funded Supplemental Nutrition Assistance Program (SNAP; formerly known as the Food Stamp Program), Child Nutrition programs including the Special Supplemental Nutrition Program for Women, Infants and Children (WIC), and elderly meal programs in combination with local food banks, soup kitchens, and food pantries. The federal food assistance programs are described in **Table 4–2**. The Food Stamp and Child Nutrition programs are federally funded entitlement programs that are available in every community to serve all people who meet the income eligibility criteria. The Summer Food Service Program, School Breakfast, WIC, and Nutrition Services Incentive Program (formerly the Nutrition Program for the Elderly) are available when a service provider in a community establishes, implements, and directs the programs. Household income is used to determine eligibility for most of the federally funded food assistance programs.

Participation in one or more food assistance programs extends the family's food purchasing power to meet the nutritional needs of family members better. In assessing family needs, each household member's participation in or eligibility for food assistance programs must be determined. When their household incomes are very low, families may not be able to meet their food needs even when they participate in one or more federal food assistance programs. In these cases, families may turn to emergency food assistance programs such as food pantries and soup kitchens. The community needs assessment should include the number of requests to food pantries and visits to soup kitchens, particularly by families with children. Although these emergency food assistance programs provide food to satisfy immediate needs, they are not designed to provide food for extended periods of time.

Over the long term, increased utilization of the federal food programs could decrease the need for families to regularly use emergency food programs and reduce the growing

TABLE 4–2   **Food Assistance Programs**

Agency	Funding and Administration	Program Services and Benefits
Special Supplemental Nutrition Program for Women, Infants and Children (WIC)	USDA (some states offer supplemental funding); Administered by state health agencies; Services provided by state or local agencies	Provides supplemental food, nutrition education, referrals, and access to health care to low-income pregnant, postpartum, and breastfeeding women; infants; and children to 5 years of age at nutritional risk. Monthly foods include milk, cheese, eggs, fruit juice, cereal, peanut butter or legumes, tuna, carrots, infant formula, and infant cereal. Provides low-income households with coupons and electronic benefit transfer (EBT) cards to purchase eligible foods for a nutritionally adequate diet at authorized food stores.
Supplemental Nutrition Assistance Programs (SNAP)		
National School Lunch Program	USDA; Administered by state welfare, social services, or human service offices	Provides nutritious low-cost lunch at full or reduced prices, or free to children enrolled in school.
School Breakfast Program	USDA; Administered by state department of education and local school districts; Services provided by all public schools, voluntary in private schools	Provides nutritious low-cost breakfast at full or reduced prices, or free to children in participating schools or institutions.
Summer Food Service for Children	USDA; Administered by state department of education and local school districts; Services provided by all public schools, voluntary in private schools	Provides free nutritious meals and/or snacks to children as a substitute for the National School Lunch and School Breakfast programs during summer vacation.
Special Milk Program WIC Farmers Market Nutrition Program	USDA; Administered generally by state department of education, but state health or social service department or an FNS regional office may be designated. Services provided by public and nonprofit private schools, public—local, municipal, county, tribal, or state—government; nonprofit private organizations, public or private nonprofit camps	Provides milk to children in schools, summer camps, and child care institutions that have no federally supported meal program.
Senior Farmers Market Nutrition Program	USDA; Administered by the state department of education; Services provided by public or private child care institutions not participating in other federally supported meal programs	Provides coupons to WIC participants to purchase fresh, unprepared, locally grown fruits and vegetables at approved farmers and farmers' markets.
Child and Adult Care Food Program	USDA; Administered by state department of education; Services provided by public or nonprofit private childcare institutions not participating in other federally supported meal programs	Provides cash reimbursements and commodity foods for meals served in child and adult day care centers, and family and group day care homes, homeless shelters, and approved after-school care programs.
The Emergency Food Assistance Program (TEFAP)	USDA; Administered by state agencies; Services provided by food banks, food pantries, soup kitchens, and private nonprofit kitchens, and private nonprofit kitchens, and private nonprofit food to the needy through distribution of food for home use or the meal preparation	Adults who are functionally impaired and are enrolled in adult day care centers or who are 60 years of age or older. Provides commodity foods to low-income persons, including elderly people, food banks, food pantries, and soup kitchens.

TABLE 4–2	*(Continued)*

Agency	Funding and Administration	Program Services and Benefits
Food Distribution Program on Indian Reservations	USDA; Administered by state agencies such as state agriculture departments, health departments, or Indian tribal organizations; Services provided by Indian Tribal council or state agency	Provides commodity foods and nutrition education to low-income families who live on Indian reservations and to Native American families who live in approved areas near reservations. Serves as an alternate to the Supplemental Nutrition Assistance Program.
Nutrition Assistance Program: Puerto Rico, American Samoa, and the Commonwealth of the Northern Marianas Islands Nutrition Services Incentive Program (Nutrition Program for the Elderly)	USDA and DHHS; Administration on Aging (AoA); private donations; Administered by state Units on Aging funded through Title III of the Older American Act (OAA); Indian tribal organizations Funded through Title VI of OAA. Services provided by senior centers, faith-based settings, schools, homes of homebound older adults	Block grant program to provide cash and coupons to participants to buy nutritious foods in place of food stamps and commodities. Provides meals for senior citizens at senior citizen centers or delivered by meals-on-wheels programs through the receipt of cash and/or commodities from USDA; nutrition screening and assessment; nutrition education; links to other in-home and community-based services, transportation, and home repair programs.
Head Start, Early Head Start	DHHS–Administration for Children and Families; Administered by DHHS regional offices; Services provided by local public agencies, private nonprofit and for-profit organizations, Indian Tribes, and school systems	Provides comprehensive medical, educational, nutrition, social, and dental services, referrals to social services, and other services to low-income children from birth to age 5, pregnant women and their families through assessment, early intervention, and prevention; provides nutritious meals and snacks.

Agency	Who Benefits
Special Supplemental Nutrition Program for Women, Infants and Children (WIC)	Pregnant women, postpartum women (6 months), breast-feeding women (up to 1 year), infants, and children (up to 5 years); must be certified to be at nutritional risk; house-hold income determined to be at or below 185% of poverty level.
Supplemental Nutrition Assistance Programs	U.S. citizen; limited benefits to legal immigrants and to able-bodied adults without dependents; eligibility and allotments are based on household size, income, assets, and other factors.
National School Lunch Program	All children attending school may participate: free meals to children from families with incomes at or below 130% of poverty level; reduced-price meals to children from families with incomes between 131% and 185% of poverty level; full price meals to children from families with incomes over 185% of poverty.
School Breakfast Program	Children under 18 years who come to an approved site; persons over 18 years who are enrolled in school program for persons with disabilities.
Summer Food Service for Children	Children attending schools or half-day pre-kindergarten programs and institutions with special milk program; milk is free to child from family eligible for free meals.
Special Milk Program WIC Farmers Market Nutrition Program	Women, infants (over 4 months), and children who have been certified to receive WIC program benefits or who are on a waiting list for WIC certification. States may serve some or all of these categories.
Child and Adult Care Food Program	Children 12 years and under and adults who attend eligible day care programs; children of migrant workers 15 years and younger; physically/mentally handicapped individuals provided care in a center where the majority are age 18 or younger; children residing in homeless shelters; snacks and suppers to youths participating in eligible after-school care program; income eligible for free or reduced-priced meals.
The Emergency Food Assistance Program (TEFAP)	Each state sets criteria for household eligibility; households may participate in another federal, state, or local food health or welfare program for which eligibility is based on income; homeless, including low-income seniors, can receive meal in congregate setting. There are no eligibility criteria for using a soup kitchen.
Food Distribution Program on Indian Reservations	Low-income households, including American Indian and non-Indian, living on a reservation or households who live in approved areas near reservations or in Oklahoma with at least one person who is a member of a federally recognized tribe. Must meet income and resource eligibility standards. Food package selected from over 70 food products. Cannot participate in the Supplemental Nutrition Assistance Program in the same month.
Nutrition Assistance Program: Puerto Rico, American Samoa, and the Commonwealth of the Northern Marianas Islands Nutrition Services Incentive Program (Nutrition Program for the Elderly)	People age 60 or older with greatest economic or social need, with special attention given to low-income minorities and rural older people; spouses of eligible people; disabled persons under age 60 who reside in housing facilities occupied primarily by the elderly where congregate meals are served, disabled persons who reside at home and accompany older persons to meals; nutrition service volunteers.
Head Start, Early Head Start	Children birth to 5 years, pregnant women and their families from low-income families receiving public assistance (TANF—Temporary Assistance for Needy Families or SSI—Supplemental Security Income) or total annual income not more than 100% of poverty level; children in foster care; at least 10% of total enrollment available for handicapped children.

burden on private food assistance programs. In addition, increased utilization could improve the stability of meeting basic food and nutritional needs of communities, families, and individuals. Many families still do not know about these programs or have inaccurate or insufficient information regarding their eligibility requirements. Complicated application forms and procedures, excessive eligibility documentation, and/or inconsistent administrative operations deter many families from applying for food assistance. Nutritionists must know eligibility requirements and be aware of administrative barriers so that they can assist potentially eligible clients in applying for benefits and navigating the food assistance system. Nutritionists should also advocate, both locally and nationally, for measures that make it easier for individuals and families to use these services.

Some families believe that there is a stigma attached to the use of food assistance programs. The negative perceptions and attitudes associated with these programs may foster shame and embarrassment, and prevent families in need from applying for food assistance. Nutritionists should be sensitive to these feelings so that they can support clients and break down negative stereotypes attributed to people using food assistance programs.

Geographic and Social Isolation

Chapter 17 discusses food insecurity in the United States in more depth.

Families who live in remote areas, distanced from settled communities or blocked from social support systems, are considered isolated. A family who does not have transportation, or the money to pay for it, may not be able to obtain adequate food at affordable prices or be able to access and/or utilize food assistance or healthcare programs. The geographically isolated include migrant and seasonal farm workers, mountain families, the rural poor, Native Americans on reservations, and homeless, displaced families without access to public transportation, even in urban areas.

Social isolation occurs when individuals or families are unable to establish supportive relationships with others. Social isolation is more subtle and difficult to recognize, as well as to overcome, than geographic isolation. Socially isolated individuals have difficulty establishing or maintaining supportive interpersonal relationships, within either their community or their family. This may occur when people move to new communities or when their cultural or ethnic background and/or their primary language differs from that of the community. Individuals and families experiencing homelessness, unemployment, marriage dissolution, mental illness, emotional breakdowns, or depression often distance themselves from their friends and family. Drug use, alcoholism, violence, and abuse dramatically change family dynamics and communication, often resulting in unstable families.

Social isolation may prevent an individual from seeking health care, food, financial or housing assistance, or other services they need. Social isolation has been identified as a contributor to inadequate food consumption for the elderly. Fewer calories are consumed at meals when eating alone than when eating with others.[29] In addition, an individual who lacks social support may find it difficult to continue ongoing health care or follow through on care plan recommendations. It may be difficult for individuals and families to access services when one family member or community decision-maker, often referred to as the "gatekeeper," controls the use of assistance programs.

Single and/or teen parents are often overwhelmed by parenting responsibilities, limited employment opportunities, low incomes, and lack of transportation, child care, and family support. Parents caring for a handicapped or chronically ill child, or adults caring for a disabled or homebound spouse or parent, are also stressed emotionally, physically, and often financially. As such, these individuals may be socially isolated and less likely to seek services. In addition, they may be unable to cope with buying and preparing nutritious meals for themselves and their children.

Nutritionists should not expect to be able to address single-handedly or resolve the social issues of isolation that may affect their clients. Nutritionists must identify the immediate needs of the individual or family and be sensitive and supportive in their response. The community needs assessment must identify other health and social services available in their community so that nutritionists can make appropriate and timely referrals. Additionally, nutritionists must recognize an individual's or family's ability to navigate service delivery systems to receive needed services and provide assistance as considered necessary. Most importantly, nutritionists must work with other members of the health and human service agency teams to address the multiple and often long-standing problems faced by many families and advocate, both locally and nationally, for solutions.

Limited or Inadequate Health Care

Regular medical care helps individuals avoid health crises and ultimately protects their nutritional status. Although it is well established that early and ongoing prenatal care is associated with positive pregnancy outcome, many pregnant women do not seek adequate prenatal care. In addition, some children and adults go

Medicaid: A U.S. government program that pays for medical assistance for certain individuals and families with low incomes. Learn more at: http://www.cms.gov/medicaid/

Medicare: A U.S. government medical benefit program for certain individuals when they reach age 65. Learn more at: http://www.medicare.gov

without needed treatment as well as ongoing preventive care. This is most often a result of no insurance, not enough money to pay physicians or hospitals, or providers not willing or unable to provide free care or accept Medicaid or Medicare payments that are less than their usual fees.

Multi-state Pregnancy Risk Assessment Monitoring System (PRAMS) data, evaluating maternal behavior trends, indicate that only 75% of women reported receiving early and adequate prenatal care. Racial and socioeconomic disparities exist in the realm of prenatal care; Hispanic and black women were more likely than non-Hispanic white women to report late entry to or inadequate frequency of care during their pregnancies.[30]

It is estimated that one in nine children in the United States lacked health insurance in 2007. Sixty percent of these children came from low-income families. Millions of children remain without health coverage due to rising health insurance premiums, declines in number of parents working for smaller employers that are offered insurance and dramatic increases in unemployment. While more than half of uninsured children are likely eligible for Medicaid or the State Children's Health Insurance Program (CHIP), their parents are sometimes unaware of the programs and may think that their children are ineligible or they cycle on and off public coverage due to fluctuations in family income.[31]

Nutritionists should know the availability of medical care services in the community and the barriers low-income families face in accessing these services. They need to work with health providers and community members to support regular medical care, including nutrition services, and ensure that it is accessible and responsive to the needs of at-risk families. It is essential to advocate for nutrition intervention, referral, and follow-up to be integrated into medical services.

■ IMPROVING SERVICES TO AT-RISK FAMILIES

A thorough and comprehensive community needs assessment is key in providing targeted nutrition services that will support and respond to the needs of at-risk individuals and families, as was discussed in Chapter 3. **Table 4–3** presents key factors to include in the assessment. This information documents needs and suggests priorities for developing community services and determining family and individual care plans. Identification of nutrition-related risk factors can be used to plan professional in-service training, mobilize resources, develop and implement health and nutrition programs, and ensure policies that respond to the nutritional needs of at-risk individuals and families and community nutrition efforts.

Action to improve services to at-risk families should be well integrated into the healthcare and nutrition service delivery system. Ideas to consider include:

- Recruit health or nutrition aides, lay health advisors, peer counselors, or volunteers that represent the populations and cultural groups in the community and train them to provide services to at-risk families.
- Coordinate one-stop service delivery by arranging with food and nutrition services, public assistance, and social services agencies to enroll eligible clients in health and social services.
- Address specific barriers that prevent eligible individuals/families from participating in assistance programs and design outreach strategies and methods to overcome these barriers.
- Streamline application processes of all programs targeting at-risk populations and utilize electronic data systems to eliminate duplication in data collection, including eligibility determination criteria.
- Schedule clinic hours so families do not need to take time off from work and lose pay to obtain services; offer locations that are accessible to clients with limited/no transportation.
- Enlist volunteer groups or clubs to adopt a service project to provide layettes, clothing, diapers, nutritious foods, or other essentials for at-risk families.
- Apply for grants to research and provide innovative services that help at-risk families work toward self-sufficiency.

Concerned health professionals, in conjunction with political leaders and concerned citizens, can collaborate with and mobilize community partners to provide integrated, comprehensive, and coordinated services to at-risk clients and families. They can participate in policy development and plans to increase awareness of problems; identify short- and long-term goals; allocate resources; and define, implement, and assess strategies to address the many complex economic and social issues that today's families face. Community coalitions can recommend and advocate for state and federal legislation that will address universal food access, housing, job training, health care, and employment.

Community needs assessment data can be presented in public meetings, legislative hearings, or other forums. An ongoing surveillance system can be used to monitor hunger, nutrition risk, diet-related health problems, and utilization of food assistance programs. Grant funding can be sought to implement outreach and nutrition education projects and to improve access to and use of various food assistance programs.

The nutritionist has a vital and critical role in effectively reaching out to those at highest risk, monitoring those at-risk, and must take a leadership and advocacy role to promote, implement, and evaluate effective services to meet the needs of at-risk populations.

TABLE 4–3   Assessing At-Risk Factors in the Community, Families, and Individuals

At-Risk Factor	Community Assessment	Family/Household Assessment	Individual Assessment
Income	Median family income; per capita income; % of population below 100% poverty level; % of population below 200% of poverty level; TANF benefit levels; availability of community-based assistance programs for food, childcare, fuel, etc., housing and basic household costs (utilities, health care, etc.)	Family/household income; family size; Number of wage earners; participation in federal/state nutrition programs; income supplements such as TANF, unemployment benefits, fuel assistance; educational expenses; childcare costs; housing and basic household costs	Individual's monthly income; lives alone or with others; household expenses, child support; participates in federal/state food assistance; income supplement such as TANF, unemployment benefits, fuel assistance; educational expenses; child care; single parent; homebound, disabled; elderly
Employment	State or local unemployment rate; median wage; predominance of minimum-wage, service-sector jobs; layoff or strike in community; jobs available; seasonal jobs (e.g., agriculture, construction, tourism)	Household member laid off or on strike	Individual unable to find work at a wage that meets basic needs; recently laid off or on strike; barriers that prevent individual from finding adequate employment (lack of child care, job opportunities)
Educational level Literacy	% of adults over age 18 that did not graduate high school; % of adults over age 18 who are low literacy proficiency; % of teen high school dropouts (by race)	Education level of head of household and mother; education obtained in country of origin	Education level; education obtained in country of origin; ability to read, speak, write English; if school age, grade level
Culture or language	Ethnic/cultural distribution in community; languages spoken, read, and/or written; availability of services representing the ethnic community; signs and information in appropriate languages; availability of traditional foods; prevailing community attitude	Ability of head of household to speak, read, write English; ability to read/write native language; use of traditional foods; use of traditional medicine; power structure in family; degree of acculturation	Ability to speak, read, write English; ability to read/write native language; use of traditional foods; use of traditional medicine
Housing	Rental unit vacancy rate; % of substandard housing; % of rental units built before 1950 (risk of lead paint); availability of subsidized housing and length of waiting list; average and range of rents for 1-2-3 bedroom units; median purchase price for a house; condo conversion in community; estimated number of homeless individuals and families	Family lives in substandard housing; problems with rodent, roaches, chipping or peeling paint or plaster; family living in a hotel, motel, shelter, car or on the street; recently moved in with friends or relatives due to the inability to obtain adequate housing; % of the family-household income spent on rent and utilities	Individual lives in substandard housing; living in hotel, motel, shelter, car or on the street; lives in room without cooking facilities or without working refrigerator or stove; % income spent on rent/utilities; inability to pay rent; evicted for nonpayment of rent
Food availability, food costs, accessibility of grocery stores	Supermarkets/grocery stores in the neighborhood offer a variety of nutritious, good-quality foods at competitive prices; Number of 'mom and pop' neighborhood markets; availability of culturally preferred foods at a reasonable price; accessible by public transportation or within walking distance; food delivery or shopping services available; availability of Farmers' Markets; average cost of full market basket of food	Family access to transportation to available grocery stores; cultural foods available at reasonable price	Individual's food needs met by himself/herself or other household members; elderly or disabled individual able to arrange for assistance with shopping for food

TABLE 4–3	(Continued)

At-Risk Factor	Community Assessment	Family/Household Assessment	Individual Assessment
Geographic or social isolation	Public transportation available; dispersed rural community; geographic barriers; condition of roads; cultural, ethnic, rural hostilities; immigrant, refugee, or migrant community; highly transient community	Supportive relationships; transportation or money for transportation; cultural or language barrier; victim of cultural, ethnic, racial prejudice; immigrant refugee, migrant family; mobile family; homeless family; family stress, unstable family, alcoholism, drug abuse, domestic abuse, violence	Single parent; teen parent; homebound living alone; physical or mental disability; lack of supportive relationships; lack of transportation or money for transportation; victim of cultural, ethnic, racial prejudice; immigrant, refugee, migrant; mobile; alcoholic, drug abuser
Access to health services	Public health, health centers, and medical practices available (e.g., obstetrics, pediatrics, family practice); sliding fee scale; number of persons receiving and eligible for Medicare and Medicaid; services near public transportation; % of no-show in a clinic or health program; preventive programs offered at no cost or reasonable cost; Medicaid payments accepted	Satisfaction of family with health services available; family members go without needed care	Satisfaction of individual with health services available; perceived barriers to utilization of services; repeatedly misses scheduled appointments
Health insurance coverage	Health insurance coverage provided by employers includes maternity care; Medicaid available to low-income married couples; coverage for prenatal care for low-income teens living with parents; % of jobs with no health insurance benefits; sliding fee scale or free health care available; Medicaid payment accepted by community physicians	Household members covered by health insurance, HMO, or Medicaid coverage; uninsured families have access to sliding fee scale or free health care; Medicaid unavailable because teen lives in parents' household; family's insurance covers preventive care, well-child care	Individual has health insurance, HMO, Medicaid coverage; types of services covered, amount of deductible; denial of health care due to lack of medical coverage or Medicaid
Health status	Infant mortality rate; hospital discharge data; leading causes of death and disability; nutritional status and nutrition-related health measurements—% of population by age groups with anemia, high serum cholesterol levels, overweight/obesity, high lead levels, cardiovascular disease, cancer, diabetes, stroke, hypertension; smoking rates; breastfeeding rates	Nutrient content of diet; knowledge, attitude and behavior related to healthy behaviors (i.e., breastfeeding, physical activity, fat intake, fruit/vegetable intake); family history of nutrition-related health conditions (cardiovascular disease, cancer, diabetes, stroke, hypertension); smoking in household	Nutrient content of diet—intake of key nutrients (calcium, iron, vitamin C, folate, etc.) and intake of fat, sugar, and salt; intake of fruits, vegetables, and whole grains; knowledge, attitude and behavior related to healthy behaviors (i.e., breastfeeding, physical activity, fat intake, fruit/vegetable intake); health parameters—weight, hemoglobin/hematocrit, cholesterol level, blood glucose, blood pressure, dental health; tobacco/alcohol/drug use

Issues for Discussion

1. Discuss the impact of cuts to federal assistance programs for those at highest risk.

2. Discuss how the different food and nutrition assistance programs can be resources for individuals across the lifespan

3. Discuss the pros and cons of one or more federal nutrition programs.

4. Discuss how you would assess the nutritional risk of a community based on the at-risk factors reviewed in this chapter.

References

1. United States Department of Health and Human Services. *Frequently Asked Questions Related to the Poverty Guidelines and Poverty.* Available at http://aspe.hhs.gov/poverty/faq.shtml#thrifty. Accessed March 24, 2010.

2. Economic Policy Institute. *EPI Issue Guide: Poverty and Family Budgets Issue Guide.* Washington, D.C.: Economic Policy Institute; 2004.

3. *Income, Poverty and Health Insurance Coverage in the United States: 2008.* Washington, DC: U.S. Census Bureau, U.S. Department of Commerce; September 2009.

4. Annie E. Casey Foundation. *Kids Count Data Book: State Profiles of Child Well-Being.* Baltimore, MD: Annie E. Casey Foundation; 2009.

5. Adler N, Stewart J. Reaching for a Healthier Life; Facts on Socioeconomic Status and Health in the U.S., 2007. The John D. and Catherine T. MacArthur Foundation Research Network on Socioeconomic Status and Health. Available at http://www.macfound.org/site/c.lkLXJ8MQKrH/b.3599935/k.66CA/MacArthur_Foundation_Home.htm. Accessed April 2, 2010.

6. Annie E. Casey Foundation. *Kids Count Indicator Brief: Reducing Infant Mortality.* Baltimore, MD: Annie E. Casey Foundation; 2009.

7. Case A, Lubotsky D, Paxson C. Economic status and health in childhood. *Poverty Res News.* 2001;55:3–5.

8. Finegold K, Wherry L. *Race, Ethnicity and Health. Snapshots of America's Families III,* No. 20. *Urban Institute,* March 2004.

9. *Chartbook on Trends in the Health of Americans. Health, U.S., 2008.* Washington, DC: National Center for Health Statistics; 2008.

10. Borbely JM. U.S. labor market in 2008: economy in recession. *Monthly Labor Rev.* March 2009.

11. *The Employment Situation—August 2009.* Washington, DC: Bureau of Labor Statistics, U.S. Department of Labor; September 2009.

12. National Center for Children in Poverty. *Most Low-Income Parents Are Employed.* New York: November 2007.

13. Shapiro I. *Unmet Need Hits Record Level for the Unemployed.* Washington, DC: Center on Budget and Policy Priorities; February 2004.

14. U.S. Census Bureau. Current Population Survey, *2008 Annual Social and Economic Supplement.* Washington, DC: U.S. Census Bureau; April 2009.

15. U.S. Census Bureau. *Educational Attainment in the U.S.: Detailed Tables.* Washington, DC: U.S. Census Bureau; March 2002.

16. Sum A, Kirsch I, Taggart R. *The Twin Challenges of Mediocrity and Inequality: Literacy in the U.S. from an International Perspective.* Princeton, NJ: Policy Information Service, Educational Testing Service; February 2002.

17. American Management Association. *Research Survey: Corporate Concerns 2001.* New York: American Management Association; 2001.

18. Reder S. *The State of Literacy in America.* Washington, DC: U.S. Department of Education; 1998:5.

19. Office of Immigration Statistics. *2008 Yearbook of Immigration Statistics.* Washington, DC: U.S. Department of Homeland Security; 2008.

20. Office of Immigration Statistics. *Estimates of the Unauthorized Immigrant Population Residing in the United States: January 2009.* Washington, DC: U.S. Department of Homeland Security; August 2009.

21. *Foreign-Born Population in the U.S.: March 2002.* Washington, DC: U.S. Department of Commerce, Economics and Statistics Administration, U.S. Census Bureau; February 2003.

22. Wardrip K, Pelletiere D, Crowley S. *Out of Reach 2009: Persistent Problems, New Challenges for Renters.* Washington, DC: National Low-Income Housing Coalition; April 2009.

23. *The 2008 Annual Homeless Assessment Report.* Washington, DC: U.S. Department of Housing and Urban Development, Office of Community Planning and Development; July 2009.

24. *America's Youngest Outcasts: State Report Card on Child Homelessness.* Newton, MA: National Center on Family Homelessness; 2009.

25. Berti LC, Zylbert S, Rolnitzky L. Comparison of health status of children using a school-based health center for comprehensive care. *J Pediatr Health Care.* 2001;15:244–250.

26. *Paradox of Hunger and Obesity in America.* Waltham, MA: Center on Hunger and Poverty and the Food Research and Action Center; July 2003.

27. Nord M, Andrews M, Carlson S. Household Food Security in the United States, 2007. Washington, DC: Economic Research Service, U.S. Department of Agriculture; October 2008.

28. Cook J, Frank D, Casey P, et al. A brief indicator of household energy security: associations with food security, child health and child development in US infants and toddlers. *Pediatrics.* 2008;122:e867–e875.

29. *Hunger Issue Brief, Hunger and Food Insecurity among the Elderly.* Food Security Institute, Center on Hunger and Poverty, Brandeis University; February 2003.

30. Williams L, Morrow B, Shulman H, Stephens R, D'Angelo D, Fowler CI. *PRAMS 2002 Surveillance Report.* Atlanta, GA: Division of Reproductive Health, National Center for Chronic Disease Prevention and Health Promotion, Centers for Disease Control and Prevention; 2006.

31. *Left Behind: America's Uninsured Children.* Washington, DC: Families USA Foundation; 2008.

Addressing Overweight in Children: A Public Health Perspective

Inger Stallmann-Jorgensen, MS, RD, LD
Edna Harris-Davis, MS, MPH, RD, LD

READER OBJECTIVES

After studying this chapter and reflecting on the contents, you should be able to:

1. List the growing problems related to overweight in children.
2. Describe the paradigm shift that occurred over the years to cause overweight in children.
3. Describe economic impacts of overweight in children on society.
4. Identify essential skills or tools that a public health nutritionist may need to help prevent or control overweight in children.
5. Describe the importance of recommendations and policy and environmental interventions.
6. Describe opportunities for public health nutritionists to address overweight in children in existing programs.
7. List three evidence-based practices to prevent or control overweight in children.
8. List some steps that families can take to help prevent overweight in children.
9. List prevention strategies that could be incorporated into existing federal programs.

■ INTRODUCTION

Obesity and obesity-related diseases are some of the biggest public health challenges of the 21st century. The rapidly increasing rate of overweight in children is especially alarming. Historically, public health has been in disarray because the medical treatment model has dominated the healthcare system and failed to provide a proactive stance to support a prevention-based model.[1] The addage that "an ounce of prevention is worth a pound of cure" needs to be taken more seriously by the food and advertising industries, community planners, school systems, businesses, public health leaders, policymakers, the health industry, and other stakeholders. Ultimately, the cry for partnerships and resources to prevent overweight and obesity will be heard because of the unparalleled rise in U.S. medical and healthcare costs for treatment of obesity and related conditions. Now is the time for public health nutritionists to accept the urgent challenge of addressing overweight and obesity through prevention-based approaches. To maximize effectiveness, overweight and obesity prevention efforts must target children and their families and focus on policy and environmental interventions.

The topic of overweight in children is a large and complex issue, and it is not possible to address every aspect of the problem and its prevention and treatment in this chapter. Rather, the aim of this chapter is to provide an overview of overweight in children and to guide the public health nutrition student and entry-level practitioner in addressing this challenging public health issue. The authors review various aspects of the problem of overweight in children and obesity, such as the health consequences, economic impact, environmental factors, and nutrition and physical activity issues. We hope that the reader will acknowledge the changes in the environment that contribute to the development of the current epidemic of overweight in children. Due to the important role of environmental interventions, we also hope that you will realize that one-on-one interventions alone will not arrest this epidemic. Rather, population-based interventions will be needed to achieve the greatest effect. We also discuss skills important to public health nutritionists, such as developing partnerships, writing grants, using media resources, and keeping current with the scientific literature. In addition, overweight in children will be addressed using a prevention-based approach by applying the public health model (assessment, policy development, and assurance) and evidence-based efforts (increase physical activity and healthy eating, and decrease television viewing). Finally, one community's experience in addressing overweight in children will be discussed.

The magnitude of the current problem of overweight in children is unprecedented; public health nutrition professionals have limited past experience with community-based interventions to address this issue comprehensively. In fact, effective strategies are few compared to the enormity of the challenge. New approaches must be conceived, tested, and applied without delay. Careful analysis of surveillance data, sound research, community resources, and priorities must be considered when problem-solving and producing effective interventions. Advocacy and education will be crucial to sound the alarm for community stakeholders and gain their support. The authors hope that public health nutritionists become empowered with the information presented and will apply this information to develop, implement, and evaluate innovative prevention-based approaches for overweight in children.

■ ASSESSMENT OF OVERWEIGHT IN CHILDREN

In the pediatric population, the body mass index (BMI) is used as a screening tool and is not a diagnosis for overweight in children. The Centers for Disease Control and Prevention (CDC) have revised and published growth charts for children 2 to 20 years of age in 2000: BMI-for-Age, Weight-for-Age, and Stature-for-Age. The BMI-for-Age nutrition status indicators for children classified as Overweight are ≥ 85th percentile to < 95th percentile and for Obese in the ≥ 95th percentile.[2] Study results have found that many overweight children will become obese adults.[3,4] However, the BMI-for-Age assessment should be applied carefully so as not to label children as overweight or obese in error. It is important to determine whether a child indeed has extra fat mass and not extra muscle mass, particularly across genders and ethnicity.[5,6]

The terms *at-risk for overweight* and *overweight* were the classification terms previously used by the CDC; *at-risk for obesity* and *obese* are terms used in the childhood overweight literature. The use of different terms may have contributed to some difficulty in interpreting and comparing data from different studies and countries. The term *at-risk*

for overweight was sometimes erroneously understood to mean that the child was at risk for becoming overweight/obese in the future, when it actually referred to a child who might be obese in regard to having excess body fat, but who should undergo a second-level screen for a more in-depth assessment.[7] However, the authors recognize the widespread past and current use of the four terms—at-risk for overweight, overweight, obese, and obesity—throughout the issue of overweight in children's literature, and that sometimes the two sets of terms are synonymous and at other times they have different meanings. Both sets of terms will be used throughout the chapter and when citing other literature to reflect the meaning intended by the original author.

■ OVERWEIGHT IN CHILDREN FROM A PUBLIC HEALTH PERSPECTIVE

Overweight Rates in the United States

There has been a rapid increase in our nation's rates of obesity in adults over the past two decades. The United States is not alone in facing this serious public health problem. Obesity has been declared one of the top ten risk conditions in the world and one of the top five in the developed world by the World Health Organization (WHO). Recent data from the 2003–2004 National Health and Nutrition Examination Survey (NHANES) found 66.3% of the U.S. adult population over 20 years of age to be overweight, as defined by a BMI of greater than 25 kg/m^2.[8] This is an 18% increase from an already high prevalence of overweight of 56% shown by NHANES III data collected during the period 1988–1994. Of perhaps greater concern is the steeper increase in the prevalence of obesity (BMI ≥30 kg/m^2), which was more than 40%.

The trend of overweight in children has increased to an even greater degree. Between NHANES I (1971–1974) and NHANES II (1976–1980) the prevalence of overweight in children was unchanged overall; however, between NHANES II and NHANES III (1988–1994), the prevalence rose within all age and gender groups. A comparison between NHANES III and the NHANES 1999–2000 data shows these trends continuing their upward trajectory for all groups, except boys aged 6 to 23 months, who showed a 0.1% (nonsignificant) decrease in prevalence. These data thus show overweight rates for 6- to 23-month-old children to be 11.6%, and for 2- to 5-year-old, 6- to 11-year-old, and 12- to 19-year-old children to be 10.4%, 15.3%, and 15.5%, respectively. These data represent increases in prevalence rates of 30%, 44%, 35%, and 48% for these respective age groups, occurring in less than two decades (see **Figure 5–1**). NHANES data from 1999 to 2004 indicated that overweight prevalence among U.S. children and adolescents continued the upward trend with the 2003 to 2004 rate at

17.1%.[9] Combining data from the four NHANES time periods (1999–2000, 2001–2002, 2003–2004, and 2005–2006), however, did not show statistically significant trends for either boys or girls. Because the time periods 2003–2004 and 2005–2006 showed no significant differences, these two datasets were combined for population estimates based on a greater sample size and four years of data, which provided a more stable measure of high-BMI for age by age, sex, and race/ethnicity. For the years 2003–2006, 11.3% of children and adolescents ages 2 to 19 were at or above the 97th percentile of BMI for age from the 2000 CDC growth charts. For the same period, 16.3% had a BMI for age at or above the 95th percentile of BMI for age, and 31.9% were at or above the 85th percentile.[10]

The increases in overweight status have not occurred to the same extent among all age groups; neither are the various ethnic groups affected equally. Most affected by the rising trend in rates of obesity are Mexican-American boys ages 6–11 and 12–19, followed by non-Hispanic African-American girls ages 6–11 and 12–19. For these groups, about one in four youths has a BMI ≥ 95th percentile. Among those with a BMI above or equal to the 85th percentile for age and sex, non-Hispanic African-American girls, ages 12–19, lead the epidemic of obesity with a rate of 44.5%; nearly half of these adolescents weigh too much.[11]

Health Effects of Overweight

The recent trends of overweight in children are especially disturbing because of the predicted health consequences later in life of overweight status beginning in childhood. Freedman et al.[12] studied the longitudinal relationship between children's BMI and their adult levels of lipids, insulin, and blood pressure. The mean time interval between first and follow-up measurements was 17 years. Over this time period, 77% of overweight children remained overweight as adults.[12] The persistence of being overweight, once it occurs, is of great concern because being overweight is more strongly linked to chronic disease than living in poverty,

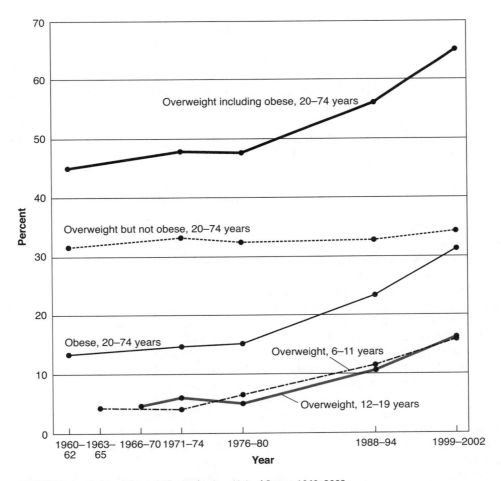

FIGURE 5-1   Overweight and Obesity by Age: United States, 1960–2002
Sources: Centers for Disease Control and Prevention, National Center for Health Statistics, National Health Examination Survey and National Health and Nutrition Examination Survey, Figure 16.

smoking, or drinking. The impact of obesity on overall health has been likened to aging by 20 years[13]: "...childhood obesity precedes insulin resistance/hyperinsulinemia and strongly predicts the risk of developing a constellation of metabolic, hemodynamic, thrombotic, and inflammatory disorders of syndrome X."[14]

Although there is well-justified concern for overweight in children tracking into adulthood and increasing the risk of adult health problems, one must not ignore the acute physical and psychological health issues that affect the overweight child. Many body functions are affected by being overweight, including the nervous, pulmonary, cardiovascular, skeletal, gastrointestinal, endocrine, and reproductive systems. In addition, overweight children suffer from mental health problems such as depression, anxiety, lowered self-esteem, and sometimes eating disorders.[15–17]

Pediatricians are diagnosing the most obese children and adolescents with hypertension, dyslipidemia, and non-insulin-dependent diabetes mellitus (NIDDM). Even if the overweight status does not track into adulthood, there may be long-lasting medical and psychosocial effects for overweight children.[18]

Health Disparities

Ethnic, cultural, gender, genetic, socioeconomic, and regional differences exist that influence which children are at greater risk for being overweight. Hispanic-American boys, African Americans, and those residing in the South are especially likely to experience higher rates of being overweight.[19,20] The ethnic differences in the degree to which certain population groups are affected by overweight prevalence may exacerbate long-term health outcomes and economic disparities that already exist in the United States.[20]

Economic Effects of Overweight

If the trend of overweight in children continues on its present course, the United States will be overwhelmed by the healthcare expenditures required to treat acute and long-term complications of this condition. Hospital costs related to overweight in children have increased from an annual cost of $35 million in 1979–1981 to the latest data (1997–1999) from the CDC of $127 million dollars.[21] A cost estimate from 2003 data suggests that each U.S. taxpayer pays $175 a year for obesity-related illnesses (heart disease, cancer, diabetes, gallbladder disease) via Medicare and Medicaid programs.[22] Hospital discharges for youths, ages 6 to 17, have doubled from 1.43% to 2.36% for obesity-related conditions such as diabetes, while obesity and gall bladder disease tripled from 0.36% to 1.07% and from 0.18% to 0.59%, respectively, within two decades (1979–1999). When diagnoses such as asthma and certain mental disorders are listed as the primary discharge diagnosis, it is common to see overweight or obesity listed as a secondary diagnosis.[21] The choice of primary discharge diagnosis may be influenced by which diagnosis will result in higher hospital reimbursements for healthcare services. Such tactics could contribute to an underestimate of the weight-related causes for hospitalization, as healthcare institutions may seek to maximize reimbursements for care.

The 2000 Actual Causes of Death report from the CDC found the leading cause of death to be tobacco use, at 435,000 annual deaths (18.1% of all deaths).[23] However, death resulting from poor diet and physical inactivity was the second-leading cause of death at 365,000, or 15.2% of all deaths per year.[23,24] Assuming that the obesity-related disease trends will continue to increase with the rise in the number of overweight children, poor diet and lack of exercise may soon be the number one cause of death in the United States. The economic cost of obesity will be increasingly challenging when considering the healthcare needs of the aging population, the already strained healthcare systems, and budget crises. Compounding these problems is society's new task of providing care for young people affected by overweight and related health problems.

The burden of being overweight stresses individuals, families, and society. For the individual, quality of life issues such as family income, rates of marriage, and educational attainment were all lower, while poverty rates were higher for women who had been obese in late adolescence and young adulthood.[16] Financially, child hospitalizations for conditions related to obesity cause parents or caregivers to be absent from work, stressing family budgets and causing loss of productivity for the parents' employer(s).

The full economic consequences of our overweight children cannot yet be known with certainty. For example, type 2 diabetes historically has been considered an adult onset condition, with negative effects on a person's health generally limited to the adult years. In adults, type 2 diabetes may show a certain pattern of development of health complications, such as peripheral neuropathy and impaired vision. The onset of such diabetic complications appears to depend to some extent on the length and severity of exposure to the diabetes condition. Thus, weight-related type 2 diabetes, which begins in youth, has the potential to cause excess morbidity, mortality, and diminished quality of life and productivity for many. It is reasonable to expect that the longer the duration of complications of being overweight, the greater the healthcare costs incurred with their treatment.[25]

On a societal level, healthcare costs related to childhood obesity could have serious implications. The new generation of young adults that is expected to "carry" the nation's productivity and pay into social security, Medicare, Medicaid, and support federal and state social programs with their tax dollars may find themselves disabled or with limited earnings potential due to overweight-related impairments in health. National and state budgets will be doubly strained as healthcare payouts to program recipients soar while the funds supplying the coffers are diminishing by a less productive workforce. In the private sector, health insurance premiums can be expected to increase to keep pace with the increased costs of health care associated with treatment for overweight and its complications. Also important are the "opportunity costs" of society not being able to fund other important social, educational, and public programs due to the drain on budgets from the healthcare costs of treating overweight individuals.

■ ENVIRONMENTAL INFLUENCES ON CHILDREN WHO ARE OVERWEIGHT

Societal Factors

Some overweight people have experienced discrimination because of the negative attitudes and judgmental behaviors of others who may see them as lazy and lacking willpower. Such attitudes have contributed to a social stigma and caused psychological pain for those suffering from the condition. Viewing overweight in children within a construct of "personal responsibility" has allowed past treatment in-terventions to focus on the child and, perhaps, the family unit. Experience has shown that this treatment model used by itself often has failed as many overweight children have grown up to be overweight adults.

Today, it is widely recognized that the microenvironment (home and family setting) and the macroenvironment (the setting in which the family is embedded) promote either healthy weight or overweight.[26] The mission of public health is to fulfill society's interest in assuring conditions in which people can be healthy.[1] Altering both the micro- and macroenvironments to prevent or treat overweight in children thus is vital to the mission of public health.

Overweight and Energy Balance

The environmental factors underlying the recent increase in obesity rates in the United States are multiple; however, diet and physical activity play a crucial role. Basic to this concept is the fact that to maintain a stable weight, energy intake and output must be balanced. When physical activity level is low, weight status thus can be maintained with a diet appropriately lower in calories. However, if an adjustment is not made by either increasing physical activity or

---

Micro- and Macroenvironments

Psychobiologic Core: Genetically programmed metabolism and behavior, which includes instinctive behavior, innate values related to survival, which are essentially immutable. Early conditioned behaviors (e.g., positive and negative reinforcement of pleasure, pain, etc.) and experiential learning, physiologic state; these are behavioral and metabolic phenotypes expressed within a given environment. The psychobiologic core also includes current health status.

Cultural: Personal life experienced, "inherited" values and beliefs (e.g., ethnic and cultural identity), self-identity within immediate social/cultural surroundings.

Societal: Roles and relationships, "acquired" values and beliefs, how society views the individual and vice versa, that is, self-identity within broader social/cultural environment, broader societal values (e.g., social trends). This layer interacts with the cultural layer, defined as how society views you affects how you view yourself.

Enablers of Choice: Most proximal factors affecting choices that are commonly identified as enhancers or barriers to change. These factors tend to be the ones most focused on in order to facilitate change.

Lifestyle: Visible physical activity and eating behavior choices made by the individual, may be a mix of who they are and who they would like to be.

Behavior Settings: Physical and social settings in which physical activity and eating behaviors take place and choices are made, the situational context within which behavior takes place.

Proximal Leverage Points: Controllers of the structure and features of the microenvironment that affect the physical activity and eating behavior choices.

Distal Leverage Points: All behavior settings and macroenvironments are influenced by additional layers of factors, either directly or indirectly (e.g., controllers of the raw materials and finished goods that consumers purchase or are exposed to, along with the laws, policies, economics, politics, etc. that affect the controllers). The distal leverage points also include some multidimensional factors that pervade all levels and that shape attitudes, beliefs, and knowledge (e.g., media).

decreasing energy intake, energy intake will exceed expenditure and will result in weight gain. The alarming rise in overweight among U.S. children begs the question: What changes have occurred in our lifestyles that could have contributed to this rapid rise in the prevalence of overweight in children?

> The 2005 and 2010 Dietary Guidelines Advisory Committee recommends that children engage in at least 60 minutes of physical activity on most (preferably all) days of the week. Physical activity may include short bouts (i.e., 10 minutes each) of moderately intense activity. In this way, exercise can be accumulated through three to six bouts over the course of the day. The accumulated total of physical activity is what is important for health.

■ DIETARY TRENDS AFFECTING OVERWEIGHT STATUS IN CHILDREN

Historical Perspective

Today's lifestyles are very different from the lifestyles of our hunter-gatherer ancestors. Genetically, we humans evolved during the Paleolithic period 2.6 million to 10,000 years ago, and were biologically adapted to survive under the prevailing conditions of that time. Today's Western-style diet is in sharp contrast to the diet of the hunter-gatherers, yet our human genome has changed little since that period to help us adapt to our present-day lifestyles. Now, most of us "dwell in mechanized urban settings, leading sedentary lives and eating a highly processed, synthetic diet."[27] Some differences in our diets were that hunter-gatherers consumed foods higher in fiber content and lower in energy density, and with a different diet composition of the long chain fatty acids. The long chain fatty acids of the n-6 and n-3 families were consumed in a ratio of about 1:1.

Today's Western-type diet can provide less of the omega-3 fatty acids with an ω-3: ω-6 ratio of 1:15–17.[28] The diet of the hunter-gatherer was rich in plant foods, supplemented by fish and lean meats and nuts. Indications are that these early ancestors did not experience obesity. Changes in agricultural practices as well as food processing and manufacturing have resulted in a vastly different food supply that has evolved over a relatively short time,

historically. The development of agricultural societies led to diets based on grains. With this change from a plant-based to a grain-based diet, vitamin and mineral deficiencies began to appear, as evidenced by studying bones and teeth. Our natural preference for foods that are calorically dense is rooted in the conditions of our ancestors, who required high levels of physical activity and high energy expenditures to obtain food for survival through hunting, fishing, and gathering.

In contrast, obtaining food today means a car ride to the grocery store and little connection between energy intake and expenditure.[27] The typical American diet today may be lower in fiber and plant foods, higher in meat, high in highly refined carbohydrates (high glycemic load), and possibly contain a much higher ratio of the ω-6 relative to the ω-3 long chain fatty acids. Sources of ω-3 fatty acids that are possibly diminished in our diet include fish, shellfish, wild game, and plant foods. Potassium intakes are much lower today, while sodium intakes are much higher than the intakes of our ancestors. In short, most people consume a diet they were not genetically designed to eat. Calcium is an important mineral to human health, yet calcium intakes are not adequate for adolescent girls, older women, and older males. Although calcium intake has increased a little for women ages 20 to 74 since NHANES III, recommendations for milk and dairy intake are not met by 70% of the population over 2 years of age according to the NHANES 1999–2000 data.[29] Researchers contend that these dietary changes, combined with sedentary lifestyles, play a significant role in the etiology of chronic diseases affecting developed countries: heart disease, diabetes, cancer, and obesity.[30,31]

Changes in the Food Environment

One of the most noticeable changes affecting our food environment during the past two decades is the rapid growth in the number of restaurants, especially of fast food establishments that are currently approaching 250,000 outlets nationally. Fast food restaurants are found throughout our communities, even inside public schools and hospitals. The effective marketing and advertising of these restaurants to adults and children have fueled the growth of this industry. Unfortunately, fast food restaurant fare is usually high in

ω-6 fatty acid: A polyunsaturated fatty acid in which the first double bond is six carbons from the methyl end of the carbon chain. Found in soybean and corn oils, and margarines and dressings made with vegetable oils.

ω-3 fatty acid: A polyunsaturated fatty acid in which the first double bond is three carbons from the methyl end of the carbon chain. Found in certain cold-water fish tissues and in vegetable sources such as flax seeds, walnuts, and olive and canola oils.

calories, fat, salt, and sugars, while low in fiber content.[32] This is especially true for menu items offered as "special value" promotions. Often, the more healthful selections on fast food menus are more expensive and are not subject to the low price offers that might otherwise encourage customers to buy them.

Fast food items are convenient and relatively low cost. These factors appeal to working and single parents, and the percentage of children eating fast food meals will likely increase.[32] The amount of food dollars spent purchasing meals at dine-in and take-out restaurants has increased significantly to comprise about 46% of total household food budgets. Fast food meals consume about 34% of the family food dollar. Meals eaten outside the home tend to have large portion sizes, have higher energy content, and include fewer fruits and vegetables than meals eaten in the home. As a result, the increase in out-of-home meal consumption may have a negative impact on diet quality and on the obesity and health risk of children and their families.[33,34] Fast food intake among adolescents is one factor that negatively impacts their intake of food groups such as fruit, milk, and vegetables and their likelihood of meeting MyPyramid recommendations.[35] Product innovations launched during the past two decades have included many products designed to lower the fat content of popular foods to address consumers' concerns about dietary fat and unwanted weight gain. Despite an explosive growth in low-fat food products in many food categories, these food supply changes have seemingly not had the desired effect on our obesity rates. Many food manufacturers offset the lower fat content of the reformulated foods by increasing sugar and carbohydrate contents to maintain product acceptance by consumers. In the end, the caloric content of the lower fat product is often similar to the original version. There is also concern that so-called low-fat foods may encourage the consumer to actually eat more calories overall because the low-fat food provides a "license to eat more."[36]

Energy intakes in children's diets have remained fairly stable since 1971–1974 (NHANES I), except for increases for children ages 1 to 2, and for adolescent girls ages 12 to 19. The macronutrient composition of children's diets has changed, however, reflecting changes in the food supply. Fat intake as a percentage of energy intake fell from 38% to 33% since 1973, while carbohydrate and protein intakes increased. Still, about 75% of children did not meet the fat intake recommendations in 1994.[34,37]

Children's diets have changed in respect to the types of carbohydrate they consume. In a 1998 roundtable and national briefing on child nutrition, the Director of the National Institute of Child Health and Human Development was quoted as saying that children's diets are characterized by "too much energy...too much sugar, and too little fiber" (fruits and vegetables) and could be described as an inverted Food Guide Pyramid.[38] Easily digestible, highly refined carbohydrates from foods and beverage sources have increased in consumption recently. A lot of scientific interest has focused on the possible role of high glycemic index (GI) foods in the childhood and adult obesity epidemic. Glycemic index (GI) is the effect of carbohydrate in a food on blood glucose, as a percentage of the effect of an equal amount of glucose. An effect of the GI of breakfast foods on subsequent unrestricted food intake at lunch has been studied. Lunch intake after a high-GI-load breakfast was greater than after a breakfast of low GI.[39] In a review of the high-GI foods and their connection to hunger and obesity, Roberts[40] concluded that, compared to similar low-GI carbohydrates, high-GI carbohydrates promote a more rapid return of the hunger sensation and increase subsequent caloric intake. High-GI foods, therefore, may contribute to maintenance of excess weight in the obese, and weight gain in susceptible individuals. Many children start their day with high-sugar-content breakfast cereals of high-GI. Over the longer term, frequent intake of high-GI foods could lead to higher energy intake and contribute to excess weight gain.[41]

High-sugar beverage intake is linked with fast food consumption because soft drinks are usually marketed and bundled with meal packages in fast food restaurants. Twice as many children and adolescents drank carbonated soft drinks if they had consumed fast foods on one of two survey days than if they had not consumed fast foods.[42] The so-called "super-sized" meal offers upgraded beverage serving size along with food portions. "Super-sizing" of meal packages may have contributed to increased intakes of sweetened beverages by children. Between 1977–79 and 1994, the proportion of children who consumed soft drinks on a given day increased by 74% for boys and 65% for girls.[34] High consumption of soft drinks among children and adolescents has been shown to be associated with higher energy intakes.[43] An association between schoolchildren's sugar-sweetened drink consumption and their BMI has been demonstrated, although more research is ongoing. For example, a study conducted prospectively over 19 months showed that for each additional serving of sugar-sweetened beverage consumed, both BMI and propensity to become obese increased. This was after controlling for anthropometric, demographic, dietary, and lifestyle variables.[44]

The typical 12-fluid-ounce can of soda is rapidly being replaced by the 20-fluid-ounce bottle at convenience stores and in vending machines, encouraging increased consumption of these drinks. Many brands offer a 32-fluid-ounce version that is packaged in a bottle shape that is easy to tote around, thereby encouraging increased consumption. Average portion sizes of soft drinks have increased by 12–18% for persons ages 2 and older.[29] Soft drink consumption (per capita) has increased about 500% over the past 50 years, with adolescents consuming between 36 grams and 58 grams of sugar daily from this source.[44]

Food portions have increased as well. Most consumers recognize portion inflation among baked goods, such as bagels and muffins, and for hamburgers, which are both larger and offered with two or three servings of meat and cheese.

Regulation of Energy Intake

Although very young children possess innate abilities to regulate energy intake based on their needs, children tend to lose some of this ability as they age and become more responsive to environmental influences, increasingly taking their behavioral cues from their surroundings. Children vary in their ability to self-regulate energy intakes,[45] but children who have experienced so-called restrictive feeding practices appear to be less able to respond appropriately to internal signs of hunger and satiety, and may be more susceptible to overeating.[46] Also, as children learn from their environment, food portion sizes will influence their intake. Children thus may over-eat when presented with excessive food and beverage portions, risking excessive weight gain over time.

The Family Eating Environment

Genetic differences are estimated to account for about 30% to 50% of the variance of BMI within a population, but these estimates do not describe the complex interactions taking place between genetics and the environment.[47] For example, parents contribute both genetics and environment to the equation, and their own eating behaviors that help shape the child's eating environment may to an extent be influenced by genetics. In turn, the child or adolescent's eating environment will help shape the development of the child's own eating behaviors. These learned eating behaviors will again influence whether any genetic predispositions toward obesity will be expressed in the child.[46]

Parents who are struggling with personal weight issues may hamper their children's ability to self-regulate energy intake. Because many adults suffer from overweight or obesity,[7] some parents are understandably concerned about their children's risk of also becoming overweight or obese. Aiming to avoid overweight in their children, parents may impose greater restrictions on their children's intake. If these same parents exhibit uninhibited eating styles themselves, they will serve as poor role models. These behaviors in combination can cause the transfer of eating styles that pose an increased risk for the development of overweight in the child. As a result, well-intentioned parents may actually produce the very outcome they sought to avoid.[45] A common strategy employed to control children's intake is to restrict their access to high-calorie foods, or to use favorite foods as a reward to shape behavior. At first, these behaviors may seem reasonable enough; however, restricting certain foods has been shown to increase the child's desire to consume these foods. When available, these desirable foods will likely be consumed in greater amounts. Again,

such family dynamics around food may set up patterns of poor self-control of energy intake in the child.[48]

An optimal environment for children to develop self-control of energy intake is when parents provide nutritious food and allow children to determine when and how much to eat. These principles of division of responsibility are discussed extensively in other resources.[49–52]

Household Food Insecurity

Although seemingly paradoxical, lower-income compared to higher-income households appear to experience increased rates of overweight for some individuals. A proposed mechanism for low socioeconomic status (SES) being related to overweight and obesity is that higher intakes of cheaper, more calorie-dense foods may lead to excessive energy intakes.[53,54] Persons from low-income, food insecure households may overeat during periods of relative abundance and gain weight as a result. Food insecurity in low-income households appears to play a role in the increased overweight rates among older Caucasian girls (8–16 years of age) compared to children from low-income households that do not experience food insecurity.[54] However, family participation in programs such as the National School Breakfast and Lunch Programs and Supplemental Nutrition Assistance Programs (Food Stamps) may be protective for these girls. Girls who participated in all three programs were 68% less likely to become overweight when compared to non-participants from families experiencing food insecurity.[55] On the other hand, a more recent study found a 42.8% increase for young girls and a 28.8% decrease for young boys in the predicted probability of obesity with participation in the Supplemental Nutrition Assistance Program (Food Stamp Program) for the previous five years. This study did not control for food insecurity within households, which may help to explain the differing results.[56] There appears to be personal characteristics such as age, race, and sex that influence the relationship between overweight and obesity in individuals within households and SES. Among boys aged 2 to 9, those of high SES had the lowest prevalence of BMI ≥ 95th percentile compared to their peers, while young girls showed only small differences according to SES.

In contrast, there was a strong inverse association between low SES and high BMI (≥ 95th percentile) for white adolescent girls, but not for boys. High-SES Black girls, in contrast to

Retrospective studies: These studies examine events that have occurred in the past or they represent attribute variables that cannot be manipulated; therefore, the researcher does not have direct control of the variables under study.

Longitudinal studies: The researcher follows a cohort of subjects over time, performing repeated measurements at prescribed intervals.

their white counterparts, were at increased risk for high BMI.[57] Additional studies that are retrospective, longitudinal, and include assessment of food security and hunger status of each household member are needed to help explain why some children are affected more than others. This is important because not all members of a household may be experiencing food insecurity to the same extent. Understanding these dynamics better will help to focus attention on those within a household who may be at a greater risk of being overweight. (Read more about food insecurity in Chapter 17.)

Breast Feeding

New mothers returning to work may decide against breast feeding or may nurse their infants for only a very limited time because of the real and/or perceived obstacles involved with breast-feeding their infants while holding a job. This is unfortunate, as breast milk is the ideal food for infants. Evidence is emerging that breast feeding may offer some protection against obesity.[58] Proposed mechanisms for this effect include more normal growth patterns (lower early weight gain) possibly associated with lower basal insulin levels in the breast-fed infant compared with an infant-fed formula, and the inherent control of food intake maintained by the breast-fed infant.[59] Breast feeding on demand is thought to teach infants to regulate their intakes appropriately, based on internal cues for hunger and satiety, and in response to their individual growth needs. Formula-fed infants may have fewer opportunities to develop this important skill, perhaps because parents or caregivers want to follow a set feeding schedule or encourage the baby to consume a certain amount of formula. Both of these feeding behaviors override the infant's internal cues and may result in overfeeding and lessening of the infant's ability to self-regulate energy intake.[46]

Study design issues and the challenges of controlling for confounders in studies that investigate the relation between infant feeding practices and later overweight have contributed to varying conclusions about the protective effect of breast feeding on risk of overweight. A literature review by the World Health Organization (WHO) concluded that breast feeding conferred a small protection against overweight later in life.[60] Differences in the nutritional content of infant formula compared to breast milk may contribute to breast feeding being protective against overweight. Breast milk nutritional content changes over time so that it contains less protein after the first few months when infant need for protein is less. It is thought that the more rapid gains in weight and length from about two months of age to the end of the first year of life of formula-fed infants may be due to the higher protein content of formula that exceeds the infant's needs after about one to two months of age. Differences in adiposity appear only at about 12 months when evidence suggests that breast-fed infants are leaner than formula-fed infants. Higher plasma levels of insulin-like growth factor-1 (IGF-1), insulin, and certain amino acids in formula fed infants compared to breast-fed infants and higher energy intake may explain these differences in growth and fat deposition.[61]

Physical Inactivity Affecting Overweight Status in Children

Physical inactivity among children is one of the major public health concerns regarding overweight children. Children learn to be physically inactive by emulating adults who are inactive and having limited access to community recreation activities, unsafe neighborhoods, and perhaps, unlimited access to television viewing and other media outlets, including computers. In addition, many newly developed communities are poorly planned and don't include "built-in" access to physical activity. Often children are bused to school because walking to school is not an option due to safety issues and distance. In many towns and cities, sidewalks were once common, but now some urban and suburban developments have shaped many residential areas into "unwalkable" communities. Although further research is needed for a better understanding of the influence of the human-built environment on physical activity, it appears clear that urban sprawl has caused some relationship between land use, transportation, and health, particularly children's health.[62]

School Physical Education

At school, children are challenged to find opportunities to be physically active on a daily basis. Often, school academic curriculums and programs take priority over physical education and recess time. Physical education (PE) curriculums and recess have slowly diminished over the last few years.

The percentage of schools that require physical education in each grade declines from around 50% in grades one through five, to 25% in grade eight, to only 5% in grade twelve. Although National Association for Sport and Physical Education (NASPE) and National Association of State Boards of Education (NASBE) discourage student exemption from physical education based on participation in other school and community activities, some states, districts, and schools allow such exemption from required physical education.[63]

Data from the Youth Risk Behavior Surveillance System (YRBSS) show that 55.7% of students nationwide were enrolled in PE classes one or more days in an average week, while only 28.4% of students nationwide attended PE classes five days in an average week. Of the 55.7% of students enrolled in PE classes nationwide, 80.3% of students actually exercised or played sports for more than 20 minutes. Improvements in PE are also needed to decrease inappropriate teaching practices, such as prohibiting physical activity as a form of punishment or physical activity games that may cause embarrassment or aggressive behavior (e.g., dodge ball).[63] Although some PE improvements are needed, a nationwide effort to establish laws or policies to increase student enrollment and participation in daily PE is desirable, especially in the older student population. The goal is for children to establish healthy lifestyle habits that may carry over into adulthood.

While the majority of children spend much of their waking hours in school, it is a threat to children's health and fitness when the school infrastructure does not mandate daily physical activity. Advocacy for increasing student participation in daily recess and physical activity should be a top priority of schools and health and community leaders to help prevent overweight in children.

Television Viewing

Television viewing and other media outlets to an extent have displaced a more natural environment of family interactions for growing children, such as learning and playing. Children who spend more time in sedentary activities tend to weigh more and be at greater risk of being overweight. Several studies conclude that children who watch four or more hours of TV are more likely to be overweight than those who watch less TV.[64-66] In addition, African-American (30%) and Hispanic-American (22%) children are both more likely than Caucasian (12%) children to spend more than five hours a day watching TV. Similarly, African-American (69%) and Hispanic-American (60%) children are more likely than Caucasian (48%) children to have a TV in their bedroom.[67] One cross-sectional study failed to find a relationship between TV viewing and overweight in adolescent girls.[68] There may be some question about leisure activities in the United States, indicating that U.S. children overall are less active than children in other countries and cultures. A participant in one focus group made a comparison between U.S. children and the children in her country. She stated, "one exercises three times a day, one goes to the river to swim in the afternoon, and here the children don't do that. They just sit to watch television and to eat."[69] The trend toward increasingly sedentary lifestyles is obvious to many older adults, as they compare the children's activity level in this current generation to that of children two or three generations earlier. Learning, playing, and being physically active were an integral part of family life, and television viewing was a special occasion. Today, television viewing, which is a sedentary behavior, is a prominent part of family life.

Not only will excessive television viewing leave less time for positive family interactions and activities, but the actual programs and advertisements also may be questionable for young viewers. Granted, there are many beneficial programs to watch on television. Unfortunately, not all programs and advertisements have children's health as a priority. One major challenge is the multimillion-dollar advertising industry that promotes products between and during television programming.[70] Appealing and enticing advertising segments are targeted at children to increase their desire to choose unhealthy foods. Food products advertised directly to young children during children's television programming have contributed to an impressive growth in sales of high-sugar breakfast cereals and snack foods. Young consumers predictably request the products or even purchase these themselves during trips to the grocery store, as they recognize their favorite cartoon characters on the colorful packages that are strategically placed at their eye level when riding in the grocery cart. Excessive television viewing by children creates a cycle of physical inactivity and high calorie consumption due to the influence of TV food advertising, which might be a perfect formula for fueling the growth in numbers of overweight children.

An important part of treating overweight in children is to decrease sedentary behavior and increase physical activity.[71] This is an important factor in the treatment process; however, children are still challenged with real barriers that exist in their physical environment. As discussed, limited access to safe physical activity in the community, unlimited television viewing, decreased physical activities in the schools, and adults who may not view physical activity as a priority are important barriers to physical activity. Thus, U.S. children live in an obesigenic society in which they continually face barriers to making healthy living choices, such as daily physical activity.

> **Obesigenic:** An environment that encourages obesity through features such as unlimited quantities of a variety of foods high in caloric density together with minimal energy expenditure.

■ ADDRESSING CHILDHOOD OBESITY/ OVERWEIGHT AS A PUBLIC HEALTH NUTRITIONIST

Public health nutritionists will soon experience a new role in their profession when addressing obesity in this nation, as the comfort level of doing what always has been done will not benefit the public. One recent study reported that the majority of health professionals working in obesity-related fields stated that they were most comfortable with education-based prevention strategies and less comfortable with environmental-based strategies.[72] Clearly, many health education strategies have not been effective during the rise of childhood obesity due to many environmental conditions that require global and societal action.[73,74] Thus, public health nutritionists may need to go beyond the traditional practice and learn to apply policy- and environmental-based strategies.[75] Public health nutritionists must become assertive in learning and applying policy and environmental interventions and be aggressive enough to demand the resources and support to implement and evaluate them. Public health nutrition leaders will be the change agents that are needed in a society that some assert is in denial about overweight in children.[76]

Chapters 7 and 8 discuss how to advocate for policies and resources. In addition, Chapter 26 focuses on social marketing for programs needed for the health and welfare of the public.

Due to the low rate of overweight in children in the past, childhood obesity was not a high priority in the healthcare arena. The traditional practice of a public health nutritionist in addressing overweight in children therefore has been mostly reactive versus proactive. In the reactive mode, parents of an overweight child may or may not seek treatment and/or counseling depending on their cultural belief system, attitude, and knowledge. If treatment was sought, usually discussions occurred in medical offices with a doctor or nurse. In the past, public health nutritionists' roles were mostly as consultants to medical professionals and/or serving as nutrition educators or counselors to families on healthy eating and exercise.

Because obesity is a multifactor issue, public health nutritionists must be proactive in learning new skills and acquiring new tools to prevent and control weight-related problems in children. Effective treatment practices are necessary for the existing population of overweight children. Treatment practices must be reliable and tailored to individuals and populations in order to be effective at changing behavior and the health status of overweight in children. Some existing treatment practices are education, behavioral therapy, and surgical procedures; however, some of these are questionable for this population.[77] The primary focus should be a multifactor population-based approach of prevention, including assessment, policy and environmental interventions; support for healthy eating, physical activity, limited TV viewing, and breast-feeding promotion; and community planning within communities, schools, worksites, faith-based groups, medical facilities, and families. This multifactor population-based approach should be included in academia and training for public health nutrition students and professionals, respectively.[78]

In addition, the public health nutritionist should be culturally competent and support the *Healthy People 2010* Objectives (HP 2010) to eliminate health disparities in chronic illnesses, such as in overweight and obesity.[79]

Read more about Healthy People 2010 at: http://www.healthypeople.gov.

Partnerships

Due to the complexity of population-based approaches in addressing overweight in children, it is essential for public health nutritionists to develop internal and external partnerships. Partnerships are useful because partners may adopt the vision of healthy children, expand resources, and build momentum and synergy to address the healthcare needs of target populations. Being aware of the knowledge, skills, and limitations of yourself and partners will enable you to close the gaps and accomplish goals set for the target population. Nutrition expertise is valuable; however, the focus must advance from educating, counseling, and telling people about the importance of healthy eating and physical activity to working with partners to change the environment so as to enable people—especially children—to eat healthy foods and to exercise or be physically active.[80,81]

Often, public health nutritionists encourage their target population to eat more fruits and vegetables, even when there are well-known barriers to consuming the recommended amount of these foods. Availability, accessibility, and affordability are real barriers to eating fruits and vegetables daily for many individuals, including children.

Acknowledgement of these barriers and knowing partners who can help overcome them will help to increase fruit and vegetable intake among children. Local media may serve as an outlet to increase fruit and vegetable intake among children through social marketing campaigns. Meetings

The 2005 and 2010 Dietary Guidelines Advisory Committee has recommended the intake of fruits and vegetables, as well as non-fat/low-fat dairy products and whole grains for children.

and discussions with local day care and school food service directors may lead to a policy change that promotes and serves more fresh fruits and vegetables during school meals and snacks; many schools have eliminated carbonated sodas and highly sugared snacks from their cafeterias and vending machines. Cooperative Extension Agents may conduct classes on purchasing fruits and vegetables in season and preservation, thus increasing fruit and vegetable availability throughout the year. Local farmers and grocers may sell their produce at different locations throughout the community. Fruits and vegetables sold at annual events (e.g., summer and fall fests) or sporting activities also may promote healthy eating. Religious groups may encourage potluck lunches or dinners that include more fruits and vegetables. Restaurants may encourage children to eat healthier by featuring fruits and vegetables acceptable to children on the menu. Finally, after-school programs may serve fruits and vegetables as snacks more often.

The marketing that creates a high demand for soft drinks causes its main ingredient—corn syrup—to be produced at high volumes. Soft drinks therefore are relatively cheap and readily available. This same principle may be applied to increase the consumption of fruits and vegetables by producing them at high volumes that cause them to be relatively inexpensive and readily available. Partnerships with the media, local farmers, grocers, community planners, schools, extension services, and USDA Food Assistance Programs all have the ability to influence the way people view fruits and vegetables. Partnerships help to remove the barriers and enable people, especially children, to obtain and consume fruits and vegetables daily. Although it may be challenging to organize partnerships, develop policies, or change the environment to increase fruit and vegetable consumption, it can be rewarding.

Evidence-based: A concept whereby analysis is based on scientific proof.

Another potential partnership for the public health nutritionist is to collaborate with research universities and/or institutes. Such partnerships may offer opportunities to develop evidence-based interventions focused on prevention of obesity or promotion of a healthy weight from which both parties may benefit. For instance, the public health nutritionist may have an existing partnership in the school system that is interested in developing programs or interventions that prevent and control obesity in children. The public health nutritionist and research investigator may collaborate with the school partner and plan, develop, implement, monitor, and evaluate the intervention. As a result, the public health nutritionist's goals and objectives may be implemented and the investigator may assist with the development of monitoring systems and evaluation tools. The investigator may also serve as an independent reviewer of data, and do monitoring, data analysis, and evaluation. Once the program is complete, the public health nutritionist and investigator may submit abstracts and manuscripts to professional conferences and journals. Also, this valuable information should be shared with community leaders and those working with the target populations. Other partnerships may also be established with existing internal partners, such as an epidemiologist, community planner, or the like.

Internal agency partnerships are also important. Often, internal partners do not know about their own agency's resources and services to the community. Sometimes internal partners may be territorial and work in silos. However, when working in the community or clinical settings, it is important to know about various internal programs and services. Individuals and communities benefit when internal partners, including the public health nutritionist, are unified and present consistent, current resources and referrals.

Another responsibility of the public health nutritionist may be to form an internal or external coalition. There are three important things to remember when forming a coalition:

1. Solicit key partners with a shared vision of the goals and objectives to accomplish.
2. Establish a mission, goals, and objectives that will advance a common vision and that benefit a majority of the goals of key partners. Often the momentum of the coalition diminishes when members are not focused, organized, or challenged with activities from which they and their constituents or target population may benefit.
3. Review the accomplishments and failures of the coalition at regular intervals and evaluate whether goals and objectives were met.

Developing partnerships is a process that demands a significant investment of time and attention. Therefore, it is essential to attend meetings, from the local town hall and county coalition meetings to state and professional meetings. At these meetings, the ultimate goal is to know the community leaders and health professionals. Leaders need to know your skills as a public health nutritionist, and your goals and vision of healthy children and adults. Over time, relationships can be developed into strong partnerships that are essential for public health nutritionists to be effective in their communities.

Coalition: An alliance, sometimes temporary, of people, factions, or parties.

Grant Writing

Many social programs have experienced budget constraints and/or cuts and are forced to become more creative with existing resources, or obtain grant funding to develop or even continue programs. Although doing more with less is the norm for many agencies, many are seeking grant funding to advance their programs. Therefore, grant applications have become very competitive, and the ability to write a favorable grant application is now an essential skill of the public health nutrition practitioner.

The public health nutritionist should possess some grant writing skills; however, working as a team to coordinate and complete the grant application is ideal. Completing a grant application is very time-consuming and labor-intensive. For this reason alone, a professional grant writer may be needed to coordinate the activities and gather materials needed to complete the grant. The role of the public health nutritionist should be to describe the vision for the project and to develop a plan of action of assessment, policy, and environmental interventions, as well as evaluation, and assurances. In addition, the public health nutritionist must act as a resource to obtain letters of support from internal and external partners.

Development of a budget is also necessary, and should be a shared responsibility between the public health nutritionist and the agency accountant. The public health nutritionist will be able to describe staffing and salary requirements needed to complete the tasks required of the action plan, and the accountant will be able to provide technical assistance for the grant budget requirements. A grant steering committee is very helpful when submitting a grant application for a large sum of money. This committee may consist of the agency epidemiologist, nurse administrator, nutrition administrator, accountant, key health professionals that may work directly with the proposed grant activities, and grant writer. The public health nutritionist can be the primary person to determine the services needed to accomplish the goals and objectives of the project. It is equally important, however, to solicit the opinions of people on the grant steering committee and internal and external partners. If possible, public health nutritionist positions and responsibilities should be included in the grant. The public health nutritionist thus should plan to write portions of the grant. Private and public funding have various requirements, so it is important to review the requirements and complete the application as specified.

Most grant applications have similar requirements. A cover sheet includes the title, the organization's information, and the budget requested. The proposal abstract provides a brief description of the project including the community problem, mission, goals, objectives, project strategies, past accomplishments, and support from internal and external partners. The proposal narrative describes the project in detail through the following: introduction, statement of community problem, project vision, mission and objectives, methods, evaluation plan, plan for financial sustainability, budget and budget justification, and overall significance.[82] Although all grant applications may not follow the same format, most applications targeted to prevent or control chronic diseases and/or illnesses require some basic information.

Many grant applications require letters of support. Sometimes public health nutritionists may appear as a salesperson when requesting a letter of support. In such cases, the request must offer a win-win solution for both parties involved. For instance, a school superintendent is asked to write a letter of support for a grant application on prevention and control of obesity in children. Before the school superintendent can write a letter of support, he or she should be able to visualize the benefits of the proposed project for the student population. Due to the existing trend of overweight in children, many leaders, including school superintendents, are eager to receive funding to address this public health issue, but are unsure of how to proceed. The public health nutritionist's role is to present the problem and some possible solutions (e.g., policy and environmental interventions), and provide suggestions as to how the school population and environment may be improved through proposed grant activities.

Advice

There are some pointers to keep in mind for each grant submitted. A peer should review the grant before you submit it. A good proofreader often catches errors or items not clearly defined. Although staffing, if allowed, may absorb most of the grant funding, it is important to establish program sustainability after the grant monies have ended. Therefore, sharing grant funding with the community and developing infrastructures to carry out the project activities after the funding has ended is ideal. In addition, many grant applications allow "matching" and in-kind contributions from various partners, which also encourage sustainability. A project should develop or enhance collaboration and partnerships, which will in turn develop momentum for the project. Also, as much as possible, the budget should be outcome driven. For instance, did the proposed project meet the objectives of decreasing the amount of fundraisers that sold high-calorie foods or increasing healthy food options in the vending machines? After two years, did students participate in more physical activity or eat healthier meals? Did students' BMI-for-age percentile and fitness level increase?

Finally, the application must follow the grant guidelines and be written concisely. This includes calling the grant agency to get technical assistance or to clarify what is required of the grant. The writing style should be clear, logical, concise, and professionally presented. A good grant application is one that shares resources, focuses on capacity building, encourages sustainability after the funding has ended, and is written concisely for grant application reviewers.

Media

Media professionals can be a useful resource for advancing the vision of healthy children. They can be seen as coworkers that present important health information to the public. Establishing good media relationships thus can enhance media advocacy interventions targeted for overweight children. The media should not sensationalize overweight in children, but instead use this public health concern to increase people's awareness of the health problem. Therefore, it is the public health nutritionist's role to enlighten audiences about the actions being taken to combat the trend of overweight in children. The public health nutritionist hence should be available as a resource for current data on overweight in children. These data may be available from a variety of resources, such as the Youth Risk Behavior Surveillance System (YRBSS), Pediatric Nutrition Surveillance System (PedNSS), and pediatric surveillance research from local universities or school data from students' annual physical exams. In addition, public health nutritionists should be actively involved in project interventions that address overweight in children, such as the School Health Index (SHI). These activities may be discussed in newsprint, on television, on radio, or on Web sites to show ways in which the problem of childhood overweight is being addressed.

Also, public health nutritionists should provide some thought-provoking ideas or challenges for the intended audiences. For instance, the nutritionist can write an article for a school newsletter that may encourage parents to get involved with developing school menus by reviewing menu items and participating in taste testing. Or, a local newspaper article may encourage local vendors to get involved in fundraising activities that do not involve food. This may initiate creative fundraising activities and eliminate the traditional bake sales and candy sales.

Working with media professionals can be stressful, especially for an entry-level public health nutritionist. However, some of this stress may be alleviated with a proactive approach and attitude. When possible, the public health nutritionist should meet with local media professionals prior to a story. It helps to get to know media professionals and relate to them as professional colleagues.

Be prepared to discuss topics that you are most familiar with and don't be afraid to say, "I don't know" on topics that you are not. A folder containing current facts, statistics, and program interventions for your population, state, district/region, county, and town/neighborhood is a valuable tool to keep at hand. This folder should be updated regularly with the latest data, including bookmarked sites on your computer. An effective delivery of the information is as important as knowing the facts. Therefore, it is a good idea to attend workshops and training opportunities on public speaking and effective communication. One organization that can help enhance your communication skills is Toastmasters International.™

Ensure that your point gets across while addressing the media professional's agenda. With preparation and organization, the public health nutritionist can assure that the message will not be lost in the excitement of obtaining the story and meeting deadlines.

There are advantages and disadvantages to working with the media. Doing a media segment on overweight in children and possible interventions will reach more people instantly than if you were working with a small community group. Also, media can be very resourceful when planning a social marketing campaign that encourages children to be physically active and to eat healthier foods. Be mindful that not everyone has access to television, radio, or print media. Also, some people in target populations may have limited language or literacy skills.

Advice

Develop a partnership with your local media professional. Invite them to a coalition meeting and discuss ways they can develop a story on successful accomplishments. Be-come familiar with their schedules and deadlines. Being proactive rather than reactive gives you time to develop a story, instead of being called 30 minutes before a story is being aired or printed. Remember that most media segments are short; therefore, it's important to be concise and focused, and to avoid jargon, acronyms, and large words. If you are unfamiliar with a topic, you may offer to research that information and follow up with the media professional. Interviews are good, but media professionals love it when health professionals can tell a story through sounds and images (e.g., children eating and talking in the lunchroom, students making a decision on snacks at the vending machine, or students exercising or not exercising during PE class). Media professionals appreciate receiving a thank-you note after a story is completed, and this helps to extend your relationship.

■ RESEARCH IN THE AREA OF OVERWEIGHT IN CHILDREN

Overweight in children is an active area of current research. Numerous articles on the topic regarding all its many facets are published each year, adding to our body of knowledge and defining new questions in need of answers. To be effective in planning successful interventions, the public health nutritionist should be familiar with the childhood overweight literature through periodic literature reviews and attendance at professional meetings, where up-to-the minute research findings are presented, often before appearing in print.

A critical review of the literature will enable the practitioner to distinguish between studies that provide information and will be useful in his or her area of practice and those that may not. The public health nutritionist should consider issues such as these in making this judgment:

- *Study design:* What was the research question or objective? Was the study designed in such a way that the question could be answered or the objective obtained? If it was an intervention study, was there a control group? Were there confounding variables that could lead to inconclusive or erroneous findings, or were such confounders considered?
- *Study subjects:* Were the subjects part of a specific ethnic group? How were subjects recruited and selected? Was the study free of bias in recruitment and selection? Was bias introduced through subject self-selection? For intervention versus control subjects, was group assignment random? Was selection done at the individual level or group level (e.g., randomization is done for individual children within a school or setting, in contrast to one or more schools being selected at random for intervention while other schools serve as the controls). Did a sufficient number of subjects par-

ticipate to draw the stated conclusions? How does a given study sample compare to the population served by the public health nutritionist?

- *Outcomes/results:* What interventions were most effective? Most cost-effective? What failed to show the desired results?
- *Application/implications:* What lessons can be applied to intervention planning, policy development, and so on for a given population? What data do the public health nutritionist already have access to (PedNSS, YRBSS, HP 2010, etc.) that can be studied with current research in mind?

Considering these issues and applying the deeper understanding in a thoughtful manner to public health activities will help ensure that our practice is evidence-based.

Being armed with a sound knowledge of the topic of childhood obesity will provide the public health nutritionist with the necessary confidence to seek and obtain support from government, community leaders, the medical community, stakeholders, the media, and community change agents as well as from his or her own public health department and supervisor in advocating for obesity prevention. It would be most helpful to have a well-stocked inventory of successful research studies to draw upon for inspiration in planning evidence-based community interventions. However, to date, there is a lack of studies with highly successful outcome measures, for a variety of reasons. Some suggested reasons include lack of adequate funding, too short a duration of intervention, or insufficient skills of key implementers. Other reasons include the inherent difficulty in achieving an effect big enough in the study sample on an outcome-based study, such as BMI. BMI will increase normally as children grow, making an intervention on BMI difficult to measure. Interventions to address overweight in children are ongoing at this writing, and it is hoped that these studies-in-progress will have benefited from weaknesses in earlier studies, resulting in outcomes that clearly demonstrate effective strategies. CATCH (Child and Adolescent Trial for Cardiovascular Health), SPARK (Sports, Play, and Active Recreation for Kids), and Planet Health are examples of recent intervention studies that provide insights into the challenges and successes of childhood obesity intervention research.

Although obesity interventions typically have been a product of academic research centers, public health nutritionists may be able to become involved in investigations through cooperation and collaboration with academic researchers. Certain issues, such as logistics, funding, and human assurance study approval for the protection of study subjects, will need to be addressed; these efforts offer great learning opportunities for the public health nutritionist who is new to research. The public health nutritionist has a unique knowledge of the study population, its barriers to a healthy lifestyle, and obesity prevention that can contribute to the formulation of appropriate research questions, and often has access to large amounts of data. The investigator, in contrast, has the research experience, access to statistical analysis, and sometimes support staff and graduate students to assist in the investigation.

■ PUBLIC HEALTH MODEL AND OVERWEIGHT IN CHILDREN

In public health, assessment, policy development, and assurance are integral parts of any intervention plan.[1] The following sections will review each component as it relates to addressing overweight in children.

Assessment

CDC School Health Index

The School Health Index (SHI) is a self-assessment and planning guide developed for grades K-12 by the CDC in Atlanta, Georgia. It consists of eight modules based on the coordinated school health program model. The modules have assessment questions in health education, physical education, health services, nutrition services, counseling, psychological and social services, healthy school environment, health promotion for staff, and family/community involvement. The current version focuses on physical activity, nutrition, and tobacco use in elementary, middle, and high schools. This tool identifies the strengths and weaknesses of a school's health promotion policies and programs. The SHI assists teachers, parents, students, and community members to develop an action plan for improving the health of the student population. Some improvements in the action plan can be implemented with little or almost no resources. Other improvements may require grant funding for implementation.[83]

The SHI is easy to administer and complete. The role of the public health nutritionist is to present current trends of poor eating habits and physical inactivity nationally, statewide, and locally. In addition, an existing partnership with local tobacco-use prevention educators is important because they may discuss trends of tobacco use in children. Once the evidence of health problems is described, the public health nutritionist should review resources, such as the SHI, and examples of policy and environmental interventions for targeted schools. Some examples of policy interventions are to: serve breakfast to all students; serve low fat milk,

CATCH: http://www.childtrends.org/Lifecourse/programs/ChildandAdolesentTrialforCardiovascularHealth.htm

SPARK: http://www.sparkpe.org

Planet Health: http://www.hsph.harvard.edu/prc/proj_planet.html

fresh fruits and vegetables, and whole grain products; limit access to vending machines during school hours and/or provide healthy options in the vending machines; provide opportunities for vigorous physical activity for all students; and offer healthy food options in school stores. Some examples of environmental interventions include: building a walking track for student, staff, and community members to use; purchasing playground equipment for students; and planning an annual community health event for community members, parents, teachers, and children.

The public health nutritionist acts as a consultant to the SHI site coordinator, who assembles and supports the SHI team members. Team members complete the assessment questions and planning guide. They develop an action plan with interventions tailored for their school. The role of the public health nutritionist is to ensure the development of an appropriate action plan that results in interventions of healthy eating practices and physical activity, especially among the student population.

The public health nutritionist should attend the planning meeting to assist SHI members in developing an action plan. Although the site coordinator should facilitate the meeting and solicit ideas and opinions, the public health nutritionist serves as a consultant by helping the team members to focus on healthy eating and physical activity. In addition, the public health nutritionist should seek, obtain, and disburse funding sources to implement some or all of the interventions. This is important because funding serves as an incentive to improve the school's health policies and programs. The SHI is an excellent tool in developing partnerships with local school staff and community, obtaining and dispersing grant funding to promote health, and monitoring and evaluating interventions that benefit children's health.

Policy Development

After an assessment is completed, areas that need improvement are identified. The next step is to develop interventions that actually empower a target population to accomplish a desired outcome. There are several types of interventions; however, for the purpose of this chapter, recommendations, policy, and environmental interventions will be discussed.

Recommendations

A recommendation is a course of action strongly advised by someone of authority, but not necessarily enforced. It is ideal to develop a policy after an assessment is complete. However, a recommendation may be used as a mechanism to get an actual policy written and/or established. A recommendation may follow the dictum of "first, do no harm." Although many people are reluctant to change, a recommendation allows them time to accept the ultimate goal of healthy children. For those who are involved, a recommendation gives people time to accept the new idea and adopt behaviors that support healthy children. In essence,

this process is similar to the Diffusion of Innovation Theory, in that a new idea is disseminated throughout the invested population in the hope that they will adopt the projected behavior (i.e., healthy eating and physical activity).

Example. After completing an assessment in one school, it was determined that fund-raising activities (e.g., candies, bake sales, etc.) may contribute to children being overweight. Because this was identified, there was a great level of reluctance among staff and administrators to develop a policy due to the revenue and cultural norm of fund-raising activities. A compromise thus was made and a recommendation was established for staff. The recommendation pointed out the increased number of overweight children in their student population and encouraged staff to consider non-food items for fund-raising activities. Although this was only a school recommendation, it created awareness among staff and was an important first step in policy development.

Policy

Policy is a law, regulation, rule, or guiding principle. It is different from a recommendation in that a policy is a guiding principle that is enforced by administrators or others. Policy may be dispersed informally, such as in a memo. Or it may be formal, including a rationale, program policy, intent, evaluation, policy review, and determination as to how it will be enforced.[84] A policy demands and expects a certain behavior. Currently, a no-smoking policy in restaurants is the norm in many cities; a vending machine or a la carte service with healthy food selections will be the norm when policies are written and enforced in school settings.

Example. In one school, the school food service director developed a policy to serve low-fat milk during mealtime. This policy decreases the fat content of the student's diet at school. Although you would expect the children to complain, it was mostly the school staff that had a difficult time adjusting to the policy. The policy also saved the school some money because whole milk cost more than low-fat milk. The students benefited from consuming low-fat milk rather than the standard whole milk served.

Environmental Interventions

Environmental interventions include changes to the economic, social, or physical surroundings. This intervention changes the physical environment to make it convenient to adopt healthy behaviors. It is important to recognize barriers to making positive changes in health behaviors among the target population. For example, barriers to exercise could include unsafe neighborhoods, lack of sidewalks and parks, and so on. The building and refurbishing of walking or biking trails in the community is an intervention that helps the target population to adopt healthy physical activity behaviors.

Example. It was identified that a walking track was needed to encourage children to walk during recess and PE classes. As a result, a walking track was built in front of the elementary school. Many parents drive or bus their children to school, so walking on the track is a good physical activity outlet for the children. Children establish many behaviors during childhood. Children who are encouraged to walk and exercise increase their chances of being physically active in their adult years.[85] In addition, school staff and community members may use the walking track.

Assurance

Interventions are essential to implement change, particularly in overweight children. It is vital, however, to evaluate the process and outcome of the interventions to assure that projected outcomes benefit the target population.

Evaluation

Evaluation is a systematic investigation of an object's merit, worth, or significance.[86] Major goals of evaluations are to assess the program's success in meeting stated objectives and identify potential improvements in program operation.[87] Process evaluation assesses the internal development of the project. It asks if certain protocols were followed, such as:

1. A school council made up of teachers, administrators, parents, health professionals, and community leaders was formed to address children's health and factors that caused them to be overweight.
2. All school nurses received training on how to measure students' BMI accurately, and how to record and report data.
3. WIC nutritionists and/or Head Start providers received training on cultural issues regarding overweight in children, educating parents on feeding young children, and overcoming barriers to healthy living for families.

Outcome evaluation assesses the external results of the program. It asks whether the program was effective and whether it accomplished its goals and objectives. For instance:

1. After teachers attend a training session, 85% of them reported not using physical activity as a form of punishment.
2. Of students who participated in 30 minutes of vigorous activity, 90% of them increased from three times per week to five times per week.
3. Of the 15% of children who were overweight, 85% either maintained their weight or lost up to 5 pounds in the last school year.

In major program interventions, evaluation tools should be standardized for several reasons.

- The tool may be used as a guide when collecting and analyzing data.

- It eliminates the use of various tools that may have insufficient validation beyond the primary program.
- A standardized tool will be validated and, thus, measures what is supposed to be measured.
- A standardized tool is efficient to use because it eliminates time spent developing a new tool.

Overall, evaluation is important because it helps to determine the program's successes and failures, and it serves as a guide for future program planning.

Survey Development

In a small program, a public health nutritionist may be asked to develop a survey or evaluation tool to see how the program is progressing and the degree to which the goals and objectives were met. To this end, the public health nutritionist should review the program goals, objectives, and strategies. A process objective may be, for example, to ensure that a trained individual will determine students' BMI during certain timeframes. A process evaluation would measure how many school nurses or nutritionists successfully completed a training on assessing overweight in children, and if a trained individual took their height and weight measurements during the specific timeframes. In the survey, a question could be: "During the first, second, third, and fourth quarter, what percentage of students' heights and weights were screened?" The outcome objective may be to decrease the number of children with a BMI greater than the 85th percentile from 15% to 10%. An outcome evaluation would measure the percentage of children who have a BMI greater than the 85th percentile. In the survey, an appropriate question would be: "What is the percentage of students who had a BMI greater than the 85th percentile?"

Surveys, observations, and other assessment tools are essential in the evaluation process because they provide a final picture of the intervention. When developing a survey, avoid "yes" or "no" questions. Formulate questions into multiple choices, instead of "Do you exercise?" ask "How many times a week do you exercise for more than 20 minutes?"

Table 5–1 is the set of sample survey questions from the *2005 State and Local Youth Risk Behavior Survey.*[88]

Surveys are also important because they can be included in grant applications and the data analyzed may be used as baseline data for the target population. Grant application reviewers like to see effective and successful programs. Without an evaluation, it is difficult to demonstrate effectiveness of an intervention in reaching desired outcomes for a population. Evaluation also provides feedback about weaknesses of the program or intervention that impede progress so that improvements can be made.

Surveys are not the only mechanism for evaluating an intervention. Observing and collecting anthropometric data are some other forms of evaluation. For instance, observing children while they eat or participate in physical activity or

TABLE 5–1	**Sample Survey Questions from the 2005 Youth Risk Behavioral Surveillance System**

1. During the past 7 days, how many times did you eat fruit? (Do not count fruit juice.)
   A. I did not eat fruit during the past 7 days.
   B. 1 to 3 times during the past 7 days
   C. 4 to 6 times during the past 7 days
   D. 1 time per day
   E. 2 times per day
   F. 3 times per day
   G. 4 times per day

2. On how many of the past 7 days did you exercise or participate in physical activity for at least 20 minutes that made you sweat and breathe hard, such as basketball, soccer, running, swimming laps, fast bicycling, fast dancing, or similar aerobic activities?
   A. 0 days
   B. 1 day
   C. 2 days
   D. 3 days
   E. 4 days
   F. 5 days
   G. 6 days
   H. 7 days

3. On an average school day, how many hours do you watch TV?
   A. I do not watch TV on an average school day.
   B. Less than 1 hour per day
   C. 1 hour per day
   D. 2 hours per day
   E. 3 hours per day
   F. 4 hours per day
   G. 5 or more hours per day

Source: Center for Disease Control and Prevention. *Youth Risk Behavior Surveillance—United States, 2005.* Available at http://www.cdc.gov/mmwr/PDF/SS/SS5505.pdf. Accessed August 25, 2010.

collecting weight and height measurements to assess BMI are some other ways to evaluate the target population.

■ OPPORTUNITIES FOR PUBLIC HEALTH NUTRITIONISTS TO INTERVENE AND PREVENT OVERWEIGHT IN CHILDREN

Public health nutritionists are challenged to think of new ways to address the problem of childhood obesity within existing venues and frameworks. To be most successful, the emphasis must be on population-based approaches and prevention, as traditional and clinical-based practices clearly have failed to adequately address the obesity epidemic. The public health nutritionist thus may examine existing nutrition, social, and other programs and seize opportunities to

advance goals. Some suggestions for opportunities are listed in the following sections.

WIC

- Develop policies and provide outreach activities to recruit pregnant women into prenatal care during the first trimester. This may improve nutrition delivery to the unborn child to avoid pregnancy under- or over-nutrition, and thereby lower the risk of future obesity.[25] Grocery store tours are conducted in some clinics to teach shopping skills for healthy eating to program participants.
- Assess monitoring systems and develop policies or protocols to target high-risk children older than 2 years who exhibit rapid weight gain, and ensure that they receive intensive guidance through culturally appropriate interventions.
- Train the healthcare team in anticipatory guidance and counseling, with regard to infant and child feeding and physical activity consistent with obesity prevention, to enable the team to serve as positive role models.
- Assess the clinic environment for inconsistencies (deliberate as well as unintended) in the healthy eating and physical activity messages, and develop policies that promote a healthy environment for staff and program participants.
- Develop policies and environmental interventions that promote, support, and protect breast feeding.

Head Start/Preschool/Day Care

- Develop policies that ensure healthy menu items and eating environments for children.
- Develop policies that ensure children participate in recommended physical activity daily.
- Train child care providers and the food service team in obesity prevention strategies through provision of nutritious food choices and daily physical activity appropriate for age and development.
- Assist with grant writing to fund environmental intervention (e.g., playground, equipment for physical activity) and policy interventions for staff and parents to attend training in healthy eating practices for children. In addition, sponsor community events that involve families and staff to adopt healthy living practices, such as reducing sedentary behavior and increasing physical activity.

School Systems

- Advocate for daily recess and active physical education for all children through school boards, parent and teacher organizations, and school administrators.
- Develop policies that limit competitive foods and beverages, and serve fresh fruits and vegetables daily on the breakfast and lunch menus.

- Develop nutrition standards for vending machines and school stores.
- Advocate for a unified message for healthy eating and physical activity throughout the school (no candy fund-raisers, no food and/or candy rewards for good behavior in the classroom, healthy snacks at parties and school events, and a campus that is friendly to physical activity, such as walkways, bicycle racks, and safe outdoor play equipment).
- Advocate for universal school breakfast and lunch program participation.
- Advocate for strengthening the nutrition education throughout the entire school curriculums, K-12, and make an impact on student behavior (50 hours/year minimum).[89]
- Develop monitoring systems to assess children's health and behaviors (e.g., height and weight, BMI, blood pressure, fruit and vegetable consumption, TV viewing, transportation modes to school, and actual physical activity during recess and PE classes).

After-School Care

- Train staff to support obesity prevention efforts (healthy snacks, physical activity for all children).
- Survey the environment for consistency of the health messages, minimizing the availability of competitive foods of poor nutritional quality, and make the environment friendly to physical activity.
- Assist with obtaining grants to provide facilities and equipment to enable and encourage physical activity (e.g., walking track, basketball court, playground equipment, etc.).

Other Possible Venues

- Advocate for child participation in federal summer feeding programs for needy children.
- Advocate for a healthful environment at various settings for children, such as Boys and Girls Clubs, YMCA/YWCA, summer camps, and other programs through provision of training opportunities and materials in obesity prevention to directors and their staff.
- See the Resources section at the end of the chapter for examples and additional possible venues.

Programs and Resources That Support Evidence-Based Practices in Preventing Overweight in Children

The CDC's Nutrition and Physical Activity Program has established three evidence-based goals to prevent and control obesity:

- To increase physical activity
- To reduce television viewing
- To improve nutrition through increased breast feeding, fruit and vegetable consumption, and healthy eating[90]

Although research is limited on successful practices in various settings, the following are a few programs and resources that may be used by a public health nutritionist when addressing overweight in children.

Physical Activity

KidsWalk-to-School   A community-based program developed by the CDC Nutrition and Physical Activity Program, KidsWalk-to-School "...encourages children to walk to and from school in groups accompanied by adults."[91] This program mobilizes community members such as school staff, the Parent Teacher Association, police departments, businesses, civic associations, and so on to work together to increase safe routes to and from school for children to walk or use their bicycles. Overall, the community becomes aware of the importance of children participating in daily physical activity, thereby changing an unwalkable community into a walkable community, which is an environmental intervention. This program supports the HP 2010 objectives related to children's trips to school by walking or bicycling.[79]

Television Viewing

TV Turnoff Network   The goal of TV Turnoff Network is to encourage children and adults to turn off the television and replace that time with quality life activities that promote healthier living and communities. It sponsors two programs: TV Turnoff Week (now known as Digital Detox week) and More Reading, Less TV. TV Turnoff Week is held during the last week of April of every year. It encourages physical activities, such as gardening, skating, dancing, walking, bicycling, or playing a sport, along with other non-physical activities. More Reading, Less TV encourages reading as a replacement to television viewing among children and adults. As mentioned earlier, there is a link between excessive TV viewing and increased BMI in children. Thus, decreasing TV viewing may encourage children to be more physically active.[92] These programs support the HP 2010 objectives related to increasing the number of adolescents watching two hours or less of television on school days.[79]

Nutrition

Breast Feeding   Because breast feeding may be an early intervention to prevent childhood obesity, breast-feeding promotion can occur in various settings. For instance, the public health nutritionist may develop a breast-feeding coalition that focuses on developing breast-feeding policies in work sites, hospitals, or public areas. In addition, coalition members may monitor and evaluate the interventions implemented. Or, a public health nutritionist may collaborate with partners or participate in coalitions to increase breast-feeding awareness and promotion through World Breast-feeding Week, health fairs, or other community events. In addition, a public health nutritionist may train other nutritionists, nurses, doctors, or other medical professionals on breast-feeding management and support ways to increase breast-feeding initiation and duration rates. In a clinical setting, a public health nutritionist may provide one-on-one breast-feeding education, counseling, and support of pregnant and lactating women to increase the breast-feeding initiation and duration rates. This initiative supports the HP 2010 objectives related to increasing the proportion of women who breast-feed their babies.[79]

Fruits and Veggies Matter The Produce for Better Health Foundation is a consumer education foundation that launched a new national campaign. This program is the nation's largest public-private nutrition education initiative. Fruits and Veggies Matter is observed monthly and encourages people to consume 7 to 13 servings a day of colorful fruits and vegetables. Researchers have studied the relationship between fruit and vegetable intake and weight maintenance and loss in the pediatric population. Some found that it is possible to decrease overweight and to increase the consumption of fruits and vegetables. Strategies to decrease energy intake while increasing fruit and vegetable intake hold promise as a dietary approach to lowering risk of overweight. Additionally, a message to increase fruits and vegetable intake has the benefit of being positive and guiding people to eat healthy foods, rather than being negative as when recommending that people do not eat high fat and sugary foods.[93,94] In addition, Fruit and Vegetable campaigns are useful because they have adaptable toolkits and other promotional items that fit various settings. In particular, *There Is a Rainbow on My Plate* is a useful guide. It is designed to educate children on the importance of healthy eating by consuming a variety of colorful fruits and vegetables. This initiative supports the HP 2010 objective related to persons two years and older consuming several servings of fruits and vegetables daily.[79]

Other Programs Beyond breast feeding, healthy eating habits among toddlers and children are vitally important, as these lay the foundation for life-long eating habits. There are many good sources of information on healthy eating practices among toddlers. One example is Children's Healthcare of Atlanta's Stress-Free Feeding curriculum,[95] which advocates a healthy eating environment that includes patience and learning healthy eating habits for both the parent and child. This initiative supports the HP 2010 objective (developmental) related to increasing the proportion of children and adolescents who consume meals and snacks that are of good overall dietary quality.[79]

The programs and resources discussed above are only a few avenues to explore and suggest to partners and perhaps focus groups. To accomplish the ultimate goal of healthy children in healthy communities, the public health nutritionist should be resourceful when suggesting programs, initiatives, and campaigns related to overweight in children.

He or she must have a toolbox of information ready when entering various settings: coalition, community, school, worksite, healthcare facility, or other organizations. This toolbox of information and resources will vary depending on the target population. Nevertheless, public health nutritionists must be creative and timely in sharing their vision and potential solutions to address childhood obesity. The authors encourage public health nutritionists and students to research other resources and participate in Internet listservs for best practices and new findings in preventing and controlling overweight in children.

■ ONE COMMUNITY'S EXPERIENCE

A local university conducted a surveillance study on 4th, 8th, and 11th graders in a small southern rural county. After reviewing the process and conducting visual observations, it was evident to the public health nutritionist and county nurse that the student population had a large number of overweight children. When grants became available on preventing heart disease and overweight in children, the baseline data were available from the university.

The public health nutritionist reviewed the grant and its requirements, and discussed the grant application with key partners in the county (the county charge nurse, school superintendent and nurse, and community leaders). A grant application was submitted, describing the county demographics, assessment of the problem, goals, objectives, strategies, time frame, stakeholders, and budget along with letters of support. The grant was awarded to work with this school district. The goals were to conduct the School Health Index (SHI) and develop policy and environmental interventions related to physical activity and nutrition.

The public health nutritionist presented the problems of obesity in children and factors involved, such as soda consumption, decreased whole milk consumption, increased sedentary behavior and decreased PE, TV viewing, and computer games. In addition, possible solutions through the use of the SHI and policy and environmental interventions were presented. An SHI site coordinator was appointed and teachers were assigned to one of eight different teams. The SHI teams completed the SHI questionnaire and met with the public health nutritionist for technical assistance in developing an action plan. This action plan served as a guide when using grant funding to ensure expenditures were appropriate and related to the goals and objectives of the project.

Many interventions were developed from the SHI. A recommendation was developed to assess all fund-raising activities to ensure that items sold were non-food items and/or encouraged healthy eating. Second, a policy was developed to sell only low-fat milk and use whole-wheat bread on school menus. Third, an environmental intervention for the school was to build a walking track to be used by students, staff, and community members to encourage daily exercise. Finally, the SHI team established a county-wide community health day featuring several events including a five kilometer (5K) marathon run, a one-mile fun walk, and a health fair that assessed community members' blood pressure, blood sugar, waist circumference, and BMI for free. In addition, children participated in a reading expo, and TV Turnoff Week was promoted. Local sponsors, including the school nutrition program, grocers, and a bottling company, donated fruits, vegetables, and water, respectively. This community event involved many partners from the hospital and health department as well as private and public donors. Television and print media promoted many activities related to healthy eating, physical activity, and the decrease of TV viewing, and covered the accomplishments of the local school staff and partners.

In addition, process and outcome evaluation tools were developed by the public health nutritionist to determine if the goals and objectives were met, as outlined in the grant application. The public health nutritionist developed an additional survey tool to capture the health status of adults who attended the health fair. The school principal developed and completed an evaluation tool to determine who used the track and how many miles were walked among students during the school year. For TV Turnoff Week, the public health nutritionist developed pre- and post-surveys to determine if participants changed their behavior during that week. From the series of events, baseline data were gathered, partnerships developed, and the potential to receive additional funds to address childhood obesity increased. A small grant mobilized the school and community to participate in healthy lifestyle choices that work toward preventing chronic diseases caused by obesity.

■ SUMMARY

Public health nutritionists may use existing nutrition and social programs as opportunities to promote evidence-based strategies to prevent obesity in children.

However, many programs are designed for specific groups (such as WIC) and do not serve or reach all segments of the population that are involved in the care of children. Because many nutrition and social programs have a narrow focus, population-based services are essential to help communities, schools, worksites, other organizations, and families to adopt healthy behaviors. Healthy eating among children cannot be addressed without including the family as a whole and the environment. As discussed earlier, almost 65% of adults are overweight or obese, and this is a risk factor for their children becoming overweight.[61,96,97]

Overweight in children is a major public health concern; however, preventive efforts must target the parents and caregivers as well as the children. "If obese parents of at-risk children reduce access to low-nutrient, calorically dense foods available in the shared family environment, model healthier eating and activity habits, and share positive food-related family experiences that reinforce eating high nutrient-dense foods, the parents may reduce the risk of their child becoming obese as well as modify their own body weight."[93] Improving family interaction through healthy eating practices and physical activity is essential to preventing childhood obesity. Healthy lifestyle behaviors can be taught in parenting classes and discussed during doctor's office visits, at worksites, at health fairs, in parent–teacher organizations, and at other sites. In addition, population-based services and partners can develop and implement policy and environmental interventions that make it convenient for families to include healthy eating practices and daily physical activity.

Healthy eating practices and physical activity are interrelated when addressing childhood obesity. Both play an integral role in decreasing the rate of overweight in the United States. Although some traditional public health nutrition roles, as nutrition educator or a consultant to medical professionals, are still valuable, the new role of public health nutrition practitioners has expanded to include stepping outside of the office and into the community. Working with partners is essential, as is obtaining financial resources to implement programs in the community or schools. The media offers endless opportunities to reach target populations with various health messages and social marketing campaigns. Policy and advocacy will be crucial in developing standard nutrition and physical activity policies within various settings.

The prevention and control of overweight and obesity in this society will be one of the greatest public health challenges in the 21st century. Public health nutritionists have rich opportunities for innovation, creativity, and personal development as this challenge demands the use of each person's unique skills: up-to-date knowledge of evidence-based care, communication and media skills, grant writing and budget know-how, research and presentation skills, advocacy and policy development, cultural competency, and relationship and coalition building. Population-based approaches should be comprehensive so that environmental changes will support healthy eating and regular physical activity and encourage optimal health for people of all ages.

Picture a future where prenatal care is provided for all pregnant women in the first trimester and health professionals provide anticipatory counseling for families to encourage breast feeding and prevent feeding problems. Working mothers are given adequate breast-feeding support before and after returning to work. Allowable WIC foods include fresh fruits and vegetables year-round in addition to the traditional WIC foods. Other food programs provide access to fresh produce at low cost for low-income families. Children learn early to love foods that will sustain their health, and feel secure that they will have enough to eat. Schools serve nutritious lunches that children enjoy, and recess time allows for daily physical activity for all children. Vending machines at school are stocked with healthful choices that supply nutrients important to children's health. After-school programs offer ample opportunities to play and consume nutritious snacks. Neighborhoods are planned with adequate green space for play and recreation, or parks are added during urban renewal projects. Children can walk or ride their bikes safely to and from school on walking trails and bike paths. Neighborhoods are planned for mixed use so that it is possible to walk to the store or other local businesses. Government agricultural support is increased for the growing of fruits and vegetables, while government subsidies for production of corn for high-fructose corn syrup manufacturing decrease. Healthy foods are inexpensive, and high fat and sugar foods are expensive. Advertisers don't advertise high-fat and sweetened foods to children during and between children's TV programming. Children participate in daily activities and their weight gain is appropriate for their growth and development. Hopefully, healthy children will become healthy adults with many quality years of life.

Issues for Discussion

1. Why is it important to have internal and external partnerships? Why is it important for public health nutritionists and internal partners to be aware of their agencies' programs and services? Discuss programs or services of a local community that you may promote to a school board to prevent or control obesity in children.

2. Physical activity and exercise are as important as healthy eating in the pediatric population. How would you include physical activity as an intervention for children if you have limited training in this area?

3. List and describe other tools or resources that a public health nutritionist may use to address overweight in children.

4. Develop a sample survey for a Parent Teacher Association to determine children's and parents' eating habits and physical activity levels. What partnerships would you develop? How would you administer the survey?

5. What power (if any) does the government have to influence factors that impact overweight in children?

6. Discuss how the media may promote overweight in children and how it may be used to prevent this problem.

7. What should the public health nutritionist consider when planning or implementing overweight-in-children prevention interventions for families in clinic settings or special programs?

8. List ways a public health nutritionist can measure the success of an intervention related to preventing overweight in children. Provide an example of one of them.

Resources

Professional Organizations

American Academy of Pediatricians
http://www.aap.org
http://www.pediatrics.org

American Dietetic Association
http://www.eatright.org

American Medical Association
http://ama-assn.org

American Nurse Association
http://www.ana.org

American Psychological Association
http://www.apa.org

American Public Health Association
http://www.apha.org

Society of Nutrition Education
http://www.sne.org

Statistical or Surveillance Systems

Behavioral Risk Factor Surveillance System (BRFSS)
http://www.cdc.gov/brfss

Kaiser Family Foundation's state health facts online
http://www.statehealthfacts.kff.org

Maternal and Child Health Bureau
http://www.mchdata.net

National Center for Health Statistics
http://www.cdc.gov/nchs

Pediatric and Pregnancy Nutrition Surveillance System
http://www.cdc.gov/pednss/

Statistical Abstract of the United States: 2004–2005
http://www.census.gov/compendia/statab/

Statistics Related to Overweight or Obesity
http://www2.niddk.nih.gov/statistics/index.htm

Youth Risk Behavior Surveillance System (YRBSS)
http://www.cdc.gov/HealthyYouth/yrbs/index.htm

Policy and Environmental Interventions

Center for Nutrition Policy and Promotion
http://www.usda.gov/cnpp

Center for Science in the Public Interest School
Nutrition Policy
http://www.cspinet.org/nutritionpolicy

The Community Tool Box
http://ctb.ku.edu

Model School Wellness Policies
http://www.schoolwellnesspolicies.org

National Association of State Boards of
Education: Fit, Healthy and Ready to Learn:
A School Health Policy Guide
http://www.nasbe.org/index.php/eli/
53-shs-resources/396-fit-healthy-and-ready-
to-learn-a-school-health-policy-guide

National Recreation and Park Association
http://www.nrpa.org

Nutrition

Center for Science in the Public Interest Nutrition Policy Project: School Foods Tool Kit. A
Guide to Improving School Foods and Beverages
http://www.cspinet.org/schoolfood

Children's Healthcare of Atlanta
http://www.choa.org

Dietary Guidelines for Americans
http://www.nal.usda.gov/fnic/dga

MyPyramid Plan
http://www.mypyramid.gov

Breast Feeding

Baby Friendly Hospital Initiative
http://www.babyfriendlyusa.org

Blueprint for Breastfeeding
HHS Blueprint for Action on Breastfeeding.
DHHS Office of Women's Health, 2000
http://www.womenshealth.gov/breastfeeding/
programs/blueprints/

Fruits and Vegetables

Fruits and Veggies Matter
http://www.fruitsandveggiesmatter.gov

Junior Master Gardner Program
http://jmgkids.us

Dairy

1% or Less Campaign-School Kit
http://www.cspinet.org/nutrition/schoolkit.
html

3-A-Day
http://www.3aday.org

Dairy Council
http://www.nationaldairycouncil.org

Exercise

Hearts N' Parks Program
http://www.nhlbi.nih.gov/health/prof/
heart/obesity/hrt_n_pk/index.htm

National Association for Sport and Physical
Education
http://www.aahperd.org/naspe

National Recreation and Park Association
http://www.nrpa.org

PE4life
http://www.pe4Life.com

The President's Council on Physical Fitness
and Sports
http://www.fitness.gov

Take 10!
http://www.take10.net

Media

Centers for Disease Control and Prevention,
Youth Media Campaign
http://www.cdc.gov/youthcampaign

TV Turnoff Network
http://www.tvturnoff.org

School Resources

Action for Healthy Kids
http://www.actionforhealthykids.org

The Center for Health and Healthcare in
Schools: School Health Issues
http://www.healthinschools.org/sh/obesity.asp

National Association of State Boards of
Education-Safe and Healthy Schools
http://www.nasbe.org

Planet Health
http://www.hsph.harvard.edu/prc/proj_
planet.html

School Health Index
http://apps.nccd.cdc.gov/shi

SPARK Program
   http://www.sparkpe.org

Team Nutrition
   http://www.fns.usda.gov/tn

Community Resources

Active Community Environments Initiative
   http://www.cdc.gov/nccdphp/dnpa/aces.
   htm

Association for Community Health Improvement
   http://www.communityhlth.org

Community Service Block Grant
   http://www.acf.hhs.gov/programs/ocs/
   csbg/index/htm

North Carolina Prevention Partners
   http://www.ncpreventionpartners.org

Task Force on Community Preventive Services
   http://www.thecommunityguide.org

Other Resources

American Public Health Association Food and
Nutrition Section: Childhood Overweight
   http://www.aphafoodandnutrition.org/
   overwt.html

Bright Futures
   http://www.brightfutures.org

Center for Science in the Public Interest
   http://www.cspinet.org

Centers for Disease Control and Prevention
   http://www.cdc.gov

Centers for Disease Control and Prevention
Evaluation and Working Group
   http://www.cdc.gov/eval/index.htm

Cooperative State Research, Education, and
Extension Service
   http://www.csrees.usda.gov

GrantsNet: Federal Grant Information
   http://www.hhs.gov/grantsnet/

Healthy People 2010
   http://www.healthypeople.gov

Institute of Medicine: Focus on Childhood
Obesity
   http://iom.edu/focuson.asp?id = 22593

Maternal and Child Health Bureau
   http://www.mchb.hrsa.gov

National Institute of Health
   http://health.nih.gov

U.S. Department of Health and Human Services
   http://www.hhs.gov

YMCA of the USA
   http://www.ymca.org

References

1. Committee for the Study of the Future of Public Health Division of Healthcare Services. Institute of Medicine. *The Future of Public Health*. Washington, DC: National Academy Press; 1988.

2. Centers for Disease Control and Prevention. *Use and Interpretation of the CDC Growth Charts*. Available at http://www.cdc.gov/nccdphp/dnpa/growthcharts/00binaries/growthchart.pdf. Accessed April 12, 2010.

3. Serdula MK, Ivery D, Coates RJ, Freedman DS, Williamson DF, Byers T. Do obese children become obese adults? A review of literature. *Prev Med*. 1993;22:167–177.

4. Freedman DS, Khan LK, Dietz WH, Srinivasan SR, Berenson GS. Relationship of childhood obesity to coronary heart disease risk factors in adulthood: The Bogalusa Heart Study. *Pediatrics*. 2001;108:712–718.

5. Ellis KJ, Abrams SA, Wong WW. Monitoring childhood obesity: assessment of weight/height2 index. *Am J Epidemiol*. 1999;150:939–946.

6. Taylor RW, Jones IE, Williams SM, Goulding A. Body fat percentages measured by dual-energy X-ray absorptiometry corresponding to recently recommended body mass index cutoffs for overweight and obesity in children and adolescents aged 3–18 y. *Am J Clin Nutr*. 2002;76:1416–1421.

7. Flegal KM, Tabak CJ, Ogden CL. Overweight in children: definitions and interpretation. *Health Edu Res*. 2006;21:755–760.

8. National Center for Health Statistics. *Prevalence of Overweight and Obesity Among Adults: United States, 1999–2002*.

9. Ogden CL, Carroll MD, Curtin LR, McDowell MA, Tabak CJ, Flegal KM. Prevalence of overweight and obesity in the United States, 1999–2004. *JAMA*. 2006;295:1549–1555.

10. Ogden CL, Carroll MD, Flegal KM. High body mass index for age among US children and adolescents, 2003–2006. *JAMA*. 2008;109:226–235.

11. Ogden CL, Flegal KM, Carroll MD, Johnson CL. Prevalence and trends in overweight among US children and adolescents, 1999–2000. *JAMA*. 2002;288:1728–1732.

12. Freedman DS, Khan LK, Dietz WH, Srinivasan SR, Berenson GS. Relationship of childhood obesity to coronary heart disease risk factors in adulthood: The Bogalusa Heart Study. *Pediatrics*. 2001;108:712–718.

13. Hill JO, Wyatt HR, Reed GW, Peters JC. Obesity and the environment: where do we go from here? *Science*. 2003;299:853–855.

14. Berenson GS. Childhood risk factors predict adult risk associated with subclinical cardiovascular disease: The Bogalusa Heart Study. *Am J Cardiol*. 2002;90(suppl):3L–7L.

15. Hassink S. Problems in childhood obesity. *Prim Care Office Prac*. 2003;30:357–374.

16. Raman RP. Obesity and health risks. *J Amer Coll Nutr*. 2002; 21(2):134S–139S.

17. Erickson SJ, Robinson TN, Haydel KF, Killen JD. Are overweight children unhappy? *Arch Pediatr Adolesc Med*. 2000;154:931–935.

18. Hill JO, Trowbridge FL. Childhood obesity: future directions and research priorities. *Pediatrics*. 1998;101(suppl):570–574.

19. Nelson JA, Chiasson MA, Ford V. Overweight children in a New York City WIC population. *Am J Public Health*. 2004;94:458–462.

20. Strauss RS, Pollack HA. Epidemic increase in overweight children, 1986–1998. *JAMA*. 2001;286:2845–2848.

21. Wang G, Dietz WH. Economic burden of obesity in youths aged 6 to 17 years: 1979–1999. *Pediatrics*. 2002;109:E81-1.

22. Editorial. Who pays in the obesity war? *Lancet*. 2004;363:339.

23. Mokdad AH, Marks JS, Stroup DF, Gerberding JL. Actual causes of death in the United States. 2000. *JAMA*. 2004;291:1263–1264.

24. Mokdad AH, Marks JS, Stroup DF. Correction: Actual Causes of Death in the United States, 2000. *JAMA*. 2005; 293:292–294.

25. Dietz WH. Overweight in childhood and adolescence. *N Engl J Med*. 2004;350:855–857.

26. Booth SL, Sallis JF, Ritenbaugh C, et al. (Working Group II). Environmental and societal factors affect food choice and physical activity: rationale, influences, and leverage points. *Nutr Rev*. 2001;59(3, part 2):S21–S39.

27. O'Keefe JH, Cordain L. Cardiovascular disease resulting from a diet and lifestyle at odds with our Paleolithic genome: how to become a 21st century hunter-gatherer. *Mayo Clin Proc*. 2004;79:101–108.

28. Simopoulos AP. The importance of the ratio of omega-6/omega-3 fatty acids. *Biomed Pharmacother*. 2002;56:365–379.

29. Briefel RR, Johnson CL. Secular trends in dietary intake in the United States. *Annu Rev Nutr*. 2004;24:401–431.

30. Simopoulos AP. Evolutionary aspects of omega-3 fatty acids in the food supply. *Prostaglandins Leukot Essent Fatty Acids*. 1999;60:421–429.

31. Conner WE. Importance of n-3 fatty acids in health and disease. *Am J Clin Nutr*. 2000;71:171S–175S.

32. Bowman SA, Gortmaker SL, Ebbeling CB, Pereira MA, Ludwig DS. Effects of fast-food consumption on energy intake and diet quality among children in a national household survey. *Pediatrics*. 2004;113:112–118.

33. American Dietetic Association. The role of dietetics professionals in health promotion and disease prevention. *J Am Diet Assoc*. 2002;102:1680–1687.

34. Nicklas TA, Baranowski T, Cullen KW, Berenson G. Eating patterns, dietary quality, and obesity. *J Amer Coll Nutr*. 2001;20:599–608.

35. Sebastian RS, Wilkinson EC, Goldman JD. US adolescents and MyPyramid: associations between fast-food consumption and lower likelihood of meeting recommendations. *J Am Diet Assoc*. 2009;109:226–235.

36. Kurzweil P. Taking the fat out of food. *FDA Consumer Magazine*. 1996 Jul-Aug;30(6).

37. Munoz KA, Krebs-Smith SM, Ballard-Barbash R, Cleveland LE. Food intakes of U.S. children and adolescents compared with recommendations. *Pediatrics*. 1997;100:323–329.

38. McBean LD, Miller GD. Enhancing the nutrition of America's youth. *J Am Coll Nutr*. 1999;18:563–571.

39. Warren JM, Henry CJ, Simonite V. Low glycemic index breakfasts and reduced food intake in preadolescent children. *Pediatrics*. 2003;112:e414.

40. Roberts SB. High-glycemic index foods, hunger and obesity: is there a connection? *Nutr Rev*. 2000;58:163–169.

41. Augustin LS, Franceschi S, Jenkins DJA, Kendall CWC, La Vecchia C. Glycemic index in chronic disease: a review. *Eur J Clin Nutr*. 2002;56:1049–1071.

42. Paeratakul S, Ferdinand DP, Champagne CM, Ryan DH, Bray GA. Fast-food consumption among U.S. adults and children: Dietary and nutrient intake profile. *J Am Diet Assoc*. 2003;103:1332–1338.

43. Harnack L, Stang J, Story M. Soft drink consumption among U.S. children and adolescents: nutritional consequences. *J Am Diet Assoc*. 1999;99:436–441.

44. Ludwig DS, Peterson KE, Gortmaker SL. Relation between consumption of sugar-sweetened drinks and childhood obesity: a prospective, observational analysis. *Lancet*. 2001;357:505–508.

45. Johnson SL. Improving preschoolers' self-regulation of energy intake. *Pediatrics*. 2000;106:1429–1435.

46. Birch LL, Fischer JO. Development of eating behaviors among children and adolescents. *Pediatrics*. 1998;101:539–547.

47. Allison DB, Faith MS. Genetic and environmental influences on human body weight: implications for the behavior therapist. *Nutr Today*. 2000;35:18–21.

48. Fisher JO, Birch LL. Restricting access to palatable foods affects children's behavioral response, food selection, and intake. *Am J Clin Nutr*. 1999;69:1264–1272.

49. Johnson SL, Birch LL. Parents' adiposity and children's eating style. *Pediatrics*. 1994;94:653–661.

50. Satter E. *How to Get Kids to Eat...But Not Too Much*. Palo Alto, CA: Bull Publishing; 1987.

51. Satter E. *Secrets of Feeding a Healthy Family*. Madison, WI: Kelcy Press; 1999.

52. Satter E. *Child of Mine: Feeding with Love and Good Sense*. Palo Alto, CA: Bull Publishing; 2000.

53. Drewnowski A, Specter SE. Poverty and obesity: the role of energy density and energy costs. *Am J Clin Nutr*. 2004;79:6–16.

54. Alaimo K, Olson CM, Frongillo Jr. EA. Low family income and food insufficiency in relation to overweight in U.S. children. Is there a paradox? *Arch Pediatr Adolsc Med*. 2001;155:1161–1167.

55. Jones SJ, Jahns L, Laraia BA, Haughton B. Lower risk of overweight in school-aged food insure girls who participate in food assistance. *Arch Pediatr Adolesc Med*. 2003;157:780–784.

56. Gibson D. Long-term food stamp program participation is differently related to overweight in young girls and boys. *J Nutr*. 2004;34:372–379.

57. Wang Y, Beydoun MA. The obesity epidemic in the United States—gender, age, socioeconomic, racial/ethnic, and geographic characteristics: a systematic review and meta-regression analysis. *Epidemiol Rev*. 2007;29:6–28.

58. Armstrong J, Reilly JJ. Breastfeeding and lowering risk of childhood obesity. Child Health Information Team. *Lancet*. 2002;359:2003–2004.

59. Dietz WH. Breastfeeding may help prevent overweight children. *JAMA*. 2001;285:2506–2507.

60. Adair LS. Methods appropriate for studying the relationship of breast-feeding to obesity. *J Nutr*. 2009;139:408S–411S.

61. Ziegler EE. Growth of breast-fed and formula-fed infants. *Nestlie Nutrition Workshop series*. 2006;58:51–59; discussion 59–63.

62. Frumkin H. Urban sprawl and public health. *Public Health Rep*. 2002;117:201–217.

63. Burgenson CR, Wechsler H, Brener ND, Young JC, Spain CG. Physical education and activity: results from the School Health Policies and Programs Study 2000. *J Sch Health*. 2001;71:279–293.

64. Andersen RE, Crespo CJ, Bartlett SJ, Cheskin LJ, Pratt M. Relationship of physical activity and television watching with body weight and level of fatness among children: results from the Third National Health and Nutrition Examination Survey. *JAMA*. 1998;279:938–942.

65. Gortmaker SL, Must A, Sobol AM, Peterson K, Colditz GA, Dietz WH. Television viewing as a cause of increasing obesity among children in the United States, 1986–1990. *Arch Pediatr Adolesc Med*. 1996;150:356–362.

66. Dowda M, Ainsworth BE, Addy CL, Saunders R, Riner W. Environmental influences, physical activity, and weight status in 8- to 16-year-olds. *Arch Pediatr Adolesc Med*. 2001;155:711–717.

67. Kaiser Family Foundation. Kids & media @ the new millennium: a Kaiser Family Foundation report. Available at http://www.kff.org/entmedia/1535-index.cfm. Accessed April 2, 2010.

68. Robinson TN, Hammer LD, Killen JD, Kraemer HC, Wilson DM, Hayward C, Taylor CB. Does television viewing increase obesity and reduce physical activity? Cross-sectional and longitudinal analyses among adolescent girls. *Pediatrics*. 1993;91:273–280.

69. Crawford P, Gosliner W, Anderson C, et al. Counseling Latina mothers of preschool children about weight issues: suggestions for a new framework. *J Am Diet Assoc*. 2004;104:387–394.

70. Borzekowski DLG, Robinson TN. The 30-second effect: an experiment revealing the impact of television commercials on food preferences of preschoolers. *J Am Diet Assoc.* 2001;101: 42–46.

71. Steinback KS. The importance of physical activity in the prevention of overweight and obesity in childhood: a review and an option. *Obes Rev.* 2001;2:117–130.

72. Antipatis VJ, Kumanyika S, Jeffery RW, Morabia A, Ritenbaugh C. Confidence of health professionals in public health approaches to obesity prevention. *Int J Obes Relat Metab Disord.* 1999;23:1004–1006.

73. Hill JO, Melanson EL, Wyatt HT. Dietary fat intake and regulation of energy balance: implications for obesity. *J Nutr.* 2000;130:284S–288S.

74. Jefferry RW. Public health strategies for obesity treatment and prevention. *Am J Health Behav.* 2001;125:252–259.

75. Schmitz MK, Jeffery RW. Public health interventions for the prevention and treatment of obesity. *Med Clin North Am.* 2000;84:491–512.

76. Ariza AJ, Greenberg RS, Unger R. Overweight children: management approaches in young children. *Pediatr Ann.* 2004;33:33–38.

77. Copperman N, Jacobson MS. Childhood obesity: interventions for the prevention and treatment of pediatrics overweight. Pediatric Perspectives Newsletter. *Mead Johnson and Company.* 2004.

78. Fox KR. Childhood obesity and the role of physical activity. *J Roy Soc Health.* 2004;124:34–39.

79. U.S. Department of Health and Human Services. *Healthy People 2010*, 2nd ed. With Understanding and Improving Health and Objectives for Improving Health. 2 vols. Washington, DC: U.S. Government Printing Office; November 2000. Information also available at http://www.healthypeople.gov/

80. Mullis RM. Entrepreneur in action. In: Boyle MA, Morris DH, eds., *Community Nutrition in Action: An Entrepreneurial Approach.* St. Paul, Minn: West Publishing;1994:434.

81. Temple SP. Professional focus. In: Boyle MA, Morris DH, eds. *Community Nutrition in Action: An Entrepreneurial Approach.* St. Paul, Minn: West Publishing; 1994:324.

82. University of Kansas. *Community Tool Box.* Available at: http://ctb.ku.edu/index.jsp. Accessed April 2, 2010.

83. Centers for Disease Control and Prevention, National Center for Chronic Disease. Healthy Youth! Welcome to the School Health Index (SHI). Available at https://apps.nccd.cdc.gov/shi/default.aspx.

84. Bogden JF. Fit, *Healthy, and Ready to Learn: A School Health Policy Guide*, Part I: Physical Activity, Healthy Eating and Tobacco-Use Prevention. Alexandria, VA: National Association of State Boards of Education; 2000.

85. Alfano CM, Klesges RC, Murray DM, Beech BM, McClanahan BS. History of sport participation in relation to obesity and related health behaviors in women. *Prev Med.* 2002;34:82–89.

86. Centers for Disease Control and Prevention. Framework for program evaluation in public health. *Morbid Mortal Wkly Rep MMWR.* 1999;48(No. RR-11):1–40.

87. Kettner PM, Moroney RM, Martin LL. *Designing and Managing Programs: An Effective-Based Approach.* Newbury Park, CA: Sage Publications; 1990.

88. National Center for Chronic Disease Prevention and Health Promotion. Welcome to the Youth Risk Behavioral Survey 2009. Available at http://www.k12.wy.us/hs/yrbs/yrbs.asp. Accesssed June 14, 2010.

89. Position of the American Dietetic Association, Society for Nutrition Education, and the American School Food Service Association. Nutrition services: an essential component of comprehensive school health programs. *J Am Diet Assoc.* 2003;103:505–514.

90. Centers for Disease Control and Prevention. *Resource Guide for Nutrition and Physical Activity Interventions to Prevent Obesity and Other Chronic Diseases*, 2003.

91. Centers for Disease Control and Prevention. KidsWalk-to-School. Nutrition and Physical Activity. Available at http://www.cdc.gov/nccdphp/dnpa/kidswalk/index.htm. Accessed April 2, 2010.

92. Center for Screen Time Awareness. Available at http://www.tvturnoff.org. Accessed April 2, 2010.

93. Epstein LH, Gordy CC, Raynor HA, Beddome M, Kilanowski CK, Paluch R. Increasing fruit and vegetable intake and decreasing fat and sugar intake in families at risk for childhood obesity. *Obes Res.* 2001;9:171–178.

94. Rolls BJ, Ello-Martin JA, Tohill BC. What can intervention studies tell us about the relationship between fruit and vegetable consumption and weight management. *Nutr Rev.* 2004;62:1–17.

95. Buechner J. *Stress-Free Feeding Curriculum and Video.* Atlanta, GA: Children's Healthcare of Atlanta; 2001.

96. Agras WS, Hammer LD, Kraemer HC. Risk factors for overweight children. *J Pediatr.* 2004;145:20–25.

97. Strauss RS, Knight J. Influence of the home environment on the development of obesity in children. *Pediatrics.* 1999 June;103(6):e85. Available at http://www.pediatrics.org/cgi/content/full/103/6/e85. Accessed April 2, 2010.

CHAPTER 6

Intervening to Change the Public's Eating Behavior

Yeemay Su Miller, MS, RD

READER OBJECTIVES

After studying this chapter and reflecting on the contents, you should be able to:

1. Describe the social, economic, and environmental factors that influence eating behavior.
2. Discuss short- and long-term intervention strategies for improving dietary behavior.
3. Compare and contrast individualized interventions versus community or population-wide interventions.
4. Understand the advantages of using an ecological model as the approach for planning effective dietary behavior change strategies.
5. Recognize and understand the relationships among eating organic, having an ecological consciousness, and supporting sustainable food and agriculture, and how these can improve overall nutritional health.

■ INTRODUCTION

The field and science of nutrition seem to be constantly changing. While this keeps the work interesting for the nutrition professional, nutrition can be quite confusing for the average person. It is no wonder that many people tend just to follow the most current diet trend or, alternatively, abstain from following any dietary recommendations because they believe the advice will change soon anyway. Even when people are motivated to make positive changes in their eating habits, the environment in which they live, work, or attend school makes continuing healthy behaviors difficult. This is why an ecological approach to intervening in eating behaviors will make the strongest impact in causing and sustaining positive change. Furthermore, we must enlist and intervene in all sectors of society: individuals, families, schools, communities, employers, healthcare providers, mass media,

> **Ecological approach:** A framework that identifies multiple levels of influence (or factors) in the design, implementation, and evaluation of health promotion programs.[1]

and government. When all these players in all the various settings work together, favorable health outcomes can be achieved.

■ CURRENT EATING TRENDS

In the past two decades, we have seen an increase in nutritional labeling information on packaged foods, greater availability of healthy choices, and more organic foods available in the marketplace and in some restaurants. The average daily consumption of vegetables, fruits, and grain products also increased during the 1990s.[2] The percentage of energy consumption from saturated fat over the last 30 years has declined; however, the total amount of fat in grams increased between 1981 and 2000.[3,4] Additionally, Americans are actually eating, on average, 250 to 300 calories more per day, much of it from carbohydrates, especially refined sugars.[3,5] Data from the National Health and Nutrition Examination Survey (NHANES) for 1971–2000 indicate similar trends in intake. According to the U.S. Department of Agriculture (USDA) survey data for 1977–1996, factors contributing to the increase in energy intake in the United States include consumption of food away from home; increased calorie consumption from salty snacks, soft drinks, and pizza[4]; and larger portion sizes.[5,6]

> Remember that for adults, overweight is a body mass index (BMI) of 25 to 29.9 and obesity is a BMI ≥ 30.

The increase in portion sizes for restaurant and processed foods and beverages has occurred concurrently with increases in the prevalence of obesity. The average fast food burger, which weighed approximately 1 ounce in 1957, weighs up to 6 ounces now; the typical serving of soda, which was 8 fluid ounces in 1957, is now 32 to 64 fluid ounces; and the average theater serving of popcorn, which was 3 cups in 1957, is now 16 cups.[7]

American adults and children consume, on average, one third of their calories from eating out. Studies link eating out with obesity and higher caloric intakes.[8,9] For example, children eat almost twice as many calories when they eat a meal at a restaurant compared to a meal at home. Meals at chain restaurants can be unexpectedly high in calories, with appetizers, entrées, and desserts sometimes providing an entire day's worth of calories on a single plate.[10]

In the 1990s, dietary fat was deemed "the enemy"; hence, the food industry responded with a reduced-fat or fat-free version of nearly every packaged food available in the market, from cheese to crackers, pepperoni, and ice cream. Although these foods are lower in fat, they are not necessarily any lower in energy density than their full-fat counterparts. This fact contributes to Americans' confusion about healthy food options. A further result of America's dietary and body fat phobia and dieting practices is that many individuals unfortunately found themselves heavier than before and with an unfavorable blood lipid profile. More specifically, people developed higher triglyceride levels (also known more recently as triacylglycerol) and decreased their levels of high density lipids (HDLs).[11–13] The reason for this may be because when individuals deliberately avoid dietary fat, the result is a much higher intake of carbohydrates. However, this increase in carbohydrate consumption is not from healthful fruits, vegetables, and whole grains, but primarily from sugars and processed "white flour" carbohydrates.

Now the pendulum on diet composition has swung in the other direction. Many dieters are shunning carbohydrate-containing foods in favor of foods high in protein and fat, such as cheese, bacon, and all types of meats. A typical meal of a person on a "low-carb" diet might be a cheeseburger with lettuce and tomato without the bun, or eating the cheese and sauce from a pizza, but not the crust. Many Americans have forgone fat gram counting in favor of carbohydrate counting, and the food industry is again catering to this diet trend. Supermarkets and some restaurant chains now sell "low-carb" milk, bread, pasta, and cereals. Restaurants offering low-carb meals have opened to the delight of many dieters. Many similar restaurants may follow suit if the popularity of this diet fad continues.

The average American purchases and consumes between 40% and 50% of meals and snacks away from home.[14] These foods tend to be higher in calories and fat, lower in fiber, and larger in portion sizes than what would be eaten at home. In addition, snacks are occupying a bigger proportion of the average American diet. In 1977, snacks comprised 11.3% of the total caloric intake; and in 1996, 17.7% of total calories were obtained from snacks.[14] This is a 60% increase during the span of 18 years. Snacks are now a booming segment of sales in the food industry, which parallels the snacking habits of Americans.

> **Blood lipid profile:** A group of blood tests that are often ordered to determine risk of coronary heart disease. The lipid profile includes total cholesterol, high density lipoproteins (HDLs), low density lipoproteins (LDLs), and triglycerides.
>
> **Triglycerides:** These store energy, which is housed in fatty tissue and is gradually released between meals to meet the body's needs. High levels of triglycerides in the blood may be associated with coronary artery disease.

Eating is a normative, acceptable behavior in almost any setting, such as in the car, at meetings, at your desk at work, in theatres, and sporting events. Eating and drinking on-the-go thus is also a normal everyday occurrence for commuters and multitaskers with packed schedules. In contrast, ordering food or coffee "to go" in some countries is an unknown concept. As an example, cars in Japan do not have drink holders. Many of us have forgone the pleasurable, slower pace needed to truly enjoy a meal. Eating too fast is a habit many individuals admit to, which contributes to overeating. Of interest is a transcontinental study, conducted in 2003, comparing the amount of time spent eating in a McDonald's in Paris and one in Philadelphia.[15] Given that portion sizes are bigger in the United States compared to other countries, one might expect meals to take longer to eat. However, in Philadelphia, people on average finished their meals in 14.4 minutes, compared to 22.2 minutes in Paris.

Hectic schedules and less time for food shopping, preparation, and cooking at home has moved convenience to the top of the list that dictates food choice. "Our nation is a car culture," which led to the birth of drive-in restaurant chains, says Eric Schlosser in his book entitled, *Fast Food Nation*. "People are so lazy they don't even want to get out of them to eat!" said Jesse G. Kirby, the founder of an early drive-in restaurant chain.[16] However, the way our physical environment has been designed—evolving into suburban sprawl or car-centric cities throughout the United States—has made it unrealistic or unsafe to shop, run errands, or just go out on foot or by bike. The good news is that the city environment is beginning to change, as the Centers for Disease Control and Prevention (CDC) and other government agencies are recognizing the need to enlist city planners, architects, researchers, and transportation engineers to redesign cities and make them pedestrian-centered.[17,18]

Because the American lifestyle will likely not change in the immediate future, more options for healthy, convenient eating are needed. Some examples include low-fat prepared foods in supermarkets, an increased number and variety of restaurants that serve "lighter fare," the display of nutrition facts on restaurant menus, and drive-through "fast food" type establishments serving predominantly healthy choices. However, an essential factor for individuals is motivation to eat better and to become educated on the benefits of doing so.

■ OBESITY IN AMERICA

Two thirds of American adults are overweight, and 50% of those overweight are considered to be obese. Obesity is an epidemic and one of the most complex public health issues that we have yet to fully understand, treat, and prevent. It will soon surpass smoking (if it hasn't already) as the strongest risk factor contributing to the top major causes of death in our country. What we do know is that nothing short of intense efforts from all sectors of society will make a difference in curbing this tidal wave of weight upon the health of Americans. According to a study of national costs attributed to both overweight and obesity, medical expenses accounted for 9.1% of total U.S. medical expenditures in 1998, and may have reached as high as $78.5 billion ($92.6 billion in 2002 dollars).[19]

The increasing prevalence of obesity has greatly increased the risk of chronic diseases for all age segments. Children and adolescents are presently showing the greatest increase, which is a sobering issue that has made some public health officials predict that this present generation of children may be the first to live shorter lifespans than their parents. The rationale thus exists behind the increase in interventions and social marketing programs specifically targeting youth.

This chapter strives to present some strategies and interventions that have shown promise in improving the nutritional health of adults and children. (Chapter 5 contains specific nutritional interventions for children.) An improvement in Americans' nutritional habits should help rein in the rise in obesity and the insurmountable healthcare costs the nation faces.

Dieting

Despite the billions of dollars that Americans continue to spend yearly on diets and weight loss drugs, products, and programs, the prevalence of obesity continues to increase at alarming rates. Clearly, dieting alone is not the answer, and actually may be causing additional harm, as well as further weight gain.

For now, diets and dieting books have moved away from counting calories as the method of controlling food intake to manage weight. Instead, the focus is on consuming directed proportions of macro-nutrients (fat, protein, and carbohydrates). Other diets promote eating disproportional and high amounts of fat and protein while keeping the carbohydrate amount quite low, at the expense of forgoing the known beneficial, cancer-preventive food groups of vegetables, fruits, and whole grains.[20] Many individuals desperately want to lose weight, and even those educated in the areas of nutrition and health will follow a diet that promises quick weight loss at the expense of health, nutrition, and even life. This is a major challenge for nutritionists, who attempt to educate the public on the harm of fad diets only to be ignored by the determined dieter.

For the obese patient and/or chronic dieter, nutritionists, behavioral therapists, physicians, and other health professionals who have influence over a patient's eating habits have a responsibility to educate the public about diets that do not work in the long term. When an individual goes "on a diet," the person often may successfully lose weight regardless of the type of diet. However, being on a diet implies that you will at some point in time come off the diet, which just leads to weight regain because no permanent dietary changes have been made. Only when an individual is ready and willing to make permanent, life-long changes is he or she able to lose weight and keep it off. Helping an individual make a few small lasting changes in his or her eating behavior is an important goal, as opposed to facilitating many major changes for immediate, quick weight loss.

Trans-Fat

The public has become increasingly aware of the harm that *trans*-fatty acids (TFAs) can do to health, and this issue has become of great concern to many. Unfortunately, the amount of TFAs in North Americans' diets has increased markedly during the past decade. This increase can wreak havoc on individuals' blood lipid profile and thereby increase the risk of heart disease. We now know that *trans*-fat is more harmful in the diet than saturated fat in raising the risk of developing cardiovascular disease. Although it is clear that saturated fat can raise low density lipoproteins (LDLs) in the blood, *trans*-fat can raise LDLs and also decreased high density lipoproteins (HDLs). In addition, TFAs, but not saturated fatty acids, tend to increase

Low density lipoproteins (LDLs): Protein molecules that carry cholesterol in the blood and around the body for use by various cells.

High density lipoproteins (HDLs): Protein molecules that carry cholesterol back from tissues or organs to the liver, where cholesterol will be degraded or recycled.

Lipoprotein (a): A cholesterol-rich particle found in human plasma that combines structural elements from the lipoprotein and blood clotting systems and that is associated with premature coronary heart disease and stroke.

the levels of the highly atherogenic lipoprotein known as lipoprotein (a).[21]

Fortunately, the government, via the Food and Drug Administration (FDA), responded in 2006 by requiring that food manufacturers of packaged goods list the *trans*-fat content on the nutrition facts label. This enables the average consumer to more easily choose among the plethora of packaged foods and select the more healthful option by a quick glance at the nutrition facts label, instead of a longer screening of all the ingredients. Labeling has become a wise marketing ploy that appeals to the health-conscious consumer, especially if the product is made *trans*-fat–free, as some spreadable butter companies and snack food manufacturers have done.

Sadly, individuals who frequent fast food establishments are likely to have a high *trans*-fat intake because partially hydrogenated oils are used for cooking and frying all of the fare. When Dr. Walter Willett, Chairman of the Nutrition Department of the Harvard School of Public Health, was asked, "What specific public health intervention do you think would make the greatest impact in helping people actually eat healthier?" He replied, "Although no single intervention will solve all our nutritional problems, a ban on the use of partially hydrogenated fats would have an enormous impact, in part because the whole population would benefit almost immediately" (Personal communication, July 20, 2004). Some cities across the United States have started to do just that.

Until TFAs are completely eliminated from use in foods, education, public pressure, and consumer demand for the use of healthy oils by food manufacturers and restaurants remain as important strategies to advocate for our health.

■ CHANGING EATING BEHAVIOR

Current public health efforts tend to focus on reducing the prevalence of specific diseases, such as cardiovascular disease or cancer, by reducing blood cholesterol levels or improving screening practices. However, these efforts need to be balanced by addressing basic behavioral and social influences on food choice that may cause or prevent disease. To elucidate, we know that individuals who consume a diet rich in vegetables, fruits, and whole grains may reduce their risk of developing cardiovascular disease and certain cancers.[19] Unfortunately, among certain ethnic and socioeconomic groups, significant variations and disparities in disease exist. This can be partly due to minimized access to healthy foods, less offerings of good supermarkets, and, therefore, decreased variety of fresh, affordable produce and low-fat products in their community.[22] In addition, these communities often have many fast food establishments and small grocery stores that sell high-fat, energy-dense foods. Furthermore, high neighborhood crime rates discourage outdoor activities and limit safe places for walking and bi-

cycling. Even when individuals are given specific dietary advice and physical activity encouragement and are motivated to make changes, the current environment may make follow-through difficult because of substantial barriers to establishing a healthy lifestyle.

The Institute of Medicine (IOM) stated, "Interventions must recognize that people live in social, political, and economic systems that shape behaviors and access to the resources they need to maintain good health."[23] Even if individual behavior changes are made, this alone is not likely to result in improved health and quality of life without an environment that enables sustenance of those changes. Persons with higher levels of education and socioeconomic status continue to be linked with better health, and are more likely to adopt more healthful behaviors.[24,25]

Making recommended dietary changes can cost more money and may require more knowledge, skill, time, or effort to prepare food. Therefore, understanding psychosocial and environmental influences on food choice and consumption is essential to creating nutrition programs, designing educational messages, and disseminating dietary recommendations that realistically help consumers make healthier dietary changes. According to a report from the IOM, Promoting Health: Intervention Strategies from Social and Behavioral Research, "The key to helping people enjoy longer, healthier lives is to understand how to promote behavioral change and create healthier environments."[26] However, some of the most meaningful changes that will have the greatest impact on the public's eating behavior are likely be the most difficult to achieve.

This chapter strives to communicate effective nutrition interventions ranging from individual behavior change strategies to the complex, long-term, costlier, difficult process of affecting policy and greater societal changes. A multilevel approach will have the greatest, most sustaining effect on improving the population's eating behavior. Using a social ecological model as the theoretical framework from which one plans, creates, researches, applies, and evaluates nutrition interventions therefore would be most effective. The Healthy People 2010 goals are based on a multilevel approach to achieving those goals, as well as the IOM's recent report on promoting healthy behavior.[27] The social ecological perspective, as it has evolved in behavioral sciences and public health, focuses on the nature of people's transactions with their physical and sociocultural surroundings.[28]

> **Social ecological model:**
> An approach in which interventions address not only individual intentions and skills, but also the social and physical environmental context of a desired behavior, considering as well all social networks and organizations that share that environment, which will have the most potential for population-wide impact.[29]

Media is a principal source of information and influence on food and nutrition for many.[30] The leverage, or power, of media is its ability to persuade; alter norms, thinking, and behavior; and thereby prompt particular ways of eating.[31] Through experience, we have come to view mass media as a powerful way to promote the consumption of many unhealthy, processed food products. However, mass media can also positively encourage a significant proportion of people to alter their dietary habits. This was exhibited by a simple "1% or less" campaign in Wheeling, West Virginia, which used paid advertising and public relations to encourage members of one community to switch from whole or 2% milk to 1% or fat-free milk.[32] The effectiveness of the campaign was evident by a 17% increase in low-fat milk sales one month after the campaign; this increase was maintained at the six-month follow-up. Pre- and post-telephone surveys revealed that 34.1% of high-fat milk drinkers had switched to low-fat milk in the intervention community compared to 3.6% in the control community ($P < 0.0001$).

This mass-media-based "1% or less" milk campaign was replicated by the California Adolescent Nutrition and Fitness Program in Spanish to reach predominantly Latino American communities in Santa Paula (in 1999) and East Los Angeles (in 2000).[33] Campaign elements included paid radio and print ads, point-of-purchase advertising, milk taste tests, community presentations, public relations, and a school-based program. After the six-week campaign, sales of 1% and fat-free milk rose 60% in Santa Paula. A six-month follow-up survey of retailers found that a large portion (25%) of this growth in sales was maintained.

The Food Industry

In 1988, the World Health Organization (WHO) recommended that sugars should account for no more than 10% of daily energy intake.[34] This recommendation has not received universal acceptance, especially from the food industry. This is no surprise given that the industry's most lucrative products are processed foods, laden with sugar and/or salt, that are calorically dense. This explains why new products like these enter the marketplace almost daily. Given the plethora of choices, selecting a granola bar or snack cracker makes food shopping a much lengthier, more complicated process. A large array of choices can also contribute to overeating. When presented with more variety, individuals eat more. When food options are more monotonous, individuals tend to eat less. Reducing easy access to energy-dense foods could help limit the opportunities for overeating.[35]

The food industry is colossal and can exert powerful influence on government policy via lobbying techniques.[36] Although the food industry may be an important factor contributing to the poor nutritional habits of consumers, industry must be enlisted now as part of the solution. In the past, industry has been a key player in curing and preventing nutritional deficiencies by vitamin and mineral fortification of foods.[36] Remember also that the food industry is quite responsive to consumer and market demands; therefore, as more grass-roots and consumer groups call for healthier food choices as a top priority, the industry can and will respond.

Schools

Schools are practical, ideal places to reach thousands of children to educate them about healthy eating behaviors. Scientific consensus panel reports have consistently recommended that children and adolescents eat at least five servings of fruit and vegetables daily and participate in daily physical activity to reduce the risk of chronic disease and premature death; however, youth are not meeting policy standards for these health behaviors.[27] Children should be a major focus of intervention efforts because many of the risk factors observed in adults can be detected in childhood, such as high blood pressure and cholesterol as well as being overweight. There is considerable evidence that middle school years and adolescence are critical periods for influencing eating behavior, as more food choices are being made independently from parents as children grow older. For example, fruit consumption decreased by 41% between grades 3 and 8 in one cohort study.[37] In a longitudinal study following adolescents from 6th through 12th grade, researchers found that healthful and unhealthful behaviors that emerged by 6th grade continued throughout high school.[38] This is evidence for promoting healthful habits to children early during middle school and elementary school.

The National Heart, Lung, and Blood Institute (NHLBI) sponsored one of the largest school-based health promotion trials, the Child and Adolescent Trial for Cardiovascular Health (CATCH), which was implemented in 96 public elementary schools from 1991 to 1995.[39] This study was designed to decrease cardiovascular risk factors in children through interventions implemented in the classroom, during physical education class, and in the cafeteria via the school food service. The most significant results were decreases in total fat and saturated fat consumption, as well as increases in physical activity in the children who received the interventions in comparison to the control schools. Five years after the intervention, follow-up studies were conducted and showed that it is possible to maintain and sustain environmental changes to promote healthy behaviors.[40,41] This is encouraging news because many positive health behavior changes seen immediately post-intervention have not always been sustained long term (2 + years). Two of the most important factors in the viability and sustainability of the CATCH intervention in the schools were staff training and a more open and supportive school climate for the health promotion program.[42,43]

Health behavior theories and the literature dictate that the most potent interventions in schools are those that have comprehensive and multiple components. The critical components to changing fruit and vegetable consumption in young children include environmental changes, classroom curriculum, parental involvement, and partnerships with local produce companies. Although limited resources in some states and school districts preclude making multilevel changes, simple environmental changes can be adopted by schools almost immediately. For example, students who received the school-based intervention called "Cafeteria Power Plus" significantly increased their fruit intake.[44] As part of the intervention, the food service staff were encouraged to increase the choices and appeal of the fruits and vegetables offered in the lunch line and snack cart. The staff also verbally encouraged the students to eat fruits and vegetables by making positive comments when students went through the line.

Schools are an efficient, practical place to influence children's eating habits, because one or two meals and many snacks per week are consumed there. In addition to government programs that were created to provide healthful nutrition, such as the National School Lunch Program and the School Breakfast Program, many schools today offer a greater variety of eating options and opportunities. Unfortunately, aspects of the school environments can overshadow and diminish the benefits these programs were designed to provide. Examples include:

- Poor quality and unpalatable food served in the cafeteria (i.e., many greasy, high-fat items and lack of healthy options)
- À la carte programs
- Snack bars/carts and vending machines that serve non-nutritious foods
- Short lunch periods
- In some schools, students' freedom to leave the premises to buy food elsewhere

Overall, few foods in this environment are low fat; quality fruits and vegetables are rare, and fruit juice is a less prevalent offering than carbonated or sweetened beverages.[45-49] Focus groups and interviews conducted with students, faculty, and staff in two New England middle schools revealed that lack of healthy options and poor quality food were the top barriers to eating healthier. Students stated that if the cafeteria offered fruits and vegetables in greater quantity and quality, they would choose to eat them instead of the less nutritious entrees or snack foods.[49]

Other in-depth focus groups conducted with schoolchildren in grades 2 through 11, randomly selected from 34 schools in Australia, elucidated the major perceived benefits and barriers to healthful eating and physical activity.[50] The most important benefits voiced by the children were the ability to think better, improved physical performance, increased energy, and mentally feeling better about oneself. The main barriers to eating healthy were convenience of less healthful alternatives, taste, peer pressure, lack of parental and school support, and few good role models. To overcome these barriers, the students in grades 5 through 11 suggested strategies that included:

- Parental support (availability of healthier foods at home)
- Planning to eat healthier by carrying nutritious foods to school
- Not taking money to school
- Reducing the availability of "junk food" at home, at school, and in the community

The core of the matter is that if non-nutritious foods and snacks are not available in schools, then students cannot purchase and eat them. Unfortunately, profits from the sale of snack foods, soda, and other sugar-sweetened beverages are used to fund scholarships and school events. Administrators admit to the challenge of relinquishing this kind of funding, especially because of the large sums of money distributed by soft drink companies, known as "pouring rights contracts."[36] In exchange for this money (which can total millions of dollars over time), schools formally agree to stock their vending machines only with that particular company's beverages and use its brand exclusively at all games and school-sponsored events. School administrators will need opposing pressure from parents and state legislatures, and also encouragement, to be creative in finding alternative funding sources for student programs that do not compromise students' health. Instead, these vending machines could and should be stocked with healthy options, such as 100% fruit juice, bottled water, flavored seltzer, low-fat and nonfat milk and yogurt, baked pita and potato chips, fresh fruit, low-fat granola bars, nuts, and trail mix.

A one-year nutrition education program in schools in England with the simple message "ditch the fizz" was effective in reducing soda intake in children ages 7 to 11.[51] The intervention classrooms received a one-hour session each school term for 12 months that educated the children on the benefits of decreased sugar consumption from soda, such as improving overall well-being and dental health. The children completed diaries at the beginning and end of the trial, reporting on drinks consumed over three days. Consumption of carbonated drinks dropped by an average of 0.6 glasses over three days among the intervention children, but increased by 0.2 glasses among the children not receiving the educational session. The intervention group dropped 0.2% in prevalence of overweight compared to the control classrooms, where the percentage of overweight and obese children increased by 7.5%. This British trial has important implications because it reiterates what other research has shown: that there is an association between consumption of sugar-sweetened drinks and obesity in children.[52-54]

The American Academy of Pediatrics (AAP) Committee on School Health published a statement to inform pediatricians, other healthcare professionals, parents, superintendents, and school board members about the nutritional concerns and health implications of soft drinks in schools:

Potential health problems associated with a high intake of sweetened drinks include: 1) overweight or obesity due to excess calories; 2) displacement of milk consumption, resulting in calcium deficiency with a resultant risk of osteoporosis and fractures; and 3) dental caries and potential enamel erosion. A clearly defined, district-wide policy that restricts the sale of soft drinks will safeguard against health problems as a result of over-consumption of these non-nutritive, highly caloric beverages.[55]

The AAP appears to be speaking out against the pouring rights contracts between schools and the beverage companies. The good news is that school districts in Los Angeles, Philadelphia, San Francisco, Chicago, and New York City as well as numerous smaller districts are leading the way by taking steps to ban the sale of soft drinks during the school day. California and Texas have issued statewide bans on soft-drink sales in elementary and middle schools. Texas, New York City, and Los Angeles have actually taken the next important step by restricting the sale of potato chips, candy, and other junk food.[56]

Peer health education programs are also important in schools because the ability to tap into social networks and cliques can increase the adoption of behavior changes, which may not otherwise occur from pure teacher-led instruction. Adolescence is a time of autonomy but also social conformity to peers. This can be advantageous if healthy norms and strategic changes can be inoculated into the group via the influential leaders of the cliques and social networks. A multicomponent, school-based intervention with a peer leader component conducted in 2002 showed the largest increase in fruit and vegetable consumption, as well as increased consumption of lower fat foods, compared to students who were exposed to classroom and environmental changes only.[57] A more recent randomized controlled trial conducted in middle schools using a socioecological model (environmental changes) to improve nutrition and physical activity resulted in significant change in physical activity for the boys. The girls in this study did not show a change in physical activity habits.[58] Furthermore, the interventions did not help decrease dietary fat intake in these school children. More research with rigorous evaluation methods is needed to reveal why particular interventions may be effective in some schools and, perhaps, not in others.

In summary, because school-aged children and adolescents spend much of their day in schools and eat numerous meals, snacks, and beverages there, offering healthy food choices is the socially responsible thing to do. (Refer to Chapter 1 on ethical responsibilities in public health.) In addition to providing a healthier food environment, students will be enabled to eat more nutritiously if: 1) access to junk food is limited; 2) healthy behavior is the group norm in the school environment; 3) peer leaders and others model nutritious choices; 4) the cafeteria offers appealing vegetables and fruits; and 5) cafeteria staff provide verbal encouragement to eat fruits and vegetables. (More about obesity in childhood is in Chapter 5.)

The 2004 reauthorization of the Child Nutrition Act took great strides forward in requiring all school districts to adopt wellness policies. The next reauthorization, scheduled for September 2010, provides an opportunity for nutrition professionals invested in improving childhood nutrition to weigh in and strengthen this requirement by offering resources for implementation of the policies and increasing the funding available for fresh, healthy school food.[59] Currently, approximately 40% of schools do not offer fresh vegetables or fruit on a daily basis.[60] President Barack Obama's 2010 budget set aside an extra $1 billion for child-nutrition programs. He said, "Let's figure out how we can get fresh fruits and vegetables in the mix. We've got to change how we think about getting local farmers connected to school districts." Many U.S. schools are making efforts to promote healthier diets.

About 9,000 schools have joined the national Farm-to-School program[61] that provides locally grown food to school cafeterias. This program sprouted from the desire to support community-based food systems, strengthen family farms, and improve student health by reducing childhood obesity. It brings local produce directly from farms to school meals so the students can learn about the path from farm to fork, in an effort to instill healthier eating habits in the children that may last for their lifetimes.

Organizational and Worksite Interventions

A review of 47 studies of worksite health promotion programs that addressed multiple risk factors revealed that almost all provided health education to their employees.[62] A smaller number of the programs (25%) implemented modifications in organizational policy or the work environment to facilitate employee behavior changes. But, imparting knowledge and skills for new health behaviors is not enough; targeting and intercepting workplace norms and eating environments is necessary to support change. Some examples of physical and environmental modifications include policies restricting or banning smoking on the premises, on-site exercise and kitchen facilities, and offering healthier fare in the cafeteria and vending machines. We have learned from existing studies that greater effort is needed to modify social factors and physical settings of the worksites. Also, having an understanding of the organizational climate and culture (e.g., attitudes, beliefs, needs, and resources of the members), including the organization's receptivity to health innovation, is important to create effective behavioral change interventions.[62]

Conducting solid formative research in the organization will elucidate perceptions and barriers to change. In addition, having all the relevant stakeholders and key figures participate in planning and conducting the health-promoting activities will help facilitate and maintain success in the organization. Management plays the important role of creating a work culture. For example, the management can provide eating norms in which employees can take a reasonable amount of time to eat a healthy lunch, as opposed to a work environment where individuals are expected to just "work through lunch" or eat at their desk. Employees, equipped with the knowledge and skills in a supportive environment with healthy norms, are much more likely to move into or remain in action and maintenance stages of change.[63,64]

Employees at their worksites are a captive audience and are ideal for intervention delivery. In particular, high traffic areas, such as the cafeteria and break rooms, are strategic places to deliver brief education. Some examples of low-intensity work-based nutrition interventions that have shown at least short-term beneficial results, such as a reduction in blood cholesterol levels,[65] include:

- Computer programs that appraise individual health risk
- Group education sessions
- Interactive activities with food sampling and recipes
- Contests (e.g., winners are individuals who exercise three times a week for one month or eat five fruits and vegetables per day for a month)
- Simple finger-prick blood glucose and cholesterol screenings accompanied by a dietitian to provide brief counseling, referrals, and follow-up plans[66]
- Printed information and materials for employees to take home

Having a personally tailored behavioral component (e.g., personalized education and/or a follow-up phone call) has been shown to promote continued employee participation in follow-up health screening compliance.[67]

Although implementation of nutrition activities has often been successful initially in numerous worksites, these health-promoting activities have generally not been sustainable two years post-intervention.[68] Upper management should increase their efforts in building capacity for sustaining health-enhancing activities in the organization that will facilitate increased commitment and follow-through by employees.

Family and Friends

The important influence of supportive family relationships and other social ties for good health is widely accepted in the scientific community.[69,70] Family members and family dynamics are interconnected and mutually influential. Whether we realize or are conscious of this, family and friends influence our consumption of certain foods by modeling healthy or unhealthy choices by peer pressure (e.g., "You have to have some apple pie, I made it especially for you."). Parents or caregivers initially play the most influential role in a young child's development of eating preferences, habits, or patterns. Parenting and feeding styles will either foster or limit a child's ability to regulate their caloric intake by altering their responsiveness to internal or external cues of hunger and satiety.[71,72] According to both Birch and Davison[73] and Golan and Crow,[74] parents play a key role in preventing or treating overweight/obesity in their children. More specifically, parents who are overweight and struggling to adopt healthier eating habits for themselves, or who are concerned about their children's risk for overweight, may adopt controlling or restrictive child-feeding practices in an attempt to prevent obesity in their children. This type of eating environment, which is inadvertently created by caring parents who only want the best for their children, may create or exacerbate an unhealthy eating pattern or genetic predisposition already present in their children.

In a longitudinal study, Caucasian girls, ages 5 to 9, with mothers who used restrictive feeding practices, ate in the absence of hunger.[75] These girls were less able to regulate their appetite and hunger needs by internal mechanisms. This point is particularly important given the rising rate of overweight and obese children and the importance of intervening to prevent parents from using restrictive feeding practices. Instead, parents need education on efficacious methods to promote healthier eating habits and physical activity with their overweight children.

How can parents foster the development of self-regulation in children? The development of self-regulation is grounded in a child's feelings of competence, autonomy, and connectedness.[76] When parents provide structure and guidelines for meals as well as the reasons behind the guidelines, this motivates compliance and internalization for children. In addition, when parents support autonomy in their children and provide a warm, positive connection with them, this motivates compliance and affirms competence.[76]

Families are imbedded in a greater ecology, and therefore are subject to outside influences. Environments provide increased opportunities and resources, thus placing constraints on parental choices.[76] An important public health goal is to identify families that are at greater risk for poorer eating habits, such as those with limited income, high levels of stress, parents with obesity, or a single working parent, and provide a family-focused intervention relevant to their circumstances. This would be an opportunity to provide social support and/or education, enabling the provision of healthy meals in the home. Acquiring an understanding of parents' beliefs and their hierarchy of goals is necessary in order to impact or change parenting practices. A review of "parent education" literature reveals three important principles for educating parents:

1. Information must be relevant to their life and family circumstances (e.g., both parents work full-time; therefore, home-cooked meals are not always realistic).
2. Information should come from a trusted source.
3. Information must be usable and accessible.[77,78]

The advice parents receive from professionals must be practical, meaning that parents need to know not only what to do, but also how to do it within the constraints of their present circumstances. The modality of the education provided must also match the parents' learning style.[76] Printed materials can be helpful to some, but a video (available in different languages) can be a better method if there is a language barrier or literacy issues.

Interventions should take advantage of and build upon the momentum created by family transitions and changes, such as a couple expecting their first baby. Pediatric healthcare providers could begin disseminating advice to new parents during their baby's infancy on how to create a child who is a "healthy eater." This would give parents the opportunity and time it takes to begin the challenging process of altering suboptimal eating habits and replacing them with more healthful patterns. The result would be a home environment more conducive to healthy eating being the norm, because parental modeling of good habits is most influential in forming a child's eating pattern. How and where does a child initially learn about healthy foods and patterns of eating? Primarily, via exposure to foods from parents or caregivers. Parents also need to understand the detriments of coercive feeding practices and be given alternatives to restricting food and pressuring children to eat. Helpful practical advice for parents could include:

- How to promote acceptance of new foods by children, which entails offering the food repeatedly (10 different instances has been suggested)[79]
- Providing parents with easy-to-use, healthy recipes and tips on simple, quick, and inexpensive meals
- Recommendations on proper portion sizes from each food group
- How to avoid food struggles with picky eaters

Feeding children healthily and handling picky eaters can be two of the more stressful or frustrating aspects of child rearing. Picky eaters (those resistant to eating many familiar foods) and children with neophobia (reluctance to try new foods) are two different and distinct consumption behaviors. It is no surprise that vegetables are the one food group

children are less apt to consume in adequate amounts, compared to children with neither pickiness nor neophobia. Given that vegetable intake among children is well below recommended levels in the United States, finding effective means to increase vegetable intake among children is important and needed.

One encouraging research study involving 192 seven-year-old girls and their parents revealed predictors of pickiness in girls, which are primarily environmental or experiential factors subject to change,[80] and not a genetically linked or normal trait of children as some may believe. Picky girls had mothers who:

- Perceived their family to have little time to eat healthful foods
- Had less variety in their vegetable intake
- Breastfed for fewer than 6 months

One explanation for this last finding is that breastfed children are exposed early in life to a diversity of flavors via breast milk (if the mother consumed a variety of foods in her diet).[80] These findings reveal important ways for dietitians, nutritionists, and other healthcare practitioners to intervene and prevent pickiness in children's eating habits. Education should include encouraging:

- Longer duration of breastfeeding
- Parental modeling of eating a greater variety of vegetables
- The use of simple methods and time-saving preparation techniques for vegetables

For adolescents, the strongest correlations for vegetable and fruit intake are home availability of these foods and taste preferences for them.[81] However, this study found that even if taste preferences for fruits and vegetables was low among these adolescents, if fruits and vegetables were available, intake increased nevertheless. Parents therefore need to be encouraged to purchase produce regularly and have fruits and vegetables available in the home and offered at all meals as much as possible.

An example of a family nutrition intervention program includes "The High 5 Low Fat" nutrition intervention as part of the Parents as Teachers Program, which targets African American parents.[82] Trained African-American parents act as role models and disseminate the information via personal visits, group sessions, and newsletters to other parents. This intervention has been shown to improve the intake of fruits and vegetables, as well as lower overall dietary fat for parents receiving the intervention.

Another example of the importance of family support in promoting better health was shown in a study conducted with individuals with diabetes in a Diné (Navajo) Native American population. Individuals with active family nutritional support showed greater control in HgA(1c) (an indicator of longer term blood glucose control) and total cholesterol and triglyceride levels, compared to individuals with less family involvement.[83] The type of support these individuals received and reported included a family member helping with shopping and cooking healthy meals, or family members who would eat low-fat, low-sugar foods with them. These persons with diabetes and this type of family support demonstrated and improved self-care behavior.

In addition, a family-focused component that was added to a worksite intervention showed that consumption of fruits and vegetables was directly associated with level of household support for healthy eating.[84] Worksite interventions, with a component involving family members, has proven more effective than targeting the worksite alone.[84–86]

We need to recognize and acquire a better understanding of the influential role and burden that society must share in helping prevent obesity and promote opportunities and easier access to healthy food choices for children and adults. "Children are most vulnerable to the persuasive appeals by food marketers which can hook them with brand new processed products that enter the market daily."[87] Strong public policies and regulations should be created to limit advertising of non-nutritious foods to children. There will be more to follow on this issue in Chapters 7 and 8.

Community Interventions

A community can be any grouping of individuals who have a shared sense of identity or a common thread that draws all of them together. Therefore, a community can be a geographic area of persons, but is not necessarily limited to this factor.[23] Examples of communities can be a certain ethnic group; a professional group, such as small business owners; or a group of individuals who are all cancer survivors. The collective strength of a community to promote its own health is beyond the ability of any single person to control or change. That is what differentiates the effectiveness of community intervention from individual behavior change. Even individuals with few social ties, but who reside in socially cohesive communities, do not appear to suffer the same adverse health consequences as do socially isolated people living in less cohesive communities.[88,89]

Valuable lessons have been learned from various community change interventions. They include the importance of the following[90]:

- Engaging the community, rather than an outside organizer or researcher, to define needs and priorities
- Identifying and building upon the strengths, assets, and resources of the community's members
- Being flexible and tailoring the change strategies to each particular community's context and milieu
- Building long-term sustainability of programs and identifying diversified sources of funding

Several community-based studies have shown that it is possible to change consumers' overall fat intake, without deliberate education on limiting fat intake, by increasing the availability and decreasing the cost of healthful products.[72] However, some large extensive communities where these studies were done showed no significant changes in dietary habits. This suggests that perhaps more focused studies within high-risk subgroups, such as minority and low-literacy populations, may be more fruitful. In fact, a number of public health agencies and their academic, managed care, community health center, and other community partners have begun to implement smaller-scale cardiovascular disease prevention projects. A good example was the 15 WISEWOMAN projects, funded by the CDC, which targeted low-income, predominantly ethnic minority women screened by the Breast and Cervical Cancer Early Detection Program. The WISEWOMAN project successfully implemented screenings for high blood pressure, blood glucose, and total cholesterol in conjunction with cancer screenings the women were already receiving. This program was deemed successful in reaching underserved women, developing a more comprehensive women's health model, strengthening linkages to primary health care, experimenting with innovative behavioral interventions, and tapping into women's roles as social support providers and family/community gatekeepers.[91]

Places of Worship

Despite continued efforts to reduce health disparities among diverse populations in the United States, certain ethnic groups are faced with higher disease risk and death rates. African Americans continue to be disproportionately affected by all causes of disease compared to other groups. Greater effort is needed to reach this segment of the population with prevention strategies. Unfortunately, African Americans are more likely to be distrustful of investigators given negative historical events (e.g., the Tuskegee experiment) and sub-par medical access and care they tend to receive. The church, therefore, has become an ideal channel and setting for reaching members of this community with health education, given the high regard and level of trust members have for their pastors. For many African-American families, life centers on the church and its activities, and therefore the church exerts a high degree of influence.[92]

Several interventions conducted in churches have shown clinically meaningful decreases in disease risk outcomes, such as body weight, blood pressure, and waist circumference.[93–95] Some of the specific successful behavioral and dietary outcomes these programs have achieved include decreased fat and sodium intake; increased fruit, vegetable, and fiber intake; and increased physical activity. One example of this type of intervention is the PRAISE! (Partnership to Reach African Americans to Increase Smart Eating!) project, conducted in 60 churches in 8 North Carolina counties, which used a community-based participatory research (CBPR) approach.[96] The CBPR approach views community participants as partners in the research process, rather than just subjects upon whom research is conducted. At least one randomized clinical trial so far has found that research designed with a CBPR approach is associated with high levels of trust and a perceived benefit of satisfaction with the research process.[97]

Meals, coffee, and refreshments are common accompaniments to fellowship in church social gatherings and meetings. These gatherings afford an opportune setting for dietary intervention, such as offering lower fat dishes and recipes and incorporating more vegetables and fruits. This is one reason the National Institute of Health (NIH) has created a program titled, "Body & Soul: A Celebration of Healthy Eating and Living."[98] This program helps empower church members to be more physically active and to eat five to nine servings of fruits and vegetables every day for better health. The combined elements of this program include pastoral leadership, health education, an environment in church that supports healthy eating, and peer counseling.

Reaching Older Adults

Innovative and effective health promotion interventions targeted at older adults, within a public health framework, are becoming increasingly important as the U.S. population ages. The benefits of healthier lifestyles for older adults include increased functional ability, delaying the onset of disease, and an improved quality of life, which are important goals in program planning for this population.[99]

Specific nutritional goals for elders should include increasing the intake of vegetables, fruits, and calcium-rich foods, just like most segments of the population.[100] Some may think that interventions targeted toward adults over age 55 seem to have a limited effect, given the difficulty of changing nearly a lifetime of eating habits and behaviors. However, a review of the literature published from 1990 to 2003 regarding nutrition interventions targeting older adults revealed many positive outcomes. Features of the most effective nutrition programs included using the appropriate behavior change theory; limiting the education to one or two key messages; providing hands-on activities, incentives, and access to health professionals; reinforcing and personalizing the health messages; and a social environment that supports healthy behavior.[101]

An example of a community intervention targeting older adults was a creative partnership established among Tri-Parish Nursing Ministries, The Arthritis Foundation, Missouri Extension Services, and the Saint Louis County Department of Health.[102] The goal was to promote the quality of life for older adults through physical activity and health education messages. Twenty-nine participants met twice a week in a local church to exercise for one hour with a trainer from PACE (People with Arthritis Can Exercise). The participants received 30 minutes of nutrition education from a Saint Louis County registered dietitian using the Missouri Extension's Health for Everybody program. The participation rate for the program was 62% at the end of six weeks. The mean age of participants was 74 years. All participants reported favorably, indicating that they enjoyed sessions and "learned something new." Unfortunately, the reasons why some participants dropped out are unknown. Feedback also revealed that participants even asked for more ways to exercise outside of class. Providing older adults with encouragement, a place to exercise, and an opportunity to learn healthy eating tips could potentially make a significant difference in improving quality of life for this segment of the population.

Individual and Group Counseling

Until greater social change occurs and the long-term solution to improve our nation's nutrition and health is realized, nutritionists and other health educators play an important role in helping individuals manage better within our current "toxic food environment," as some have termed it.[36] Educating individuals and equipping people with tools and strategies is critical to resist or combat the powerful "eat more" marketing messages that we are constantly bombarded with by the food and restaurant industries.[36]

Brief counseling that incorporates principles of motivational interviewing and patient-centered behavioral change strategies have shown promise in medical settings.[103] For example, a randomized study of 206 adult patients with type 2 diabetes combined patient-centered self-management with interactive computer technology to improve dietary behaviors and decrease serum cholesterol levels.[103] This study integrated feasible, appealing behavioral interventions into the clinic flow of a primary care office. The intervention involved a sequence of the following: a 15-minute touch-screen computer assessment, which helped subjects identify dietary goals and barriers to accomplishing these goals; immediate scoring and two tailored feedback/goal printouts summarizing the information (one for the patient and one for the physician); a 20-second motivational message emphasizing the importance of the goal the patient had selected; a 15 to 20 minute meeting with a health educator to review the patient's goal and collaboratively develop barriers-based problem-solving strategies; and lastly, two brief follow-up phone calls from the health educator to check on progress. This sequence was repeated at a regular three-month follow-up visit. The intervention group showed greater improvements in total and saturated dietary fat intake as well as serum cholesterol levels, compared to the control group. Additionally, results were maintained at 12-month follow-up and the intervention proved to be cost-effective.

Outside the medical setting, motivational interviewing (MI) techniques,[104] which have traditionally been used for counseling patients with addictive behaviors, are showing promise in community settings with counselors via telephone to improve eating behaviors and increase physical activity.[99]

> **Motivational interviewing:** A directive, client-centered counseling style for eliciting behavior change by helping clients to explore and resolve ambivalence. Compared with nondirective counseling, it is more focused and goal-directed. Motivation to change is elicited from the client and not imposed by the counselor.[105]

The U.S. Preventive Services Task Force (USPSTF) has extensively reviewed the literature between 1966 and December 2001 regarding the effectiveness of counseling to promote a healthy diet among patients in primary care settings.[106] They found that dietary counseling produces modest changes in self-reported consumption of saturated fat, fruits and vegetables, and possibly dietary fiber. More intensive interventions were more likely to produce greater changes than brief interventions, but may be more difficult to apply in typical primary care visits. Interventions using interactive health communications, including computer-generated telephone or mail messages, can also produce moderate dietary changes.

Since that extensive review by the USPSTF, two additional studies on counseling to produce dietary change have been published, which are consistent with the review's conclusion. The results showed increases in the consumption of fruits and vegetables, as well as a decrease in dietary fat intake. Between the two studies, patients exhibited significant improvements following either two 45-minute counseling sessions, including computer interaction,[107] or two 15-minute individual counseling sessions by research nurses.[108]

Role of Government

Individual counseling in a healthcare setting and public health interventions in a variety of settings play significant roles in bringing preventative nutrition to the forefront. However, those methods as presently implemented are still limited in their effectiveness. In contrast, laws and regulations have proven to play a decisive and more effective role in advancing the public's health. Public health's contribution is particularly evident in the prevention and control of communicable diseases and in the realm of injury prevention, which were the leading causes of death at the beginning of the 20th century. Today, chronic disease is the leading cause of death and disability.[109] Our strength in protecting the public has still primarily been in our means of responding to acute threats such as the Severe Acute Respiratory Syndrome (SARS) outbreak or, perhaps, terrorism since the attack on September 11, 2001. It is imperative for this country to move from a palliative medical model to one that is prevention-based if we are to make noticeable improvements in Americans' quality of life and control rising healthcare costs. The role of law has been fully applied to the prevention and control of chronic diseases and their

risk factors (e.g., tobacco control and smoking prevention). There has been a noteworthy impact on public health, such as a major decrease in smoking rates across the country for most segments of the population.

We have reached a point in healthcare history where we need to fully explore and create comprehensive legal frameworks for preventing and controlling the growing epidemics of obesity, heart disease, stroke, diabetes, and other chronic diseases and their related major risk factors.[110] "These frameworks will be a crucial addition to the tools available to the public health workforce, especially state and local health department program managers, as well as state and national policy makers. They also can assist program managers' interaction with city mayors, legislators, governors, and other policy makers."[110] Legal steps or laws may take the form of constitutional provisions, statutory enactments, regulations, ordinances, government-initiated litigation, court rulings, or policies adopted by public-sector bodies, such as schools and zoning boards. For example, we have seen bans on the sale of sodas and junk foods adopted by certain California schools and zoning boards, as mentioned earlier in this chapter.

Law also can include policies or treaties adopted by international bodies, such as the International Code of Marketing of Breast-Milk Substitutes ("The Code") passed in 1981 by the World Health Organization (WHO). It states that governments should provide information about the superiority of breast feeding. The Code also outlines measures that would control use of inappropriate marketing practices that can undermine "a mother's ability to breastfeed her baby."[111] The enactment of this code was necessary in an effort to mitigate the aggressive marketing of infant formula by companies in developing countries, where infant mortality rates increased when mothers were disingenuously persuaded to formula-feed instead of breast-feed.

In 1995, the AAP issued a statement regarding the food industry's marketing effects on children: "Advertising directed at children is inherently deceptive and exploits children less than eight years of age." This strong statement should have set in motion the steps necessary by the federal government to ban junk food advertisements directed at children. Norway, Sweden, Australia, Italy, and New Zealand have either banned advertising directed at children altogether or have legislative guidelines restricting it.[56]

Anti-junk food ads that promote healthy eating via a government-sponsored public service campaign could be another important strategy to combat the tens of thousands of commercials that the average child sees each year, enticing them to consume high-fat, high-sugar products that are continually being churned out in the marketplace.[109]

Legislation that would require calories on chain restaurant menus and menu boards now has the support of the restaurant industry as well as health groups thanks to an agreement struck among senators who were previously supporting separate state labeling bills. Besides requiring calories on menus, menu boards and drive-through displays, the new legislation would require chains with 20 or more outlets to provide additional nutrition information upon request.

Similar bills or regulations have been adopted in New York City, Philadelphia, Massachusetts, California, and a number of major counties. Bills in Oregon, Maine, and Connecticut have passed their state legislatures and are awaiting final action.

"This legislation will help individuals make more informed, healthier choices by making calorie information easily accessible at thousands of restaurants throughout our state and the country," stated California Governor Arnold Schwarzenegger when he signed the law in 2008. Kelly Brownell of Yale University's Rudd Center for Food Policy and Obesity goes further with his statement, "...providing the [menu] data is a 'right-to-know' issue, regardless of what people do with the information. It is no different than knowing what materials your clothes are made of or the nutritional content and ingredients of packaged food."

Mainstream Media

Between the years 2004 and 2009 alone, at least 19 documentary films have been produced on topics ranging from the state of our water supply, agricultural practices of our national farmers large and small, animal production farms, soil, coffee trade, and our industrial food production systems. *Fresh*, *King Corn*, *Food, Inc.*, and *The Future of Food*, are just a few examples of film titles that have removed the veil covering the public's eyes as to our government's priorities: subsidies for agriculture and the farmers who overproduce, as well as the food manufacturing industries' lobbying powers and influence to maximize profits, which can be in direct opposition to preserving health and well-being for American consumers. Two examples are Morgan Spurlock's documentary film entitled, *Supersize Me*, about the deleterious effects of a month eating only fast food, and Eric Schlosser's book and film entitled, *Fast Food Nation*, which gave the public a wider perspective on slaughterhouse practices, food processing, and how corporate policies affect employees within the fast food industry. Given that illiteracy still exists, movies in the mainstream media are opportunistic channels to inform and reach the lay public who either cannot read or who may not necessarily seek out nutrition and health information that ultimately can im-

pact their health positively. Because these movies are both entertaining and educational, they can be effective nutrition education tools to stimulate thought, community dialogue, personal action, and policy change. The American Dietetic Association's Hunger and Environmental Nutrition Dietetic Practice Group introduced the "Film Feastival" concept at the 2007 Food & Nutrition Conference & Expo (FNCE) held in Philadelphia. This concept entails showing one or two feature films, adding a panel of experts, mixing in film-related food such a locally grown produce, and an ordinary classroom has transformed into a appealing educational event.[112] Popular, well-researched books such as Michael Pollan's *In Defense of Food* and *Omnivore's Dilemma*, Mark Bittman's *Food Matters*, and Barbara Kingsolver's *Animal, Vegetable, Miracle* is another type of opportunity to educate ourselves on where our food comes from and how it is produced. Change is possible and does happen when parents (motivated for their children and future generations) and citizens organize themselves to pressure decision-makers to improve the choices in the supermarket and various eating venues.

Eating Eco-Consciously

The "Going Green" movement to preserve our natural environment and prevent the long-standing industrial damage to it has spilled into the nutrition world. As people have become more eco-conscious, interest has increased in sustainable food and agriculture to mitigate effects of climate change, and in the availability and quality of our natural resources: soil, water, genetic biodiversity in plants, and renewable energy sources.[113]

In addition to the continual rise of organic food purchases, people are trying to eat more locally grown produce to support the small farms and farmers as well as minimize their carbon footprint on the Earth from transportation costs of foods traveling from all parts of the globe. We are learning that the real cost of being able to buy our food cheaply comes at the expense of compromising the health of workers in these massive industrial farms who endure very poor working conditions. Americans, with their traditionally high meat consumption, not only increase their risk of heart disease, cancer, and stroke but the animals suffer from the extremely congested feed lot farms they are raised in with no light or space to move within. Seventy percent of all antibiotic use in the United States is on animals because their cramped conditions make them susceptible to continuous infections.[114] The majority of meat available for purchase in supermarkets is produced and controlled by only a few companies in the United States.

Our environment is being polluted due to livestock production, which accounts for approximately 80% of greenhouse gas production, more than the all car emissions on our planet.[115] The policies that need to be implemented to reduce greenhouse gas emissions could also bring about substantial reductions in health concerns such as heart disease, cancer, obesity, diabetes, road deaths and injuries, and air pollution.[116,117]

Industrialization of our food supply has contributed to the degradation of the environment and our health. What many are learning is that what we choose to eat has ramifications far beyond our personal weight, health, and risk for future disease. In addition, our meals may have profound political, economic, psychological, and ethical implications for our Earth and everyone living on it.

Local Grassroots and Governmental Efforts

Community efforts occurring at the local and academic levels often begin first before local and federal legislation occur. We can be inspired by the grassroots efforts to improve school lunches, documented in *Lunch Lessons* by Ann Cooper and Lisa M. Holms.[118] Some restaurants, college food service, and other public venues where food is served have moved to providing smaller, more reasonable portions as well as nutritional information at the point of service.

Personal action is not enough, however. The agricultural sector of the government has the greatest potential to contribute to large-scale, population-level dietary improvements beyond the conscientious efforts of each person to eat more organically, sustainably, and locally grown foods.

Two points of intervention in the agricultural sector have the potential to be leveraged to preserve soil health and promote healthy diets for people: 1) agricultural policies and 2) agricultural production practices. Agricultural policies and practices affect diet through their influence on food availability, price, and nutrient quality, which in turn affects food choices available to consumers. Agricultural policies amenable to intervention include input, production, and trade policies; agricultural production practices amenable to intervention include crop breeding, crop fertilization practices, livestock-feeding practices, and crop systems diversity.[119]

The hopeful bright horizon amidst these somber facts is that a growing public concern and awareness of the above may result in an overall healthier diet in the future as more people choose to eat less meat or pay more for meat from free-range animals, and more organic foods, home or locally grown produce, and less processed packaged items.

Genetically Modified or Engineered Foods

It has been estimated that approximately 70% of the current processed or packaged food items contain a genetically modified organism or ingredient.[120] This estimate is based on the fact that the highest yield crop items that U.S. farmers produce are soy, corn, cottonseed, and canola, which are genetically engineered food items almost ubiquitous in our food supply. One would be hard pressed to find products on our supermarket shelves that do not include some form of soy, corn cottonseed, or canola oil.

The introduction of genetically engineered foods into our diet was done quietly and without the mandatory labeling that is required in many other of the world's industrialized countries.

Unfortunately, precaution is not the default legal position in our country, so hazards and risks are defined on a case-by-case basis in the courts. This is in contrast to Canada and the European Union's commitment to a Precautionary Principle, where instead of a judicial system of "guilty until proven innocent," their philosophy is: "When an activity raises threats of harm to the environment or human health, precautionary measures should be taken even if some cause-and-effect relationships are not fully established scientifically."[121]

These countries believe that scientific experts' opinions cannot be solely depended upon to determine what the public would consider as acceptable types of risks. Only the people themselves can decide what they consider as an acceptable level or if even any amount of risk is acceptable, given the ethical and social consequences in the advancing area of food bioengineering.[122] Even if the most rigorous risk assessments are conducted, uncertainty of the long-term consequences and unanticipated effects cannot be eliminated.[122] What has complicated the ability to test safety of genetically modified organisms and predict health outcomes is the varying amounts in each food item. If some negative health impacts are seen, often it is difficult to trace them back to one particular genetically engineered ingredient in a particular food.

Proponents of the field of biotechnology of food have created the means of efficiency and higher yield

Genetically Modified Organism (GMO) or **Genetically Engineered Ingredient:** Created from a laboratory process that artificially inserts foreign genes into the DNA of food crops or animals. Those genes may come from bacteria, viruses, insects, animals, or even humans. According to the World Health Organization, GMOs are "organisms in which the genetic material (DNA) has been altered in such a way that does not occur naturally." This technology is also referred to as *genetic engineering biotechnology*, or *recombinant DNA technology*. Although banned by food manufacturers of many European Union countries, the U.S. Food and Drug Administration does not require any safety evaluations, nor is there a requirement to label foods as containing GMOs. GMOs have been in the food supply since 1996 and are now present in the vast majority of processed foods in the United States.

Sources: World Health Organization. (2002). Foods derived from modern technology: 20 questions on genetically modified foods. Available at http://www.who.int/foodsafety/publications/biotech/20questions/en/index.html

http://www.responsibletechnology.org/GM Free/Home/index.cfm

of biotech corn, which has created surpluses for not only the United States but enough to export to several other countries. U.S. crops have been genetically engineered to be pest- and herbicide-resistant, so higher yields ultimately has allowed U.S. food prices to be lower in cost and thus more affordable; U.S. food costs are a smaller percentage of our overall household expenditures when compared to those living in most other countries. Many would agree this is true but argue at the hidden costs to our nation's health, the sustainability of our environmental resources, and our personal health.

What We Can Do

For those concerned about choosing foods that are better and safer for their health as well as the environment, here are a few actions steps:

- Buy organic. Organic foods are not allowed to contain genetically modified (GM) ingredients. Buying products that are certified organic or that say non-GMO are two ways to limit one's risk of eating GM foods. Another is to avoid products containing any ingredients from the seven food crops that have been genetically engineered: soy, corn, cottonseed, canola, Hawaiian papaya, and a little bit of zucchini and crook neck squash. This means avoiding soy lecithin in chocolate, corn syrup in candies, and cottonseed or canola oil in snack foods.
- Buy locally grown produce. Shop at farmer's markets and farm stands.
- Join a Community Supported Agriculture (CSA) program.
- Buy in season produce and preserve them to enjoy later.
- Avoid highly processed foods and eat a more plant-based diet with more fresh fruits, vegetables, beans/legumes, and whole grains.
- Compost your yard and kitchen waste.
- Plant your own garden for the freshest produce.
- Stay informed on these topics of the current food industry.
- Ask your grocer to carry local produce and eat at restaurants that serve locally produced foods.

Advocate and organize to promote these steps to all in your sphere of influence.

Price Adjustments, Taxation, and Subsidies

Many factors influence our food choices; however, the top four considerations of why we eat what we do are taste, convenience, cost, and nutritional value.[123] Studies reveal that simply lowering the price of healthier foods, including fruits, vegetables, and salad bars in cafeterias, as well as healthy snacks in vending machines in schools and worksites, has proven to be a highly effective method to increase the sales of these items. At minimum, this change in cost can positively change the proportion of sales of healthier choices versus less nutritious ones.[124–126] Price reductions of healthier foods in cafeterias or vending machines in 12 worksites and 12 secondary schools led to increased sales volume, which provided a constant level of profit, indicating a win-win situation for both consumers and food companies. This type of pricing strategy was pilot-tested in a midwestern suburban high school cafeteria during an entire school year.[127] Seven foods were targeted during the intervention: three popular higher fat foods (french fries, cookies, and cheese sauce) and four lower fat foods (fresh fruit, low-fat cookies, low-fat chips, and cereal bars). Prices ranged from 35¢ to $1.00. Prices on the higher fat foods were raised by approximately 10% and prices on the lower fat foods were reduced by approximately 25% for the school year. Sales data collected from school food services showed the revenue from the seven foods were within 5% of revenues estimated for usual price conditions. Therefore, students purchased based on price, which included a larger quantity of lower fat foods at lower prices, as revenue remained relatively unchanged.

In addition, French's 2003 study[126] examined the impact of a 50% price reduction on fresh fruit and baby carrots in two secondary school cafeterias. Compared with usual price conditions, price reductions resulted in a fourfold increase in fresh fruit sales and a twofold increase in baby carrot sales. These studies demonstrate the efficacy of price reductions in increasing purchases of more healthful foods in community-based settings, such as worksites and schools.

Paralleling the successful 1960s anti-smoking campaign, taxation on non-nutritious food and soda has been proposed as perhaps the most efficacious method to limit unhealthy food purchases and encourage better choices.[128–130] This strategy was originally suggested in the WHO's *1988 Healthy Public Policy Report*, which stated, "Taxation and subsidies should discriminate in favor of easy access for all to healthy food and improved diet."[131] In other words, taxations on unhealthy food could and should be used to subsidize fruits, vegetables, and whole grains.

Implementation of a minimal tax (one or two cents) has already begun in at least 18 states and in some major U.S. cities on items such as soda, gum, candy, and other snack foods.[56,130] Revenue generated from these nominal taxes has totaled $1.5 billion in just one year.[56] This money could be used for health promotion programs as well as subsidies for produce companies. There are dissenters, however, who believe that these types of economic or governmental measures are "food policing."[132] The question becomes, "How do we determine what foods are clearly 'unhealthy,' and therefore should be subject to taxation?" The United States faces the arduous task of creating and passing legislation for food and health policies that protect the health of Americans.

Another idea, in addition to taxation of unhealthy food, parallel to the anti-smoking campaign is the banning of junk food commercials and advertisements to children, just as the federal government banned cigarette ads from television in 1971.[56] Food advertising to children has infiltrated every aspect of a child's life—in school, on the Internet, at sports arenas, and on radio and television. Children are now exposed to 40,000 TV ads a year, up from 20,000 in the 1970s, according to a report by the Henry J. Kaiser Family Foundation."[133]

Social Marketing

As discussed more thoroughly in Chapter 26, social marketing is a powerful tool for reaching an enormous number of people via a well-designed campaign. To improve personal and social welfare, social marketing campaigns apply commercial marketing strategies to influence the voluntary behavior of target audiences.[134] The three main attributes of a successful social marketing campaign are the following:

1. Its primary goal is to influence the voluntary behavior of target market members.
2. It offers benefits for changing behavior and reduced barriers to perform the behavior.
3. It primarily benefits members of the target audience, or society at large, rather than the organization that initiated it.[134]

This is what makes social marketing distinctly different from commercial marketing.

The VERB Campaign

VERB is a multiethnic media campaign sponsored by the CDC, the goal of which is to increase and maintain physical activity among "tweens," that is, children aged 9 to 13 years.[135] Young people are encouraged to get off of the sofa, choose their "cool verb," and be active in sports and other hobbies (dance, swing, swim, play, etc.). It is an excellent example of successful social marketing that is reaching youth and changing their behavior. Parents and other influential community members (i.e., teachers, youth program leaders, and coaches) are the secondary audiences of the VERB initiative. VERB is not an acronym but a word that indicates action: "It's what you do."

VERB has successfully applied sophisticated commercial marketing techniques to address the public health problem of the sedentary lifestyles of American children. The social marketing principles address product, price, place, and promotion. Additionally, this initiative has been successful because it is quite focused and consumer-centric, and is designed specifically for and by kids of a specific age range.[136] Having an adequate budget to carry this message into all media that children use is necessary to "break through the clutter" of competing media messages. VERB spent a total of $125 million in one year, which predominantly went to paid advertising on television programs most watched by tweens. VERB's financial resources are a major factor contributing to the campaign's success; unfortunately, many other well-designed campaigns do not have this amount of funding.

The VERB campaign strives for high brand awareness and affinity among tweens. The theory is that when tweens bond positively with VERB, they will be more receptive to messages about physical activity. Then many, if not most, will take the next step and be active. In the first year of VERB (launched in June 2002), marketing efforts were dedicated to creating and introducing the VERB brand to tweens. As a previously nonexistent brand, VERB initially had no value to tweens. VERB has now been successfully "sold" to tweens as "their brand for having fun," because the campaign associates itself with popular kids brands, athletes, celebrities, and activities and products that are appealing, fun, and motivating. When asked about VERB, the majority of children familiar with it respond with, "It's cool."[136]

More than 450 partners are involved in this initiative to promote more physical activity in children. As the VERB brand continues to be promoted and spreads throughout the country, eventually it should become a well-established, popular brand. A social marketing program that models VERB strategies to promote healthier eating should be the next campaign initiated in the effort toward obesity prevention.

Powerful Bones, Powerful Girls

Another initiative to note is the National Bone Health Campaign (NBHC): Powerful Bones, Powerful Girls. This initiative is a multi-year campaign to promote optimal bone health in girls aged 9 to 12, and thus reduce their risk of osteoporosis later in life.[137] The goal is to educate and encourage girls to establish lifelong healthy habits, especially increased calcium consumption and weight-bearing physical activity to build and maintain strong bones.

The following are some features of Powerful Bones, Powerful Girls that have contributed to its success in reaching its target audience:

- Paid print and radio advertising for girls and parents
- Participation in the Radio Disney Live World Tour 2001
- An award-winning Web site for girls—this girl-friendly Web site helps girls understand how weight-bearing physical activity and calcium can be a fun and important part of everyday life. The site's key features include interactive games and quizzes, recipes for tasty foods with calcium, and ideas to help girls get plenty of weight-bearing physical activity.
- A downloadable calendar—this free calendar for girls and parents allows girls to track their calcium intake and physical activity, with their parents' input

- Collaboration with the Girl Scouts of the USA, Girls Inc., and the National Association of School Nurses

Fuel Up/Lift Off! LA/Sabor y Energia!

A Los Angeles County Department of Health Services social marketing campaign, Fuel Up/Lift Off! LA/Sabor y Energia! is targeted at obesity control in predominantly African-American and Latino-American communities.[138–140] Primary interventions include demonstrations and training in strategies to integrate physical activity and healthy food choices into routine business activities. Examples include incorporating activity breaks with music into lengthy meetings, offering healthy food choices when refreshments are served, and hosting walking meetings. A randomized, controlled trial tested the feasibility of including physical activity breaks as a part of lengthy meetings. The trial demonstrated success in the feasibility of engaging more than 90% of a sample of predominantly middle-aged and older women in 10 minutes of moderate physical activity, regardless of their fitness level or overweight status. It is worth noting that 10 minutes of activity is one-third of the federally recommended daily allowance of physical activity. If these women could add another 20 minutes of walking (e.g., after work) on a daily basis, then they would be reaching the recommended goal of 30 minutes per day of physical activity to achieve better health and prevent many chronic diseases.[141–143]

Health Communication Technology

Printed educational materials and face-to-face communication are two basic and simple methods to increase knowledge and understanding of health risks and how to make healthful behavior changes. However, these two traditional methods for health education are now supplemented by or even being replaced by DVD, CD-ROM, the Internet, e-mail, wireless communication options such as cellular telephones, handheld computers, and instant messaging. Newer technologies have opened up an unprecedented range of options for communicating and facilitating health behavior change strategies.[144] Advancements in computer software have simplified the process of producing personalized printouts tailored to an individual's needs or stage of change. The question of whether tailored or general printed materials are more effective has no definitive conclusion as of yet. Research thus far shows mixed results, with some studies finding tailored material to be more effective than non-tailored and other research showing that either type has equal effects on changing behavior.[144–146]

For those seeking a program for weight loss, individuals are able to enroll and participate in one without even leaving home or having face-to-face contact with anyone. A copious number of Internet programs can provide sound nutrition and exercise advice from qualified fitness professionals and registered dietitians. The top-rated sites may include these features:

- Personal nutrition, exercise, and behavioral assessments
- Customized meal planning tools, healthy recipes, online food journal, and exercise logs
- Scientifically sound, up-to-date nutrition information and weight loss tips
- Personalized exercise plan appropriately matched to ability, interest, and fitness level
- Information addressing emotional and behavioral issues (e.g., stress) related to food, along with coping strategies and support
- An online "community" and chat rooms to motivate and provide support on a regular basis

Nine studies examining the effectiveness of online support groups for weight loss have shown mixed but mostly nonsignificant results. The results of one particular study suggest that Internet support does not appear to be as effective as minimal or frequent intensive in-person therapist support for facilitating the long-term maintenance of weight loss.[147]

Thousands of electronic health-related peer-to-peer support groups in the form of mailing lists, chat rooms, and discussion forums are available on the Internet. Internet access has created opportunities to access health

Listservs: Contact with a specific group or organization through regular e-mail broadcasts.

information on any topic and has led some to self-diagnosis. This can be either a favorable or an unfortunate phenomenon, depending on whether the individual is then prompted to seek qualified medical advice in person. Numerous online support groups exist that serve as important social networks, especially for people with stigmatizing diseases such as AIDS, alcoholism, and certain cancers.[148] For individuals suffering from chronic pain, rare diseases, or conditions for which modern medicine has no effective remedy, and/or for those who are socially isolated with no family, these virtual friends and support groups can be life-giving. The primary medium for virtual communities today is the Internet in the form of emailing lists, newsgroups, listservs or discussion forums, Web-based discussion forums, and live chat rooms. As of April 2004, Yahoo! groups listed almost 70,000 electronic support groups in the health and wellness section. Anecdotal evidence shows that electronic peer-to-peer self-help groups might be beneficial social support interventions.

In contrast, a systematic review of studies examining the beneficial health effects of online peer-to-peer interaction failed to find robust evidence on the health benefits of virtual communities and peer-to-peer online support.[148] In 31 studies, investigators evaluated complex interventions, combining, for example, educational or cognitive behavior therapy components with peer-to-peer communications.

Integrative approaches like this make it challenging to draw conclusions on the effectiveness of pure electronic peer-to-peer interactions used daily by millions of people participating in Internet discussion groups or listservs. However, this study did not find any harm or negative health effects on participants who engaged regularly in virtual communities.[138]

The use of nutrition education CD-ROM programs for particular populations, such as those receiving food assistance programs, is increasing and showing promising results. One randomized study with Women, Infants and Children's (WIC) program participants in North Carolina employed an interactive CD-ROM program consisting of a targeted video soap opera, dietary assessment, and individually tailored diet feedback with strategies for making changes.[149] After receiving the intervention just once, participants significantly increased their self-efficacy and scored higher on low-fat eating and infant-feeding knowledge as compared to controls. It remains to be tested whether repeated use of this program can be instrumental in impacting behavior change for these participants.

Another CD-ROM program, entitled *Little by Little*, was created and tested with a low-income population of women in California with the aim to increase fruit and vegetable consumption and decrease fat intake.[150] This CD-ROM intervention program includes a brief assessment of fruit and vegetable intake as well as messages and tips on how to increase it. This tool proved effective in improving fruit and vegetable intake and helped advance participants through the study's Stage of Readiness for Change continuum, as compared with the control group. This *Little by Little* CD-ROM could prove quite useful in increasing fruit and vegetable intake of clients in public health and clinical settings.

Additional Favorable Health Effects

The numerous goal-specific interventions discussed in this chapter can also have reverberating positive health benefits that are not captured only because a particular outcome was not measured or studied. As one example, the goal of a British school-centered intervention was to slow the rise in obesity in children by decreasing soft drink consumption.[44] However, given the significant inverse relationship between soft drink consumption and bone mineral density[151] as well as the strong association between carbonated drink consumption and bone fractures,[152] interventions that decrease soda consumption in children could, in turn, improve bone health in young girls and lower their subsequent risk of osteoporosis.

■ CONCLUSION

As time passes, we will continue to learn and improve upon current strategies for intervening in dietary behaviors. At present, however, the most effective interventions are likely based on the social ecological theory. This theoretical model utilizes a multilevel approach, while altering the environment where individuals reside or work to be more conducive to and supportive of healthy eating. While recognizing the continued importance of intervening at all levels of society (from individual to population-wide), we must focus more attention and utilize the power and influence of media and governmental policy for effective and enduring change. Better health and quality of life can be achieved for every individual when all sectors of society work together in minimizing barriers to health and capitalizing on each other's strengths.

Issues for Discussion

1. Even when the study results of nutrition interventions appear efficacious, how strongly should we consider that self-reports of dietary intake are often wrought with random errors and recall bias, especially when revealing such personal behavior as eating?

2. Individuals who agree to participate and are captured in health interventions tend to be Caucasian, educated, English-speaking, and more health conscious.[153] How do we better engage marginalized individuals who need health-promoting interventions the most?

3. How transferable and practical do you feel these research intervention strategies are to implement in your own school, home, or work setting?

4. Has an interest in eating more "eco-consciously" paved a path that can lead to a healthier, safer, and more nutritious diet for the individual?

References

1. McLeroy KR, Bibeau D, Steckler A, Glanz K. An ecological perspective on health promotion programs. *Health Educ Q.* 1988;15:351–377.

2. Ory MG, Jordan PJ, Bazzarre T. The Behavior Change Consortium: setting the stage for a new century of health behavior-change research. *Health Educ Res.* 2002;17:500–511.

3. Kennedy ET, Bowman SA, et al. Dietary fat intake in the US population. *J Am Coll Nutr.* 1999;130:284S–288S.

4. Centers for Disease Control and Prevention. Trends in intake of energy and macronutrients—United States, 1981–2000. *Morbid Mortal Wkly Rep MMWR.* 2004;53:80–82. Available at http://www.cdc.gov/mmwr/preview/mmwrhtml/mm5304a3.htm. Accessed April 6, 2010.

5. Nielsen SJ, Siega-Riz AM, Popkin BM. Trends in energy intake in US between 1977 and 1996: similar shifts seen across age groups. *Obes Res.* 2002;10:370–378.

6. Nielsen SJ, Popkin BM. Patterns and trends in food portion sizes, 1977–1998. *JAMA.* 2003;289:450–453.

7. Nicklas TA, Baranowski T, Cullen KW, Berenson G. Eating patterns, dietary quality, and obesity. *J Am Coll Nutr.* 2001; 20:599–608.

8. Duffey KJ, Gordon-Larsen P, Jacobs DR Jr, Williams OD, Popkin BM. Differential associations of fast food and restaurant food consumption with 3-y change in body mass index: the Coronary Artery Risk Development in Young Adults Study. *Am J Clin Nutr.* 2007;85:201–208.

9. Ayala GX, Rogers M, Arredondo EM, et al. Away-from-home food intake and risk for obesity: examining the influence of context. *Obesity.* 2008;16:1002–1008.

10. Science in the Public Interest. Menu labeling legislation gains support from chain resturants. June 10, 2009. Available at http://www.cspinet.com/new/200906101.html. Accessed April 6, 2010.

11. Kris-Etherton PM, Binkoski AE, Zhao G, et al. Dietary fat: assessing the evidence in support of a moderate-fat diet; the benchmark based on lipoprotein metabolism. *Proc Nutr Soc.* 2002;61:287–299.

12. Sacks FM, Katan M. Randomized clinical trials on the effects of dietary fat and carbohydrate on plasma lipoproteins and cardiovascular disease. Review. *Am J Med.* 2002;30(suppl 9B):13S–24S.

13. Hu FB, Willett WC. Optimal diets for prevention of coronary heart disease. Review. *JAMA.* 2002;288:2569–2578.

14. Food Marketing Institute. 2007 news publication, "Facts and Figures." Available at http://www.fmi.org/news_releases/index.cfm?fuseaction = mediatext&id = 873. Accessed April 13, 2010.

15. Guggenbühl N. Obesity: it's super-size mania. *Belgian J Health Food.* 2003;60:9–10.

16. Schlosser E. *Fast Food Nation: The Dark Side of the All-American Meal.* New York: Houghton Mifflin; 2001:17.

17. Frumkin H. Urban sprawl and public health. *Public Health Rep.* 2002;117:201–217.

18. Jackson RJ, ed. *Am J Public Health* (entire issue). 2003;93: 1376–1589.

19. Finkelstein EA, Fiebelkorn IC, Wang G. National medical spending attributable to overweight and obesity: how much and who's paying? *Health Affairs.* 2003;W3;219–226.

20. Milner JA, McDonald SS, Anderson DE, Greenwald P. Molecular targets for nutrients involved with cancer prevention. *Nutr Cancer.* 2001;41:1–16.

21. Stender S, Dyerberg J, Holmer G, Ovesen L, Sandstrom B. The influence of trans fatty acids on health: a report from the Danish Nutrition Council. *Clin Sci (Lond).* 1995;88:375–392.

22. Sloane D, Diamant A, Lewis L, et al. Improving the nutritional resource environment for healthy living through community-based participatory research. *J Gen Intern Med.* 2003;18:568–575.

23. Institute of Medicine. *Health and Behavior.* Washington, DC: National Academy Press; 2001.

24. Kaplan GA, Keil JE. Socioeconomic factors and cardiovascular disease: a review of the literature. *Circulation.* 1993;88:1973–1998.

25. Syme S, Berkman L. Social class, susceptibility, and sickness. *Am J Epidemiol.* 1976;104:1–8.

26. Institute of Medicine, Smedley BD, Syme SL, eds. *Promoting Health: Intervention Strategies from Social and Behavioral Research report.* Washington, DC: National Academy Press; 2000.

27. U.S. Department of Health and Human Services. *Healthy People 2010.* Washington, DC: Department of Health and Human Services; 2000.

28. Stokols D. Establishing and maintaining healthy environments: toward a social ecology of health promotion. *Am Psychol.* 1992;47:6–22.

29. Stokols D. Translating social ecological theory into guidelines for community health promotion. *Am J Health Promot.* 1996; 10:282–298.

30. Making sense of global markets: beer in the USA. *Euromonitor International.* March 1, 2004.

31. Nestle M, Wing R, Birch L, et al. Behavioral and social influences on food choice. *Nutr Rev.* 1998;56(II):S50–S74.

32. Reger B, Wootan MG, Booth-Butterfield S. Using mass media to promote healthy eating: a community-based demonstration project. *Prev Med.* 1999;29:414–421.

33. Yancey AK, Kumanyika SK, Ponce NA, et al. Population-based interventions engaging communities of color in healthy eating and active living: a review. *Preventing Chronic Disease.* 2004; Jan. Available at http://www.cdc.gov/pcd/issues/2004/jan/03_0012.htm. Accessed April 6, 2010.

34. World Health Organization Regional Office for Europe. *The Adelaide Recommendations: Healthy Public Policy.* Geneva, Switzerland: WHO; 1988.

35. Goldfield GS, Epstein LH. Can fruits and vegetables and activities substitute for snack foods? *Health Psychol.* 2002; 21:299–303.

36. Nestle M. *Food Politics: How the Food Industry Influences Nutrition and Health.* Berkeley: University of California Press; 2002.

37. Tillotson JE. Pandemic obesity: is it time for change in economic and development policies affecting the food industry? *Nutr Today.* 2003;38:242–246.

38. Lytle LA, Seifert S, Greenstein J, McGovern P. How do children's eating patterns and food choices change over time? Results from a cohort study. *Am J Health Promot.* 2000;14:222–228.

39. Kelder SH, Perry CL, Klepp KI, Lytle LL. Longitudinal tracking of adolescent smoking, physical activity, and food choice behaviors. *Am J Public Health.* 1994;84:1121–1126.

40. Perry CL, Stone EJ, Parcel GS, et al. School-based cardiovascular health promotion: the child and adolescent trial for cardiovascular health (CATCH). *J Sch Health.* 1990;60:406–413.

41. Hoelscher DM, Feldman HA, Johnson CC, et al. School-based health education programs can be maintained over time: results from the CATCH institutionalization study. *Prev Med.* 2004;38:594–606.

42. Osganian SK, Hoelscher DM, Zive M, Mitchell PD, Snyder P, Webber LS. Maintenance of effects of the eat smart school food service program: results from the CATCH-ON study. *Health Educ Behav.* 2003;30:418–433.

43. Parcel GS, Perry CL, Kelder SH, et al. School climate and the institutionalization of the CATCH program. *Health Educ Behav.* 2003;30:489–502.

44. Perry CL, Bishop DB, Taylor GL, et al. A randomized school trial of environmental strategies to encourage fruit and vegetable consumption among children. *Health Educ Behav.* 2004;31:65–76.

45. American Food Service Association. *School Food Service and Nutrition Operations Study.* Alexandria, VA: American Food Service Association; 1999.

46. Story M, Hayes J, Kalina B. Availability of foods in high schools: is there cause for concern? *J Am Diet Assoc.* 1996;96:123–126.

47. Harnack L, Snyder P, Story M, Holliday R, Lytle L, Neumark-Sztainer D. Availability of a la carte food items in junior and senior high schools. *J Am Diet Assoc.* 2000;100:701–703.

48. Kubik MY, Lytle LA, Hannan PJ, Perry CL, Story M. The association of the school food environment with dietary behaviors of young adolescents. *Am J Public Health.* 2003;93:1168–1173.

49. Bauer KW, Yang YW, Austin SB. "How can we stay healthy when you're throwing all of this in front of us?" Findings from focus groups and interviews in middle schools on environmental influences on nutrition and physical activity. *Health Educ Behav.* 2004;31:34–46.

50. O'Dea JA. Why do kids eat healthful food? Perceived benefits of and barriers to healthful eating and physical activity among children and adolescents. *J Am Diet Assoc.* 2003;103:497–500.

51. James J, Thomas P, Cavan D, Kerr D. Preventing childhood obesity by reducing consumption of carbonated drinks: cluster randomized controlled trial. *BMJ.* 2004;328:1237.

52. Ludwig DS, Peterson KE, Gortmaker SL. Relation between consumption of sugar-sweetened drinks and childhood obesity: a prospective, observational analysis. *Lancet.* 2001;357:505–508.

53. Gillis LJ, Bar-Or O. Food away from home, sugar-sweetened drink consumption and juvenile obesity. *J Am Coll Nutr.* 2003; 22:539–545.

54. Bellisle F, Rolland-Cachera MF. How sugar-containing drinks might increase adiposity in children. *Lancet.* 2001;357:505–508.

55. American Academy of Pediatrics Committee on School Health. Soft drinks in schools. *Pediatrics.* 2004;113(1 Pt 1):152–154.

56. *Time Magazine.* Special issue: overcoming obesity in America; June 7, 2004.

57. Birnbaum AS, Lytle LA, Story M, Perry CL, Murray DM. Are differences in exposure to a multicomponent school-based intervention associated with varying dietary outcomes in adolescents? *Health Educ Behav.* 2002;29:427–443.

58. Sallis JF, McKenzie TL, Conway TL, et al. Environmental interventions for eating and physical activity: a randomized controlled trial in middle schools. *Am J Prev Med.* 2003;24: 209–217.

59. Healthy Schools Campaign. *Child Nutrition Act.* Available at http://www.healthyschoolscampaign.org/getinvolved/action/childnutrition/act.php. Accessed April 6, 2010.

60. *Time Magazine for Kids.* World Report Edition, From Farm to You. Oct 23, vol 15, no.7.

61. Heaney CA, Goetzal RZ. A review of health-related outcomes of multi-component worksite health promotion programs. *Am J Health Promot.* 1997;11:290–308.

62. Emmons KM, Thompson B, McLerran D, et al. The relationship between organizational characteristics and the adoption of workplace smoking policies. *Health Educ Behav.* 2000;27:483–501.

63. Biener L, Glanz K, McLerran D, et al. Impact of the Working Well Trial on the worksite smoking and nutrition environment. *Health Educ Behav.* 1999;26:478–494.

64. Kristal AR, Glanz K, Tilley BC, Li S. Mediating factors in dietary change: understanding the impact of a worksite nutrition intervention. *Health Educ & Behav.* 27:112–125.

65. Glanz K, Sorensen G, Farmer A. The health impact of worksite nutrition and cholesterol intervention programs. *Am J Health Promot.* 1996;10:453–470.

66. Karlehagen S, Ohlson CG. Primary prevention of cardiovascular disease by an occupational health service. *Prev Med.* 2003;37: 219–225.

67. Tilley BC, Vernon SW, Myers R, et al. The Next Step Trial: impact of a worksite colorectal cancer screening promotion program. *Prev Med.* 1999;28:276–283.

68. Patterson, RE, Kristal AR, Biener L, et al. Durability and diffusion of the nutrition intervention in the Working Well Trial. *Prev Med.* 1998;27(5 Pt 1):668–673.

69. House JS, Landis KR, Umberson D. Social relationships and health. *Science.* 1988;241:540–545.

70. Uchino BN, Cacioppo JT, Kiecolt-Glaser JK. The relationship between social support and psychological processes: a review with emphasis on underlying mechanisms and implications for health. *Psych Bull.* 1996;119:488–531.

71. McCaffree J. Childhood eating patterns: the roles parents play. *J Am Diet Assoc.* 2003;103:1587.

72. Nestle M, Wing R, Birch L, et al. Behavioral and social influences on food choice. *Nutr Rev.* 1998;56:S50–S74.

73. Birch LL, Davison KK. Family environmental factors influencing the developing behavioral controls of food intake and childhood overweight. *Pediatr Clin North Am.* 2001;48:893–907.

74. Golan M, Crow S. Parents are key players in the prevention and treatment of weight-related problems. *Nutr Rev.* 2004;62:39–50.

75. Birch LL, Fisher JO, Davison KK. Learning to overeat: maternal use of restrictive feeding practices promotes girls' eating in the absence of hunger. *Am J Clin Nutr.* 2003;78:215–220.

76. McHale SM. Family dynamics: challenges and opportunities for preventing childhood obesity. Workshop presentation, December 9, 2003. The Prevention of Childhood Obesity: Understanding the Influences of Marketing, Media, and Family Dynamics. Available at http://www.iom.edu/Activities/Children/Obes Prevention/2003-DEC-09.aspx. Accessed April 19, 2010.

77. Grusec JE, Goodnow JJ, Kuczynski L. New directions in analyses of parenting contributions to children's acquisition of values. *Child Dev.* 2000;71:205–211.

78. Dunst CJ, Trivette CM. Empowerment, effective help-giving practices and family-centered care. *Pediatr Nurs.* 1996;22: 334–337, 343.

79. Birch LL. Development of food acceptance patterns in the first years of life. *Proc Nutr Soc.* 1998;57:617–624.

80. Galloway AT, Lee Y, Birch LL. Predictors and consequences of food neophobia and pickiness in young girls. *J Am Diet Assoc.* 2003;103:692–698.

81. Neumark-Sztainer D, Wall M, Perry C, Story M. Correlates of fruit and vegetable intake among adolescents. Findings from Project EAT. *Prev Med.* 2003;37:198–208.

82. Haire-Joshu D, Brownson RC, Nanney MS, et al. Improving dietary behavior in African Americans: the Parents As Teachers High 5, Low Fat Program. *Prev Med.* 2003;36:684–691.

83. Epple C, Wright AL, Joish VN, Bauer M. The role of active family nutritional support in Navajos' type 2 diabetes metabolic control. *Diabetes Care.* 2003;26:2829–2834.

84. Sorensen G, Hunt MK, Cohen N, et al. Worksite and family education for dietary change: the Treatwell 5-A-Day program. *Health Educ Res.* 1998;13:577–591.

85. Sorensen G, Stoddard A, Peterson K, et al. Increasing fruit and vegetable consumption through worksites and families in the Treatwell 5-A-Day study. *Am J Public Health.* 1999;89:54–60.

86. Macario E, Sorensen G. Spousal similarities in fruit and vegetable consumption. *Am J Health Promot.* 1998;12:369–377.

87. Schwartz, MB, Puhl R. Childhood obesity: a societal problem to solve. *Obesity Rev.* 2003;4:57–71.

88. Seeman T, Berkman L, Kohout F, LaCroix A, Glynn R, Blazer D. Intercommunity variation in the association between social ties and mortality in the elderly: a comparative analysis of three communities. *Ann Epidemiol.* 1993;3:325–335.

89. Kawachi I, Berkman L. Social cohesion, social capital and health. In: Berkman L, Kawachi I, eds. *Social Epidemiology.* New York: Oxford University Press; 2000.

90. Minkler M, Wallerstein N. Improving health through community organization and community building. In: Glanz K, Lewis FM, Rimer BK, eds. *Health Behavior and Health Education: Theory, Research, and Practice,* 2nd ed. San Francisco: Jossey-Bass; 1997:241–269.

91. Viadro CI, Farris RP, Will JC. The WISEWOMAN projects: lessons learned from three states. *J Womens Health (Larchmt).* 2004;13: 529–538.

92. Yanek LR, Becker DM, Moy TF, Gittelsohn J, Koffman DM. Project Joy: faith based cardiovascular health promotion for African American women. *Public Health Rep.* 2001;116(suppl 1):68–81.

93. Demark-Wahnefried W, McClelland JW, Jackson B, et al. Partnering with African American churches to achieve better health: lessons learned during the Black Churches United for Better Health 5-A-Day project. *J Cancer Educ.* 2000;15:164–167.

94. Campbell MK, Motsinger BM, Ingram A, et al. The North Carolina Black Churches United for Better Health Project: intervention and process evaluation. *Health Educ Behav.* 2000;27:241–253.

95. Resnicow K, Jackson A, Braithwaite R, et al. Healthy Body/Healthy Spirit: a church-based nutrition and physical activity intervention. *Health Educ Res.* 2002;17:562–573.

96. Ammerman A, Corbie-Smith G, St. George DMM, Washington C, Weathers B, Jackson-Christian B. Research expectations among African American church leaders in the PRAISE! Project: a randomized trial guided by community-based participatory research. *Am J Public Health.* 2003;93:1720–1727.

97. Corbie-Smith G, Ammerman AS, Katz ML, et al. Trust, benefit, satisfaction, and burden: a randomized controlled trial to reduce cancer risk through African-American churches. *J Gen Intern Med.* 2003;18:531–541.

98. United States Department of Agriculture. Body & Soul: A Celebration of Healthy Eating & Living. Available at http://foodstamp.nal.usda.gov/foodstamp/resource_finder_details.php?id=409. Accessed April 19, 2010.

99. Clark PG, Nigg CR, Greene G, Riebe D, Saunders SD, Study of Exercise and Nutrition in Older Rhode Islanders Project Team. The Study of Exercise and Nutrition in Older Rhode Islanders (SENIOR): translating theory into research. *Health Educ Res.* 2002;17:552–561.

100. Bernstein A., Nelson ME, Tucker KL, et al. A home-based nutrition intervention to increase consumption of fruits, vegetables, and calcium-rich foods in community dwelling elders. *J Am Diet Assoc.* 2002 Oct;102:1421–1427.

101. International Longevity Center, USA, Ltd. Maintaining healthy lifestyles: a lifetime of choices. Workshop Report. December 1999.

102. Chapel DL, McCulla MM, Reinsch B, Warren C. Moving right along: a creative partnership to engage older adults in physical activity and nutrition programs. Abstract. Preventing Chronic Disease. 2004 Apr. Available at http://www.cdc.gov/pcd/issues/2004/apr/03_0034d.htm. Accessed April 6, 2010.

103. Glasgow RE, La Chance PA, Toobert DJ, Brown J, Hampson SE, Riddle MC. Long term effects and costs of a brief behavioral dietary intervention for patients with diabetes delivered from the medical office. *Patient Educ Couns.* 1997;32:175–184.

104. Rollnick S, Miller WR. What is motivational interviewing? *Behav Cogn Psychother.* 1995;23:325–334.

105. Resnicow K, Jackson A, Wang T, et al. A motivational interviewing intervention to increase fruit and vegetable intake through black churches: results of the Eat for Life trial. *Am J Public Health.* 2001;91:1686–1693.

106. Pignone MP, Ammerman A, Fernandez L, et al. Counseling to promote a healthy diet in adults: a summary of the evidence for the U.S. Preventive Services Task Force. *Am J Prev Med.* 2003;24:75–92.

107. Stevens VJ, Glasgow RE, Toobert DJ, Karanja N, Smith KS. One-year results from a brief, computer-assisted intervention to decrease consumption of fat and increase consumption of fruits and vegetables. *Prev Med.* 2003;36:594–600.

108. Steptoe A, Perkins-Porras L, McKay C, Rink E, Hilton S, Cappuccio FP. Behavioural counselling to increase consumption of fruit and vegetables in low income adults: randomised trial. *BMJ.* 2003;326:855–860.

109. Mensah GA, Goodman RA, Zaza S, et al. Law as a tool for preventing chronic diseases: expanding the spectrum of effective public health strategies. In: *Preventing Chronic Disease.* 2004; Jan. Available at http://www.cdc.gov/pcd/issues/2004/jan/03_0033.htm. Accessed April 6, 2010.

110. Gostin LO. Public law in a new century. 1. Law as a tool to advance the community's health. *JAMA.* 2000;83L:2837–2841.

111. Institute of Medicine. *The Future of Public Health.* Washington, DC: National Academy Press; 2002.

112. *Today's Dietitian Magazine.* Food (and film) for thought (and action). October 2009, vol 11, No. 10.

113. Benbrook C, McCullum-Gómez C. Organic vs conventional farming. *J Am Diet Assoc.* 2009;109:809,811.

114. McCullum-Gomez C, Scott A-M. *Perspectives on the Benefits of Organic Foods.* Hunger and Environmental Nutrition Dietetic Group, September 2009. American Dietetic Association, Eat Right. Available at http://www.eatright.org/About/Content.aspx?id=6812. Accessed April 6, 2010.

115. Tagtow A, Harmon H. Sustainable food systems: perspectives from the United States, Canada, and the European Union. *J Hunger Environ Nutr* 2008;3:103–105.

116. Friel S, Dangour AD, Garnett T, et al. Public health benefits of strategies to reduce greenhouse-gas emissions: food and agriculture. *Lancet.* 2009;374:2016–2025.

117. Roberts I. The health co-benefits of climate change policies: doctors have a responsibility to future generations. *Clin Med.* 2009;9:212–213.

118. Cooper A, Holmes LM. *Lunch Lessons, Changing the Way We Feed Our Children.* New York: HarperCollins; 2006.

119. Hawkes C. Promoting healthy diets and tackling obesity and diet-related chronic diseases: what are the agricultural policy levers? *Food Nutr Bull.* 2007;28(2 suppl):S312–S322.

120. World Health Organization. (2002). Foods derived from modern technology: 20 questions on genetically modified foods. Available at http://www.who.int/foodsafety/publications/biotech/20questions/en/index.html. Accessed April 20, 2010.

121. Kogan, LA. Precautionary Preference. Institute for Trade Standards and Sustainable Development, 2005. Available at http://www.nftc.org/default/Trade%20Policy/WTO_Issues/Kogan-ITSSD%202005.pdf. Accessed April 12, 2010.

122. United States. President's Commission for the Study of Ethical Problems in Medicine and Biomedical and Behavioral Research. *Splicing Life: A Report on the Social and Ethical Issues of Genetic Engineering and Human Beings.* Washington, DC: President's Commission for the Study of Biomedical and Behavioral Research, 1982:126.

123. Glanz K, Basil M, Maibach E, Goldberg J, Snyder D. Why Americans eat what they do: taste, nutrition, cost, convenience, and weight control concerns as influences on food consumption. *J Am Diet Assoc.* 1998;98:1118–1126.

124. Jeffery RW, French SA, Raether C, et al. An environmental intervention to increase fruit and salad purchases in a cafeteria. *Prev Med.* 1994;23:788–792.

125. French SA, Jeffery RW, Story M, Hannan P, Snyder P. A pricing strategy to promote low-fat snack choices through vending machines. *Am J Public Health.* 1997;87: 849–851.

126. French SA. Pricing effects on food choices. *J Nutr.* 2003;133:841S–843S.

127. Hannan P, French SA, Story M, Fulkerson JA. A pricing strategy to promote purchase of lower fat foods in a high school cafeteria: acceptability and sensitivity analysis. *Am J Health Promot.* 2002;17:1–6.

128. Temple NJ, Balay-Karperien AL. Nutrition in cancer prevention: an integrated approach. Review. *J Am Coll Nutr.* 2002;21:79–83.

129. Jacobson MF, Brownell KD. Small taxes on soft drinks and snack foods to promote health. *Am J Public Health.* 2000;90:854–857.

130. Wilson N, Mansoor O. Getting the fat tax on the table. *N Z Med J.* 2000;113:451.

131. World Health Organization. Technical Report Series. *Diet, Nutrition and the Prevention of Chronic Diseases.* Geneva, Switzerland: WHO; 2003:916.

132. Byers T. Reflections on the war on cancer. *J Am Coll Nutr.* 2002;21:77–78.

133. American Dietetic Association. Position paper: total diet approach to communicating food and nutrition information. *J Am Diet Assoc.* 2002;102:100.

134. Glanz K, Lewis FM, Rimer BK, eds. *Health Behavior and Health Education: Theory, Research, and Practice,* 3rd ed. San Francisco: Jossey-Bass;2002.

135. Centers for Disease Control and Prevention. *VERB: It's What You Do.* (Historical Document). Available at http://www.cdc.gov/youthcampaign. Accessed April 6, 2010.

136. Rosenthal E. Marketing and Media Influences. Workshop presentation. December 9, 2003. The Prevention of Childhood Obesity: Understanding the Influences of Marketing, Media, and Family Dynamics. Available at http://www.iom.edu/Activities/Children/ObesPrevention/2003-DEC-09.aspx. Accessed April 19, 2010.

137. Centers for Disease Control and Prevention. Best Bones Forever! Available at http://www.bestbonesforever.gov/. Accessed April 6, 2010.

138. Sloane DC, Diamant AL, Lewis LB, et al. Improving the nutritional resource environment for healthy living through community-based participatory research. *J Gen Intern Med.* 2003;18:568–575.

139. Kumanyika S. Obesity treatment in minorities. In: Wadden TA, Stunkard AJ, eds. *Obesity: Theory and Therapy,* 3rd ed. New York: Guilford Publications; 2002:xiii,377.

140. Yancey AK, Miles OL, McCarthy WJ, et al. Differential response to targeted recruitment strategies to fitness promotion research by African-American women of varying body mass index. *Ethn Dis.* 2001;11:115–123.

141. National Cancer Institute. Introducing the next generation of 5-A-Day. Available at http://www.5aday.gov. Accessed April 6, 2010.

142. Foerster SB, Kizer KW, Disogra LK, Bal DG, Krieg BF, Bunch KL. California's "5-A-Day-For Better Health!" campaign: an innovative population-based effort to effect large-scale dietary change. *Am J Prev Med.* 1995;11:124–131.

143. National Cancer Institute. *5-A-Day for Better Health Program.* NIH publication 01–5019; September 2001.

144. Brinberg D, Axelson ML, Price S. Changing food knowledge, food choice, and dietary fiber consumption by using tailored messages. *Appetite.* 2000;35:35–43.

145. Brug J, Steenhuis I, van Assema P, de Vries H. The impact of a computer-tailored nutrition intervention. *Prev Med.* 1996;25:236–242.

146. Campbell MK, DeVellis BM, Strecher VJ, et al. Improving dietary behavior: the effectiveness of tailored messages in primary care settings. *Am J Public Health.* 1994;84:783–787.

147. Harvey-Berino J, Pintauro S, Buzzell P, et al. Does using the internet facilitate the maintenance of weight loss? *Int J Obes Relat Metab Disord.* 2002;26:1254–1260.

148. Eysenbach G, Powell J, Englesakis M, Rizo C, Stern A. Health related virtual communities and electronic support groups: systematic review of the effects of online peer to peer interactions. *BMJ.* 2004;328:1166.

149. Campbell MK, Carbone E, Honess-Morreale L, Heisler-Mackinnon J, Demissie S, Farrell D. Randomized trial of a tailored nutrition education CD-ROM program for women receiving food assistance. *J Nutr Educ Behav.* 2004;36:58–66.

150. Block G, Wakimoto P, Metz D, et al. A randomized trial of the *Little by Little* CD-ROM: demonstrated effectiveness in increasing fruit and vegetable intake in a low-income population. *Preventing Chronic Disease.* 2004 Jul. Available at http://www.cdc.gov/pcd/issues/2004/jul/04_0016.htm. Retrieved April 6, 2010.

151. McGartland C, Robson PJ, Murray L, et al. Carbonated soft drink consumption and bone mineral density in adolescence: the Northern Ireland Young Hearts project. *J Bone Miner Res.* 2003;18:1563–1569.

152. Wyshak G. Teenaged girls, carbonated beverage consumption, and bone fractures. *Arch Pediatr Adolesc Med.* 2000;154:610–613.

153. Bull SS, Gillette C, Glasgow RE, Estabrooks P. Work site health promotion research: to what extent can we generalize the results and what is needed to translate research to practice? *Health Educ Behav.* 2003;30:537–549.

PART

III

Shaping the Policies That Affect the Public's Health

In Part III, we shift gears to investigate how science and needs assessment translate into public policy. It is through governmental policy that public health nutritionists are directed to educate and serve the public. Chapters 7 and 8 describe how nutrition policy is created, advocated for, and influenced by the public, health practitioners, lobbyists, and legislators. These chapters highlight the need for dietitians and nutritionists to get involved in advocating for and influencing the passing of important nutrition policy. Chapter 9 demonstrates how the USDA acts on nutrition policy once it is made, and illustrates the complexity of that role in fulfilling the challenges of public health nutrition.

Creating Public Policy

Bruce Rengers, PhD, RD

READER OBJECTIVES

After studying this chapter and reflecting on the contents, you should be able to:

1. Define public policy.
2. Discuss some of the characteristics of public policy and why it is important.
3. Describe the conflicting aspects of public policy.
4. Discuss the evolution of nutrition policy in the United States.
5. Identify the steps involved in the creation of public policy.
6. Delineate the steps by which legislation is created in Congress.
7. Describe the role various levels of government play in creating public health policy.

■ INTRODUCTION

To accomplish something in an organized and efficient manner you must have a goal and a plan of action. This is the reason for creating policy. Policy may be defined as "a course of action or principle adopted or proposed by a government, party, business, or individual,"[1] though some have suggested that a truly accurate definition of policy may be impossible to create.[2] This definition of policy may vary depending on the goals and needs of those trying to define the concept. In a very general sense, a policy is a set of rules to solve a problem, real or perceived. Most policies consist of two parts[3]: 1) a statement or goal of what is to be accomplished, and 2) a set of practical rules, guidelines, programs, or regulations to accomplish the stated goal.

This chapter is about public policy, specifically public health policy as it relates to nutrition. Policy is labeled *public policy* when it is created by government. Public policy is created at all levels of government. It is how government functions. The government creates policies to regulate its own actions and to govern the actions of citizens, businesses, and other entities under its control. Ultimately, what a government does is a reflection of its public policy. Some would say that what government does is public policy, regardless of what may be written or stated.

Birkland[2] describes public policy as having several attributes, including being made in the public's interest, that it is interpreted and implemented by public and private actors, that it is a reflection of what the government intends to do, and what the government chooses not to do. Policy is also more than simply the sum total of all of the government's laws and regulation. Policy is also created daily by people as they implement policy.[2]

Public policy may be created by the legislative, executive, or judicial branch of government.[4] Generally, policy is created by legislation that is introduced and passed by the legislative branch.[3] This legislation or policy is then translated into a set of practical rules by the executive branch to accomplish the intent of the legislation. Policy, however, also may be informal, indirect, and even unwritten. For example, a governing political party may have a philosophical belief of government involvement in food regulation. This philosophy becomes the government's guiding public policy.[5] Special interest groups, organizations, and certain individuals may also play an important role in determining public policy.

Government policy is reflected as much in what

> A special interest group or organization may convince policy makers to create or avoid legislation that would affect their interests.[3,4]

government won't do as in what it will do.[3] Many unwritten and informal policies are more about what government will not be involved in. If the government identifies a problem, such as advertising directed at children, and then takes no action to regulate such advertising, this is a reflection of government policy. The decision not to become involved may be based on philosophies of downsizing government, reducing spending, decreasing regulation, responding to special interest groups, or even a distrust of the evidence that says such advertising may be harmful. Because these philosophies direct the actions of the government, they become part of public policy.

■ CHARACTERISTICS OF PUBLIC POLICY

Policy is generally created in response to a problem, perceived or real.[3,4] In an ideal world, policy would be created from objective assessments to identify potential problems and then prevent them. This, however, is rarely how public policy is created. Government officials generally create policy in response to emerging or existing problems that are important to the public, special interest groups, or professional or scientific groups. These emerging problems may be real or only perceived problems.[4] Sometimes popular belief or philosophies may result in identification of a concept as a problem or as a cause of a problem, when in fact there is little evidence to support the belief. It has been stated that more public policies fail from working to solve a perceived problem that is not real than from creating the wrong plan to solve a real problem.[4,6] Many policy issues are emotional, and solutions are created based on philosophical beliefs rather than actual understanding of the facts.[7]

Public policy is often controversial. Because it generally affects a great number and variety of people and interests, it tends to be more controversial than less expansive private policies.[2] But because public policy also affects a great number of people, it is more important than private policy. Public policy generally results in some form of control that limits the freedoms of some or all so that the majority may experience a greater benefit.[8] There are those who believe government should limit its role and allow society to function with minimal interference.[3] Under this philosophy of limited involvement, economics and the free market create an environment where individuals have responsibility for their own actions and situations.

This is in contrast to a social justice philosophy, which acknowledges that so-ciety may share in the responsibility for a person's health.[3] Although it may be true that a person who overeats is responsible for his or her diet, there also may be societal factors that strongly influence a person's diet. For example, a person working for low wages in a decaying neighborhood without grocery stores or public transportation may have few options other than to buy high-calorie prepared foods from a local convenience store. Public policy may be needed to alter those conditions in order for a person to have a reasonable ability to choose a healthy diet and lifestyle. Some argue that it is the role of government to create conditions that make healthy choices easier and unhealthy choices harder.[3,9] The mission of public health is to assure conditions in which people can be healthy.[10] To assure these conditions requires policies that result in government intervention. The decision to limit personal choices and freedoms cannot be taken for granted, however, and the benefit from such public policies must be balanced against economic costs and losses of individual freedom.[8]

In the United States, we are conflicted with these two philosophies of public policy. For example, we want the government to ensure that our food supply is healthful, yet we also want the personal freedom to purchase unhealthful food. We want the government to guard us against becoming obese, yet we also want the freedom to make dietary and lifestyle choices that will lead to obesity. We want it both ways—freedom to make harmful choices, yet protection from harm when we do make those choices.

While many argue for less government, public policy is necessary in a complex society,[11] especially to safeguard health. To use a simple example, in a nation with little population and only a few cars, no significant public policy may be necessary with respect to automobiles. In a nation with millions of automobiles crowded into a dense area, public policies are needed with respect to driving, parking, passenger safety, road building and maintenance, car manufacturing, auto emissions, and even car disposal.

The same idea can easily be applied to other health issues in a society. For example, as societies become larger it becomes more important that a family not dump its sewage and other waste into the local water supply used by many others. Or, as our food supply changes and we become removed from production, policies are needed to ensure an adequate and safe food supply. Obviously, in a democratic society there must be a balance between the need to create a healthier society and the need to maintain personal freedoms.[8]

As an example of minimal government interference, one viewpoint could be that an obese person is obese because he or she chooses to overeat, and it is the individual's responsibility to eat less. An obese person is, therefore, responsible for the consequences of overeating. No action is required by the government.

The Code of Federal Regulations (CFR) is the codification of the general and permanent rules published in the Federal Register by the executive departments and agencies of the federal government. It is divided into 50 titles that represent broad areas subject to federal regulation.

As a result of a need for public policy in a complex society, public policy touches almost every aspect of our lives.[3] One only need visit the government documents section of a library or peruse the Code of Federal Regulations to see that there are numerous public policies that affect our daily lives. Public policy is a reality. Life in a complex society without policies would be difficult and disorderly. Policy development for community living is a universal requirement.[11]

■ U.S. PUBLIC HEALTH POLICY

Government has many reasons to be interested in the health of its citizens. A democratic government is elected by its citizens, and therefore has an interest in the welfare of the citizens who have created it.[12] Beyond the needs of individual health, the collective health of a country's citizens is vital to a country's economic health and independence as a nation. Health is a social as well as individual responsibility.[10]

The mission of public health, as stated by the Institute of Medicine (IOM) in its report entitled, *The Future of Public Health*, is "fulfilling society's interest in assuring conditions in which people can be healthy."[10] Many of the major improvements in the health of the American people have come about because of changes in public health policy. By one estimate, 25 of the last 30 years added to the U.S. life expectancy rate have been a result of changes brought about by public health policy.[13]

In its review of the U.S. public health system, the IOM noted that the United States has generally come to take the successes of public health for granted and that the nation has lost sight of its public health goals.[10] To date, the nation lacks a comprehensive public health policy.[12] Instead, the IOM[12] described a situation where public health policy tends to be antiquated, inconsistent, redundant, and at times ambiguous. Despite greater knowledge about health and the factors that affect health, technical knowledge plays a smaller role today in creating public policy than it did in the past.[10] Health policy is determined more by crises, hot issues, and the concerns of organized interest groups than careful analysis of objective data and technical knowledge about health.[10]

The IOM gave many reasons for the disarray of the U.S. public health system and challenged public health officials and policy makers to refocus on the three essential functions of public health: assessment, policy development, and assurance.[10] Although the responsibilities for public health are spread throughout the Federal Government, the Department of Health and Human Services (DHHS) is generally considered the principle agency of the federal public health infrastructure. It is also the principal contact for other federal agencies, as well as state and local agencies, with respect to public health issues.[12] Policy development is a critical function of DHHS in maintaining public health.[12] The U.S. Department of Agriculture (USDA), however, was designated as the lead for nutrition policy by the 1977 Farm Bill. Most federal nutrition programs are administered by USDA at the federal level.[3]

Nutrition Policy: A Brief History

As with the national health policy in general, there is no single or unifying public policy that guides the activities of government agencies with respect to nutrition in the United States.[3] Nutrition policy is fragmented amongst numerous laws, agencies, programs, and branches of the government.[3] Nutrition policy is often conflicting and inconsistent. Much of it is antiquated, having been created in the past when different nutritional problems affected the public.[3]

At the beginning of the twentieth century, little was known about nutrition. The main nutritional concerns of most people and the government were related to getting enough food to eat and avoiding foods that would make people sick. Early nutrition policy was, therefore, primarily agricultural policy. The government created policies to provide the population with a consistent and plentiful food supply at low cost. Because getting adequate calories was a major concern, emphasis was placed on providing foods that were a dense source of calories. These agricultural policies of the past had a major impact on shaping food supply that continues to this day.[3]

With the discovery of vitamins in the early part of the twentieth century, nutrition experts began to create guidelines encouraging people to eat certain groups of foods. In 1917, the USDA created the Five Food Groups to encourage people to eat food that provided all of the then-known nutrients. This guide was modified over time into a variety of forms to ensure that people were getting adequate diets. It wouldn't be until much later that nutrition guidelines from the government would start mentioning moderating, or limiting intakes of certain types of foods, such as those high in fat or sodium.

During the first half of the twentieth century, other nutrition policies were enacted, including fortification of salt with iodine, food distribution programs to feed children and other hungry people during the depression of the 1930s, the first Nationwide Food Consumption Survey, and establishment of the National School Lunch Program. In 1941, the first set of "Recommended Dietary Allowances (RDAs)" was published, making recommendations for levels of certain nutrients in the diet. The emphasis was still about getting an adequate diet.

During the 1960s, the attention of the public health community started to change from an emphasis on infectious diseases to one on chronic diseases. Many accomplishments had been made in controlling communicable disease, and chronic diseases had become the main causes of death in the United States. Public interest in nutrition and its effects on long-term health was also heightened by the publication of books in the popular press by Adelle Davis, Rachel Carson, and others, which stirred interest and controversy in the long-term effects of food, food additives, and nutrients on health. Continued interest in ensuring that people got enough food led to the establishment of the Food Stamp Program (now called Supplemental Nutrition Assistance Program [SNAP]), School Breakfast Program, and the Special Supplemental Food Program for Women, Infants and Children (WIC) during the 1960s and 1970s.

In 1977, the Senate Select Committee on Nutrition and Human Needs issued the first edition of the Dietary Goals for the United States. It was one of the first governmental attempts at making nutritional recommendations, based on theories about the effects of diet on chronic disease.[3] This started a change in dietary recommendations that addressed moderation of certain foods and making choices between foods within a food group.[3] The focus of recommendations and policy was changing from just getting an adequate diet to making qualitative choices related to diet. Moderation and choosing one type of food over another because of its effects on chronic disease became important.

Since the Dietary Goals for the United States were released, many government documents have been created that make recommendations about diet with respect to chronic diseases. The Surgeon General's Report on Nutrition and Health presented the first comprehensive review of the scientific evidence associating diet with chronic disease.[14] Nutrition and Your Health: Dietary Guidelines for Americans, created by DHHS and USDA and jointly published every five years since 1980, recommended dietary changes to help people avoid certain chronic diseases. The Dietary Guidelines were intended to be the foundation of all federal nutrition policies and programs and a vehicle for the government to speak with one voice on nutrition and health.[15] Unfortunately, many federal policies, such as agricultural polices, do not follow the Dietary Guidelines and promote foods high in components such as saturated fat and sodium that are overconsumed by the public.

The Healthy People initiative led by the DHHS Office of Disease Prevention and Health Promotion has become the latest model for policy development, including nutrition policy. Healthy People 2010 was developed by DHHS with input from all its operating divisions, state and local government partners, more than 350 national membership organizations, nongovernmental organizations, corporate sponsors, and public input. It was a cooperative effort of government and nongovernment entities to create policy goals for the United States. Healthy People 2010 contains a number of goals related to nutrition and is used by many public health agencies in creating nutrition policies. It has been suggested that Healthy People 2010 may be DHHS's most effective non-legislative policy vehicle for improving public health.[12] The creation of Healthy People 2020 is now underway.

Nutrition Policy: Goals and Methods

If the goal of public health policy is "fulfilling society's interest in assuring conditions in which people can be healthy,"[10] then nutrition policy would have the goal of assuring conditions in which people can be healthy through diet. There are two general ways that are used to try to influence what people eat: through education and through modification of the food supply.[3] In a very simplistic example, if a group of people were found to have a nutritional problem with inadequate amounts of vitamin A in the diet, the approach would be to teach them about the need for and sources of vitamin A, and assure that they have a culturally acceptable, inexpensive, and appealing source of vitamin A available. (Another approach to finding a culturally acceptable and appealing source of vitamin A would be to create a new source for the vitamin through fortification of food, as has been done with some nutrients in the United States. This approach only works, however, when the lacking substances are known nutrients that can be easily added to common foods that are readily available.)

The problem becomes more complicated when the major nutritional problems being encountered are ones of excess, as with calories, sodium, and certain types of fat, or when whole food groups need to be increased, such as with fruits and vegetables. How does government create policies to discourage the consumption of certain foods and encourage the consumption of others?

The preferred policy method by many is *education*: training the public on which foods should be consumed and which foods should be avoided or eaten in moderation.[3] This may be accomplished through consumer education campaigns, food assistance programs, and official documents of the government giving dietary advice, such as the Dietary Guidelines. Using education to influence food choices is a less powerful way to influence dietary behavior than actually trying to modify the food supply. Many prefer education, however, because it has less of an effect on personal freedom (you can still choose to eat excess high-calorie foods laden with sodium and saturated fat), and it has less impact on the economies of those producing and selling the foods to be avoided. Education may also be about prohibiting claims that provide false information or unfairly influence certain segments of the population. For example, it may be desirable to restrict unsubstantiated claims for foods and nutrients or to limit advertising of certain foods to children.

A more powerful way to influence dietary choices is through modifying the food supply.[3] Foods that are healthful should be more readily available and less expensive than those that would be considered less healthful or that are currently eaten in excess. Some have argued that the current obesity epidemic is due to a toxic environment where the wrong types of foods are readily available in supersized amounts.[16] Portion sizes of foods in restaurants have increased, the number of convenience foods has multiplied, and vending machines make low-nutrient foods readily available almost everywhere. Changes in the food supply, coupled with education, is generally considered a more successful strategy for dietary change.[3]

Government policies have a great impact on what foods are available to the public and at what price. Many of the current food policies come from a time when providing adequate food at a cheap price was the goal of U.S. agricultural and nutrition policy. The conditions and health issues that existed when those policies were created are not the same as exist now. From a nutrition policy point of view, these policies need to be reevaluated to create food policies that support the production, marketing, and low price of foods that are associated with a healthier diet rather than support the production of less healthy foods. This is not a readily acceptable option to many, however, because it means dramatic changes in economic realities for those whose livelihoods depend on current government food and agricultural policy.[17]

Beyond agricultural policy, there are ways to control the food supply that have been tried or suggested. Some of these suggestions include altering school lunch menus to meet the Dietary Guidelines, offering low cost or free fruits and vegetables to schools, adding fruits and vegetables and limiting the fat content in WIC food packages, limiting vending machines and pouring rights for soft drinks in schools, taxing empty-calorie foods, and removing candy from the checkout stands of supermarkets. The Institute of Medicine recently published a report on ways local governments can create policies to promote healthier food consumption by communities.[18] Suggestions included requiring restaurants to post calorie information, using tax credits and incentives to attract supermarkets to underserved neighborhoods, zoning to prevent fast food restaurants near schools, and junk-food taxes.

Another way the government attempts to modify the food supply, at least for a select part of the population, is through redistribution. The government purchases foods for those who lack resources to purchase healthy or adequate amounts of food. Food stamps, WIC, and commodities programs are examples of these types of programs. Nutrition policy is also required for nutrition monitoring and surveillance, research, food assistance, licensure, and food safety and quality.[12]

■ POLICY FORMULATION

Policy formation is a complex, dynamic, and sometimes difficult process.[4] In an ideal world, nutrition policy would be formed using an accurate assessment of a community and its nutritional needs, the latest scientific information about nutrition, information about effective strategies, and community values. Policy would be evaluated on a regular basis and revised as needed, and would be created proactively to prevent as well as to solve problems. Nutrition policy would be integrated with other public policies, and all public policies would be supportive of the same goals. This is rarely the way public policy is created, however.

Public policy is created in a political environment.[3,8] Although public health officials prefer to look at problems and solutions in an objective manner, valuing technical expertise and scientific data, most policy makers work in a political environment where public values, popular opinions, and organized special interest groups have considerable influence.[10] There are many players in the public policy development process, and some are considered more important than others.[4] There are special interest groups, congressional committees and subcommittees, agencies of the executive branch of government, professional organizations, political parties, private and nonprofit organizations, economic and religious groups, individuals, and the media. Each of these has its own perspectives and philosophies that influence what is perceived as problems and what solutions should be created to solve problems. Scientific evidence may or may not coincide with the views of these groups. In the political process, all views become important, and public health officials must work to put forward solutions to problems that are objective and consistent with scientific observations. To many politicians, the opinion of public health officials may be just another opinion, and not necessarily an important, informed opinion.

Policy is generally created to solve a specific problem—often an emerging problem—that has generated public concern.[3,4] As stated earlier in this chapter, the problem may be real or it may simply be something that is perceived to be a problem. The more severe the problem is perceived to be and the more public interest the problem generates, the more likely it will result in new policy.[5]

> **Incrementalism:** Policy making in small steps, rather than with large comprehensive reforms.

Most policies are created in an incremental fashion.[3,5] Public officials prefer incrementalism because it allows them to draw on past experience, work within an existing framework, and avoid major changes that could create large unforeseen problems and political fallout.[3,5] On the other hand, incrementalism stifles innovation and may add to the complexity of existing policy. If multiple small changes are made to a policy to solve immediate problems, sometimes the overall integrity of the original policy starts to break down. This is often observed in federal food programs, where incremental policy changes continue to add policy requirements without making changes to the overall program to accommodate these changes.

Once policies are created there is a reluctance to change them, especially as they become accepted practice. Old policies that become ineffective because the conditions for which they were created have changed often stay in force because of resistance to change.[19] Changing old policies is especially difficult when economic interests are dependent on the old policy. As noted by the IOM and others, much of

U.S. public health policy was created at a time when conditions were quite different from what they are today.[3,10]

Most political scientists identify at least four steps for creating public policy[5]:

1. Agenda setting
2. Policy formulation
3. Policy implementation
4. Policy evaluation

Agenda Setting

The first steps in creating new policy are to identify the problem to be solved, create broad goals to resolve the problem, and then position the issue on the policy maker's agenda. A number of potential problems may make it difficult or impossible to move beyond these steps in policy creation, however.

Identify the Real Problem and Create Goals

Identifying the real problem may be easier than it sounds. For example, one of the goals of Healthy People 2010 is to increase breast-feeding rates. There are many theories about why women are unable or reluctant to breast-feed their infants for six months or a year, but which of these theories may be the real reason(s) and, therefore, most important for policy development? Changes to which of them would have the greatest impact on breast-feeding rates? Public opinion, people's belief structures, and special interest groups may be passionate about their views on what prevents breast-feeding rates from increasing, but the real reasons may not be readily apparent. Creating policy to solve the wrong problem would have limited impact on breast-feeding rates.

Promoting Policy Maker Initiatives

Once problems have been identified and policy goals set, then public health officials need to create a plan to get their recommended policy on the policy maker's agenda. Although the value of creating a policy to deal with a nutrition issue may be obvious to public health officials, it may not be to policy makers. In addition, getting a policy issue on the political agenda may be difficult and time-consuming. In general, policy issues are more likely to get on the political agenda when a great number of people believe the problem is real, and when people believe the consequences of the problem are likely to be severe, immediate, and affect them personally.[5]

Even when a problem is perceived by many people to be a threat, it still may not get on the political agenda.

Policy makers must believe that the problem is something that warrants government intervention.[3,5] There must also be room on the political agenda, and the issue must have enough priority over other issues. In a year when there are many significant problems facing policy makers, even an important issue may not make the political agenda.[5] Special interest groups that are opposed to a policy may also have enough clout to prevent a worthy policy issue from making the political agenda.[5]

Lawmakers and the public must believe that a new policy is actually a legitimate policy for the government to make. What the public believes is legitimate for policy makers to tackle changes over time. Currently, some public health officials are talking about creating a junk food tax to try to discourage consumption of soft drinks and other foods that are high in sugar.[18] Some people in society believe this is a legitimate action of the government while others do not.

Perceptions of what is legitimate change with time. One only has to look at how non-smoking policies have changed over time. Thirty years ago the notion of smoke-free bars and restaurants would have been unthinkable, but now most of the public embraces laws in cities and states prohibiting smoking in bars and restaurants.

Policy Formulation

Once an agenda has been set and a public health problem is placed on that agenda, the next step is formulation of an actual policy to address the issue. Alternative proposals are created. Information is collected about each of the proposals, and then a case is made for the proposal that seems to be the best solution for the problem.

Policy formation is about compromising and bargaining. Generally, one solution to a problem will not be accepted and championed to succeed without substantial changes and compromises. More likely, many different solutions and versions will be presented and debated. The solution that is eventually successful will often be modified before it reaches its final form. These modifications may weaken or strengthen the policy. Modifications are generally based on the ideologies and interests of various players in the political process, who have an interest in the outcome and effects of the proposal.

Policy Implementation

After a new policy has been created, it must be implemented. New policies are rarely written with adequate detail to allow their implementation.[5] The policy must be interpreted with rules and regulations written to spell out how a policy will be implemented. Responsibility and financial resources must be assigned so that the policy can be instituted.

The usual process for policy creation at the federal level is for Congress to pass legislation that then goes to various government cabinets, usually the USDA or DHHS for nutrition policy, where the new law is interpreted through creation of rules and regulations that reflect practical application of the law.

It may be tempting to believe that once a law has been passed, public health officials should feel confident that the policy is now in place and will be effective. The implementation phase is very critical for the success of public policy.[5] Sometimes laws are passed establishing a new policy, but no funding is given for implementation, or those who write the rules and regulations do so in such a way as to make the policy weak or ineffective.[5] How a policy is implemented is critical to its success and must be guided by those who have the knowledge and expertise to create rules to make the policy successful.

Policy Evaluation

The final stage in policy development is policy evaluation. Despite the best efforts of everyone involved in policy development, new policies are rarely perfect. Once a policy has been implemented, it needs to be evaluated for success. If the policy is successful, it should be evaluated to see how it can be changed to make it more successful. Few policies retain the same level of value, simply because the environment and conditions for which they were created change with time. Sometimes a sound nutrition policy is formulated that later becomes a policy that promotes poor nutrition. As an example, when the WIC program was originally created, its policies regarding the amount of juice in the food package made sense. Later, as obesity became a more urgent problem in the United States, the amount of juice in the WIC food package was considered a nutritional problem. Policies need to be continuously evaluated so that they may be modified or discontinued as times change.

■ POLICY CREATION AT THE FEDERAL LEVEL

The federal government was created to have a separation of powers. There are three branches of the federal government, each with its own responsibility and power. The legislative

branch (Congress) is responsible for creating laws, the executive branch (the President) for enforcing laws, and the judicial branch (the courts) for interpreting laws.[12]

In the United States, most public policy is created by legislation.[3] Congress has the authority to pass laws that initiate, modify, and authorize, and appropriate funding for all programs and services administered by the federal government. The legislative process is started when a member of Congress introduces a bill for consideration. If the bill is introduced in the Senate, it is given a designation starting with S., followed by an identifying number; if the bill is introduced in the House of Representatives, it is given a designation starting with H.R., followed by an identifying number. The leadership of the Senate or House then assigns the bill to a subcommittee or committee that will consider the bill. Because of the numerous bills that are introduced to Congress each year, many die from low priority in subcommittees and committees.[20]

Congressional committees have considerable power in determining what will move forward to possibly become law and what will be tabled.[4,20] If the bill is of interest to the members of the assigned committee, is of sufficient priority, and the political climate is right, the committee may hold hearings on the bill. The committee may decide to amend the bill by adding or deleting parts. The clean bill (amended version) is voted on and is "reported out" either to a committee if it was in a subcommittee or to the entire Senate or House if the bill was in a committee. If the bill was started in the Senate, it will be debated by the Senate, possibly amended, and then voted on. The bill would then go to a committee in the House for consideration. The House committee would then consider the bill, possibly amend it, and send it to the House for amendments and a vote. To save time, versions of the same bill may be introduced into both the Senate and House at the same time. These are referred to as companion bills.

If a bill is successfully voted on and passed by both the Senate and the House, the bill is often sent to a conference committee made up of members of both the Senate and House. This is necessary when there are differences in versions of a bill passed by the Senate and House. The conference committee attempts to resolve any differences between the two versions of the bill. The conference version of a bill must be sent back to both the Senate and House for a final vote before the bill is sent to the President.

The President has three choices when receiving a bill: First, he may sign the bill within 10 days and it becomes law. Second, he may veto the bill and send it back to Congress. This effectively kills the bill unless two-thirds of the members of both the Senate and House vote in favor of the bill to override the veto. Third, the President may do nothing with the bill when it is received.

If the President does nothing with the bill after it has been sent to him by Congress, there are two possibilities. If

111TH CONGRESS
1ST SESSION

H.R. 2590

To amend title XVIII of the Social Security Act to reduce the occurrence of diabetes in Medicare beneficiaries by extending coverage under Medicare for medical nutrition therapy services to such beneficiaries with pre-diabetes or with risk factors for developing type 2 diabetes.

IN THE HOUSE OF REPRESENTATIVES

MAY 21, 2009

Ms. DEGETTE (for herself, Mr. CASTLE, Mr. BECERRA, and Mr. KIRK) introduced the following bill; which was referred to the Committee on Energy and Commerce, and in addition to the Committee on Ways and Means, for a period to be subsequently determined by the Speaker, in each case for consideration of such provisions as fall within the jurisdiction of the committee concerned

---

A BILL

To amend title XVIII of the Social Security Act to reduce the occurrence of diabetes in Medicare beneficiaries by extending coverage under Medicare for medical nutrition therapy services to such beneficiaries with pre-diabetes or with risk factors for developing type 2 diabetes.

1   *Be it enacted by the Senate and House of Representa-*

2   *tives of the United States of America in Congress assembled,*

3   **SECTION 1. SHORT TITLE.**

4   This Act may be cited as the "Preventing Diabetes

5   in Medicare Act of 2009".

Congress is in session, the bill will become law in 10 days (excluding Sundays) even without the President's signature. If Congress is not in session, the bill does not become law. This is known as a "pocket veto."

Although most public policy in the United States is created by legislation through Congress, the other two branches of government can and do create public policy.[21] Legislation passed by Congress must be turned into practical rules and regulations so that they may be carried out.[20] This is the duty of federal employees in the executive branch of government. The rules and regulations created to implement policy will have a great impact on whether the original intent of a policy can be accomplished. These employees have considerable policy making power, because they create the rules and regulations of policy implementation.

The executive branch of government also is responsible for the enforcement of legislation. Decisions about how forcefully or even whether to enforce legislation have significant impact on policy. Public policy is what government actually does or does not do. If enforcement is lax, then the intended outcome of legislation or policy will be lost.

The agenda of a U.S. president and his political party can have significant impact on how legislation is turned into practical policies and how they are enforced and funded. Members of the executive branch of government, including the President, have a large role in advocating for budget allocations, enforcing policy, and acting as advisors to members of Congress on technical issues.

The President may also create public policy through executive orders. Executive orders are sometimes used to avoid public debate and opposition on an issue. Executive orders are usually considered to equivalent to federal statutes and do not require the approval of Congress. President Clinton created policy when leaving office by making an executive order that the WIC program would screen children under age 2 for immunizations.

The judicial branch of the federal government makes public policy through court decisions that decide the intent and meaning of laws, whether a public health agency is operating within its scope of legislative authority, and whether public health statutes and regulations are constitutionally permissible.[12] The U.S. Supreme Court has made many decisions of importance to public health, including upholding the power of the government to protect the public's health.[12]

■ POLICY DEVELOPMENT AT ALL LEVELS OF GOVERNMENT: FEDERAL, STATE, AND LOCAL

Policy development is important at all levels of government in order for public health agencies to fulfill their role in assuring health.[10] Each level of government has its own unique contributions to make in policy development and in providing public health services. From a historical and constitutional perspective, states have the primary responsibility for the health of citizens of the United States.[10] Local governments, in turn, receive their authority from state governments. The federal government has, over time, developed a larger role in the promotion of health and now has many technical and leadership roles that influence state and local health policies.

It is important that all levels of government work together to create effective health and nutrition policy.[12] By the very nature of having so many divisions of government, policies can become fragmented, overlapping, redundant, and at times contradictory. To deliver a convincing policy message in an organized and efficient way, all levels of government must work together.

Health problems, including nutritional problems, are seldom confined to one set of boundaries in the United States. For example, obesity may be more prevalent in some parts of the nation, but overall it is a problem in all parts of the nation. Food is grown in various parts of the country but is then distributed to the entire country. Most processed foods are universally distributed across the nation. Television advertising and the lifestyle effects of television are universal throughout the United States. Food franchises, food labeling, and the effects of federal nutrition programs are nearly the same everywhere in the nation. The factors that improve or detract from our nutritional health are generally widespread and not confined to a single state, county, or city. To make changes in policy that affect nutritional health requires a concerted policy effort by all levels of government giving a unified message.

Role of the Federal Government in Policy Development

The federal government plays a vital role in health and nutrition policy development. Many nutrition problems, such as obesity, increased prevalence of certain cancers, and heart disease, are faced by everyone in our nation, and they are affected by behaviors and conditions that exist throughout the country. These problems require national policy attention as well as state and local attention, if they are to be solved.

The federal government's policies affect the nutritional health of U.S. citizens in several ways[10,12]:

1. Federal policies greatly affect the food supply in the United States, including the quantity, types, and pricing of available foods. Because the food supply affects nutritional health, any changes in agricultural policy would need to come from the federal level.
2. Because most food production, processing, packaging, labeling, and marketing are done at the national level, federal policies are necessary to bring about any changes.
3. The major food and nutrition programs in the United States are all administered and funded by the federal government. These programs impact a significant portion of the public. The policies of these programs determine what foods are given and what nutritional information is provided. For most states, the majority of the nutritionists and dietitians working in public health are employed by these programs. For some states, these programs constitute almost their entire public nutrition policy. Because federal programs, such as WIC, purchase such large quantities of foods such as cereals and infant formulas, program regulations affect manufacturing and marketing practices of the foods to the entire population.
4. The federal government plays an important role in assessing nutritional health of the population of the United States. The National Health and Nutrition Examination Survey, Behavioral Risk Factor Surveillance System, and other surveys give the nutrition public health community the nutritional data upon which to base policy decisions.
5. The federal government has built up a resource of scientific and technical assistance that may be used by states to identify nutrition and health issues and to help create effective policies for solving the problems.
6. Because most nutritional problems are national, the federal government must play a role in policy leadership to identify, monitor, and resolve nutritional issues.
7. The federal government has the technical and financial resources for research to understand and solve nutrition problems.
8. Finally, the federal government has financial resources to assist states with public policies to solve public health nutrition problems. A good example of this is the money states are receiving from the CDC to create policies and programs to prevent obesity.

Role of Public Agencies in Policy Development

In the context of this chapter, agencies are governmental units that oversee nutrition programs. These agencies can exist at all levels of government, from the federal to the local level. At the federal level, the USDA is the agency that has been given the primary responsibility for nutrition programs and policy. Nutrition programs such as Food Stamps (SNAP), the Commodity Supplemental Food Program, WIC, and the National School Lunch Program are administered at the federal level by the USDA. Operation of these programs is delegated to state agencies, which in many cases then delegate the programs to local agencies where services are actually provided.

Nutrition programs are created through legislation that is written with broad goals and a basic design for a program. It is the responsibility of agencies to translate these broad goals and designs into practical rules and regulations that allow for the actual operation of programs. This arrangement permits legislatures to create broad policies to accomplish goals, and then allows agency staff to use their expertise to create the rules that provide for actual delivery of services. Agency staff have more expertise in nutrition and in techniques to improve nutrition behavior than legislative staff, so this is a good arrangement.[3] Agency staff can work out details in programs that allow them to be effective and to work in an efficient manner.

Agency staffs have great influence on public policy because they write rules and regulations for programs. If rules and regulations are written poorly, then programs will be ineffective and the goals of legislated policy will not be achieved. If the rules and regulations are well written, then the program may have great success. Whatever the intent by legislators, the end result depends in great measure on those designing the details of the programs.[5]

Agency staff are also responsible for enforcement, interpretation, and prioritization of rules and regulations. This can have a significant impact on policy. Most government programs have large numbers of rules with many details. It is virtually impossible to follow all rules to the letter. Which rules agency staff decide to focus their energy on or to enforce will substantially impact public policy by what the program accomplishes.

Agency staff members also have a role in advising policy makers at various levels of government. Agency staff can make recommendations for legislation and budgets. Because many agency staff are experts in their subject areas, such as nutrition, they can advise policy makers about proposed policies and proposed budgets, and can recommend new policies. For example, if agency staff monitoring health statistics find that fruit and vegetable consumption in school-age children is lacking, they can make recommendations for legislation to encourage fruit and vegetable consumption. Likewise, if a legislator decides that a new program is needed to address obesity, agency staff can help develop the legislation and make recommendations for how the legislation is written, methods for decreasing obesity, and how much money should be allocated. Agency staff often make recommendations for policy when new legislation is being created and when programs are being reauthorized by Congress.

Role of State Government in Policy Development

State governments are responsible for the health of their citizens.[10] This responsibility was given to the states by the U.S. Constitution. States may delegate some of this responsibility to local governments, but the ultimate responsibility rests with the states.[10,21] Since the 1960s, the federal government has been playing a larger role, providing resources and expertise to help state governments fulfill their responsibility for the health of their citizens.[12] Because states have the ultimate responsibility for their citizens' health, however, they must be involved in the process of policy development related to health issues.

In its report, *Future of Public Health*, the IOM remarked that states must be the central force in public health.[10] States have a responsibility to collect and analyze information on the health of their citizens, to set policies and standards, to carry out national and state mandates, and to respond to health issues. The IOM recommended that each state have a health council that reports on health issues in the state and makes policy recommendations to the governor and legislature for policy development.

Policy does not just happen, and legislatures are generally not looking for new public health policies to create. Because many states do not have a single lead nutritionist responsible for policy development, it is the responsibility of all nutrition professionals in a state to assess their state's nutritional health and determine what legislation is needed. This includes nutritionists at the state-agency level and their professional associations. Nutritionists also need to monitor all legislative activities for policy changes that could affect the nutrition of the public.

State personnel are sometimes restricted in their government positions from advocating for legislation, at least while functioning as a government employee. Local dietetic associations and nutrition alliances, such as anti-hunger groups or nutrition networks, may be effective in proposing and advocating for nutrition policy changes.

State governments offer an advantage in policy development in that most state legislators are more accessible than are federal legislators. Legislators may be more responsive to small groups of advocates. Nutritionists at the state level have been successful at getting legislation introduced and passed regarding licensure of dietitians, pro-breast-feeding policies, issues affecting school nutrition, and reimbursement for certain types of nutrition counseling.

Role of Local Government in Policy Development

Local governments vary considerably in their form and configuration as well as how they deal with health issues. There are a great many units of local government with a wide range of structures, functions, and size.[10] Some local governments are larger than some state governments, and others are so small that they have few resources and staff for health functions.

Local government is where nutrition services occur. State governments often delegate portions of their responsibility for health to local government units because it is local governments that are able to actually provide health services. Many nutrition programs, while administered at the state level, provide services through units of local governments.

Policy development needs to occur at the local level, as at all levels of government.[10] Local governments may be the most accessible of all when trying to create policy. One passionate nutritionist with good organizational and people skills can do great things with respect to nutrition policy while working with the school board, local health department, physicians, and city government. It may be possible to get legislation created and passed around nutrition education or vending machines in the school, breast-feeding issues, or senior nutrition programs. Policies created at the local level can become models and open doors to get similar policies passed at the state level. Of course, it is always important that local policies target goals similar to national nutrition policies.

Much like agency personnel, local nutrition professionals have a great impact on actual nutrition policy as it is administered. A nutritionist working for a federal nutrition program at the local level can determine how well that program functions and interacts with other health programs. A local nutritionist working for WIC, who reaches out to the community and builds a quality WIC program, helps create effective nutrition policy. Likewise, a nutritionist who works to build coalitions with Head Start, preschools, daycare programs, nurse partnerships, and other programs can create an environment where nutrition issues are addressed and the nutritional health of the community benefits. A nutritionist in the same community who creates barriers to WIC services and builds walls with other programs will have the opposite effect on nutrition in the community.

An excellent example of how a local government can affect nutrition policy was when the government of New York City decided to ban *trans*-fats in foods served at certain restaurants in 2009.[22] This not only had an impact on the people of New York but resulted in companies reformulating food products for the entire nation. New York's example and success also led other state and local governments to pursue similar policies.

■ LEADERSHIP ROLES FOR NUTRITIONISTS

The purpose of public health policy is to create conditions in which people can be healthy. Public policy should create conditions where it is easier to be healthy and harder to make decisions that contribute to a person being less healthy. Policy makers at all levels of government are responsible for policy development.

Good nutrition policy does not just happen. Policy development is a long and complex process, affected by many players and filled with compromises. There is no "nutrition czar" in the United States to watch out for needed nutrition policy legislation. It is the role of every nutritionist to be involved and to work for good nutrition policy. Nutritionists need to be informed and work together to bring about changes for better nutrition. This is especially true as the United States faces one of its most challenging nutritional epidemics, that of obesity.

Members of The American Dietetic Association can sign up to be a member of a listserv called "On the Pulse" to receive nutrition policy updates. To do this, go to http://www.eatright.org/Member/83_11027.cfm.

Issues for Discussion

1. Why is public policy important? Discuss public policy in relation to obesity.

2. Nutritional concerns have changed significantly since the beginning of the 20th century. Yet nutrition policy remains conflicting, inconsistent, and fragmented among numerous laws, agencies, programs, and branches of government. Discuss how nutrition policy could be improved in the United States.

3. Public policy is created in a political setting. Explain who you think the best group or groups are to create public policy. Why?

References

1. *The New Oxford Dictionary of English*. Oxford, UK: Oxford University Press; 1998.

2. Birkland TA. *An Introduction to the Policy Process: Theories, Concepts, and Models of Public Policy Making*, 2nd ed. Armonk, NY: M.E. Sharp; 2005:17–20.

3. Sims L. *The Politics of Fat: Food and Nutrition in America*. Armonk, NY: M.E. Sharp; 1998.

4. Block LE. Health policy through the looking glass. In: Harrington C, Estes CL, eds. *Health Policy: Crisis and Reform in the U.S. Health Care Delivery System*, 3rd ed. Sudbury, MA: Jones and Bartlett; 2008:258–369.

5. Anderson G, Hussey PS. Influencing government policy: A framework. In: Pencheon D, Guest C, Melzer D, Muir GJA, eds. *Oxford Handbook of Public Health Practice*. Oxford, UK: Oxford University Press; 2001:146–154.

6. Ackoff RL. *Redesigning the Future: A Systems Approach to Societal Problems*. New York: Wiley; 1974.

7. Pencheon D, Guest C, Melzer D, Muir Gray JA, eds. Introduction. In: *Oxford Handbook of Public Health Practice*. Oxford, UK: Oxford University Press; 2001:126–127.

8. Gostin L. Public health law in a new century: Part III: Public health regulation: a systematic evaluation. *JAMA*. 2000;283:3118–3122.

9. Milio N. A framework for prevention: changing health-damaging to health-generating life patterns. *Am J Public Health*. 1976;66:435–439.

10. Institute of Medicine, Committee for the Study of the Future of Public Health. *The Future of Public Health*. Washington, DC: National Academy Press; 1988.

11. Foege W. Leadership and policy development. In: Rowitz L, ed. *Public Health Leadership: Putting Principles into Practice*. Gaithersburg, MD: Aspen; 2001:126–147.

12. Institute of Medicine, Committee on Assuring the Health of the Public in the 21st Century. *The Future of the Public's Health in the 21st Century*. Washington, DC: National Academy Press; 2002.

13. Bunker JP, Frazier HS, Mosteller F. Improving health: measuring effects of medical care. *Milbank Q*. 1994;72:225–258.

14. McGinnis JM, Nestle M. The Surgeon General's report on nutrition and health: policy implications and implementation strategies. *Am J Clin Nutr*. 1989;49:23–28.

15. McMurray KY. Setting dietary guidelines: The U.S. process. *J Am Dietetic Assoc*. 2003;103:S10–S16.

16. Murray B. Fast-food culture serves up supersize Americans. *APA Monitor*. 2001;32:33.

17. Nestle M. *Food Politics. How the Food Industry Influences Nutrition and Health*. Berkeley and Los Angeles: University of California Press; 2002.

18. Institute of Medicine of the National Academies. *Local Government Actions to Prevent Childhood Obesity*. Washington, DC: National Academy Press; 2009.

19. Koh YM. Shaping your organization's policy. In: Pencheon D, Guest C, Melzer D, Muir Gray JA, eds. *Oxford Handbook of Public Health Practice*. Oxford: Oxford University Press; 2001:128–135.

20. Hart S, Jackson N. Primer on policy: the legislative process at the federal level. In: Harrington C, Estes CL, eds. *Health Policy: Crisis and Reform in the U.S. Health Care Delivery System*, 3rd ed. Sudbury, MA: Jones and Bartlett; 2008:370–372.

21. Mensah GA, Goodman RA, Zara S, et al. Law as a tool for preventing chronic diseases: Expanding the spectrum of public health strategies [Part 2], Preventing Chronic Disease. Available at http://www.cdc.gov/pcd/issues/2004/apr/04_0009.htm. Retrieved April 8, 2010.

22. Department of Health and Human Services. In New York City, Trans Fat Ban Is Working. July 20, 2009. Available at http://www.womenshealth.gov/news/English/629180.htm. Accessed April 8, 2010.

CHAPTER 8

Advocating and Influencing Health and Nutrition Policies

BRUCE RENGERS, PHD, RD

READER OBJECTIVES

After studying this chapter and reflecting on the contents, you should be able to:

1. Describe the importance of being an advocate for public health policy.
2. Justify the role of politics in policy development.
3. Identify factors that influence policy development.
4. Delineate methods to build support for new policies.
5. Discuss the importance of building an infrastructure of support for policy development.
6. Name some individual skills needed for being an effective public health advocate.

■ INTRODUCTION

Advocacy is the act of supporting or promoting a cause. Public health and nutrition professionals must advocate for nutrition policy. Nutrition policy does not just happen. We tend to take for granted nutrition policies from the past and to allow market forces and special interest groups to determine nutrition policies for the future. For nutrition and public health professionals, it is a primary responsibility to advocate for effective public policies that will improve the nutritional health of people in the United States.[1]

Public policy is how government creates conditions to maintain or improve the health of its citizens (see Chapter 7). Every aspect of our lives is influenced by public policy, including what we eat and our nutritional health.[2] Government has an interest in keeping its citizens healthy. Using public policy, government can have a powerful effect on a nation's health. Keeping citizens healthy results in a more productive society, lower healthcare costs, and an improved general well-being of society.

Good policy development is a result of a careful assessment of problems, objective knowledge about problems, establishment of priorities based on data, and allocation of resources for maximum benefit.[3] It is tempting to think that public health policy in the United States is generally created in this manner; however, this is often not the case. Policy development in the United States has been described as "complex, dynamic, confusing, and at times mysterious."[4] Development of public policy has been driven by crises, hot issues, and the concerns of well-organized interests.[5] As a result of this undisciplined and subjective process, public health policy in the United States has been described as outdated, fragmented, conflicted, and ineffective,[3] and the U.S. public health infrastructure as being in disarray.[5]

Policy development is one of the core functions of public health.[5] Leaders of public health have a responsibility to develop sound policy[6] and to use every opportunity to influence policy to improve the health of citizens.[1] Public policy is the primary tool public health officials have to maintain and improve the public health. If public health officials do not lead in policy development, then policy development will be dominated by well-organized special interest groups, motivated by profit,[7] and by those with agendas unfounded in science. The net effect will be ineffective policy, a waste of resources, and detrimental effects on the public's health. Because of a lack of effective leadership and support, current public health policy lags behind scientific knowledge and consumer concerns.[2]

Leadership and advocacy in nutrition policy development is the responsibility of all nutritionists.[8-10] Although those employed in leadership roles in public health nutrition have specialized roles for leading in policy development, it is the responsibility of all nutritionists to advocate for effective nutrition policy. Marianne Smith Edge, former president of The American Dietetic Association (ADA), noted that gains in policy and advocacy for nutrition issues have been the result of many individuals and their willingness to get involved.[8] ADA's State Issues Task Force recommended that all ADA members be trained in leadership and policy development[9] and ADA has the position that registered dietitians and dietetic technicians, should be leaders in advocating for nutrition funding and policy initiatives at the local, state, and federal levels of government.[10] ADA and its members have become increasingly more active in trying to change public policy to promote nutritional health.[11]

It takes many people working together to influence the political process for effective policy change. The Institute of Medicine (IOM)[5] noted that one of the difficulties of policy development in public health has been public health officials trying to work in isolation, without a broad base of support. Public health officials must learn to work in a political environment, using the political process to accomplish their goals.

Policy development for improved nutrition can occur at all levels of government: federal, state, and local. Advocacy for new policies often starts at the local level since this is where politicians are elected. Visits to the local offices of politicians are a good way to start building support for a new or proposed policy. In addition, the value of local policies should not be overlooked. When local policies are put in place to improve nutrition, they can serve as models for state or federal policy and they can help to build support for state and federal policy. The recent policy change in New York City to ban *trans*-fats in certain restaurants, bakeries, and fast food outlets led to national changes in the use of *trans*-fats nationwide.[12]

■ POLITICS IN POLICY DEVELOPMENT

Most public policy in the United States is created by legislation through passage of laws.[2] This process involves politicians and the political process. Many people view politics with cynicism, as something that is undesirable. Yet politics is a necessary way to bring about change.[13] *Politics* is the use of power to shape policy and accomplish goals.[13] Science and logic may help to identify a public health problem, but it is generally emotion and power in the political process that determine what will be done about a problem.[14]

The IOM noted that many public health officials view politics as a contamination of the policy development process.[5] Substantial tension between professional expertise and politics has been observed throughout the U.S. public health system.[5] Public health officials are accustomed to using professional judgment, technical expertise, and scientific information to identify and solve problems.[5] This is how public health officials have been trained. It is a central

tenet of their professional ethic to use objective, scientific information to solve problems.[5] Public policy, however, is developed in a political atmosphere that is anything but objective and rational. This dichotomy of perspective has led to isolation and difficulty in creating new health policy. The IOM and others[5,9] recommend that public health professionals learn how to use the political process to accomplish needed goals. This includes developing political skills and a broad base of support to use in the political process.

Influencing Legislation

The first step in creating new public policy is to get the proposed policy on the agenda of lawmakers. This may be the most difficult part of the policy-making process.[2] Legislators have many issues and many individuals and interest groups vying to capture their attention. Organized interest groups whose purpose is to create legislation have proliferated.[2] In a given year, far more bills are proposed than can possibly be turned into policies.[2] Also, health issues must compete with policy issues unrelated to health, as well with other health issues.[15]

To create new federal policy, a sponsor or sponsors must be found to introduce a bill to the House of Representatives or Senate. If the bill is introduced, it is then assigned to a committee or subcommittee that has responsibility for food and nutrition issues. Committees and subcommittees are the "gatekeepers" for legislation, and they determine which bills will get testimony and which will pass on to the full House or Senate. Many bills die in committees because they are of low priority in a packed agenda. Policy makers can concentrate on only a few new policies during a legislative session.[15]

A number of factors help determine which bills are likely to get put on the policy agenda and successfully move on to become law.[15] Bills are more likely to be successful at being placed on the policy agenda if:

- A greater number of people perceive the policy issue to be a problem.
- The problem is perceived to have greater severity.
- The problem is more immediate and novel.
- More people are affected by the problem personally.
- The political atmosphere is supportive of the policy.
- The policy appeals to the public.

In democracies, public opinion and special interest groups have a substantial impact on whether a bill for new policy will be put on the legislative agenda.[14] It is, therefore, important for public health officials to know how to influence public opinion and to obtain the support of organized interest groups. Working effectively with the media to

> Read more about nutrition policy, terms, and procedures at these sites: http://www.loc.gov and http://thomas.loc.gov.

form public opinion is an important relationship and skill to cultivate.[15]

It is important that the public view particular new policies as legitimate functions of the government in order to gain their support for the policies. If the public views taxation of junk food as overly intrusive control by the government, then they are not going to support such a policy change. What the public views as legitimate for government policy, however, changes with time. The early stages of policy development may be about educating the public to understand why a policy is important so that they see it as a legitimate action by the government.

Public support alone will not always be enough to get a bill on the policy agenda.[15] The policy in question must be one that members of Congress also consider appropriate for government action. For example, legislators may not believe it is the government's role to discourage certain types of foods through taxation. In their view, people should be able to make choices about food without government interference. If this is the prevailing political view, then it is unlikely that such a policy would ever be placed on the policy agenda for consideration.

Well-organized and financed special interest groups can also sway policy makers away from following public opinion in some situations. This is especially true when the policy only affects a small number of people, large economic interests are involved, or the issue is very technical in nature.[15] Even if public opinion can get legislation passed, influential interest groups can have substantial impact on the fine print of legislation that substantially changes the actual intent or effectiveness of a new policy.[2]

Once a proposed policy is on the policy maker's agenda, continued support is needed until it is passed as law. Compromising, bargaining, expert testimony, and guidance of the bill through the legislative process are all required. There is potential at every step of policy development for something to go wrong and for the policy to be derailed.[15] The process of creating public policy rarely allows the original policy, as it was introduced, to remain unmodified. Public health officials must be willing to compromise and bargain to create a policy with the greatest public and political acceptance.[15] Compromising, however, must be balanced with a need to maintain the original intent of the policy.

Building Support for New Policies

The Policy

The first step in building support for a new policy is to create a defensible, sound policy.[6,16] Health policies must be based on accurate and complete scientific information. Cause and distribution of the health issue need to be known as well as effective strategies for intervention.[5] Public health leaders must know the scientific literature and be able to present a strong case in favor of the policy. Is there sufficient scientific information to justify the policy? Sometimes, complete information is not available when creating policy. The potential risk of creating policy with inadequate information needs to be weighed against the need for the policy.[16]

Public health leaders must also be able to assess the feasibility of the new policy, the costs and benefits of having the policy, the costs and benefits of not having the policy, and the compatibility of the policy with public values.[5,17] The human rights burden, the effects of the new policy on personal freedoms, fairness of cost distribution, and reasonableness between means and end must also be considered.[18] It is the responsibility of the policy developer to justify the costs and burdens of new policy against its benefits.[18]

Public Opinion

Public policy tends to follow public opinion.[15] It is, therefore, very important to build public support for new policies. This can be done through the media, public officials, celebrities, and public awareness campaigns.[15] Public opinion can also be developed by building coalitions or alliances, citizen participation in policy development, communication with the public at large, and communication with elected officials.[5] The IOM noted that the public health system in the United States tends to be isolated and recommended that public health officials work at building a broad base of support.[5]

To be effective in building public support, public health officials need to cultivate a relationship with the public through regular communication, not just when policy issues are being discussed. Public health officials need to build ongoing credibility and a positive relationship with the public. The community, as well as elected officials, must see public health personnel as technical experts and as advocates for the community and supportive of community values.[5] Both technical knowledge and public values determine how public health is practiced.[5] Rather than having a paternalistic approach to communication, public health needs to encourage debate[14] and empower communities to create solutions to their own health issues.[6]

Timing of Policy Proposals

A new policy may not become part of the political agenda even when it is well supported. Timing is critical.[15] Policy agendas may be filled with other issues that are considered higher priorities. Reintroduction of the health policy in a different legislative session, when fewer priority items are on the agenda, may increase the likelihood of getting the proposed policy on the political agenda.

It is important to judge the political climate when introducing new policy. What is the prevailing philosophy concerning the health issue and proposed solution? Who in the legislative committee will be in favor or strongly opposed to the new policy? If the political climate is not supportive, it may be impossible to get the new policy on the legislative agenda. Waiting another year until the players or climate changes may be the best option.

Sometimes it takes multiple tries to get a new policy on the legislative agenda. Then once on the agenda, it may also take multiple tries to get the legislation passed. Repeated attempts help gather support and decrease opposition in many cases. Policy may also need to be created incrementally or in small steps over time.[2,15] To get legislation for dietetic licensure in one state, the sponsors of the legislation had to agree to exempt dietitians employed in certain practice settings. This wasn't the intent of the original policy, but it allowed a licensure bill to become law. In the following years, the legislation was amended to include some of the dietitians originally excluded. Through incremental change over time, the original intent of the policy was eventually accomplished.

Lobbying

Lobbying is the process of trying to influence the members of a legislature.[19] Lobbying is an art, not a science.[19] It can be done by professional lobbyists or it can be done by individuals or groups trying to advance their cause. By one estimate, there are 12,500 professional lobbyists in Washington, D.C.,[20] which makes for a lot of people trying to influence policy makers' decisions.

Lobbyists serve several functions in their roles. They attempt to educate legislators on issues important to their cause, stimulate public debate on issues, and encourage participation in the political process while trying to gather public support for their legislative issues.[2] "Lobby" has also come to have a negative connotation, referring to pressure groups that run sophisticated campaigns to influence legislators by a variety of persuasive methods.[19]

Public health professionals, health professionals, and consumer advocate groups have taken up lobbying as a way to influence legislation on public policy. Some have been reasonably successful.[19] In general, public health lobbyists are fewer in number and are less well-financed than those from commercial interests. It is a challenge to overcome the influence of lobbyists from well-funded groups that may not favor certain policy changes important for health.

Government programs are generally prohibited from lobbying, as are government employees in many circumstances. Because government programs need the benefits of lobbying, they sometimes form private groups that will lobby for them. For example, many state and local WIC programs are members of the National WIC Association (NWA). NWA is a private, nonprofit organization that advocates for WIC and issues related to the WIC program. NWA provides information to legislators, makes recommendations on funding and policy changes related to WIC, and works to build community support for the program.

Groups That Are Part of the Political Process

Political Action Committees   *Political Action Committees* (*PACs*) are organized for the purpose of raising and spending money to elect or defeat political candidates.[21] Most PACs have specific legislative agendas and work to elect political candidates sympathetic to their cause. Health-related groups have created PACs so that their members can contribute money to help elect candidates that support their issues. As an example, the American Dietetic Association has an active PAC.

Coalitions   A *coalition* is a group of people and organizations that have come together to influence outcomes related to a specific problem.[6] For example, a coalition of interested citizens and health groups may come together to find ways to reduce the increasing prevalence of obesity in a community. Many communities have nutrition or hunger coalitions to solve nutrition and hunger issues.

Coalitions can be an excellent way for public health officials to design and propose new public health policies. They bring together community and health-related groups as well as public and private organizations for public health issues. Building coalitions for policy development in public health was one of the recommendations made by the IOM to allow for more community involvement in public health.[5]

Alliances   *Alliances* are groups of healthcare and public health organizations that combine forces to address public health issues in a specific geographic area.[6] Alliances can also bring together public and private groups to work on a common issue. Coalitions and alliances allow for synergism in solving problems. Collectively, the group can do more than all of the partners separately.

Professional Organizations   Organizations of health professionals, such as the American Dietetic Association (ADA), the Society for Nutrition Education (SNE), or the American Public Health Association (APHA), have a strong role in advocating for public health issues. These organizations can create policy statements that support legislation. They can hire lobbyists, and they have the ability to mobilize members to lobby legislators on specific legislation. They can be technical resources when legislation is being created and provide expert testimony. Belonging to a professional organization that advocates for nutrition and public health is an important responsibility every nutritionist has to the nation's health.[9]

Health Advocacy Organizations   *Health advocacy organizations* generally focus on a specific health issue. They help advocate for public health in the same way as professional organizations. For example, the American Diabetes

Association would be active in advocating for health issues related to diabetes. They can be an important partner in an alliance or coalition working for public policy change.

Consumer Advocacy Groups   *Consumer advocacy groups* can have a very powerful influence on legislatures. The American Association of Retired People (AARP) is one of the largest advocacy groups in the United States, and as such has tremendous influence with legislatures. It represents a very large and growing block of voting citizens.

The Center for Science in the Public Interest (CSPI) is another consumer advocacy group that has had considerable impact on nutrition policy in the United States. CSPI's goals include providing useful, objective information to the public and policy makers on food and nutrition; representing citizens' interests before government units; and ensuring that science and technology are used for the public good.[22] CSPI has brought significant attention to nutrition issues, especially in controversial areas, through use of the media.

Political Parties   *Political parties* have a major role in determining public policy.[15] This is done by formal party manifestos prior to elections,[1] or in an informal way through the philosophical beliefs under which the political parties operate. A political party that is supportive of health policy can be indispensable in helping to draft health legislation and to get it on the policy agenda. A political party opposed to health legislation can be a formidable hurdle.

The National Academies and Institute of Medicine   *The National Academy of Science (NAS)* is a private, nonprofit society that was given a charter by Congress in 1863. NAS has a mandate to advise the federal government on scientific and technical matters. The Institute of Medicine (IOM) was established under the charter of the NAS in 1970 to provide independent, objective, evidence-based advice to policy makers, health professionals, the private sector and the public.[23] The IOM conducts policy studies on health issues as part of the National Academies composed of the National Academy of Sciences, National Academy of Engineering, and the National Research Council. Congress often refers health issues to the IOM when a nonpartisan, impartial review and recommendation are needed. Documents from the IOM are invaluable in advocating for change in public health and nutrition policy.[23]

Media   The *media* helps shape the public's view of reality and can have strong effects on public opinion.[15] Anyone who has ever worked with the media is aware of how important it is to develop a positive and mutually beneficial relationship with the media. How the media "frames" an issue can make a major difference in whether the public will support or reject proposed policy. The media needs news stories of interest to entice the public, and public health officials need the media to educate the public. Public health officials must become dependable sources of accurate information for the media so that the media may frame them as knowledgeable experts when health issues arise.

■ IMPORTANCE OF BUILDING AN INFRASTRUCTURE OF SUPPORT

To be able to build an ongoing base of support, it is necessary to cultivate relationships with the public and politicians,[24] in essence, to create an infrastructure of support. Policy development should be an ongoing process to improve the health of the community, rather than a crisis-driven necessity when health issues arise. For public health officials to be effective advocates for policy change, they need to have the support of the community, other health professionals, and politicians. The IOM has made several recommendations for building a base of political support[5]:

- Public health officials should develop relationships with legislatures and other public officials and educate them on public health issues.
- Public health agencies should train staff in community relations and citizen participation.
- Public health agencies should develop relationships with physicians and other private sector representatives, including professional societies and academic medical centers.
- Public health agencies should seek stronger relationships and common goals with other professional and citizen groups involved with health issues.
- Agencies should undertake education of the public on health issues.
- Agencies should review the quality of contacts between employees and clients to ensure the public is treated with cordiality and respect.

The IOM noted that these relationships need to be cultivated and fostered on an ongoing basis.[5] Building these relationships is part of the political process necessary to accomplish goals. It has been suggested that political skills must be consistently used in order to maintain them.[7]

Advocacy Activities and Skills for Individuals

Individuals may be the most important advocates for public health and nutrition. All of the organizations and groups listed previously are made up of collections of individuals. It is the actions of those individuals that make groups effective.[8] Margaret Mead made the statement, "A small group of thoughtful people could change the world. Indeed, it is the only thing that ever has." It is important not to feel powerless when confronting major health or nutrition problems. Passionate, persistent individuals have made remarkable differences in the face of poor odds.

There are many ways that an individual can advocate for nutrition policy, either as a private individual or as a professional. The following suggestions apply to individuals advocating on their own or as part of groups made up of individuals:

- Know your elected officials and develop professional relationships with them.[24] Read about their voting records, and get to know their philosophies and voting records related to health issues. Attend town hall meetings and make your opinions heard. Some professional associations, such as state affiliates of the ADA, have legislative luncheons where you can meet your elected officials. Attend these luncheons and talk to your elected officials. Be assertive, but polite, friendly, and tactful. Write letters, email, telephone, and visit your elected officials telling them your views on public health and nutrition issues. Even when it is unlikely that the official will be swayed to change his or her mind on an issue, it is still good to let him or her know your views. It may soften his or her opposition.
- Vote in elections to influence who will represent your views in government.
- Be informed about the issues, current legislation, your community, and the arguments of those opposed to your views.
- Join a professional association or advocacy group(s) that advocates for public health. Many voices are generally louder than one. Be active in the group and encourage policy involvement.
- Respect others and their points of view even when they are diametrically opposed to your own.
- Conflicts arise. Don't take them personally. Learn from your opponent's position; it may strengthen your own position. Accept that some people may reject you for your position on an issue.
- Write letters to the editor of the newspaper when you have a strong position on a health or nutrition issue.
- Identify and know your audience. Adjust your message to better target their concerns and needs.[24]
- Be persistent. Learn from your own mistakes and move on with that knowledge to do a better job next time.

Writing for Advocacy

There are a number of situations where advocacy is best done in writing. These could include letters to the editor of a newspaper, letters to elected officials, and written testimony for policy change.

For most writing it is important to remember that no one has to read what you have written.[25] Unless your letter is well written and catches the reader's attention, it may be ignored. Think before you write and organize your thoughts. Make your position clear early in the letter and find a way to get your reader's attention. Focus on one or two ideas and be brief. Most people are not motivated to read long essays.

Collect key statistics, research the literature, and make sure you are knowledgeable about current events related to your topic before you start writing.[25] Make sure that you are able to back up every fact and assertion with documentation and evidence. Accuracy is very important.

Use small words and short sentences, and don't be offensive. Write while the issue is still in the public's attention. After writing, let the letter wait for a few hours or overnight before sending it. Reread the letter to make sure it says what you really intended and in a way you intended. Remember that what you write may be read by many thousands of people and will be remembered into the future. It may be helpful to have someone else read your letter and give you feedback before mailing it.

The government often requests written comments on new policies and policy changes. These requests for comments are printed in the *Federal Register* for comment periods of 30 to 90 days. This is one of those unusual times when someone is required to read your letter and comments. Federal employees are required to read and compile all comments received during a comment period. These compiled comments are then used to support approval, change, or rejection of proposed policies. Most people don't make a habit of reading the *Federal Register*, but news reports will often comment on certain proposed changes related to food or nutrition. The *Federal Register* can be accessed online for easy reading at http://www.gpoaccess.gov/fr/index.html. Organized special interest groups will comment on proposed policy, so it is important that public health advocates also comment.

Media

Most people do not like talking in front of a crowd or on television. Media, however, is a very important tool in advocacy. The media can help form public opinion by reporting on issues related to nutrition and public health. How media frames an issue will help determine public reaction.

> **Federal Register:** A daily publication that compiles every regulation, and change in regulation, proposed and enacted upon by any branch of the U.S. government.

Many organizations actively look for media exposure to build their credibility in the eyes of the public. For example, universities often want faculty to comment on public health issues related to their research. Public health departments may want staff to discuss health issues when public involvement is needed. Nutritionists can use the media to discuss current issues, build credibility, and educate the public on nutrition principles.

With the media, there is always a danger of being misquoted or quoted out of context. There is also the possibility of a reporter, with an agenda, making the interview negative and combative. You should receive training in media interviews to help avoid such situations, but it is equally important that health officials not shy away from media attention for fear of negative consequences.

Public Testimony

Legislatures and government agencies often require public hearings on proposed legislation before a formal vote is taken or major policy changes are made. For example, a committee of a state senate may hold public hearings on a farmer's market bill before taking a vote. Again, most people are not eager to speak in public, but this can be a very important way of advocating for good nutrition or public health policy. It is also an example where public and private partnerships are very important for advocacy. A state agency may propose new legislation to offer fresh fruit snacks in schools but be limited by its government association from testifying in favor of the legislation. The local dietetic association or health coalition can be very helpful advocates by rallying members to testify in favor of the legislation.

■ THE FUTURE OF PUBLIC HEALTH

The future of public health will be determined by those with the greatest influence on public policy development. It is critical that public health officials work to become effective advocates of public health. Good public policy does not happen on its own. Without effective leadership from public health officials, public health will be determined by those with the greatest economic interest or political need. Effective skills and strategies in policy development must be developed by public health professionals. These skills require development of a broad base of support in the community and credibility as technical experts. As individuals, those with concerns for public health must remember that it is the actions of many individuals that result in positive changes for public health. Each public health professional as an individual and as part of organized groups must advocate for optimal health for all.

Issues for Discussion

1. Briefly describe the steps required to create new public health policy.

2. Describe examples of how the media has helped shape the public's view of reality on public health policy.

3. Building a base of public support is important to get a public health policy through the legislature. Explain how to develop public support in respect to a policy on obesity.

References

1. Wall P. Influencing government policy: a national review. In: Pencheon D, Guest C, Melzer D, Muir Gray JA, eds. *Oxford Handbook of Public Health Practice*. Oxford, UK: Oxford University Press; 2001:156–161.

2. Sims L. *The Politics of Fat: Food and Nutrition in America*. Armonk, NY: M.E. Sharp; 1998.

3. Institute of Medicine, Committee on Assuring the Health of the Public in the 21st Century. *The Future of the Public's Health in the 21st Century*. Washington, DC: National Academy Press; 2002.

4. Block LE. Health policy through the looking glass. In: Harrington C, Estes CL, eds. *Health Policy: Crisis and Reform in the U.S. Healthcare Delivery System*, 3rd ed. Sudbury, MA: Jones and Bartlett; 2008:358–369.

5. Institute of Medicine, Committee for the Study of the Future of Public Health. *The Future of Public Health*. Washington, DC: National Academy Press; 1988.

6. Foege W. Leadership and policy development. In: Rowitz L. *Public Health Leadership: Putting Principles into Practice*. Gaithersburg, MD: Aspen; 2001:126–142.

7. Dodd CJ. Can meaningful health policy be developed in a political system? In: Harrington C, Estes CL, eds. *Health policy: Crisis and Reform in the U.S. Healthcare Delivery System*, 3rd ed. Sudbury, MA: Jones and Bartlett; 2008:373–382.

8. Edge MS. Get involved and make a difference. *J Am Dietetic Assoc.* 2004;104:159.

9. Ochs M, McKnight P. Preliminary report of the State Issues Task Force: trends affecting the dietetics profession. *J Am Dietetic Assoc.* 2003;103:1595–1596.

10. Position of the American Dietetic Association: the roles of registered dietitians and dietetic technicians, registered in health promotion and disease prevention. *J Am Dietetic Assoc.* 2006;106:1875–1884.

11. Pavlinac JM. Let's make 2009 a year to remember. *J Am Dietetic Assoc.* 2009;109:1331.

12. Okie S. New York to *trans* fats: you're out. *N Engl J Med.* 2007;356:2017–2021.

13. Koh YM. Shaping your organization's policy. In: Pencheon D, Guest C, Melzer D, Muir Gray JA, eds. *Oxford Handbook of Public Health Practice*. Oxford, UK: Oxford University Press; 2001:128–134.

14. Pencheon D, Guest C, Melzer D, Muir Gray JA, eds. Introduction. In: *Oxford Handbook of Public Health Practice*. Oxford, UK: Oxford University Press; 2001:126–127.

15. Anderson G, Hussey PS. Influencing government policy: a framework. In: Pencheon D, Guest C, Melzer D, Muir Gray JA, eds. *Oxford Handbook of Public Health Practice*. Oxford, UK: Oxford University Press; 2001:146–154.

16. Cooper MJ, Zlotkin SH. An evidence-based approach to the development of national dietary guidelines. *J Am Dietetic Assoc.* 2003;103:S28–S33.

17. Frommer M, Leeder S, Rubin G, Tjhin M. Translating goals and targets into public health action. In: Pencheon D, Guest C, Melzer D, Muir Gray JA, eds. *Oxford Handbook of Public Health Practice*. Oxford, UK: Oxford University Press; 2001;136–144.

18. Gostin L. Public health law in a new century: Part III: Public health regulation: a systematic evaluation. *JAMA.* 2000;283:3118–3122.

19. Muir Gray JA. The public health professional as political activist. In: Pencheon D, Guest C, Melzer D, Muir Gray JA, eds. *Oxford Handbook of Public Health Practice*. Oxford, UK: Oxford University Press; 2001:262–267.

20. Fund J. Happy Heather of K Street. *The Wall Street Journal*, August 25, 2009. Available at http:// online.wsj.com/article/SB 10001424052970203706604574372843757253038.html. Accessed May 3, 2010.

21. Misiroglu G. *The Handy Politics Answer Book*. Canton, MI: Visible Ink Press; 2003.

22. Center for Science in the Public Interest. Mission Statement. Available at http://www.cspinet.org/about/mission.html. Accessed April 9, 2010.

23. Institute of Medicine of the National Academies. Available at http://www.iom.edu. Accessed April 9, 2010.

24. Patrick MS. Sending the right message: how ADA's public policy workshop can work for you and nutrition policy in America. *J Am Dietetic Assoc.* 2008;108:776–777.

25. Jessop E. Writing to effect change. In: Pencheon D, Guest C, Melzer D, Muir Gray JA, eds. *Oxford Handbook of Public Health Practice*. Oxford, UK: Oxford University Press; 2001:428–434.

Role of the United States Department of Agriculture in Public Health Nutrition

BEVERLY J. McCABE-SELLERS, PhD, RD
MARGARET L. BOGLE, PhD, RD

READER OBJECTIVES

After studying this chapter and reflecting on the contents, you should be able to:

1. List the major agencies within the United States Department of Agriculture (USDA) that contribute to the practice of public health nutrition.

2. Identify the primary USDA programs that provide food assistance and nutrition education.

3. Discuss the agencies whose roles are to provide research data to support human nutrition in public health.

4. Discuss the major vehicles by which USDA agencies contribute to nutrition policy and promotion of health.

5. Discuss the historical perspective of nutrition education within the USDA.

■ INTRODUCTION

The United States Department of Agriculture (USDA) is a large and complex federal organization with seven undersecretaries who administer a diverse set of agencies and programs. Since the 1994 reorganization of the federal government, three undersecretaries supervise agencies, centers, and services that impact on public health nutrition: 1) Food, Nutrition, and Consumer Services (FNCS); 2) Food Safety; and 3) Research, Education, and Economics (REE). These agencies will be discussed for their individual major roles but, in reality, a large amount of interdependence and collaboration are needed to achieve their mutual mission and their goals of meeting the food and nutritional needs of Americans.

■ OVERVIEW OF FOOD, NUTRITION, AND CONSUMER SERVICES

The Food, Nutrition, and Consumer Services (FNCS) has two major agencies: the Food and Nutrition Service (FNS) and the Center for Nutrition Policy and Promotion (CNPP). FNCS's stated mission is to:

...ensure access to nutritious, healthful diets for all Americans. Through food assistance and nutrition ed-

ucation for consumers, FNCS encourages consumers to make healthful food choices. Rather than simply providing food, FNCS works to empower consumers with knowledge of the link between diet and health, providing dietary guidance based on research.[1]

Food and Nutrition Service

The Food and Nutrition Service (FNS) increases food security and reduces hunger in partnership with cooperating organizations by providing children and low-income people access to food, a healthy diet, and nutrition education in a manner that supports U.S. agriculture and inspires public action.

FNS administers some 15 domestic food service programs that serve about one in five Americans at some point during the year.[2] The programs work individually and in concert to provide a nutrition safety net for children and low-income adults and are a major component of the federal safety net. Together these programs account for about half of total USDA outlays. A total of $23.3 billion was dis-

> Read more about each of the food assistance programs online at the USDA's Food and Nutrition Services Web site at http://www.fns.usda.gov/fns/.

tributed during the first half of fiscal 2004 (October 1, 2003 to March 31, 2004), and by the end of 2004 the USDA was projected to exceed the record $41.8 billion spent on food assistance in fiscal 2003.[3] These expenditures are up again after a decline in the 1990s, largely due to a decline in participation in the Supplemental Nutrition Assistance Program (FSP) to a low of $16 billon (18.2 million people) in 1999.[4] Five programs account for almost 95% of the USDA's food assistance expenditures. These are the Supplemental Nutrition Assistance Program, the National School Lunch Program, the Special Supplemental Nutrition Program for Women, Infants and Children (WIC), the School Breakfast Program, and the Child and Adult Care Food Program.

Supplemental Nutrition Assistance Program

Since 1980, the Supplemental Nutrition Assistance Program has been the largest federal food assistance program and a mainstay of the federal safety net.[5] The program's intent is to enable people with low income to obtain a nutritionally adequate diet through coupons or Electronic Benefit Transfer (EBT) payments. These coupons or payments allow for the purchase of food and nonalcoholic beverages in authorized stores. These stores are then reimbursed by the federal government for the full value of the food. States administer the program in accordance with federal regulations and share the administrative expenses with the federal government.[4]

> Current eligibility criteria appear on the Food and Nutrition Service's Web site at http://www.fns.usda.gov.

To qualify for FSP benefits, a household without an aged or disabled member must have a gross income less than 130% of the official poverty guidelines. The household's net income must fall below the poverty line and must meet asset limits. In determining the benefit level, FNS assumes that a household will contribute 30% of its countable income toward food purchases. In addition, the Thrifty Food Plan for a family of four is determined by FNS to calculate the basic expenditure by which a family of four could purchase a nutritionally adequate diet with minimum costs.[4]

Most people who receive food stamps rely on the program for support over a relatively long period of time because of high re-entry rates.[5] Individuals' economic circumstances, such as employment status and income level, are an important determination of participation patterns.

Single women with children, older people, and people with disabilities have longer periods of participation.[5] Although no significant increase in food insecurity and hunger occurred in the 1995–1999 time period for those participating in the FSP, food insecurity and hunger did increase significantly (from 19.6% to 23.9%) for those low-income families not receiving food stamps in this same period.[6] (Read more about food insecurity in the United States in Chapter 17.)

A major goal of the Supplemental Nutrition Assistance Program is to protect against food insecurity and hunger. Olson et al.[7] studied factors that protect against and contribute to food insecurity among 316 rural families with household incomes of less than 200% of the federal poverty level. Mothers who used more food and financial skills, such as budget making, meal preparation, and stretching groceries, were more likely to have food-secure households than those who used fewer of these skills. Reports of depression and of difficulty paying for medical expenses were related to increased risks of food insecurity. This report reinforces the need for teaching financial management and food preparation and purchasing skills to low-income families. Training in these skills is currently being provided by the Expanded Food and Nutrition Education Program (EFNEP) administered through State Cooperative Services. The report also highlights how health disparities of rural populations contribute to greater food insecurity.

> Read more about the federal poverty levels and their impact in Chapters 4 and 20.

Special Supplemental Nutrition Program for Women, Infants and Children

The WIC program, administered by the USDA's Food and Nutrition Service, was established as a pilot program in 1972 and made permanent in 1974.[8] The program is based on two premises: 1) inadequate nutritional patterns and health behaviors of low-income women and children mean they are more vulnerable to adverse health outcomes; and 2) food interventions during critical times of growth and development can help prevent future medical and developmental problems.[9,10] Data from the 1994–1996 Continuing Survey of Food Intakes by Individuals (CSFII) suggest that WIC recipients have higher intakes of all nutrients than income-eligible nonparticipants.[11] A secondary data analysis of the cross-sectional survey of preschoolers from the 1994–1996 and 1998 CSFII confirmed beneficial effects, especially for the targeted nutrients.[12] One study in Idaho[13] examined the impact of WIC on the eating behaviors of preschool children and found significant improvement in eating behavior after six months on the WIC program, with improved overall Healthy Eating Index (HEI) scores including scores for vegetables, fruits, and meats.

The WIC program is a broad-based and comprehensive food and nutrition program providing three main benefits to participants: 1) supplemental foods, 2) nutrition education, and 3) referrals to healthcare and social service providers The specific aims of the WIC program are to augment available health care in order to prevent nutrition-related health problems and to improve the health of participants. The program serves not only as a secondary prevention program by providing risk appraisal and risk reduction, but also as a tertiary prevention program by providing treatment or rehabilitation to those with a diagnosed health condition.[14]

Supplemental Foods

WIC food supplements to pregnant women are designed to improve nutritional status during pregnancy, improve pregnancy outcomes, and promote a better nutritional status for mothers and infants. Supplements for lactating women are designed to provide special nutrients needed for lactation, improve lactation performance, and promote a better nutritional status for the mother and infant. WIC food supplements for postpartum mothers who are not breast feeding are intended to improve nutritional status during the postpartum period to better meet the physical demands of postnatal care and improve nutritional status and health for any future pregnancy. The general consensus that "WIC works" has been questioned because most WIC research studies fail to control for selection into the program. Bitler and Currie[15] evaluated the selection problem using data from the national Pregnancy Risk Assessment Monitoring System and found that relative to Medicaid mothers, all of whom are eligible for WIC, participation was associated with improved birth outcomes, even after controlling for multiple factors.

See http://www.cms.gov/Medicaid/ to learn about those who qualify for Medicaid. Also, see Chapter 4 to read about those at highest nutritional risk in the United States.

The reduction or prevention of iron deficiency anemia is a primary goal of WIC food supplements for infants and children. Other goals are to improve diets and to support physical growth and mental development. These goals are perhaps even more important than previously thought, because the cross-sectional National Health and Nutrition Examination Survey III (1988–1994) demonstrated an increased prevalence of iron deficiency among overweight children and highlighted the need to screen for iron deficiency in children.[16] WIC participation has a significant positive effect on children's intakes of iron, folate, and vitamin B_6,[8,17] even after controlling for self-selection bias.[18] Iron is one of five nutrients specifically targeted by the WIC program; the four other nutrients besides iron are protein, calcium, and vitamins A and C.[17] A 1991 USDA study recommended that folate, vitamin B_6, and zinc should also be targeted.[19]

Nutrition Education

The WIC program also provides nutrition education to improve the nutritional status of participants. At least one-sixth of WIC administrative funds must be spent by local agencies on nutrition education and counseling. Local agencies also must offer at least two nutrition education sessions to each participating woman in each six-month certification period. With increased recognition of the value of breast feeding, specific programs and earmarked funds, such as for the purchase of lactation aids like breast pumps, are intended to foster successful breast feeding.

Referrals for Health Care

Referrals to healthcare providers are intended to promote good health care by increasing the use of prenatal and postpartum care, and by improving access to routine preventive services such as immunization, smoking cessation, and family planning. Social service referrals to substance abuse treatment, housing assistance, Medicaid, and food stamps assistance are intended to meet a full range of health and nutrition needs of low-income women and their children.

Center for Nutrition Policy and Promotion

The second major agency within FNCS is the Center for Nutrition Policy and Promotion (CNPP). It was created on December 1, 1994 as the focal point within the USDA where scientific research is linked with the nutritional needs of the public. CNPP works to improve the health and well-being of Americans by developing and promoting dietary guidance that links scientific research to the nutrition needs of consumers. Center staff help to define and coordinate nutrition education policy within the USDA and translate nutrition research into information and materials for consumers, policy makers, and professionals in health, education, industry, and the media. An issue of the agency's publication, *Family Economics and Nutrition Review*, illustrates some of the major projects of CNPP.[20] The issue includes research reports on factors influencing children's consumption of meals served in the Summer Food Service Program,[21] factors affecting food security among first-time WIC participants,[22] and contributors to food insecurity among rural families.[7] Basiotis et al.[23] addressed the HEI for 1999–2000 as a means of charting dietary patterns of Americans and another way of assessing the nutritional quality of U.S. diets.

Healthy Eating Index

The Healthy Eating Index (HEI) was developed by CNPP to assess and monitor the quality of the U.S. diet.[24-26] The Interactive Healthy Eating Index (IHEI) program is an online dietary assessment tool that allows a consumer to calculate his or her own HEI score for a given day or days and provides information on the individual's diet quality. The program links to related nutrition messages and nutrient information. The Physical Activity Tool is a recent addition to the IHEI that assesses an individual's physical activity status and provides energy expenditure information and educational messages. The IHEI thus enhances the link between good nutrition and the health benefits of regular physical activity.

> The Interactive Healthy Eating Index program is available online at http:// www.cnpp.usda.gov/ HealthyEatingIndex.htm. Accessed on 4/20/10.

Dietary Guidelines for Americans and MyPyramid

In conjunction with the Department of Health and Human Services, CNPP participates in the review and update of the nutrition science underlying revisions of the Dietary Guidelines for Americans (DGA).[27-29] **Table 9–1** summarizes DGA activities. The process for updating the Dietary Guidelines includes an evidence-based review of the latest science, which results in recommendations of the Dietary Guidelines Advisory Committee (DGAC). The committee consists of leading health and nutrition experts from across the country.[20,29] The process is open, and minutes of meetings of the DGA Committee are posted online through a federal Web site (http://www.usda.gov/cnpp/dietary_guidelines.html). Written and oral public comments

and feedback about the proposed guidelines are solicited through *Federal Register* notices. A new revision of the Dietary Guidelines for Americans was released in summer of 2010 and is discussed in Chapter 2. A revision of the food guidance system, commonly known as the MyPyramid (formerly called the Food Guide Pyramid), has been carried out by CNPP in conjunction with the 5th revision of the Dietary Guidelines and was released in April 2005. A new revision of the Dietary Guidelines was released in 2010.

CNPP also maintains and updates the Thrifty Food Plan, which serves as the nutritional basis for determination of benefits in the Supplemental Nutrition Assistance Program. Carlson et al.[30] outlined

> All of CNPP's projects are available on the Internet at http://www.cnpp.usda.gov.

three additional food plans that specify the type and quantity of foods that people could consume at home to have a nutritious diet at various cost levels. Each food plan has 12 market baskets, one for each of 12 age-gender groups. These plans were developed when the USDA's 1989–1991 CSFII and the Food Price Database were merged.

■ OVERVIEW OF THE FOOD SAFETY AND INSPECTION SERVICE

The Food Safety and Inspection Service (FSIS) is the public health agency within the USDA responsible for ensuring that the nation's commercial supply of meat, poultry, and egg products is safe, wholesome, and correctly labeled and packaged.[31] It provides both education and inspection services. The USDA is responsible for nutrition labeling and inspection of foods not covered by the Food and Drug Administration. Although not a direct research agency, research does play an important role in FSIS's ability to fulfill its public health mission and to guarantee that the foods it regulates continue to be safe. The agency funds research in food safety and food safety education at various universities and institutes around the country. FSIS is now an important element in homeland security. (Read more about food safety in Chapter 16 and homeland security in Chapter 18.)

■ OVERVIEW OF RESEARCH, EDUCATION, AND ECONOMICS

The USDA-Research, Education, and Economics (REE) agency was created to provide federal leadership in creating and disseminating knowledge spanning the biological, physical, and social sciences related to agricultural research, economic analysis, statistics, extension, and higher education.[32] REE has four major service areas: 1) Agricultural Research Service (ARS); 2) Cooperative State Research, Education, and Extension Service (CSREES); 3) Economics Research Service (ERS); and 4) National Agricultural Statistics

TABLE 9–1	USDA Food Guides and Tools	
Name		**Year Established**
Dietary Guidelines for Americans revised every five years (1985–2010)		1980
Food Pyramid—Visual Tool		1988
Healthy Eating Index—Assessment Tool		1995
Individual Healthy Eating Index—Online Consumer Tool		2006
MyPyramid		2005
Physical Activity Guidelines for Adults		2008

Service (NASS). Congress created CSREES through the 1994 Department Reorganization Act, which combined the former Cooperative State Research Service (CSRS) and the former Extension Service (ES) into a single agency (CSREES).

Agricultural Research Service

In 2004, the Agricultural Research Service celebrated its 50th anniversary as the principal research arm of the USDA and of human nutrition research. ARS is organized into 22 national programs that coordinate, communicate, and empower more than 1,200 research projects carried out by the ARS. The vision statement and the mission statement of the Human Nutrition National Program are:

Vision:
Provide a nutritious food supply, promote nutritional health, and quality of life, reduce morbidity and mortality associated with chronic diseases influenced by dietary intake and develop sound dietary recommendations which can be used to establish more effective nutrition assistance programs.

Mission:
...to conduct basic and applied research to identify and understand how nutrients and other bioactive food components affect health. The ultimate goal of the food-based agricultural research is to identify foods and diets, coupled with genetics and physical activity that sustain and promote health throughout the life cycle. (http://www.ars.usda.gov/research/programs/programs.htm?NP_CODE-107)

Important programs that are closely related to ARS's role in public health nutrition include:

- National Agricultural Library (NAL)
- Eight research locations concentrating on human nutrition
- Food consumption surveys
- Food composition databases
- Food and nutrition research publications

National Agricultural Library

> The online National Agricultural Library is at http://www.nal.usda.gov.

Beyond the traditional functions of a national library of agriculture, the NAL provides six online information centers, one of which is the Food and Nutrition Information Center (FNIC). Founded in 1971, FNIC's mission is to collect and disseminate information about food and human nutrition. In 1977, the Food and Agriculture Act (Farm Bill) established FNIC as a permanent entity within the National Agricultural Library. Five special projects have their own Web sites accessible through http://www.nal.usda.gov/fnic/general/general.html:

1. Child Care Nutrition Resource System (CCNRS): Provides information to people working in the USDA's Child Nutrition Programs.
2. Food Stamp Nutrition Connection: A resource system for Supplemental Nutrition Assistance Program nutrition education providers.
3. Healthy School Meals Resource System (HSMRS): Provides information to people working in the USDA's Child Nutrition Program.
4. International Bibliographic Information on Dietary Supplements (IBIDS): Databases that provide access to bibliographic citations and abstracts from published, international, scientific literature on dietary supplements. The USDA and agencies from NIH are working collaboratively to establish a dietary supplement database.
5. WIC Works Resource System: Serves as an encompassing resource for WIC nutritionists and other WIC professionals nationwide.

National Programs in Human Nutrition

The mission of the National Programs in Human Nutrition is carried out in eight locations that serve as major centers for human nutrition research. Each location has special research interests and extensive collaborations and partnerships with universities.

1. Arkansas Children's Nutrition Center (Little Rock, AR; founded in 1995) has primary studies in brain development and function, dietary factors affecting development, and bone development.
2. Beltsville Human Nutrition Research Center (Beltsville, MD; founded in 1941) focuses on defining the role of food and its components in optimizing human health and reducing the risk of nutrition-related diseases. It also houses the Nutrient Data Laboratory and the Food Surveys Research Group, which have a long history of important contributions to public health nutrition research.
3. Children's Nutrition Research Center at Baylor College of Medicine (Houston, TX; founded in 1979) studies the role of maternal, infant, and child nutrition in optimal health, development, and growth, including childhood dietary habits.
4. Grand Forks Human Nutrition Research Center (Grand Forks, ND; founded in 1977) has long served as the world's leading research center in basic and applied mineral nutrition.
5. Western Human Nutrition Research Center (Davis, CA; founded in 1980) strives to improve health through the study of diet, genetics, and environmental interactions.
6. Jean Mayer Human Nutrition Research Center on Aging at Tufts University (Boston, MA; founded in

1980) was founded to study the relationship between nutrition and aging.

7. Lower Mississippi Delta Nutrition Intervention Research Initiative (NIRI) (Little Rock, AR; founded in 1995) is focused on community intervention research through community-based participatory research in rural communities in Arkansas, Louisiana, and Mississippi. The Delta NIRI was established by congressional mandate to improve health and well-being in the Lower Delta through research in nutrition and intervention methodology.

8. Plant, Soil, and Nutrition Laboratory at Cornell University (Ithaca, NY; founded in 1940) was established to study the influence of soils on nutritional quality of plant foods and has a proud history of outstanding research, including the award of a Nobel Prize to one of its scientists.

Food Surveys Research Group

Housed within the Beltsville Human Nutrition Research Center, the Food Surveys Research Group (FSRG) has conducted food surveys on Americans since the 1930s. These surveys have summarized nutrient intakes and monitored trends in food intakes. The Continuing Survey of Food Intakes by Individuals (CSFII) was conducted by the USDA in 1977–1978, 1985–1986, 1989–1991, and 1994–1996 before becoming combined with the National Health and Nutrition Evaluation Survey (NHANES) in 2000 as the "What We Eat in America" dietary component of NHANES 2000. Combining the two surveys has allowed data to be collected on an annual basis, rather than sporadically depending on the availability of monies. The first data from the combined survey are available on the Internet.

The FSRG has continued to develop, evaluate, and create new dietary assessment tools. In previous CSFII surveys, the Multiple Pass Method was used with pencil and paper using a five-step system to obtain free-flowing recall, remember forgotten foods, assign eating occasion, obtain more details, and allow one last opportunity to recall foods. Over a seven-year period, the original method was transferred to a computer-assisted interviewing instrument. The Automated Multiple Pass Method (AMPM) is the cornerstone of a Dietary Intake Data System consisting of three computer systems and an extensive food and nutrient database.[33,34] The Food and Nutrient Database for Dietary Studies (FNDDS) includes food descriptions, food portions, and their weights and nutrients; a listserv[35] provides emailed alerts when new data or instruments become available.

Join the Food Survey Research Group listserv at http://riley.nal.usda.gov/nal_display/index.php?info_center=4&tax_level=2&tax_subject=279&topic_id=1388.

Effective, efficient, and validated dietary methodology allows the collection of accurate information on what people eat in research studies and over time as free-living individuals. Study of specific nutrients requires accurate and available food composition data of each nutrient in a sufficient number of foods. For large surveys, the food composition data need to include all the foods that the participants are likely to be consuming. The nutrient databases thus need continuous updating as new food products come on the market, new food varieties are developed, and new technologies for nutrient analysis are developed. (Read more about food intake surveys in Chapter 3 and managing data in Chapter 20.)

Food Composition Databases

Food composition databases are planned and developed by the USDA Nutrient Data Laboratory (NDL), ARS, and Beltsville Agricultural Research Center (BARC), and are considered to be the authority of composition data on foods available in the United States. NDL develops methods to acquire, evaluate, compile, and disseminate composition data on available foods. **Table 9–2** provides a selected list of datasets created and compiled into national databases. Two major databases have been the USDA Nutrient Data Laboratory (formerly Nutrient Database for Standard Reference), now in its 22nd release, and the Primary Data Set (PDS) for USDA Nationwide Food Surveys. These have served as the numerical foundation of essentially all public and private work in the field of nutrition. These data were originally published in the form of *Agriculture Handbook 8* (AH-8), which is no longer available in print form. In order to provide timely release of nutrient data, the database is available for download from the Internet to a hard drive, CD, or handheld personal digital assistant (PDA), or they can be purchased on CD.

The Standard Reference Database contains over 7,000 foods. SR data are also included in the Child Nutrition (CN) Database, which is maintained for the School Lunch Program and other child nutrition programs. In 2003, NDL released the USDA Database for the Flavonoid Content of Foods and the USDA Table of Nutrient Retention Factors Release, and in 2004 it released the USDA Database for the Choline Content of Common Foods and the USDA Database for Proanthocyanidin Content of Selected Foods.

Visit the USDA databases at http://www.nal.usda.gov/fnic/foodcomp/Bulletins/timeline.htm.

Underlying human nutrition research and, subsequently, public health nutrition policymaking and practice are quality food composition data.[36] Public health applications include assessing food and nutrient availability and intakes in populations, evaluation of programs to protect and improve nutritional status, research on diet and disease interrelationships,

TABLE 9–2 | **Selected Tables of Food Composition Published by the USDA, ARS Nutrient Data Laboratory**

Year(s)	Food Component(s)	Medium
1927	Vitamin content of food	Print
1939	Thiamin added	Print
1942	Nutritive value of the national food supply	Print
1944–1952	Amino acid content of food	Print
1950	Agricultural Handbook No. 8 containing proximate composition, 3 minerals, and 5 vitamins in 750 foods	Print
1959	Fatty acids	Print
1961	Vitamin B$_{12}$	Print
1963	Cholesterol	Print
1966	Vitamin E	Print
1973	Pantothenic acid, Vitamin B$_6$, Vitamin B$_{12}$	Print
1981–1988	Handbook No. 8 Series of various foods, fatty acids and cholesterol, stearic acid, total fat, omega-3 fatty acids and other fat components, fast foods, amino acids in fruits and vegetables, dietary fiber	Print
1987, 1990	Sugar content of selected foods	Print
1983	Iron	Print
1990–1994	Vitamin K, Vitamin D, selenium	Print
1995	*Trans*-fatty acid	Print/Electronic
1996	Carotenoids	Transition from print to electronic software to allow free and easy access to updates and new additions to Standard Reference database
1993, 1998	Isoflavonoids (Iowa State University)	Electronic
1998, 2000	Isoflavonoids, database	Electronic
2002	Choline, proanthocyanidin	Download software to handheld personal digital assistant (PDA)
2003	Dietary Supplement Database	Electronic
2004		Electronic

Home and Garden Bulletin No. 72 was again released in print form due to popular demand. All other food composition publications are available either online or on CD.

health education and promotion activities, assessment of risk from food-borne contamination, and preserving information on traditional foods. None of these applications can occur without a national nutrient database. Development and maintenance of a high-quality nutrient database continues under the leadership of USDA research scientists.

Collaboration of the food industry with the USDA Nutrient Data Laboratory is an essential element in capturing the latest food products. It is expensive to develop high-quality food composition data and is usually affordable only by governments. Representative sampling of perishable foods across a country, standardized procedures, and up-to-date technology are required for a valid food composition database.

According to Burlingame,[37] five conventional criteria are critical to quality food composition databases. Quality first

begins with a *sampling plan* that may require a year of planning and that specifies the number of samples at every stage including sample preparation, discrete sample analyses, replicates, and variability. *Representativeness* is the traditional term used to describe the suitability of data to be entered into a database. The third factor is *completeness*, a term suggesting all foods and all food components for all user groups. In reality, certain foods or food components are missing from every database. Choices and priorities have to be made to achieve a comprehensive database for most user groups. Foods in industrialized countries undergo constant change with the continuing introduction of new processed foods, many of which may be gone within a year. Continued development of new food varieties with more disease resistance, higher yields, or richer nutrients (phytochemicals) also changes the food supply. The fourth quality factor is *harmonization* of databases, which attempts to achieve international standards for defining elements in databases. The final quality criterion is *documentation*. Although detailed documentation cannot be published, database compilers have the responsibility to fully record details and have these readily available.[37]

Applications of these databases have been enhanced and increased by the development of Web sites that allow ready and free downloading of new releases of the Standard Reference database onto computer hard drives and handheld computers. Anyone with access to a personal computer can find the 90+ nutrients or components of some 7,000 foods.

ARS Publications

A major movement to increase efficiency and ease dissemination of research findings in a timely manner has been the increasing publication of online materials for both lay and professional audiences. *Agricultural Research* is the ARS bimonthly magazine that highlights research activities by ARS scientists, including development of new and improved varieties of fruits and vegetables that will provide more protective factors, community intervention projects, improved control of pests in crops, new methodology to study human nutrition, improved water quality projects, and other diverse topics. Quarterly newsletters such as *Food and Nutrition Research Briefs* provide updates on research and services from ARS scientists.

Cooperative State Research, Education, and Extension Service

The unique mission of Cooperative State Research, Education, and Extension Service (CSREES) is to advance knowledge for agriculture, the environment, human health and well-being, and communities by supporting research, education, and extension programs in the land-grant university system and other partner organizations. Although not performing actual research, education, or extension, CSREES helps fund these activities at the state and local level and provides program leadership in these areas.

Eleven targeted areas of interest and the 59 resulting programs include 4 areas closely related to public health: Economics and Commerce; Families, Youth, and Communities; Food, Nutrition, and Health; and Natural Resources and Environment.[32] Knowledge is advanced through two key mechanisms: 1) national program leadership that helps states identify and meet research, extension, and educational priorities in areas of public concern; and 2) federal assistance that provides annual funding to land-grant universities and competitively grants funds to researchers at universities.

To read more about the emphasis areas of the CSREES, visit http://www.csrees.usda.gov/nea/food/food.html.

An extensive network of state, regional, and county extension offices in every U.S. state and territory has a focus on critical issues affecting people's daily lives and the nation's future. The aim is to empower people and communities to solve problems and improve their lives on the local level. An example of such programs is the USDA's 102-year-old youth development program called 4-H (Heart, Hand, Head, and Health).

Food, Nutrition, and Health

The Food, Nutrition, and Health National emphasis area is committing increased dollars and resources to remedy the negative effects of poor dietary choices and unhealthy lifestyles, food-borne illnesses, and the potential for terrorist-related and other threats to the food supply. Not to be forgotten, however, is that millions of Americans struggle to obtain sufficient food, and U.S. food suppliers attempt to keep up with changing food trends. Program leadership and funding opportunities work to strengthen the nation's capacity to address important issues surrounding diet, health, food safety, food security, and food science and technology. Six major programs in this area are:

1. Food safety and biosecurity
2. Food sciences and technology
3. Health
4. Hunger and food security
5. Nutrition
6. Obesity and healthy weight

Food Safety Food safety activities illustrate the wide diversity supported by CSREES. Food safety concerns cover a broad spectrum from on-farm production to post-harvest processing, distribution, food preparation, selection, and consumption. Consumer education strives to increase understanding of disease-causing microorganisms, their products, naturally occurring toxicants, and chemical contamination in meat, poultry, seafood, and fresh fruits and vegetables. Protecting the national food supply, which can be threatened by both incidental and deliberate contamination, is another focus for research, education, and extension programs. Development of new technology such as thermal processing, irradiation, hydrostatic processing, and ohmic processing are just a few examples of adding value in processing, packaging, marketing, and distributing of wholesome and safe food.

Food Security *Food security* has been defined as:

> . . . having access, at all times, to enough food for an active, healthy life for all its household members . . . including availability of nutritionally adequate and safe foods and assured ability to acquire personally preferred foods in a socially acceptable way.[38]

CSREES engages in a variety of education and awareness activities to increase public knowledge about nutrition, food safety, and community food security, such as a grant program that funds private nonprofit organizations to address community food security issues, as well as collaborating through partnerships across the USDA.

Community-Based Nutrition Education

In partnership with the Cooperative Extension Systems, CSREES delivers community-based nutrition education programs designed to help individuals, families, and communities make informed choices about food and lifestyles that support health and economic and social well-being. Four broad program areas are the foundation of CSREES nutrition education programs: food security, food safety, dietary guidance, and health. The Expanded Food and Nutrition Education Program (EFNEP) helps low-income families improve their diets for better health, to increase physical activity, and to save money. The EFNEP program is offered to all limited resource families who are eligible for food stamps. EFNEP Success Stories evaluate how EFNEP benefits have helped low-income audiences achieve good nutrition through knowledge and behavior change, and EFNEP Impact Reports include data and evaluations on the various EFNEP components.

> Research the EFNEP online at http://www.csrees.usda.gov/ProgView.cfm?prnum=2300.

CSREES Partnerships   CSREES has a partnership with the National Cancer Institute and the Produce for a Better Health Foundation to develop and promote the 5-A-Day for Better Health Program. Another USDA partnership is with the Department of Health and Human Service's *Healthy People 2010* to set and promote health goals for the United States. Other partnerships exist among CSREES and other USDA agencies.

Economic Research Service

The Economic Research Service (ERS) studies the economics of food, farming, natural resources, and rural America. For example, the agency provides analyses of the economic issues affecting the safety of the U.S. food supply, including estimating: 1) the cost of specific food-borne diseases ($3 billion in 2010 for just two organisms), and 2) the costs and benefits of programs aimed at improving food safety, including conducting a nationally representative survey of meat and poultry plants on the costs of the Hazard Analysis Critical Control Plan (HACCP). Another food safety report[39] examined changes in hamburger preparation behavior, the reasons for the changes, the medical costs saved as a result of the changes, and the implications for future food safety education. Other examples of economic analysis include the study of how economics influence eating choices, body weight outcomes,[40] and the economic assessment of costs and benefits of food labeling.[41]

Food Assistance and Nutrition Research Program

Although the ERS does not administer food assistance programs, it does administer the Food Assistance and Nutrition Research Program (FANRP), which was established by the U.S. Congress in 1998 to conduct research and evaluation on topics relevant to USDA food assistance programs including program outcomes, program operations and integrity, vulnerable populations, the relationship between food assistance programs and the general economy, and food security in the United States. An example of an FANRP evaluation is The WIC Program: Background, Trends, and Issues, Report Number FANRR27.[42] FANRP's research emphasis is on the role of USDA food assistance and nutrition programs in promoting a healthy, well-nourished population. FANRP conducts intramural research such as the WIC report[42] and also sponsors extramural research. Extramural funding efforts include: 1) support of improved nutrition data, for example, funding of an annual collection of national data on household food security; 2) the FANRP Competitive Grants and Cooperative Agreements, which support policy-relevant research on food assistance programs and nutrition issues; and 3) support for the Small Grants Program, which encourages research innovation and broader scholarly participation in food assistance and nutrition research. Information about these is available online at http://www.ers.usda.gov/Briefing/FoodNutritionAssistance/.

ERS Publications   ERS publishes reports and periodicals that address the economic analysis of the impact of food assistance programs. Twice a year, ERS publishes *The Food and Assistance Landscape*, which provides a brief overview of the USDA's domestic food assistance programs including program statistics, expenditures, participation levels, and related economic indicators such as unemployment rates, income growth, and food price inflation. Another series, titled *Issues in Food Assistance*, addresses a variety of topics including effects of legislative changes, social changes, and operational issues on the Supplemental Nutrition Assistance Program, food insecurity, and other aspects of the well-being of low-income households. A lay magazine, *Amber Waves*, covers a wide variety of ERS research topics including food assistance, nutrition, and food safety.

ERS reports document the importance of USDA food assistance and nutrition programs. Its reports examine our understanding of how well the programs operate as a "food safety net." A four-volume series, *Effects of Food Assistance and Nutrition Programs on Nutrition and Health*, is a comprehensive review and synthesis of research on the impacts of USDA food assistance and nutrition programs on

> Another series of online information covers WIC and child nutrition issues. Find it at http://www.ers.usda.gov/publications/fanrr34/.

numerous important outcomes including food expenditures, household nutrient availability, dietary intake, nutritional status, food security, birth outcomes, breast-feeding behaviors, immunization rates, use and cost of healthcare services, and selected non-health outcomes, such as academic achievement, school performance (children), and social isolation (elderly).

ERS studies also examine issues related to participation decisions. For example, the Supplemental Nutrition Assistance Program Access Study was a national study of Supplemental Nutrition Assistance Program accessibility at the local office level, and described the nature and prevalence of local office practices hypothesized to influence participation; households' stated reasons for not participating or ending their participation; and characteristics, attitudes, and experiences associated with participation behavior. It then analyzed the association between local office practices and household participation behaviors.[43] Results provide information to policy and program officials on how programs can become more effective and efficient.

■ HISTORY OF NUTRITION EDUCATION AT THE USDA

The USDA has a rich history of providing science-based nutrition information and education to the public.[44] The Organic Act of 1862 directed the newly formed Department of Agriculture to "acquire and diffuse among the people of the United States useful information on subjects connected to agriculture and rural development."[44] In the 1930s, the USDA's focus was on providing "common-sense knowledge of nutrition," followed by the RDAs in the early 1940s, which emphasized maintaining health for the war effort. In the 1950s, nutrient adequacy was emphasized, and the USDA focused on providing the right kind of information for an adequate diet.[44] In 1969 the White House Conference on Food, Nutrition, and Health was held, and the focus became linking nutrition education to the promotion of optimal health with food. The president of the American Dietetic Association testified in favor of the amendment of the Food Stamp Act in 1969 and the expansion and improvement of the National School Lunch Act in 1969.[45]

In the 1970s, the Food and Agriculture Act of 1977 named the USDA as the "lead government agency for nutrition research, extension, and teaching."[44] A call for the development of more effective systems for delivering nutrition information to the public was linked to the growing evidence relating some food components to risks for chronic disease. Increased public interest in diet and disease risks led to the first set of USDA Dietary Guidelines for Americans. **Table 9–3** outlines three USDA Nutrition Education Programs with Legislative Authorization that began in the 1970s: 1) Nutrition Education and Training Programs (NET), 2) WIC, and 3) EFNEP.

The 1980s brought increased interest in nutrition education research for the development of improved materials and methods to better inform the general public about good nutrition. Evaluation of nutrition education tools was increased to measure comprehension and perceived usefulness by the targeted audiences.

In the 1990s, a revised *Dietary Guidelines for Americans* was released. A greater coordination of nutrition education efforts and survey efforts was called for by the Nutrition Monitoring and Related Research Act.[46,47] The focus shifted from a simple nutrition information provision to promoting behavioral change and motivating consumers to adopt eating practices to promote optimal health. The latest revision of the *Dietary Guidelines for Americans* was released in 2010.

Nutrition, Agriculture, and Health of Americans

The health of rural populations is essential to the production and maintenance of an adequate and safe food supply. The USDA thus has long been committed to improving the nutritional health of Americans through a program of research and education to maintain a food supply of high nutritional quality and to encourage consumption of a healthful diet.

Nutrition is a bridge between agriculture and the health of American consumers in a two-way process. Science-based nutrition messages can motivate Americans to make healthful changes in their diets that will create new demands in the kinds and amounts of food people buy in the marketplace.[44] Market responses to consumer demands can lead, in turn, to the creation of new products and other changes in the food system. Examples include the development of low-fat and reduced calorie foods, leaner meats, and calcium-enriched orange juice and other beverages.[44] Well-targeted nutrition education and health promotion activities can encourage Americans to adopt new agricultural products into healthy eating habits and eventually lead to positive health outcomes and reduced healthcare costs.

History of the USDA's Research Role in Public Health Nutrition

The founding of food and nutrition science policy was nurtured by the establishment of the Land-Grant College System by the Hatch Act of 1887, shortly after the creation of the Department of Agriculture in 1862.[48] The first federal funding of human nutrition research occurred in 1893–1894. An early beneficiary of the USDA Land Grant program at the University of Connecticut at Storrs was Dr. Wilbur O. Atwater, whose "Atwater values for carbohydrates, protein, and fat" are among the first nutrition facts taught in introductory nutrition courses and are used on a daily basis by dietitians and nutritionists.[48] Dr. Atwater, credited as the father of American food science, was appointed the Director of the Office of Experiment Stations, which was funded by the USDA.[49] The contributions of Atwater and other pioneers of the 19th

TABLE 9–3 USDA Nutrition Education Programs with Legislative Authorization

Program	Target Population	Agency Responsible	State Collaborators	Delivery
Nutrition Education and Training Program (NET)	Children, all incomes	FCS	State education departments	Training of school food service and teachers, school nutrition education curricula, training for child care providers and parents
Special Supplemental Nutrition Program for Women, Infants and Children (WIC)	Low-income pregnant and breast-feeding women, infants, and children up to age 5	FCS	State health departments and WIC clinics	Individual counseling or group lessons along with WIC food package or vouchers for supplemental foods; two contacts per 6-month certification period
Expanded Food and Nutrition Education Program (EFNEP)	Limited-resource families with young children; low-income youth	CSREES	State land-grant universities; county cooperative extension offices	One-on-one home visits or group classes by trained paraprofessional aides; in-depth 6-month program
Education Program (EFNEP)	Limited-resource families with young children; low-income youth	CSREES	State land-grant universities; county cooperative extension offices	One-on-one home visits or group classes by trained paraprofessional aides; in-depth 6-month program

century are the cornerstone of current nutrition science and policy. These principles of rigorous quantitative analysis, using appropriate standard reference materials, are still applied today in the USDA nutrient data laboratory in Beltsville and in collaborating universities' laboratories.[50-52]

The first tables of average nutrient values of foods were published in 1896 as *The Chemical Composition of American Food Materials*, USDA Bulletin 28.[48] The third version, by Atwater and Bryant in 1906 included analysis of more than 4,000 food items and served as a standard reference for dietitians and nutritionists for more than four decades (see Table 9–1).[45] The Nutrient Data Laboratory and the Food Survey Group of the Agricultural Research Service continue collaboration to plan, develop, and monitor nutrient databanks and methodology that underlie all nutrition surveys and nutrition intervention research in the United States.

The 1994–1996 CSFII was the USDA's 10th survey since the 1930s, producing the nutrient intakes of a stratified representative sample of Americans and providing standards against which regional and local nutrition studies have been compared.[53]

With the merging of the CSFII Survey and the National Health and Nutrition Examination Survey in 1999, continuous monitoring of the health and nutrient intake of Americans is now being carried out with the nutrition methodology

developed and tested by the Food Survey Research Group. This merger of the USDA and NIH in nutrition monitoring for better health and disease prevention in Americans is a model from which Americans may benefit enormously, as the combined expertise of these departments promotes improved nutrition and health and helps prevent disease. The USDA has focused largely on promotion of health through supporting food production, food technology, nutrition research, and nutrition education.

Issues for Discussion

1. Is a single pyramid the best graphic model to represent the 2010 Dietary Guidelines for Americans in its food and physical activity recommendations?

2. How does a nutritionist translate research findings from large national studies into effective interventions for individuals?

3. Should nutrition interventions such as "healthy weights" be implemented on a community level or an individual level?

4. What are factors impacting participation in food assistance programs such as WIC, the Supplemental Nutri-

tion Assistance Program, and the School Lunch Program? Conversely, what impacts does participation in food assistance programs have on health?

References

1. Bost EM. *Food, Nutrition, and Consumer Services.* Available at http://www.fns.usda.gov/fns. Accessed April 13, 2010.

2. Lin BH, Smallwood D. Research designs for assessing the USDA's food assistance and nutrition programs outcomes: Part I: Evaluation of ongoing national programs. *Nutr Today.* 2003;38:139–145.

3. Oliveira V. Food assistance landscape, September 2004. In: *Food Assistance and Nutrition Research Report No. FANRR28-5.* Alexandria, VA: Economic Research Service, United States Department of Agriculture; 2004. Available at http://www.ers.usda.gov/Publications/FANRR28-5. Accessed May 7, 2010.

4. Wilde P, Cook P, Gundersen C, Nord M, Tiehen L. The decline in food stamp program participation in the 1990's. In: *Food Assistance and Nutrition Research Report No. 7.* Washington, DC: USDA, Economic Research Service; 2000.

5. Gleason P, Schochet P, Moffett R. *The dynamics of food stamp program participation in the early 1990's.* Report submitted to the U.S. Department of Agriculture, Food and Nutrition Service. Princeton, NJ: Mathematica Policy Research; 1998.

6. Nord M, Andrews MA, Carlson S. Household food insecurity in the United States, 2001. In: *Food Assistance and Nutrition Research Report No. 29.* Washington, DC: Economic Research Service, U.S. Department of Agriculture; 2002.

7. Olson CM, Anderson K, Kiss E, Lawrence FC, Seiling SB. Factors protecting against and contributing to food insecurity among rural families. *Fam Econ Nutr Rev.* 2004;16:12–26.

8. Oliveira V, Gundersen C. WIC and the nutrient intake of children. In: *Food Assistance and Nutrition Research Report No. 5.* Washington, DC: USDA Economic Research Service; 2000:1–22.

9. Rush D. *Evaluation of the Special Supplemental Food Program for Women, Infants, and Children (WIC).* Volume 1: Summary. Washington, DC: U.S. Department of Agriculture; 1986.

10. Rush D, Sloan N, Leighton J, Alvir J, Horwitz D. (1988). The national WIC evaluation: evaluation of the special Supplement Food Program for Women, Infants, and Children. *Am J Clin Nutr.* 1988;48:S389–S519.

11. Rose D, Habicht JP, Devaney B. Household participation in the food stamp and WIC programs increases the nutrient intakes of preschool children. *J Nutr.* 1998;128:548–555.

12. Siega-Riz AM, Kranz S, Blanchett D, Haines PS, Gulkey DK, Popkin BM. The effect of participation in the WIC program on preschoolers' diets. *J Pediatr.* 2004;144:229–234.

13. Dundas ML, Cook K. Impact of the Special Supplemental Nutrition Program for Women, Infants and Children on the healthy eating behaviors of preschool children in eastern Idaho. *Top Clin Nutr.* 2004;19:273–279.

14. Committee on Scientific Evaluation of WIC Nutrition Risk Criteria, 1996

15. Bitler MP, Currie J. Does WIC work? The effects of WIC on pregnancy and birth outcomes. *J Policy Anal Manage.* 2005;24:73–91.

16. Nead KG, Halterman JS, Kaczorowski JM, Aulinger P, Weitzman M. Overweight children and adolescents: a risk group for iron deficiency. *Pediatrics.* 2004;114:104–108.

17. Oliveira V, Chandran R. Children's consumption of WIC approved foods. In: *Food Assistance and Nutrition Report No. 44.* Washington, DC: Economic Research Service, United States Department of Agriculture; 2005.

18. Heckman J. Sample selection bias as a specification error. *Econometrica.* 1979;41:1.

19. United States Department of Agriculture, Food and Nutrition Service. *Review of WIC Food Packages: Technical Paper, Economic Research Service.* Washington, DC: United States Department of Agriculture; 1991.

20. Hentges EJ. Front and Center: Making a difference with dietary guidance: From science to promotion. *Fam Econ Nutr Rev.* 2004; 16:1.

21. Cotugna N, Vickery CE. Children rate the Summer Food Service Program. *Fam Econ Nutr Rev.* 2004;16:3–12.

22. Herman DR, Harrison GG, Abdelmonem AA, Jenks E. The effect of the WIC program on food security status of pregnant, first-time participants. *Fam Econ Nutr Rev.* 2004;16:21–29.

23. Basiotis PP, Carlson A, Gerrior SA, WenYen J, Lino M. The Healthy Eating Index, 1999–2000: charting dietary patterns of Americans. *Fam Econ Nutr Rev.* 2004;16:39–48.

24. Basiotis PP, Carlson A, Gerrior SA, Juan WY, Lino M. *The Healthy Eating Index: 1999–2000.* (CNPP-12). Washington, DC: U.S. Department of Agriculture, Center for Nutrition Policy and Promotion; 2002.

25. Kennedy ET, Ohis J, Carlson S, Fleming K. The Healthy Eating Index: design and application. *J Am Dietetic Assoc.* 1995;95: 1103–1108.

26. United States Department of Agriculture, Center for Nutrition Policy and Promotion. *The Healthy Eating Index* (CNPP-1). Washington, DC: United States Government Printing Office; 1995.

27. United States Department of Agriculture, Center for Nutrition Policy and Promotion. The Food Guide Pyramid. Washington, DC: United States Department of Agriculture; 2010.

28. United States Department of Agriculture and United States Department of Health and Human Services. *Dietary Guidelines for Americans.* Available at http://www.cnpp.usda.gov/dietaryguidelines.htm. Accessed April 20, 2010.

29. United States Department of Health and Human Services and the United States Department of Agriculture. *Dietary Guidelines for Americans, 2005.* Washington, DC: U.S. Government Printing Office; 2005.

30. Carlson A, Linn M, Gerrior SA, Basiotis PP. *The Low-Cost, Moderate-Cost, and Liberal Food Plans: 2003 Administrative Report.* (CNPP-13). Washington, DC: Center for Nutrition Policy and Promotion; 2003.

31. United States Department of Agriculture, Food Safety and Inspection Service. Fulfilling the vision: Updates and initiatives in protecting public health. (2004). Available at http://www.fsis.usda.gov/About_FSIS/Fulfilling_the_Vision/index.asp. Accessed April 13, 2010.

32. National Institute of Food and Agriculture (NIFA), United States Department of Agriculture. Available at http://www.csrees.usda.gov/. Accessed April 13, 2010.

33. Bliss RM. Researchers produce innovations in dietary recall. *Agric Res.* 2004;52:10–12.

34. Raper N, Perloff B, Ingwersen L, Stainfeldt L, Anand J. (2004). An overview of USDA's Dietary Data System. *J Food Compos Anal.* 2004;17:545–555.

35. Food Surveys Research Group. Food Surveys Research Group Listserv. Available at http://www.ars.usda.gov/main/site_main.htm?modecode=12-35-50-00. Accessed July 1, 2009.

36. Harrison GG. Fostering data quality in food composition databases: Applications and implications for public health. *J Food Comp Anal.* 2004;17:259–265.

37. Burlingame B. Fostering quality data in food composition databases: visions for the future. *J Food Comp Anal.* 2004; 17:251–258.

38. Anderson SA. Core indicators of nutritional state for difficult to sample populations. *J Nutr.* 1990;120:1559–1600.

39. Ralston K, Brent CP, Starke Y, Riggins T, Lin CTJ. Consumer food safety behavior: a case study in hamburger cooking and ordering. In: *ERS Agricultural Economic Report No. AER804*. Washington, DC: Economic Research Service, United States Department of Agriculture; 2002.

40. Mancino L, Lin BH, Ballenger N. The role of economics in eating choices and weight outcomes. In: *Agriculture Information Bulletin Number 791*. Washington, DC: USDA, Economic Research Service; 2004.

41. Golan E, Kuchler F, Mitchell L, Greene C, Jessup A. Economics of food labeling. In: *Agricultural Economic Report No. AER793*. Washington, DC: United States Department of Agriculture; 2001.

42. Oliveira V, Racine E, Olmstead J, Ghelfi I. The WIC program: background, trends, and issues. In: *Food Assistance and Nutrition Report No. FANRR27*. Alexandria, VA: Economic Research Service, U.S. Department of Agriculture; 2002.

43. Bartlett S, Burstewin N, Hamilton W, Kling R, Andrews M. *Food Stamp Program Access Study: Final Report*. (E-FAN-03-013-3) Alexandria, VA: Economic Research Service; 2004.

44. Kennedy E. *The State of Nutrition Education in USDA: A Report to the Secretary by the State of Nutrition Education in USDA Working Group*. Washington, DC: USDA Center for Nutrition Policy and Promotion; 1996.

45. Cassell JA. Carry the Flame: The History of the American Dietetic Association. Chicago, IL: American Dietetic Association; 1990.

46. Interagency Board for Nutrition Monitoring and Related Research. *Nutrition Monitoring in the United States: The Directory of Federal and State Nutrition Monitoring Activities*.

47. Interagency Board for Nutrition Monitoring and Related Research, Life Sciences Research Office, FASEB. *Third Report on Nutrition Monitoring in the United States: Executive Summary*. Washington, DC: Government Printing Office; 1995.

48. DuPont J. The third century of nutrition research policy-shared responsibility. *Nutr Today.* 1999;34:234–241.

49. McBride J, Wilbur O. Atwater: father of American nutrition science. *Agric Res.* 1993;41:5–11.

50. Harnly JM, Doherty RF, Beecher GR, et al. Analytical determination of flavonoids (S Aglycones) in foods. In: *Proceedings of the 28th National Nutrient Databank Conference, From Farm to Fork-Practical Applications for Food Composition Data.* June 23–26. Iowa City, IA: University of Iowa; 2004.

51. Holden JM, Andrews K, Ahao C, et al. Development of the dietary supplement ingredient database, phase II progress. *Proceedings of the 28th National Nutrient Databank Conference, From Farm to Fork-Practical Applications for Food Composition Data.* June 23–27. Iowa City, IA: University of Iowa; 2004.

52. Teague AM, Sealey WM, McCabe-Sellers BJ, Mock DM. Biotin is stable in frozen foods. *FASEB J.* 2004;18:A118.

53. Borrud L. *What's on the CD-ROM...the 1994–96 Continuing Survey of Food Intakes by Individuals and Diet and Health Knowledge, USDA, ARS, BHNRC, Foods Survey Research Group.* In: What We Eat in America Research Results Survey Conference, September 14–15, 1998, Washington, DC; 1998.

DHHS publication [PHS] 92-1255-1. Hyattsville, MD: Human Nutrition Information Services; 1992.

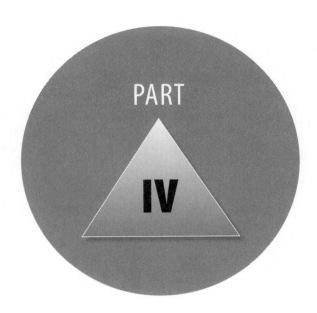

PART

IV

Promoting the Public's
Nutritional Health

CHAPTER 10

Growing a Healthier Nation: Maternal, Infant, Child, and Adolescent Nutrition

SHORTIE MCKINNEY, PhD, RD, LDN, FADA
BETH LEONBERG, MS, RD, CSP, FADA, LDN
BONNIE SPEAR, PhD, RD

CHAPTER 11

Importance of Public Health Nutrition Programs in Preventing Disease and Promoting Adult Health

JUDITH SHARLIN, PhD, RD

CHAPTER 12

Assuring Nutrition for Older Adults

JOSEPH M. CARLIN, MS, RD, LDN, FADA

CHAPTER 13

Providing Nutrition Services in Public Health Primary Care

ARLENE SPARK, EdD, RD, FADA, FACN

CHAPTER 14

The Baby Boomers: Identification of Wellness Needs

STACEY CHAPPA, RD
SHIRLEY CHAO, MS, RD, LDN
SARI EDELSTEIN, PhD, RD

CHAPTER 15

Maintaining Nutrition and Food Service Standards in Group Care

THELMA B. BAKER, PhD, RD, LD

Part IV includes those chapters that illustrate the programs and services public health nutrition provides for different groups of Americans. Through needs assessment, scientific study, and policy, many groups have been identified as qualified to receive public health nutrition. Chapter 10 discusses these programs and services, along with the challenges of serving children, adolescents, and women. In Chapters 11 through 15, the reader is then educated about the public health nutrition programs that affect adults and a special subset of adults: the baby boomers and the elderly. Each group has different needs and challenges, but all will need to be provided for by public health nutrition now and in the future.

CHAPTER 10

Growing a Healthier Nation: Maternal, Infant, Child, and Adolescent Nutrition

Shortie McKinney, PhD, RD, LDN, FADA
Beth Leonberg, MS, RD, CSP, FADA, LDN
Bonnie Spear, PhD, RD

READER OBJECTIVES

After studying this chapter and reflecting on the contents, you should be able to:

1. Discuss the need for public health nutrition services for women, infants, children, and adolescents.
2. Identify the health maladies that can occur without public health nutrition services in these groups.
3. Describe the nutrient requirements for each group.
4. Forecast how adolescent mothers may fare in society without public health programs.
5. Clarify the reasons for supplying maternal, child, and adolescent public health nutrition programs.

■ INTRODUCTION

Receiving adequate food and nutrition throughout the various stages of growth and development is crucial to lifelong health and optimal functioning. Numerous studies have documented the physiological and mental deficits that can occur when pregnant women, infants, and children are not provided with the nutritional resources and advice they need for optimal health. With medical interventions becoming more sophisticated than ever, society must find ways to support the provision of nutrition and health care to these vulnerable groups to minimize the strain on our already overburdened healthcare system. Numerous negative outcomes, such as preterm births, small-for-gestational-age infants, fetal alcohol syndrome, gestational diabetes, anemia, obesity, stunting, nutrient deficiencies, and eating disorders, can result when adequate food and nutrition are not provided during pregnancy and the early stages of life.

Pregnancy, infancy, childhood, and adolescence are all life stages in which nutrients are needed for the development of important body systems. In addition, the preconceptional period for women of childbearing age is a time when nutrition education can help promote an optimal environment for a healthy pregnancy.

■ HEALTHY PEOPLE OBJECTIVES

The *Healthy People (HP) 2010*[1] objectives were established to promote improved health across the nation. Maternal and child health programs provide key interventions to help achieve these objectives. This chapter will review the important issues that public health professionals should consider. The importance of the mother and maternal–child programs is well recognized in the HP 2010 guidelines. Objective 16 of HP 2010 focuses on a variety of issues related to healthy pregnancies, infant birth rates, child growth and development, and preventable health consequences during development. Objective 18 focuses on food and nutrition goals. Most of the nutrition goals apply to mothers and children and their diets, and some objectives specifically address children's issues. **Table 10–1** lists the HP 2010 objectives that relate to nutrition issues in pregnancy, lactation, infancy, childhood, and adolescence.

As a result of the growing overweight/obesity epidemic, many of the HP 2000 nutrition objectives were not reached, and some categories moved even further away from the target goals. For example, the prevalence of overweight increased rather than decreased. The overall nutrition and overweight objective for 2010 is to "…reduce the proportion

TABLE 10–1	*Healthy People 2010*: Nutrition-Related Maternal–Child Health Objectives
Fetal, Infant, Child, and Adolescent Deaths	
16-1.	Reduce fetal and infant deaths.
16-4.	Reduce maternal deaths.
16-5.	Reduce maternal illness and complications due to pregnancy.
Prenatal Care	
16-6.	Increase the proportion of pregnant women who receive early and adequate prenatal care.
Risk Factors	
16-10.	Reduce low birth weight (LBW) and very low birth weight (VLBW).
16-11.	Reduce preterm births.
16-12.	Increase the proportion of mothers who achieve a recommended weight gain during their pregnancies.
Developmental Disabilities and Neural Tube Defects	
16-14.	Reduce the occurrence of developmental disabilities.
16-15.	Reduce the occurrence of spina bifida and other neural tube defects (NTDs).
16-16.	Increase the proportion of pregnancies begun with an optimum folic acid level.
Prenatal Substance Exposure	
16-17.	Increase abstinence from alcohol, cigarettes, and illicit drugs among pregnant women.
16-18.	Reduce the occurrence of fetal alcohol syndrome (FAS).
Breast feeding, Newborn Screening, and Service Systems	
16-19.	Increase the proportion of mothers who breast-feed their babies.
Weight Status and Growth	
19-3.	Reduce the proportion of children and adolescents who are overweight or obese.
19-4.	Reduce growth retardation among low-income children under age 5 years.
Food and Nutrient Intake	
19-5.	Increase the proportion of persons aged 2 years and older who consume at least two daily servings of fruit.
19-6.	Increase the proportion of persons aged 2 years and older who consume at least three daily servings of vegetables, with at least one-third of them being dark green or orange vegetables.
19-7.	Increase the proportion of persons aged 2 years and older who consume at least six daily servings of grain products, with at least three being whole grains.
19-8.	Increase the proportion of persons aged 2 years and older who consume less than 10% of calories from saturated fat.
19-9.	Increase the proportion of persons aged 2 years and older who consume no more than 30% of calories from total fat.
19-10.	Increase the proportion of persons aged 2 years and older who consume 2,400 mg or less of sodium daily.
19-11.	Increase the proportion of persons aged 2 years and older who meet dietary recommendations for calcium.
Iron Deficiency and Anemia	
19-12.	Reduce iron deficiency among young children and females of childbearing age.
19-13.	Reduce anemia among low-income pregnant females in their third trimester.
19-14.	Reduce iron deficiency among pregnant females.
Schools, Worksites, and Nutrition Counseling	
19-15.	Increase the proportion of children and adolescents aged 6 to 19 years whose intake of meals and snacks at school contributes to good overall dietary quality.
Food Security	
19-18.	Increase food security among U.S. households, and in so doing reduce hunger.

Source: U.S. Department of Health and Human Services, *Healthy People 2010*. Available at http://www.healthypeople.gov. Accessed Februray 25, 2010.

of children and adolescents who are overweight or obese" (Goal 19-3).[1] Eleven percent of children and adolescents were at or above the gender- and age-specific 95th percentile of the body mass index (BMI) during baseline measurements between 1988 and 1994. The target percentage for overweight or obese children and adolescents in 2010 is 5%. The overweight/obesity epidemic is more prevalent among African Americans and Mexican Americans, and reaching this objective will be more challenging for these populations. The differential between the existing and targeted rates of overweight, as well as nutrient and food pattern goals, is substantial.[2]

■ MATERNAL HEALTH

The health of the mother is especially important to the health of the child. The nutritional status of the mother before she conceives establishes the quality of the environment in which the fetus will develop and is a key determinant in the life of the newborn. The mother's nutritional health also affects her ability to breast feed the infant and provides postnatal nurturing. The interconceptional period before the woman becomes pregnant again is vital to the health of both the mother and the next baby she will conceive. If she becomes pregnant too soon or does not have sufficient food intake before she becomes pregnant, her limited body stores will put both the mother and the fetus at risk. Beyond pregnancy and infancy, the mother's health impacts her interactions with her family and her ongoing ability to feed her children and provide them with an optimal maternal–child experience as they move to adulthood. Health professionals who work with women of childbearing age have the potential to make significant impacts on the entire society by focusing on ways to improve the health of the mother.

Preconceptional Period

The preconceptional period is the time before a woman becomes pregnant. Women who are trying to become pregnant are more likely to be aware of their food intake and the importance of nutrition in relation to the success of their eventual pregnancy. But most women are pregnant for six to eight weeks before they know it. This early pregnancy period is especially important in fetal development, and women who have health problems, nutritional deficiencies, or who consume alcohol or illicit drugs have a much higher risk of poor pregnancy outcomes. For this reason, health messages directed at women in the preconceptional period need to focus on information about the importance of a healthy diet before becoming pregnant so any future baby will be healthy. Women are most likely to receive this advice during visits to their gynecologist, family physician, or family planning clinic.

The primary nutrition messages for women in their childbearing years relate to weight management, nutritional intake, and alcohol intake. Women who are at extremes of either underweight or obese are at higher risk of delivering preterm or experiencing health problems during pregnancy. For this as well as other reasons, these women should be advised to maintain their weight in the normal range. With increasing numbers of women in the overweight and obese categories, this issue will take on more importance in relation to pregnancy and childbirth. Adequate nutritional intake in the preconceptional period is important to ensure that the woman enters pregnancy with fully replete body stores; this is especially important for women who are in the interconceptional period. Nutrient intake should be kept in the recommended range to avoid both deficiencies and excesses. Women should be evaluated for dietary practices that may put them at increased risk for either extreme. Alcohol intake during the first trimester is associated with higher rates of fetal alcohol syndrome. Because no level of alcohol has been identified as being safe, women should be advised to keep their alcohol intake levels low if they decide to drink alcohol during this time period. The following are guidelines for nutritional assessment and intervention for women in their childbearing years that should be conducted by the health professional:

1. Screen and assess women for preconceptional nutritional status. A self-administered questionnaire can be used to collect pertinent data, which is then reviewed by a healthcare professional. Criteria for referral to the dietitian can be established.
2. Nutrition information should be provided to all women. Women categorized as healthy and with no nutritional problems can be given a standard pamphlet to review. Women with low-risk problems can be counseled by the healthcare provider who is monitoring her care. Women identified as high risk should be referred to the dietitian for more intensive nutrition counseling.
3. Specific nutritional guidance should include:
   - Maintaining a healthy weight in the normal BMI range
   - Consuming a healthy diet that meets the Dietary Guidelines
   - Maintaining adequate intake of all nutrients, with special attention to iron, folic acid, calcium, vitamin C, vitamin D, and protein
   - Stopping smoking due to its impact on infant development
   - Avoiding alcohol
   - Monitoring medical conditions, such as diabetes and hypertension

Prenatal Care

Once a woman learns she is pregnant, she needs to be evaluated and provided with appropriate guidance to assist her in staying healthy and delivering a healthy full-term baby. Nutritional assessment and advice, though similar to the preconceptional period, becomes more precise to the woman's particular status and needs.

Weight Gain

Prepregnancy weight, in conjunction with height, provides the baseline for determining weight gain ranges for the pregnant woman. Recommendations of the Institute of Medicine (IOM) of the National Academy of Sciences are based on the BMI of the woman when she became pregnant. Women are placed into one of four categories (underweight, normal weight, overweight, or obese) based on their BMI. Women in the normal weight category (BMI 19.8–26) should gain between 25 and 35 pounds during pregnancy. Underweight women (BMI < 19.8) should gain between 28 and 40 pounds. Overweight women (BMI > 26–29) should gain between 15 and 20 pounds; obese women (BMI > 29) should gain at least 15 pounds. If a woman is carrying twins, she should gain 35 to 45 pounds.

Once the woman has been placed into a weight category, her weight should be measured and plotted at each prenatal visit. Weight gain should be lowest during the first trimester (range 2–5 pounds). Weight gain higher than this indicates that too many calories are being consumed. During the second and third trimesters, most women should gain one pound per week, on average. Underweight women should gain slightly more (1.07 lb.) and overweight women should gain only two-thirds of a pound weekly. Maternal weight gain is an important factor in reducing the incidence of preterm delivery.[3]

Although excessive weight gain can be harmful, weight loss and dietary restrictions are not recommended. A woman may be advised to slow her rate of weight gain, but women should never be told to lose weight while pregnant.

Weight gain components include the fetus, fat stores, extracellular fluid, blood volume, uterus, amniotic fluid, placenta, and breast tissue (listed in order from highest to lowest weight for a term pregnancy). After delivery of a full-term infant weighing 7.5 to 8.5 pounds on average, most mothers will retain 10 to 20 pounds. By six weeks postpartum, most women are 5 to 10 pounds heavier than preconception levels.[4] Some reports indicate that women who breast-feed are able to lose fat tissue more readily than women who formula-feed their infants.[5] Appropriate strategies should be used to help mothers to lose the weight gain of pregnancy.[6] This weight retention contributes to the high nationwide obesity rates for women.

Nutrient Intake

In order to support the recommended level of weight gain, the pregnant woman needs to eat and drink wisely. Although health professionals know that pregnant women should not "eat for two," many women tend to eat more than advised. Review of food intake during pregnancy can help the pregnant woman eat the food she needs to maintain a healthy pregnancy and deliver a healthy baby, while ensuring that she does not consume more than she needs.

Calories

The Dietary Reference Intakes (DRIs) for pregnant women vary by trimester. The Estimated Energy Requirements (EER) for a woman in the first trimester is the same as a non-pregnant woman due to the low level of additional energy needed to sustain the pregnancy. A pregnant woman needs an additional 340 kcal/day in the second trimester and 452 kcal/day in the third trimester. These calorie goals may need to be adjusted for women who are in the underweight or overweight/obese weight categories.

These additional calories need to be used wisely to ensure that they are nutrient-rich foods that contribute to the other nutrients that need to be consumed in levels higher than for a non-pregnant woman. Recommended intake for nearly all nutrients is higher in pregnancy. Vitamin/mineral supplementation should be evaluated on an individual basis. Supplements cannot replace the combination of nutrients found in food. Some women tend to rely on the supplements and are less careful about their food intake. Nutrients that may require supplementation include iron, calcium, and folic acid. Additional nutrients may be indicated in some cases, such as an adolescent or a woman who is carrying multiple fetuses.

> Visit the Food and Nutrition Information Center to accesss DRIs online at http://www.nal.usda.gov/fnic/etext/000105.html and find the nutrition requirements of non-pregnant, pregnant, and lactating women.

Protein

Protein intake is especially important in pregnancy. Growth and development of the fetus, as well as the tissues to support the pregnancy, rely on adequate protein for tissue development. The DRI for protein in pregnancy is an additional 25 g/day for all three trimesters. This level of additional protein is relatively easy for most women to consume. This is a key example of wise food selection. If one cup of non-fat milk is consumed, protein, calcium, vitamin D, and numerous other nutrients are significantly increased with only 100 kcal added to the diet. Dairy products are not appropriate for all women, however, particularly those who are lactose intolerant, but other solutions can be developed for them.

Smoking

Smoking cessation should be advocated as part of the nutrition education session. Smoking is totally contraindicated during pregnancy due to the profound impact it has on development of the fetus. Less oxygen is available to the fetus of a mother who smokes, so the baby is likely to be small for gestational age (SGA). SGA babies are at higher risk of complications of birth and have higher rates of problems during the first year of life. Pregnant women who smoke need to be referred to an appropriate smoking cessation program if they are willing to try to stop smoking.

Teratogenic: Causing birth defects.

Alcohol

Alcohol abstinence is an essential element of pregnancy. Alcohol is a known teratogenic agent and is linked to fetal alcohol syndrome (FAS). Infants born with FAS exhibit numerous permanent developmental problems, including mental retardation. Infants who have been exposed to alcohol in utero may have fetal alcohol effects even if they are not diagnosed with FAS. Most pregnant women willingly abstain from alcohol to eliminate any risk of FAS.

Special Conditions

Adolescent Pregnancy

Recommended weight gains during pregnancy may be slightly higher for the teenager than for the adult. The current recommendation is that pregnant adolescents should gain weight within the upper range of that currently recommended for adults (i.e., 30–35 lb.).[7] For adolescents with a below-normal pre-pregnancy weight, a 35- to 40-lb weight gain may be desirable.[7,8]

Pregnant adolescents who are of young gynecologic age (the number of years between the onset of menses and the date of conception) or who are undernourished at the time of conception have the greatest nutritional needs. A young woman who conceives soon after her first menstrual period is at greatest physiologic risk. It was once thought that adolescents with advanced physiologic maturity had no more physical complications during pregnancy than adult women, but the Camden Study[9] showed that both these adolescents and their infants are at increased risk. This longitudinal study sought to explain why, with increasing maternal weight gains in adolescent mothers, the infant birth weights remained low. This increased risk of fetal growth restriction may be attributed to disruption in the fetal-placental blood flow and in the transmission of nutrients to the fetus as a result of the physiology associated with maternal growth.

Aside from the consequences to the outcome of pregnancy, adolescents who begin their childbearing early (while still growing themselves) may be at particular risk for overweight and obesity. The Camden Study[10] has documented that the excessive accrual of subcutaneous fat stores at central body sites often, later in life, leads to the development of cardiovascular disease, non–insulin-dependent diabetes mellitus, and hypertension.

A clinically practical method of ensuring nutritional adequacy is to encourage the pregnant adolescent to gain the recommended amount of weight by consuming nutrient-rich foods. Most important, contact with health professionals during prenatal care provides the opportunity to teach adolescents about feeding themselves and their families.[11] Because of the economic instability of the pregnant adolescent, it is impossible to assume that she will have an adequate food supply. Health professionals can help provide access to and information about resources, such as food stamps, food banks, and the Special Supplemental Nutrition Program for Women, Infants and Children (previous known as the WIC Program).

Gestational Diabetes

Gestational diabetes is a form of diabetes that develops in some women when they become pregnant, but resolves once the pregnancy ends. Many of these women will go on to have type 2 diabetes later in life, particularly if they become obese. Gestational diabetes can have harmful effects on both the mother and the infant. The mother has an increased risk of preeclampsia and delivering by Cesarean section. Infants born to women with all types of diabetes have a higher risk of becoming too large in utero (macrosomia: weighing more than 10 pounds). The infant also is at higher risk to be stillborn, to have hypoglycemia at birth, and to develop hypertension, diabetes, and obesity as an adult.

Preeclampsia: A hypertensive disorder of pregnancy that is characterized by the presence of protein in the urine and swelling, putting both mother and infant in danger.

Women in moderate to high risk categories need to be screened for gestational diabetes using a glucose tolerance test. This is usually done by weeks 24 to 27 of pregnancy. Once diagnosed, an intervention plan is developed to bring the diabetes under control. Interventions generally start with diet and exercise and move to include medications as necessary to control blood glucose levels. Women with gestational diabetes need to be counseled and monitored by a dietitian.[12]

Professional guidelines for nutritional assessment and intervention in pregnancy include:

1. Screen and assess the nutritional status of pregnant women. A self-administered questionnaire can be used to collect pertinent data, which is then reviewed by a healthcare professional. Criteria for referral to the dietitian can be established.
2. Nutrition counseling should be provided to all pregnant women. Counseling strategies can be based on:
   - Women categorized as healthy and with no nutritional problems can be provided routine prenatal nutrition advice as part of their routine care.

- Women with low-risk problems can be counseled by a healthcare provider who is monitoring their care using materials provided by the dietitian.
- Women identified as high risk should be referred to the dietitian for more intensive nutrition counseling. High-risk women may include those who are not gaining sufficient weight; those who are gaining excessive amounts of weight; women with preexisting health conditions, such as diabetes, that require dietary intervention; and women who develop diseases requiring nutrition advice.

3. Specific nutritional guidance for women during pregnancy can include:
   - Maintaining a healthy weight gain as appropriate for her BMI category. Weight should be plotted at every prenatal visit to monitor growth.
   - Increasing calorie and protein intake during the second and third trimesters.
   - Consuming a healthy diet that meets the Dietary Guidelines. Emphasis should be placed on fruits and vegetables, whole grains, dairy products, and protein foods.
   - Maintaining adequate intake of all nutrients, with special attention to iron, folic acid, calcium, vitamin C, vitamin D, and protein. Supplements should be recommended if needed.
   - Maintaining physical activity as advised.
   - Consuming adequate amounts of fluid.
   - Stopping smoking due to its impact on infant development.
   - Abstaining from alcohol.
   - Learning about infant feeding methods; strong consideration should be given to breast feeding with an emphasis on the benefits for both the mother and baby.
   - Monitoring medical conditions, such as diabetes and hypertension.
   - Providing nutrition intervention as needed.

■ INFANCY

The first 12 months of a child's life are a critical period for establishing health and health-related habits. Key issues include the parent's decision to breast feed or formula feed; monitoring growth and development; introducing appropriate complementary foods when the infant is developmentally ready; and providing adequate amounts of key nutrients such as vitamin D, iron, and fluoride. This section provides an overview of these key issues and describes several initiatives aimed at helping infants get a good start.

Breast Feeding

Breast milk is the undisputed optimal food for both term and pre-term newborn infants.[13] The unique characteristics of breast milk and breast feeding confer many advantages, including health, nutritional, immunological, developmental, psychological, social, economic, and environmental benefits. The American Academy of Pediatrics (AAP) Breastfeeding Working Group,[14] American Dietetic Association (ADA),[15] and World Health Organization[16] (WHO) support exclusive breast feeding of infants for the first six months. The AAP further recommends that breast feeding be continued for the first 12 months and beyond for as long as it is mutually desired by the mother and toddler.

Although breast-feeding rates are on the rise in the United States, they remain below nationally established goals. In 2001, 69.5% of mothers initiated breast feeding and 32.5% continued to breast feed at six months.[17] The HP 2010 goals target 75% initiation of breast feeding, with 50% continuing to breast feed at 6 months, and 25% continuing to breast feed at 12 months.[18] The rates of breast feeding are different across demographic groups within the United States. Mothers who are less educated, single, young, have other children, work, or are African American or Hispanic American may be less likely to breast feed. However, from 1993 to 1998, breast-feeding promotion was credited with significantly increasing the rates among vulnerable groups in 10 states from 57.0% to 67.5%. The groups most changed included low-income and African-American women, participants in Special Supplemental Nutrition Program for Women, Infants and Children (previously known as the WIC Program), and mothers of infants admitted to the neonatal intensive care unit.[19]

There are very few instances when breast milk and/or breast feeding are not recommended.[20] These include infants with galactosemia or certain other metabolic disorders, infants whose mothers abuse illegal drugs, or those mothers with certain other medical conditions, as recommended by the infant's pediatrician. In the United States, breast feeding is not recommended for infants of mothers with human immunodeficiency virus (HIV).

Formula Feeding

Infant formula is the appropriate food for infants who are weaned from the breast before 12 months and for infants who are not breast-fed. Infant formulas sold in the United States must meet safety and nutritional guidelines that are established and updated periodically by the U.S. Food and Drug Administration.[21,22] The WHO International Code of Marketing of Breast-Milk Substitutes recommends that infant formulas should not be advertised or promoted to the general public and that manufacturers should not provide samples of products to pregnant women, mothers, or members of their family.[23] In agreement, the AAP has stated their disapproval of direct advertising because it may negatively impact breast-feeding initiation or continuation.[20]

Infant formulas are available as ready-to-feed liquid, or as concentrated liquid or powder to which water must be added. The majority of infant formulas are made from modified cow milk; however, soy-based and specialty formulas designed for medical conditions are also available. Cow milk–based infant formulas are available either as iron-fortified or low iron. Both the AAP and the Centers for Disease Control and Prevention (CDC) recommend that infants less than 12 months old be fed only iron-fortified infant formula.[24,25] Soy-based formulas are appropriate for infants with galactosemia, hereditary lactase deficiency, documented lactose intolerance following acute gastroenteritis, and for vegetarian infants. However, the routine use of soy-based formulas has not been demonstrated to be effective in preventing or managing colic or in preventing the development of food allergies, and is not appropriate for pre-term infants weighing less than 1,800 grams.[26] Infants who develop symptoms of food allergy may benefit from using a soy-based formula or a hypoallergenic formula in which the protein is partially or totally hydrolyzed.[27]

In the last decade, infant formula manufacturers have begun to examine the benefits of adding a variety of nutrients and biological factors to mimic the composition and quality of breast milk.[28] These include long-chain polyunsaturated fatty acids, nucleotides, and prebiotics/probiotics. At this time, the benefits of these and other ingredients are still being studied.

Growth and Development

Infancy is a period of rapid growth and development. Most infants double their birth weight by the 6th month and triple it by the 12th month.[29] However, there are normal differences in growth between healthy breast-fed and formula-fed infants during the first year of life. Breast-fed infants tend to gain weight more rapidly than formula-fed infants in the first 2 to 3 months, but less rapidly from 3 to 12 months.[2] These differences in weight gain and growth tend to disappear in the second year.[30]

Growth can best be assessed by plotting weight and length for age, and weight for length on an appropriate National Center for Health Statistics Growth Chart (as discussed in Chapter 3). These charts have been constructed using data from large population groups over time and are a way to assess an individual's growth against group norms. However, each infant will establish and follow his or her own growth curve.

Find the Start Healthy Feeding Plan at http://www.gerber.com/feedingplan/.

Rapid development during the first year is responsible for the infant changing from a newborn who needs head support to feed and is capable of a simple suck-swallow-breathe pattern during feeding, to an older infant who can easily feed herself with her fingers and can drink from a cup. The Start Healthy Feeding Plan reflects a recent evaluation of many years of research and graphically represents the advancement of developmental and feeding skills throughout infancy.[31]

Healthcare providers can monitor growth and development by comparing an infant's progress against these tools. Periodic visits allow the provider to establish a relationship with the infant and his caregivers, through which a dialogue can be held. At the appropriate times, questions about the child's development and feeding will provide the basis for anticipatory guidance or counseling to help provide a smooth transition between developmental stages as the child grows.[32]

Complementary Foods

Research has demonstrated that exclusive breast feeding can meet the nutrient needs of infants through the first six months. Most infants are developmentally ready for the introduction of complementary foods and beverages by four to six months.

Solids

In the United States, an infant's first solid food is typically iron-fortified, single-ingredient (rice) infant cereal. Recent research has affirmed the importance of a good source of iron for breast-fed infants by four to six months in meeting daily requirements.[33] This can be provided by iron-fortified infant cereal and later by meats. Following cereal, single-ingredient pureed fruits and vegetables are offered to the infant, with at least two to four days between introductions of each new food. Whether fruits or vegetables should be offered first has long been a subject of debate, but a recent review of the literature indicates the order in which they are introduced isn't critical.[31] It is well-established that it can take 10 to 15 exposures to a new food for it to be accepted by an infant or toddler, and parents should be encouraged to present the food repeatedly to encourage acceptance.[34,35]

This chapter introduces the reader to the many public health nutrition issues of feeding infants and children. Additional training and research on the appropriate feeding practices of infants and children should be a part of the continuing education of those healthcare providers counseling parents of young children.

Juice

Juice manufacturers have successfully marketed 100% fruit juice as a healthy beverage. However, some fruit juices, such as prune, apple, and pear, contain a significant amount of sorbitol (a sugar alcohol) and proportionally more fructose than glucose. Infants can absorb only a portion of the sorbitol (as little as 10%) and fructose in these juices.[36] The unabsorbed carbohydrate is fermented in the lower intestine, causing diarrhea, abdominal pain, or bloating. These symptoms are commonly reported in infants and toddlers who drink excessive amounts of juice. The AAP has concluded that fruit juice offers no nutritional benefit for infants younger than six months and no benefit over whole fruits for infants older than six months. They recommend that juice not be introduced to infants before six months, should not be given in a bottle or easily transported covered cup, should not be given at nap- or bedtime, and should be limited to four to six ounces daily for infants and children up to six years old.[37]

Key Nutrients

Vitamin D

Rickets is a disease of vitamin D and/or calcium deficiency, characterized in infants by poor bone growth leading to bowing of the legs or knock knees. Although the incidence of rickets in developed countries is very low, cases have continued to be reported regularly over the last 20 years. Most cases have occurred in breast-fed infants of dark-skinned mothers who had minimal exposure to sunlight[38-40] and in toddlers on vegetarian diets.[41] Although rickets can be prevented by regular exposure to sunlight, increasing concern over the long-term effects of early sun exposure on the development of skin cancer have led to new recommendations for vitamin D supplementation of all infants. The AAP now recommends that all breast-fed infants receive 200 IU of vitamin D daily, unless they are weaned, to at least 500 mL per day of vitamin D–fortified formula or milk.[42] They further recommend that formula-fed infants who consume less than 500 mL of formula daily receive 200 IU of vitamin D daily.

Iron

Iron deficiency anemia in infancy has been associated with significant developmental deficits, including language difficulties, poor motor skills and balance, and poor attention, responsiveness, and mood, which may be only partially reversible with subsequent supplementation.[43] Fetal iron stores are exhausted by four to six months of age, making it necessary that iron be supplied by the diet.[20] This need corresponds well with the introduction of high-iron complementary foods, such as iron-fortified infant formula, iron-fortified infant cereals, and/or meats. The AAP recommends that full-term breast-fed infants need a supplemental source of iron beginning at four to six months and that only iron-fortified formula should be used for weaning or supplementing breast milk for infants up to 12 months.[20,24] The immature gastrointestinal (GI) tract of infants is unable to digest and absorb cow's milk during the first year, and its ingestion is responsible for GI blood loss leading to anemia.[44] The AAP recommends the avoidance of regular cow, goat, or soy milk for the milk-based part of the diet before 12 months of age.[20]

Fluoride

Exposure to appropriate levels of fluoride is effective in reducing the prevalence of dental caries. Most public water supplies are fluoridated to provide 0.7 ppm to 1.2 ppm of fluoride. The need for fluoride supplementation depends on the total amount of fluoride available to the infant from all sources, including infant formula, water, and commercial and home-prepared baby foods. Breast milk contains little fluoride, even in areas with fluoridated water.[45] The amount of fluoride in commercial concentrated or powdered infant formula depends on the amount of fluoride in the formula and in the water used for mixing. Infants fed formula made with fluoridated water may receive up to 1.0 mg/day of fluoride.[46] Ready-to-feed infant formulas are manufactured with non-fluoridated water. The AAP, the American Academy of Pediatric Dentistry, and the CDC recommend no fluoride supplementation for infants less than 6 months old.[20,47,48]

For infants older than six months whose community drinking water contains < 0.3 ppm fluoride, they recommend supplementation of 0.25 mg sodium fluoride/day.

Guidelines for nutritional assessment and intervention in infancy are recommended in the following steps.
Birth to six months:

1. Breast feed for the first four to six months. Supplement with iron and vitamin D.
2. If breast feeding is not selected, provide a fortified infant formula that approximates breast milk. Ensure that the formula is prepared under sanitary conditions and according to directions.
3. Begin complementary foods when the infant is developmentally ready.
4. Measure length and weight growth status and plot on NCHS growth charts.

Six months to one year:

1. Continue breast milk or formula.
2. Continue to introduce foods as directed by pediatrician or dietitian.
3. Include infant in family meals.
4. Provide finger foods and child-sized utensils to encourage self-feeding.
5. Measure length and weight growth status and plot on NCHS growth charts.
6. Provide opportunities to develop physical abilities.

7. Refer to Special Supplemental Nutrition Program for Women, Infants and Children when indicated.

8. Provide appropriate care for disease or other health conditions.

■ CHILDHOOD AND ADOLESCENCE

Beyond infancy, children move through various stages of growth and development on their journey to becoming young adults. Each age level has different nutrient needs. Toddlers have a slower growth rate that continues through childhood until the growth spurt of adolescence starts. Children also move from being dependent on parents to provide healthy food choices to making all their own food choices when they are in late adolescence. An important role for parents and other caregivers is to provide a wide variety of healthy foods and let the children decide which foods and the amount to eat. Mealtime struggles can create an unpleasant environment for everyone and do little to encourage children to eat more foods.

Assessment of Growth

Growth assessment is the best way to determine if children are well nourished. When children are getting enough to eat and do not have health problems, they should be growing normally. Plotting height (or length for very young children) and weight on the NCHS standardized growth charts can help determine if a child's growth is appropriate.

The CDC/NCHS BMI tables are available at http://www.cdc.gov/growthcharts/.

Weight and height can be plotted on growth grids to determine whether individuals are maintaining their growth pattern or growth channel. The relationship between weight and height can be evaluated by using the CDC/NCHS BMI tables. Appropriate weights for height, according to age and sex, lie between the 10th and 85th percentiles, a range that allows for individual differences in body build.[49]

Use of BMI, which is highly correlated with body fatness, can also indicate weight status. BMI is calculated by dividing body weight (expressed in kilograms) by the square of height (in meters), that is, $BMI = kg/m^2$. Children with BMIs below the fifth percentile should be assessed for organic diseases or eating disorders. Children with BMIs between the 85th and 95th percentiles are at risk for overweight, and a nutritional screening/assessment should be performed to determine health risk. Children with BMIs ≥ 95th percentile for age and gender are overweight and should have an in-depth medical assessment[50] that includes data on family history, blood pressure, total cholesterol level, any major change in BMI, and concern about weight.[49,51]

A skinfold evaluation yields a further degree of precision. For example, a low skinfold measurement in an individual who is above the 85th percentile BMI indicates a state of being overweight, but not overfat. An assessment of muscle and arm circumference can confirm the muscular composition. However, a skinfold in the 90th percentile or greater with a BMI greater than the 95th percentile suggests overfat or truly overweight.

Excessive or less-than-normal growth can be detected by plotting height changes on the CDC growth charts. The major cause of short stature during adolescence is genetically late initiation of puberty, although other conditions, such as chronic disease or skeletal and chromosomal abnormalities, also can account for certain children being shorter than normal. Hormonal imbalances leading to abnormal growth are rare.

Nutrient Requirements

Energy

Energy requirements are designed to maintain health, promote optimal growth and maturation, and support a desirable level of physical activity. Children who limit energy intake or have food security issues that limit energy intake may limit ultimate adult growth. In 2002, the National Academy of Sciences released new guidelines for energy requirements.[52] Estimated Energy Requirements (EER) are based on energy expenditure, requirements for growth, and level of physical activity. Variability in the EER exists for both males and females because of variations in growth rate and physical activity.

To derive the EER, the adolescent's gender, age, height, weight, and physical activity level (PAL) were utilized in calculations, with an average of 25 kcal/day added for energy deposition. In order to determine adequate energy (kcal) intake, an assessment of physical activity is required. The energy requirements allow for four levels of activity (sedentary, low active, active, and very active). This physical activity reflects the energy expended in activities beyond the activities of daily living.

Protein

Protein needs, like those for energy, correlate more closely with the growth pattern than with chronological age. The 2004 Dietary Reference Intakes for protein are based on the amount of protein needed for growth and positive nitrogen balance.[52] The DRIs provide for both the Estimated Average Requirements (EAR) and the Recommended Dietary Allowances (RDA). The DRIs recommend using the EAR when assessing nutrient intakes of groups. The EAR provides for adequate intake of 50% of the population. The RDA is recommended for assessing the intake of an individual. Average intakes of protein for adolescents are well above the RDA for all age groups. In fact, when comparing protein intakes of adolescents from the United States with teens from other countries, studies show that U.S. adolescents have a much higher intake of protein. There is little evidence to show that insufficient protein intake is common in the adolescent population. However, if energy intake is inadequate for any reason (i.e., food security issues, chronic illness, or attempts to lose weight), dietary protein may be used to meet energy needs and will, therefore, be unavailable for synthesis of new tissue or for tissue repair. This may result in a state of insufficient protein, which will lead to a reduction in growth rate and a decrease in lean body mass. Current dieting patterns in some adolescent girls can result in restricted calorie intakes that are potentially harmful, especially when protein sources are used to meet energy needs. However, excessive intakes of protein can also have an impact on nutritional status. For example, a high protein intake can interfere with calcium metabolism as well as increase fluid needs. These increased fluid needs may put adolescent athletes at high risk for dehydration.

Minerals and Vitamins

Micronutrients (vitamins and minerals) play an important role in the growth and health of adolescents. Inadequate fruit and vegetable consumption has been linked to certain types of cancer and other diseases. Because of the many health benefits associated with fruits and vegetables, national recommendations support increased consumption of these foods. The U.S. 2010 Dietary Guidelines recommend 2 cups of fruit and 2½ cups of vegetables per day.[18] Unfortunately, surveys show that, for adolescents, there are significant gaps between actual intake and these recommendations. The 2003 Youth Risk Behavior Survey (YRBS) revealed that only 22.0% of all adolescents ate ≥ 5 servings of fruits/vegetables a day: 20.3% of gjrls and 23.6% of boys.[53]

Despite the low levels of fruits and vegetables, most children get sufficient amounts of vitamins and minerals until they reach adolescence, when requirements increase dramatically due to growth demands. Because of increased energy demands during this period, increased quantities of thiamine, riboflavin, and niacin are required for the release of energy from carbohydrates. With tissue synthesis, there is an increased demand for vitamin B_6, folic acid, and vitamin B_{12}. There is also an increased requirement for vitamin D (for rapid skeletal growth), and vitamins A, C, and E are needed for new cell growth. Although there are few reports of low serum vitamin C levels in teens, those who habitually avoid fruits and vegetables and those who smoke cigarettes may be at increased risk for deficiency.

Calcium

Because of accelerated muscular, skeletal, and endocrine development, calcium needs are greater during puberty and adolescence than in childhood or during the adult years.

At the peak of the growth spurt, the daily deposition of calcium can be twice that of the average during the rest of the adolescent period. In fact, 45% of the skeletal mass is added during adolescence.[54]

Calcium requirements are expressed as Adequate Intakes (AIs). The AI is believed to cover needs of all individuals in a group, but lack of data or uncertainty in the data preclude specifying, with confidence, the percentage of persons covered by this intake.[55] This is especially true for adolescents. The National Institutes of Health Consensus Development Conference Statement on Optimal Calcium Intake[56] recommended 1,200 to 1,500 mg of calcium per day for adolescents aged 11 to 24 years. In its statement, the committee acknowledged that there appears to be a certain threshold level of dietary calcium that is necessary to allow growing adolescents to achieve their genetically predetermined peak bone mass. Dietary survey data indicate that adolescents, particularly girls, are at greatest risk for inadequate calcium intake.[57] Calcium intake tends to decline among girls 10 to 17 years of age. Consumption surveys show an average intake for girls to be 780 to 820 mg per day. In adolescent boys, the average intake is 800 to 920 mg per day.

Several human and animal studies have suggested a specific role for calcium in modulating body fat. Zemel et al.[58] demonstrated that increased dietary calcium inhibited adipocyte intracellular calcium, resulting in increased stimulation of lipolysis and inhibition of lipogenesis during energy restriction. National Health and Nutrition Examination Survey (NHANES) III data showed an inverse relationship between calcium and BMI, indicating that individuals with higher calcium intake had lower BMIs. Skinner et al.[59] showed the same effect in children. In examining children ages 9 to 14, she found that those who consumed more calcium tended to weigh less and have lower body fat than those with low calcium consumption. In this study, the intake of calcium accounted for 4.5% to 9.0% of the variance in body fat. Skinner suggested that children could reduce their body fat if they increased their calcium intake with one glass of skim milk or 8 oz of yogurt per day. Even the slightest decrease in body fat could help in preventing comorbidities associated with overweight/obesity.

Iron

Iron is a key indicator nutrient throughout childhood and adolescence. Iron deficiency anemia is fairly common, with 4% to 7% of children exhibiting low hemoglobin and hematocrit. During adolescence iron requirements are increased. Dallmon et al.[60] noted that in boys there is a sharp increase in the requirements for iron from approximately 10 to 15 mg/day. This increase reflects not only the expanding blood volume, but also a rise in hemoglobin concentration that occurs with sexual maturation in boys. After the growth spurt and sexual maturation, growth increases rapidly and so does the need for iron. In girls, the growth spurt is not as great, but menstruation typically starts about one year after peak growth. The mean requirement for iron reaches a maximum of approximately 15 mg/day at peak growth, but settles to a mean of approximately 13 to 15 mg/day because of the need to replace menstrual iron losses.

In girls with marginal intakes, iron deficiency anemia may result from growth demands. Conversely, iron deficiency may be a limiting factor for growth during adolescence. Additionally, anemia in adolescence may impair the immune response. A study of Native American children aged 1 to 14 indicated that the cell-mediated immune response and the bactericidal capacity of leukocytes (in vitro methods) were significantly depressed in those with hemoglobin concentrations below 10 mg/day.[60]

Reports from dietary surveys indicate that iron intakes of adolescents with normal dietary patterns were between 12.5 and 14.2 mg/day for girls compared to between 13.6 and 18.0 mg/day for boys. The average U.S. diet contains an estimated 6 mg iron/1,000 kcal.[25] Adolescent girls, who typically have lower caloric intakes than boys, may have more difficulty in obtaining adequate levels of iron from their diets.

NHANES III found iron deficiency in 14.2% of the 15- to 18-year-old girls and 12.1% of the 11- to 14-year-old boys.[57] Iron deficiency is prevalent in adolescents of both genders and in teens of all ethnicities and socioeconomic levels. In its recommendations to prevent and control iron deficiency in the United States, the CDC includes guidelines for prevention, screening, and treatment of iron deficiency anemia.[25]

Nutrition Education

School settings are ideal for nutrition education. The majority of U.S. children between the ages of 5 and 17 are enrolled in school, and this provides a unique learning community through which children are able to participate in nutrition-based education. A familiar environment and the support of teachers and peers strengthens the impact of nutrition education. Programs are likely to be more widely accepted by the participants when they are culturally and socially sensitive. Multidimensional strategies including health/physical education, parental involvement, and food service involvement along with nutrition education helps to promote learning and behavior change. Children seem most interested in teaching methods that use discovery learning, student learning stations, cooperative groups, situation analysis, and cross-age and peer teaching. Extensive research on school-based methods to improve nutritional intake supports their continued use, but confirms that behavioral change is slow. Nutrition education needs to be part of the comprehensive school health education program to strengthen and advance positive food and nutrition messages.

Physical Activity

Physical Activity and Health: A Report of the Surgeon General is a comprehensive overview of research related to physical activity and health.[61] The report 1) summarizes the benefits of physical activity; 2) reinforces the importance of promoting physical activity; 3) states that many children and adolescents are at risk for health problems because of inactive lifestyles; and 4) states that everyone should participate in a moderate amount of physical activity (e.g., 15 minutes of running, 30 minutes of brisk walking, 45 minutes of playing volleyball) on most, if not all, days of the week. The 2003 YRBS[62] indicated that 30% of teens did not participate in at least 20 minutes of vigorous physical activity at least three times a week. The rate of inactivity increased with each grade level, from 28.2% in 9th grade to 40.2% in 12th grade. This same pattern was seen with ethnicity (Caucasian 31%, African American 41.2%, Hispanic American 36.5%).

Read *Physical Activity and Health: A Report of the Surgeon General* at http://www.cdc.gov/nccdphp/sgr/sgr.htm.

These findings are disturbing in view of the numerous health benefits that children and adolescents derive by being physically active on a regular basis. Physical activity can lead to improved body composition (e.g., increased lean muscle mass, reduced total body fat) and can help reduce other coronary heart disease (CHD) risk factors among adolescents. For example, increased physical activity levels can favorably alter blood lipid profiles in adolescents at high risk for CHD (e.g., children and adolescents who are obese or who have type 1 or 2 diabetes mellitus) and can reduce blood pressure, especially in adolescents whose blood pressure is elevated. Physical activity plays a substantial role in the development of bone mass during adolescence and can help maintain the structure and functional strength of bone throughout life.[63,64]

Efforts to increase physical activity levels among children and adolescents have been most successful in school settings. However, little attention has been focused on promoting physical activity among children and adolescents in settings other than schools, including healthcare settings (i.e., health professionals counseling children and adolescents about physical activity during health supervision visits).[65]

Health professionals, families, peers, and communities can influence children's and adolescents' physical activity levels. Parents who participate in physical activity themselves and who support and encourage physical activity in their adolescents have a positive influence on adolescents' physical activity levels. In addition, older children and adolescents whose friends are physically active tend to be more physically active themselves.

Little is known about which factors motivate children and adolescents to become physically active, remain physically active, and increase their physical activity levels as they become older. In addition, it is not clear why these factors differ for girls and boys or for different racial and ethnic groups. However, it is clear that girls are less likely than boys to participate in vigorous physical activity, participate in strengthening or toning activities, or participate on sports teams. Strategies different from those used to promote physical activity in and young and adolescents boys may be needed to promote physical activity in young and adolescent girls.[63] Strategies that take into account children's and adolescents' race or cultural background could also be beneficial. The 2003 Surgeon General's Report recommends the following intervention strategies to promote physical activity in children and adolescents:

- Make physical activity enjoyable.
- Help adolescents succeed and increase their confidence in their ability to be physically active.
- Support adolescents' efforts to be physically active.
- Help adolescents learn about the benefits of physical activity and help them develop positive attitudes toward it.
- Help adolescents overcome barriers that keep them from being physically active.

Family Mealtime

Increasing emphasis is being placed on family mealtime because of its positive impact on food intake and child development. Project EAT surveyed middle school and high school students from ethnically and socioeconomically diverse communities.[66] Results show that almost one-third of participants reported only eating one to two meals with their family each week, or never eating family meals. Children eating more than three family meals per week were significantly less likely to skip breakfast and to report poor consumption of fruits, vegetables, and dairy foods, compared to children eating less than three family meals per week. African Americans and Hispanic Americans were less likely to skip breakfast and to report poor fruit consumption compared to Caucasian children. A higher frequency of family meals is associated with significantly lower odds of the following variables: cigarette, alcohol, and marijuana use; low grade point average; high depressive symptoms; and suicidal ideation. Family meal frequency had a strong positive association with intake of energy; percentage of calories from protein; calcium; iron; vitamins A, C, E, B_6; folate; and fiber.[32]

Read more about Project EAT at http://www.epi.umn.edu/research/eat/.

Another family meal study involved children of participants in the ongoing Nurses' Health Study II. Subjects who ate family dinner every day consumed an average of 0.8 more servings of fruits and vegetables than those who never ate family meals or did so only on some days. Additionally, consumption of fried food and soda was inversely associated with frequency of family meals. Participants who ate family meals more often reported slightly higher energy intakes and also higher intakes of several nutrients including: fiber; calcium; folate; vitamins B_6, B_{12}, C, and E; and iron. In addition, they consumed less trans-fat and saturated fat as a percentage of energy intake.[67] Family mealtime may be a potentially protective factor in the lives of children for nearly all these variables.

Read more about the Nurses' Health Study II at http://www.channing.harvard.edu/nhs/.

Childhood overweight and obesity are critical public health threats, but are addressed in an earlier chapter. Please refer to Chapter 5 to learn about their cause and recommended treatments.

School-Based Growth Screening

Until recently, most schools did not assess weight status using BMI. In many school districts, the school nurse measured height and weight and plotted them on a growth chart; however, no additional referral or reporting procedures were required.

In response to the increasing epidemic of childhood obesity across the nation, many state and local governments have implemented programs to measure children's growth and educate and inform parents about their child's weight status. These screening programs are designed to provide a mechanism by which parents of high-risk children are:

- Informed about their child's risk of overweight
- Educated on the risks of childhood overweight on health
- Referred for available community and school-based interventions

Screening programs provide an excellent way for parents and children to more easily access the needed resources to address childhood overweight in an effective manner and facilitate collaboration between school, family, primary care providers, and interested community partners. For example, the Pennsylvania Growth Screening Program requires that school nurses and/or teachers measure height and weight and calculate BMI, record these results in the child's school health record, plot results on the CDC growth charts, and inform parents of children who are at risk for overweight (85th to less than 95th percentile on the BMI-for-age chart) or who are overweight (above 95th percentile on the BMI-for-age chart). Results are submitted on an annual basis to the Division of School Health for surveillance and program planning purposes. This program is providing a comprehensive way to identify overweight children and those at risk for becoming overweight, and then link them with available interventions.[68]

Early Childhood Specifics

After the rapid growth of infancy, the toddler and preschool child's growth slows. Toddlers (age 1–3) gain about half a pound a month and grow ¼ inch to ½ inch. Preschool children gain about 4 to 5 pounds and grow 2 inches per year. Children generally lose some of the body fat accumulated as an infant, their bodies elongate, and they begin to look more like children. All baby teeth should be in place by age 2. Brain development continues to be important, with brain growth 75% complete by age 2, and attaining adult size during the elementary school years.

Total energy needs continue to increase to support body maintenance and a slow rate of growth, but calories per kilogram declines until the growth spurt of adolescence. Along with the gradual increase in total calories, the need for protein, vitamins, and minerals also increases.

Eating Patterns

Young children develop lifelong eating patterns in response to the food environment in which they live. This is easily demonstrated by the diverse foods eaten by children of different cultures. Children learn to prefer the foods that they are exposed to at mealtimes. Parents and other adults have an important role to play as food and nutrition gatekeepers by ensuring that a wide variety of nutritious foods are served. Foods rejected by children should continue to be offered on other occasions. Children are naturally neophobic about new foods, and frequency of exposure to food promotes increased preference. Food choices of other children in the home or in childcare settings also influence what children like to eat. Children often go on food jags where they want to eat the same foods; fortunately, these periods generally don't last long enough to impact their nutritional intake.

Young children respond well to small frequent meals; snacks contribute as much as 20% of daily calories. Portion sizes need to be kept in balance with the child's appetite. Children like foods with interesting shapes, colors, and contrasting temperatures. Foods that might cause choking if swallowed whole, such as grapes, popcorn, hard candy, and hot dogs, should be avoided. Parents and caregivers can help promote a healthy variety of food choices by maintaining a positive attitude towards food and minimizing mealtime conflicts.[69]

Guidelines for nutritional assessment and intervention in early childhood, ages 1 to 5, may include the following:

1. Screen and assess growth status and plot on NCHS growth charts.
2. Provide a wide variety of healthy foods with emphasis on nutritious choices such as whole grains, fruits, vegetables, dairy foods, and lean meats and protein alternatives.
3. Continue to serve new foods even if not initially preferred.

4. Avoid using food as a reward or punishment.
5. Provide opportunities for physical activity through active play.
6. Avoid low nutrient-dense foods as snack choices.
7. Evaluate nutrition services in childcare facilities to ensure standards are met.
8. Provide appropriate care for disease or other health conditions.
9. Teach children to wash their hands before eating.

Childcare Programs

Many parents have jobs outside of the home, which means that many children are in childcare programs during the preschool years. Generally, these programs provide some level of food service to the children they serve. The ADA position paper on childcare programs recommends that childcare menus provide one-third of a child's nutritional requirements in the meals and snacks provided.[70] Fats, salt, and sugar should be maintained at modified levels. Childcare centers are advised to use the services of a dietitian in planning the menus and to include nutrition education in the classroom. Cleanliness in food production and service are important to minimize food-borne illness. The Child and Adult Care Food Program administered by the USDA provides assistance to childcare programs in setting food standards and gives financial support to provide nutritious foods for low-income children.[71]

> Read more about The Child and Adult Care Food Program administered by the USDA at http://www.fns.usda.gov/cnd/care/cacfp/cacfphome.htm.

Lead Exposure

Concerns about lead in the environment have resulted in numerous bans on the use of lead in such things as gasoline and paint. Although these efforts have had a positive impact, the lingering lead in the environment continues to contribute to lead poisoning in young children. Many young children are exposed to lead in their homes. Lead is present in old paint and water pipes. Lead absorption is highest during stages of rapid growth such as early childhood. Lead intake is harmful to children because it contributes to iron deficiency and anemia. Low levels of lead toxicity can be difficult to diagnose because the symptoms, such as diarrhea, irritability, and fatigue, are nonspecific. Early identification is important due to the permanent damage that can occur, leading to nerve damage and mental retardation.[72]

Food Allergies

Food allergies are caused when the body's immune system reacts to a whole food protein. Allergic responses can range from inflammation of the nasal passages to skin rashes to anaphylactic shock. Food allergies can be difficult to identify, particularly if the response is delayed. Non-allergenic adverse reactions to foods can be misidentified as food allergies. Most children outgrow food allergies. Foods likely to cause allergies include eggs, milk, fish, peanuts, and soybeans. Children with severe allergic reactions need to be evaluated by a physician and will require careful monitoring of their food intake.

School-Aged Child Specifics

By the time a child enters school, he or she should weigh twice as much as he or she did at age 1. During the elementary school years, children continue to grow at a steady rate, gaining approximately 2.5 inches per year and 5 to 7 pounds. Children's appetites will ebb and wane as their growth patterns change, with increased food intake during a growth spurt. Families continue to play an important role in food choices, but peer pressure and media influences begin to play a strong role in food decisions.

Children mature physically and mentally during this time span. They become progressively stronger and their motor coordination increases. Body image becomes important in relation to peers, as children don't want to be seen as different. Their independence grows and they learn how to make decisions for themselves. This can lead to conflicts over food choices and emotional struggles with parents.

School Meals

The USDA National School Lunch Program provides financial support to schools to provide nutritious lunches to low-income children. In addition, these programs mandate food and nutrition criteria for schools to use in planning school meals. The USDA allows for several methods for schools to meet the nutrient requirement for school lunches. The traditional meal planning approach includes five components; newer strategies include computerized nutrient analysis. Nutrition education displays are often provided in the school lunchroom. The USDA's Team Nutrition was established to provide resources and technical support to help schools improve healthy eating and physical activity patterns.[73]

Read more about The School Lunch and Breakfast Programs administered by the USDA at http://www.fns.usda.gov/cnd/.

The School Breakfast Program extends free nutritious food to the breakfast period. More schools in low-income neighborhoods should be encouraged to participate in this program. Many low-income children go to school hungry or eat low nutrient foods before starting school. A healthy breakfast has been shown to improve school performance.

Guidelines for nutritional assessment and intervention in school-aged children, ages 6 to 10, should include:

1. Screen and assess growth status and plot on NCHS growth charts.
2. Children identified as at risk for overweight or who are overweight should be referred for further evaluation and possible treatment.
3. Provide a wide variety of healthy foods with emphasis on nutritious choices, such as whole grains, fruits, vegetables, dairy foods, and lean meats and protein alternatives.
4. Ensure that children eat breakfast before going to school.
5. Promote regular physical activity at school and at home.
6. Reduce sedentary activity with an emphasis on reduction of screen time.
7. Provide nutrition education in school.
8. Ensure regular meals and snacks.
9. Encourage reduced levels of low nutrient-dense beverages.
10. Support school lunch and breakfast programs.
11. Provide appropriate care for disease or other health conditions.

Food Advertising

Television and magazines probably have a greater influence on children's eating habits than any other form of mass media. It is estimated that, by the time the average child reaches the teen years, he or she has viewed 100,000 food commercials, most of them for products with high concentrations of fat and simple carbohydrates. More than 65% of food advertisements promote beverages (primarily alcohol) and sweets.[2,74] Food advertisements use a variety of techniques to appeal to children such as cartoon characters, catchy songs, colorful images, and appealing colors and tastes. Many advertisers use prizes and other incentive items to encourage food purchases. Advertisements for low nutrient-dense foods, such as soda, candy, and snacks, have a dominant presence in the time slots in which children's programming is aired.

Recently, food manufacturers have been under tremendous pressure to modify their advertising to children. Some fast food outlets and food manufacturers have started to respond with plans to eliminate some advertising directed at children. Efforts such as these will help to improve the unhealthy food environment in children's television.

Adolescence Specifics

Adolescence is a time of dramatic change in the life of every human being. The relatively uniform growth of childhood is suddenly altered by an increase in the velocity of growth. This sudden spurt is also associated with hormonal, cognitive, and emotional changes. All of these changes create special nutritional needs. Adolescence is considered an especially nutritionally vulnerable period of life for several reasons. First is the greater demand for nutrients due to the dramatic increase in physical growth and development. Second is the change of lifestyle and food habits of adolescents that affect both nutrient intake and needs. Third are those adolescents with special nutrient needs, such as those who participate in sports, have a chronic illness, diet excessively, or use alcohol or drugs.[75]

Physiologic Changes

Puberty, the process of physically developing from a child to an adult, is initiated by physiological factors and includes maturation of the entire body. Adolescence is the only time following birth when the velocity of growth actually increases. The adolescent gains about 20% of adult height and 50% of adult weight during this period.

This growth continues throughout the approximately five to seven years of pubertal development. A great percentage of this height will be gained during the 18- to 24-month period of the growth spurt. The growth spurt or peak height gain velocity occurs at different ages for different individuals, as does the initiation of puberty. In general, girls began the pubertal process approximately two years earlier than boys. Although growth slows following the achievement of sexual maturity, linear growth and weight acquisition continue into the late teens for young women and early twenties for men. Most girls gain no more than one to two inches following menarche, although girls who have early menarche tend to grow more after its onset than do those having later menarche.

In the process of total body maturation, the composition of the body changes. Prepubertal boys and girls tend to be similar, with body fatness averaging about 15% and 19%, respectively. Girls gain more fat than boys during puberty, and in adulthood they have about 22% to 26% body fat, compared with around 15% to 18% in men. During puberty, boys gain twice as much lean tissue as do girls.

Psychological Changes

Adolescence is a period of maturation for both mind and body. Along with the physical growth of puberty, emotional and intellectual development is rapid. Adolescents' capacity for abstract thinking, as opposed to the concrete thought patterns of childhood, enables them to grow cognitively during adolescence. Many of these tasks have implications for their nutritional well-being.

Cognitive and emotional development can be divided into early, middle, and late adolescence. Determining the adolescent's stage can be very helpful in providing nutritional counseling as well as in designing educational programs.[76] In early adolescence, the adolescent:

- Is preoccupied with body and body image
- Trusts and respects adults
- Is anxious about peer relationships
- Is ambivalent about autonomy

The nutritional implications are that adolescents in this stage are willing to do or try anything that will make them look better or improve their body image. However, adolescents at this stage want immediate results, so nutrition counseling should be geared to short-term goals and to addressing nutritional concerns that impact the teen's appearance, performance (e.g., dance, sports), or both. A teen in middle adolescence:

- Is greatly influenced by his or her peer group
- Is mistrustful of adults
- Sees independence as being very important
- Experiences significant cognitive development

During this stage, the teen will listen to peers more than to parents or other adults. Teens are becoming more in charge of the foods they eat. The drive toward independence often results in temporary rejection of the family dietary patterns. At this age, adolescents often experiment with vegetarianism. Nutritional counseling should include making wise decisions when eating away from home. The teen in late adolescence:

- Has established a body image
- Is oriented toward the future and is making plans
- Is increasingly independent
- Is more consistent in his or her values and beliefs
- Is developing intimacy and permanent relationships

By late adolescence, teens are thinking about the future and are interested in improving their overall health. Nutritional counseling during this stage can address long-term goals. Adolescents in this stage still want to make their own decisions but are open to information provided by healthcare professionals. Nutritional counselors should not only present current recommendations but also explain the rationale behind them.

As adolescents strive for independence, they often take risks. Many of these risks are important to becoming independent (e.g., trying out for a sports team, applying to college, dating), but many risk behaviors can be dangerous. Resnick et al.[77] found that serious behaviors, termed *acting out behaviors*, can be grouped together and include the following: drug use, school absenteeism, and unintended injury risk, such as drinking and driving, not wearing seatbelts, and not using a bicycle helmet. The second group of serious behaviors, termed *quietly disturbed behaviors*, are of concern to nutritionists because these behaviors include the following: poor body image; disordered eating, including binging, bulimia, and chronic dieting; fear of loss of control over eating; emotional stress; and suicidal ideation.

Food Habits

Recommendations for fulfilling the nutritional needs of adolescents arise from a small research base. Often, the amounts recommended are extrapolated from studies in adults or children. Part of the difficulty lies in the fact that studies of requirements must consider not only age, but also stage of physical maturity. The DRIs, which include the RDAs, AIs, and Tolerable Upper Intake Levels (ULs) for adolescents, can be accessed online.

Childhood and Adolescence: Read more about the DRIs, RDAs, AIs, and ULs at http://www.fcs.uga.edu/pubs/PDF/FDNS-E-65.pdf.

Adolescents search for identity, strive for independence and acceptance, and are concerned about appearance. Irregular meals, snacking, eating away from home, and following alternative dietary patterns characterize the food habits of adolescents. These habits are further influenced by family, peers, and the media.

Irregular Meals and Snacking

Meal patterns of adolescents are often chaotic. Teenagers miss an increasing number of meals at home as they get older. Breakfast and lunch are often the meals most frequently missed, but social and school activities may cause a teen to miss an evening meal as well. Adolescent girls tend to miss more meals than their boy counterparts.[32]

Although concern has been expressed about the habit of snacking, teenagers may obtain substantial nourishment from foods eaten outside traditional meals. Thus, the choice

of foods is more important than the time or place of eating.

As a result of health and science education at school, most adolescents know what they should and should not eat.[32,78] However, overcoming barriers to act on that knowledge is the concern. Teens identify the biggest barrier as time. Teens perceive themselves as too busy to worry about food, nutrition, meal planning, or eating right. Additionally, adolescents tend to form different associations with healthy foods and junk foods. Adolescents form mainly negative associations with healthy foods, but positive associations with junk foods.[79] In order for adolescents to change their eating habits to better behaviors, counseling must center on fitting proper nutrition into allowable time, making selection of healthy foods easier, and making healthy foods appealing to teens and their peers.

During the time of peak growth velocity, adolescents usually need to eat large amounts of food often. They are able to use foods with a high concentration of energy; however, they need to be increasingly careful of the amounts and frequency of eating when growth has slowed. Habits of overeating adopted during adolescence may ultimately contribute to adult obesity and a number of related diseases.

Fast Foods

The use of fast foods for meals or snacks is especially popular with busy adolescents. So-called fast foods include foods from vending machines, self-service restaurants, convenience groceries, and franchised food restaurants. Fast foods tend to be low in iron, calcium, riboflavin, and vitamin A, and there are few sources of folic acid. The vitamin C content of fast foods is also low unless fruit or fruit juice is consumed. Although most places offer a selection of healthy foods, many of the food items provide more than 50% of their calories from fat. Adolescents should be counseled on how to make wise and healthy choices when eating out in a restaurant.

Adolescents as Food Purchasers

For marketers, being a teenager is a matter of lifestyles and spending habits, not age. Marketing to teens has become a multi-billion-dollar business. It is estimated that the nation's approximately 23 million teens spend nearly $100 billion annually.[80] Teenagers spend $15 billion annually on fast food and other food and snacks. Teens not only spend money themselves, but also wield a tremendous influence over purchases made by their parents.[80]

Teens are frequent visitors to different stores. In a 30-day period, the top two types of stores teens visited were food stores, with more than 200 million visits to convenience stores and supermarkets. Teens eat in fast food restaurants often, with most visits occurring either immediately after school or at a weekday dinnertime.

Guidelines for nutritional assessment and intervention in adolescence may include:

1. Screen and assess growth status and plot on NCHS growth charts.
2. Refer adolescents identified as at risk for overweight or who are overweight for further evaluation and possible treatment.
3. Provide a wide variety of healthy foods with emphasis on nutritious choices such as whole grains, fruits, vegetables, dairy foods, and lean meats and protein alternatives.
4. Promote daily physical activity that fits with the adolescent's interests.
5. Reduce sedentary activity with an emphasis on reduction of screen time.
6. Provide nutrition education in school.
7. Ensure regular meals and snacks.
8. Encourage reduced levels of low nutrient-dense beverages and promote intake of milk and dairy foods.
9. Provide appropriate care for disease or other health conditions.

Situations with Special Needs

Vegetarian Eating Practices   Adolescents tend to be attracted to vegetarian eating practices, especially during middle or late adolescence, because of their concerns about animal welfare, ecology, the environment, or personal health. Additionally, concerns about body weight motivate some adolescents to adopt a vegetarian diet, because this is a socially acceptable way to reduce dietary fat. Vegetarian eating is often seen in adolescents with anorexia nervosa, who adopt the diet in an attempt to hide their unnecessary restriction of food intake.[49]

Vegetarian diets are consistent with the Dietary Guidelines for Americans and can meet the DRIs/RDAs for nutrients. With planning, vegetarian diets can provide a variety of nutrient-dense foods that promote health, growth, and development. Diets need to be planned to provide adequate energy, protein, calcium, iron, zinc, and vitamins B_{12} and D. The bioavailability of calcium, iron, and zinc should also be ensured. When adolescents become vegetarians, parents are often concerned about the diet's nutritional adequacy, especially about meeting protein requirements. Parents need reassurance that a vegetarian diet can meet their adolescent's nutrition needs, and they should receive information on the principles of healthy vegetarian eating for adolescents. But both parents and adolescents should be informed that overly restricted or inappropriately selected vegetarian diets can result in significant malnutrition. Some vegetarian adolescents have suffered from a delayed growth spurt, iron-deficiency anemia, and vitamin B_{12} deficiency.[49,81]

Eating Disorders   Eating disorders rank as the third most common chronic illness in adolescent females, with an incidence of up to 5%. The prevalence has increased dramatically over the past three decades.[82,83] Large numbers of adolescents who have disordered eating do not meet the strict *Diagnostic Statistical Manual of Mental Disorders*, version IV (DSM-IV)[84] criteria for either Anorexia Nervosa or Bulimia Nervosa but can be classified as Eating Disorders Not Otherwise Specified (EDNOS). In one study,[85] more than half of the adolescents evaluated for eating disorders had subclinical disease but suffered a similar degree of psychological distress as those who met strict diagnostic criteria. Diagnostic criteria for eating disorders such as DSM-IV may not be entirely applicable to adolescents. The wide variability in the rate, timing, and magnitude of both height and weight gain during normal puberty, the absence of menstrual periods in early puberty along with the unpredictability of menses soon after menarche, and the lack of abstract concepts limit the application of diagnostic criteria to adolescents.[82,83]

Just as adolescents are at increased risk for developing eating disorders, they are also more vulnerable to the complications of these disorders. The impact of malnutrition on linear growth, brain development, and bone acquisition can be long-standing and irreversible. Yet, with early and aggressive treatment, there is also potential for a better outcome than in adults who have more long-standing disease.[86]

Early identification of adolescents with disordered eating habits has been linked to improved long-term outcome, but this is difficult to accomplish. Often, parents will bring an affected teen in for another reason, such as gastrointestinal complaints, amenorrhea, or unexplained weight loss. A screening for disordered eating can easily be done, and this should include questions about fear of becoming fat, amount of dieting, use of laxatives, fasting or frequent meal skipping to lose weight, fear of certain foods (e.g., foods containing fat or sugar), vomiting, binging, and excessive exercise.

Because adolescence is the greatest period of risk for development of an eating disorder, efforts must be made to reduce the incidence of malnutrition, or at least provide early intervention to prevent its serious complications.[87]

Adolescence is one of the most challenging periods in human development. Because of the extent of the physical and psychological changes taking place, a number of important issues arise that influence the nutritional well-being of the teenager. Knowledge of the developmental processes is a prerequisite to understanding the nutritional aspects of this period of life. Understanding the nutritional and physical activity needs of adolescents will help nutrition professionals provide counseling and programs that can impact the future health of these individuals.

■ PUBLIC HEALTH INITIATIVES

Special Supplemental Nutrition Program for Women, Infants and Children

For more than 30 years, the WIC Program (now known as the Special Supplemental Nutrition Program for Women, Infants and Children) has provided supplemental foods and nutrition education for low-income women, infants, and children up to five years of age. The ultimate goal of WIC is to improve the nutritional status of low-income pregnant or lactating women, infants, and young children who have been identified as being at nutritional risk. The primary method of achieving that goal is through the provision of specific nutrient-dense foods paid for through program checks or vouchers by eligible pregnant or lactating women and mothers/caregivers of infants and children.[88]

The WIC is funded at the federal level by the U.S. Department of Agriculture, and is administered by states through public and private organizations, such as county and regional health departments. Breast-feeding promotion and support are central to the WIC program, and it has been credited with improving breast-feeding rates among vulnerable populations.[89] WIC program participation includes regular nutrition risk screening, growth assessment, and counseling by healthcare providers. During the infant's first year, WIC supplemental food packages for breast-feeding mothers provide milk, iron-fortified breakfast cereals, 100% juice containing vitamin C, eggs, and either dried beans/peas or peanut butter. Mothers of exclusively breast-fed infants also receive cheese, tuna, and carrots. Breast-fed infants do not receive food packages until they are weaned. Food packages for infants who are weaned provide iron-fortified infant formula for the first six months with the addition of iron-fortified infant cereal and infant juices at four to six months.

WIC provides nutritional services to a very large proportion of the population. WIC benefits are received by 24% of children ages one to four, 35% of all pregnant and postpartum women, and 50% of all infants in the United States.[90] Food availability and food insecurity are problems for many WIC recipients, with approximately one-third of all WIC recipients on food stamps. Any barriers that decrease food resources for these individuals make them more vulnerable to food insecurity as well as nutritional risk.[91]

Numerous studies have been conducted to evaluate WIC. Many have focused on specific outcomes such as the incidence of low-birth-weight infants,[92] nutritional assessment of pregnant women,[93] and the nutrient intakes of infants and young children.[94] Recently, some studies have investigated barriers to WIC usage. Woelfel et al.[95] identified several key barriers to the use of WIC services. Their survey of over 3,000 WIC recipients rated 68 potential barriers to WIC use as measured by likelihood of not picking up WIC checks. Of greatest interest are the top 11 items that were identified by more than 20% of respondents. Based on these findings, dietitians and nutritionists who are involved with WIC programs, or who are interested in enhancing the success of WIC programs, can take specific steps to determine if these barriers exist in their local setting and decrease their incidence, if present. These barriers can be broken into three broad categories: office procedures, the WIC food package, and nutrition education.

Office Procedures

The office setting is a key area for change. The most frequently reported barrier relates to the long waiting times to receive WIC services.[95,96] When combined with three related items from the top 11 (more than an hour to recertify, overcrowded waiting rooms, and no activities for children), office procedures become a logical target for improvement. The image of unhappy, crying children waiting with their mothers in a cramped waiting room does not create a positive response. WIC providers can make the greatest impact on clients' use of WIC services by identifying reasons for long waiting times and improving contributing processes. Less wait time results in fewer clients and children in the waiting room. In addition, all WIC sites should provide enjoyable activities for infants and children. Creatively developed activities could become nutrition education opportunities for children and caregivers.

WIC Food Package

Dissatisfaction with the WIC food package has been recognized by many practitioners. The food package barriers include problems with the actual food items and purchasing issues. Mothers report that they do not receive enough formula and juice; this may indicate a need for improved education on appropriate amounts of formula and juice to feed children and a review of procedures for mixing formula. Excessive consumption of energy-dense beverages, such as juice, in early childhood could contribute to child obesity problems. Dissatisfaction with the types and amounts of foods included in the WIC package often come from ethnic subgroups who do not consume some WIC foods. Mothers also report difficulties in purchasing some foods due to problems with package size and store policies about WIC. If clients are having problems identifying the correct size cereal package to select or are uncertain about store policies, dietitians can design a learning activity that simulates the options available in the store.[97]

WIC Nutrition Education

To be effective, nutrition education must engage the client in the learning process in a meaningful way. Less than optimal nutrition education could result from a variety of reasons, ranging from staff training and available nutrition education materials to inappropriate techniques, as well as insufficient nutrition staff and requirements for time efficiency. Very often, the WIC nutritionist is an entry-level position for a nutritionist, dietitian, or other health professional or paraprofessional, and suffers from frequent turnover. These frontline nutrition educators need to be provided with the skills and resources to be most effective in making meaningful connections with their clients and to be a stimulating and vibrant part of the WIC experience. WIC nutritionists need to evaluate objectively the effectiveness of their customary nutrition education programs and involve clients in determining pros and cons of current practices and ways to improve.

Improvements in WIC office procedures, the WIC food package, and WIC nutrition education can have a significant impact on the nutritional status of WIC clients. The more barriers encountered by WIC recipients, the less likely they are to obtain the nutritious food needed to improve nutrition status. Most of these areas of barrier reduction are within the control or influence of dietitians. WIC nutrition practitioners can make the greatest impact by identifying and eliminating barriers in their locale.[97]

Bright Futures

Launched in 1990 by the Health Resources and Services Administration's Maternal and Child Health Bureau, Bright Futures is an initiative aimed at improving health promotion and preventive services for infants, children, and adolescents. Bright Futures has produced a series of guidelines and supportive materials for health supervision focused on the areas of oral health, nutrition, physical activity, and mental health. The nutrition guidelines include recommendations for nutrition supervision from infancy through adolescence, common nutrition issues and concerns, and nutrition tools.[32] In 2002, collaboration with the AAP led to the establishment of the Bright Futures Education Center and Pediatric Implementation Project, whose objective is to support the implementation of the guidelines.

Read more about Bright Futures at http://www.brightfutures.org.

Start Healthy, Stay Healthy

In 2002, the ADA began a partnership with Gerber Products Company to launch a research and education initiative focused on infant and toddler feeding. The Start Healthy Feeding Guidelines for Infants and Toddlers are based on existing recommendations of authoritative organizations, careful analysis of the feeding and nutrition literature, and evaluation of the nutrient needs of infants and toddlers.[31] Its recommendations are grouped into five areas: nutrients and foods, infant and toddler development, healthy feeding relationships, safe feeding, and physical activity. These recommendations are being disseminated to healthcare professionals through professional publications and presentations and to parents through education materials.

Read more about Start Healthy, Stay Healthy at http://www.gerber.com/starthealthy.

Start Healthy, the Guide to Teaching Your Little One Good Eating Habits delivers the following six messages:

1. Establish healthy eating habits right from the beginning—by breast-feeding.
2. Healthy eating starts with a positive parent-child partnership.
3. If he or she rejects a new food, try, try again!
4. Build your baby's taste buds with variety.
5. Five servings of fruits and vegetables a day are important.
6. The other side of the healthy habits equation: Activity!

■ SUMMARY

Public health nutrition programs that provide services to women in the childbearing years, pregnant and lactating women, infants, children, and adolescents are vital to the health of the nation. Nutritionists, dietitians, and other health professionals have important roles to play in improving the health of the nation by ensuring that these vulnerable groups get the services they need to grow and develop to their full potential. Attainment of the Healthy People 2010 goals that relate to maternal, child, and adolescent issues can be used as an indicator of how successful public health programs are in providing the necessary services. Many of the programs mentioned in this chapter have Web sites that provide extensive information (**see Table 10–2**).

TABLE 10–2   **Maternal Child Health Internet Resources**

Organization	Web Site
American Medical Association Adolescent Health Online	http://www.ama-assn.org/ama/pub/category/1947.html
Breastfeeding Legislative Updates	http://www.house.gov
Breastfeeding Policy	Search under breastfeeding
Bright Future Lactation Resource Centre	http://www.aap.org/policy/re9729.html
Bright Futures	http://www.bflrc.com
Bureau of Maternal and Child Health Library	http://mchb.hrsa.gov/programs/training/brightfutures.htm
	http://mchlibrary.info
CDC/NCHS BMI tables	http://www.cdc.gov/growthcharts
Center for Health and Health Care in Schools	http://www.healthinschools.org
Coalition for a Healthy and Active America	http://www.chaausa.org
DHHS HRSA Maternal and Child Health Bureau	http://www.mchb.hrsa.gov
Dietary Guidelines, 2010	http://www.health.gov/dietaryguidelines/dga2010
Food Allergy & Anaphylaxis Network	http://www.foodallergy.org
Healthy People 2010	http://www.healthypeople.gov
Human Milk Banking Association of North America	http://www.hmbana.org
International Lactation Consultants Association	http://www.ilca.org
Kidnetic	http://www.kidnetic.com

continues

TABLE 10-2 (Continued)	
Organization	**Web Site**
Kids Count	http://www.kidscount.org
La Leche League	http://www.lalecheleague.org
National Academies Press, Dietary Reference Intakes	http://www.nap.edu
National Center for Education in Maternal and Child Health	http://www.ncemch.org
National Center for Health Statistics (source of growth charts)	http://www.cdc.gov/nchs
National Early Childhood Technical Assistance Center	http://www.nectac.org
Neonatology on the Web	http://www.neonatology.org
School Meals Programs	http://www.fns.usda.gov/cnd/
Start Healthy, Stay Healthy	http://www.gerber.com/content/usa/bin/pdf/Feeding_Plan.pdf
Support Breastfeeding.com	http://www.supportbreastfeeding.com
Team Nutrition	http://www.fns.usda.gov/tn/
U.S. Breastfeeding Committee	http://www.usbreastfeeding.org
U.S. government's food and nutrition site	http://www.nutrition.gov
USDA Center for Nutrition Policy and Promotion	http://www.usda.gov/cnpp
USDA Food and Nutrition Information Center	http://www.nal.usda.gov/fnic
USDA Women, Infants and Children (WIC) Program	http://www.fns.usda.gov/wic/

The stages of growth and development covered in this chapter are the most nutritionally challenging periods in human development. Knowledge of the developmental processes is a prerequisite to understanding the nutritional aspects of these life stages. Understanding these groups' nutritional and physical activity needs will help nutrition professionals provide counseling and programs that can impact the future health of these individuals and the nation.

Issues for Discussion

1. After reading the chapter's description of some of the problems with the WIC/SNAP program, how would you plan to go about making changes?

2. After your plan is in place for changing WIC, strategize how you would institute the changes.

3. What types of problems might you expect from both staff and clients if you change public health programs?

References

1. U.S. Department of Health and Human Services. *Healthy People 2010*. Available at http://www.healthypeople.gov. Accessed January 17, 2010.

2. Story M, Neumark-Sztainer D, French S. Individual and environmental influences on adolescent eating behaviors. *J Am Dietet Assoc*. 2002;102:s40–s51.

3. Schieve LA, Cogswell ME, Scanlon KS. Maternal weight gain and preterm delivery: differential effects by body mass index. *Epidemiology*. 1999;10:141–147.

4. Gunderson EP, Abrams B, Selvin S. Does the pattern of postpartum weight change differ according to pregravid body size? *Int J Obesity*. 2001;25:853–862.

5. Kramer FM, Stunkard AJ, Marshall KA, McKinney S, Liebschutz J. Breast-feeding reduces maternal lower body-fat. *J Am Dietet Assoc*. 1993;93:429–433.

6. Wosje KS, Kalkwarf HJ. Lactation, weaning and calcium supplementation: effects on body composition in postpartum women. *Am J Clin Nutr*. 2004;80:423–429.

7. Institute of Medicine, Committee on Nutrition Status During Pregnancy and Lactation. Nutrition during pregnancy, Pt. 1. *Weight gain*. Washington, DC: National Academy Press; 1990.

8. Story M, Stang J. *Nutrition and the Pregnant Adolescent*. Minneapolis, MN: Center for Leadership Education and Training in Maternal and Child Health, University of Minnesota; 2000.

9. Scholl TO, Sowers M, Chen X, et al. Maternal growth and fetal growth: pregnancy course and outcome in the Camden Study. In: Jacobson MS, Rees JM, Golden NH, Irwin CE, eds. *Adolescent Nutritional Disorders: Prevention and Treatment*. New York: The New York Academy of Science; 1998.

10. Hediger ML, Scholl TO, Schall JI. Implications of the Camden Study of Adolescent Pregnancy: interactions among maternal growth, nutrition status, and body composition. In: Jacobson MS, Rees JM, Golden NH, Irwin CE, eds. *Adolescent Nutritional Disorders: Prevention and Treatment*. New York: The New York Academy of Science; 1998.

11. American Dietetic Association (ADA). Position on nutrition care for pregnant adolescents. *J Am Diet Assoc*. 1994;94:449.

12. Kaiser LL, Allen L. Position of the American Dietetic Association: nutrition and lifestyle for a healthy pregnancy outcome. *J Am Dietet Assoc*. 2002;102:1479–1490.

13. Lawrence RA, Lawrence RM. *Breastfeeding: A Guide for the Medical Profession*, 5th ed. St. Louis, MO: Mosby, Inc.; 1999.

14. Breastfeeding Working Group, American Academy of Pediatrics. Breastfeeding and the use of human milk. *Pediatrics*. 1997;100:1035–1039.

15. American Dietetic Association. Position of the American Dietetic Association: Breaking the barriers to breastfeeding. *J Am Dietet Assoc*. 2001;101:1213–1220.

16. World Health Organization (WHO) Expert Consultation. The Optimal Duration of Exclusive Breastfeeding. 2001. Available at http://whqlibdoc.who.int/hq/2001/WHO_NHD_01.09.pdf. Accessed January 18, 2010.

17. Ryan AS, Wenjun Z, Acosta A. Breastfeeding continues to increase into the new millennium. *Pediatrics*. 2002;110:1103–1109.

18. U.S. Department of Health and Human Services and U.S. Department of Agriculture. *U.S. Dietary Guidelines for Americans, 2010*, 7th ed. Washington, DC: U.S. Government Printing Office; January 2010.

19. Ahluwalia IB, Morrow B, Hsia J, Grummer-Strawn LM. Who is breastfeeding? Recent trends from the pregnancy risk assessment and monitoring system. *J Pediatr*. 2003;142:486–491.

20. Kleinman RE, ed. *Pediatric Nutrition Handbook*, 5th ed. Elk Grove Village, IL: American Academy of Pediatrics; 2004. Breastfeeding: 55–78. Formula Feeding of Term Infants: 87–95. Iron Deficiency: 299–312. Nutrition and Oral Health: 789–800.

21. *Congressional Record*. 99th Congress 2nd Session, Senate S 14042–14047. Washington, DC: U.S. Government Printing Office; 1986:132(130).

22. Life Sciences Research Office, Food and Drug Administration. Assessment of nutrient requirements for infant formulas. *J Nutr*. 1998;128:11S.

23. World Health Organization (WHO). *International Code of Marketing of Breast-milk Substitutes*. Geneva, Switzerland: WHO; 1981.

24. Committee on Nutrition, American Academy of Pediatrics (AAP). Iron fortification of infant formulas. *Pediatrics*. 1999;104:119–123.

25. Centers for Disease Control and Prevention (CDC). Recommendations to prevent and control iron deficiency in the United States. *MMWR*. 1998;47(No. RR-3):1–36.

26. Committee on Nutrition, American Academy of Pediatrics (AAP). Soy protein-based formulas: recommendations for use in infant feeding. *Pediatrics*. 1998;101:148–153.

27. Committee on Nutrition, American Academy of Pediatrics. Hypoallergenic infant formulas. *Pediatrics*. 2000;106:346–349.

28. Carver JD. Advances in nutritional modifications of infant formulas. *Am J Clin Nutr*. 2003;77(suppl):1550S–1554S.

29. Butte NF, Wong WW, Hopkinson JM, Smith EO, Ellis KJ. Infant feeding mode affects early growth and body composition. *Pediatrics*. 2000;106:1355–1366.

30. Butte NF, Hopkinson JM, Wong WW, Smith EO, Ellis KJ. Body composition during the first 2 years of life: an updated reference. *Pediatr Res*. 2000;47:578–585.

31. Butte NF, Cobb K, Dwyer, J, Graney L, Heird WC, Rickard KA. The Start Healthy Feeding Guidelines for infants and toddlers. *J Am Dietet Assoc*. 2004:104:442–454.

32. Story M, Holt K, Sofka D, eds. *Bright Futures in Practice: Nutrition*, 2nd ed. Arlington, VA: National Center for Education in Maternal and Child Health; 2002.

33. Devaney B, Ziegler P, Pac S, Karwe V, Barr SI. Nutrient intakes of infants and toddlers. *J Am Dietet Assoc*. 2004;104:S14–S21.

34. Birch LL, Gunder L, Grimm-Thomas K. Infants' consumption of a new food enhances acceptance of similar foods. *Appetite*. 1998; 30:283–295.

35. Sullivan SA, Birch LL. Pass the sugar, pass the salt: experience dictates preference. *Dev Psychol*. 1990;26:546–551.

36. Lifschitz CH. Carbohydrate absorption from fruit juices in infants. *Pediatrics*. 2000;105:e04.

37. Committee on Nutrition, American Academy of Pediatrics. The use and misuse of fruit juice in pediatrics. *Pediatrics*. 2001;107: 1210–1213.

38. Kreiter SR, Schwartz RP, Kirkman HN, Charlton PA, Calikoglu AS, Davenport ML. Nutritional rickets in African American breast-fed infants. *J Pediatr*. 2000;137:153–157.

39. Pugliese MT, Blumberg DL, Hludzinski J, Kay S. Nutritional rickets in suburbia. *J Am Coll Nutr*. 1998;17:637–641.

40. Welch TR, Bergstrom WH, Tsang RC. Vitamin D-deficient rickets: the reemergence of a once-conquered disease. *J Pediatr*. 2000; 137:143–145.

41. Carvalho NF, Kenney RD, Carrington PH, Hall DE. Severe nutritional deficiencies in toddlers resulting from health food milk alternatives. *Pediatrics*. 2001;107:e46.

42. American Academy of Pediatrics, Section on Breastfeeding and Committee on Nutrition. Prevention of rickets and vitamin D deficiency: new guidelines for vitamin D intake. *Pediatrics*. 2003;111:908–910.

43. Nokes C, van den Bosch C, Bundy DA. The effects of iron deficiency and anemia on mental and motor performance, education achievement, and behavior in children: a report of the International Nutritional Anemia Consultative Group. Washington, DC: ILSI Press; 1998.

44. Ziegler EE, Jiang T, Romero E, Vinco A, Frantz JA, Nelson SE. Cow's milk and intestinal blood loss in late infancy. *J Pediatr*. 1999;135:720–726.

45. Hale TW. *Medications and Mothers' Milk*, 11th ed. Amarillo, TX: Pharmasoft Publishing; 2004.

46. Institute of Medicine. *Childhood Obesity*. Washington, DC: National Academy Press; 2004.

47. American Academy of Pediatric Dentistry. Clinical guideline on fluoride therapy. *Pediatr Dent*. 2003;25:67–68.

48. Centers for Disease Control and Prevention (CDC). Recommendations for using fluoride to prevent and control dental caries in the United States. *MMWR*. 2001;50(RR-14):1–42.

49. Story M, Holt K, Sofka D, eds. *Bright Futures in Practice: Nutrition*. Arlington, VA: National Center for Education in Maternal and Child Health; 2000.

50. Barlow SE, Dietz WH. Obesity evaluation and treatment: expert committee recommendations. *Pediatrics*. 1998;102:1–11.

51. Dietz WH. Use of the body mass index (BMI) as a measure of overweight in children and adolescents. *J Pediatr*. 1998;132:191–193.

52. National Academy of Sciences. *Recommended Dietary Allowances*. Washington, DC: National Academy Press; 2004.

53. Centers for Disease Control and Prevention (CDC). *Obesity Still on the Rise, New Data Show*. National Center for Chronic Disease Prevention and Health Promotion, Division of Nutrition and Physical Activity Web site. Available at http://www.cdc.gov/nccdphp/sgr/npai.htm. Accessed May 15, 2010.

54. Lytle L. Nutritional issues for adolescents. *J Am Dietet Assoc*. 2002;102:S8–S12.

55. Institute of Medicine. *Food and Nutrition Board. Dietary Reference Intakes for Calcium, Phosphorus, Magnesium, Vitamin D, and Fluoride*. Washington, DC: National Academy Press; 1997.

56. National Institutes of Health (NIH) Consensus Conference. Optimal calcium intake. NIH consensus development panel on optimal calcium intake. *JAMA*. 1994;272:1942–1948.

57. Alaimo K, et al. *Dietary intake of vitamins, minerals, and fiber of persons ages 2 months and over in the United States: Third National Health and Nutrition Examination Survey, Phase 1, 1988–91*. Advance Data from Vital and Health Statistics, No. 258. Hyattsville, MD: National Center for Health Statistics; 1994.

58. Zemel MB. Role of dietary calcium and dairy produce in modulating adiposity. *Lipids*. 2003;38:139–146.

59. Skinner JD, Bounds W, Carruth BR, Zeigler P. Longitudinal calcium intake is negatively related to children's body fat indexes. *J Am Dietet Assoc*. 2003;103:1626–1631.

60. Dallmon, PR. Iron deficiency: does it matter? *J Intern Med.* 1989; 226:367–372.

61. Centers for Disease Control and Prevention (CDC). *Physical activity and health: a report of the Surgeon General.* Washington, DC: National Center for Chronic Disease Prevention and Health Promotion, President's Council on Physical Fitness and Sports; 1996.

62. Centers for Disease Control and Prevention. Youth risk surveillance—United States 2003. *MMWR.* 2004;53(SS-2):1–29.

63. Patrick K, Spear B, Holt, Sofka D, eds. *Bright Futures in Practice: Physical Activity.* Arlington, VA: National Center for Education in Maternal and Child Health; 2001.

64. Sallis JF, Patrick K. Physical activity guidelines for adolescents: consensus statement. *Pediatr Exerc Sci.* 1994;6:302–314.

65. Corbin CB, Pangrazi RP. *Physical Activity for Children: A Statement of Guidelines.* Reston, VA: National Association for Sport and Physical Education; 1998.

66. Eisenberg ME, Olson RE, Neumark-Sztainer D, Story M, Bearinger LH. Correlations between family meals and psychsocial well-being among adolescents. *Arch Pediatr Adolesc Med.* 2004;158:792–796.

67. Gillman MW, Rifas-Shiman SL, Frazier AL, et al. Family dinner and diet quality among older children and adolescents. *Arch Fam Med.* 2000;9:235–240.

68. Pennsylvania Nutrition and Activity (PANA). *Pennsylvania Growth Screening Process.* Harrisburg, PA: 2004.

69. Nicklas TA, Johnson R. Position of the American Dietetic Association: Dietary guidance for healthy children ages 2 to 11 years. *J Am Dietet Assoc.* 2004;104:660–677.

70. Briley ME, Roberts-Gray C. Position of the American Dietetic Association: Nutrition standards for child-care programs. *J Am Dietet Assoc.* 1999;99:981–988.

71. Stang J, Bayerl C. Position of the American Dietetic Association: child and adolescent food and nutrition programs. *J Am Dietet Assoc.* 2003;103:887–893.

72. Farley, D. Dangers of lead still linger. *FDA Consumer.* 1998;Jan/Feb:16–21.

73. Briggs M, Safii S, Beall DL. Position of the American Dietetic Association, Society for Nutrition Education, and American School Food Service Association: nutrition services: an essential component of comprehensive school health programs. *J Am Dietet Assoc.* 2003;103:505–514.

74. Brown JD, Witherspoon EM. The mass media and American adolescents' health. *Proceedings of the Health Futures of Youth! Pathways to Adolescent Health Conference.* Annapolis, MD; September 14, 1998.

75. Spear BA. Adolescent growth and development. In: Rickets VI, ed. *Adolescent Nutrition: Assessment and Management.* New York: Chapman and Hall; 1996:3–24.

76. Sigman-Grant M. Strategies for counseling adolescents. *J Am Dietet Assoc.* 2002;102:S32–S39.

77. Resnick MD, et al. Health and risk behaviors of urban adolescent males involved in pregnancy. *Fam Soc: J Contemp Hum Serv.* 1993;74:366.

78. Story M, Resnick MD. Adolescents' views on food and nutrition. *J Nutr Educ.* 1986;18:188.

79. Chapman G, Maclean H. "Junk food" and "healthy food": meanings of food in adolescent women's culture. *J Nutr Educ.* 1993;25:108.

80. Channel One Network. *Teen Fact Book.* New York: Channel One Network; 2000.

81. Sanders T. Vegetarian diets and children. *Pediatr Clin N Am.* 1995;42:955–965.

82. Kreipe RE, Birndorf DO. Eating disorders in adolescents and young adults. *Med Clin N Am.* 2000;84:1027–1049.

83. Spear BA, Stellefson-Myers E. Position of the American Dietetic Association: nutrition intervention in the treatment of anorexia nervosa, bulimia nervosa, and eating disorders not otherwise specified (EDNOS). *J Am Dietet Assoc.* 2001;101:810–819.

84. American Psychiatric Association (APA). *Diagnostic and Statistical Manual of Mental Disorders,* 4th ed., text rev. Washington, DC: APA Press; 2000.

85. Bunnell DW, Shenker IR, Nussbaum MP, Arden MR, Jacobson MS. Subclinical versus formal eating disorders: differentiating psychological features. *Int J Eat Disord.* 1990;9:357–362.

86. Golden NH. The adolescent: vulnerable to develop an eating disorder and at high risk for long-term sequelae. *Ann NY Acad Sci.* 1997;817:94–97.

87. Striegel-Moore R. Risk factors for eating disorders. In: Jacobson MS, Rees JM, Golden N, Irwin C, eds. *Adolescent Nutritional Disorders: Prevention and Treatment.* New York: Annals of the New York Academy of Sciences; 1997:98–109.

88. U.S. Department of Agriculture, Food and Nutrition Services. *WIC.* Federal Register: 7 CFR Part 246. Washington, DC: National Archives and Records Administration; January 1, 2003.

89. Wright AL, Schanler RJ. The resurgence of breastfeeding at the end of the second millennium. *J Nutr.* 2001;131:421S–425S.

90. Fox HB, McManus MA, Schmidt HJ. *WIC Reauthorization: Opportunities for Improving the Nutritional Status of Women, Infants, and Children.* Washington, DC: National Health Policy Forum; 2004.

91. Conrey EJ, Frongillo EA, Dollahite JS, Griffin MR. Integrated program enhancements increased utilization of farmers market nutrition program. *J Nutr.* 2003;133:1841–1844.

92. Kowaleski-Jones L, Duncan GJ. Effects of participation in the WIC program on birthweight: evidence from the National Longitudinal Survey of Youth. *Am J Pub Health.* 2002;92:799–804.

93. Swensen AR, Harnack LJ, Ross JA. Nutritional assessment of pregnant women enrolled in the Special Supplemental Program for Women, Infants, and Children (WIC). *J Am Dietet Assoc.* 2001;101:903–908.

94. Ponza M, Devaney B, Ziegler P, Reidy K, Squatrito C. Nutrient intakes and food choices of infants and toddlers participating in WIC. *J Am Dietet Assoc.* 2004;104S:S71–S79.

95. Woelfel ML, AbuSabha R, Pruzek RM, Stratton H, Chen SG, Edmunds LS. Barriers to use of WIC services. *J Am Dietet Assoc.* 2004;738–743.

96. Rosenberg TJ, Alperen JK, Chiasson MA. Why do WIC participants fail to pick up their checks? An urban study in the wake of welfare reform. *Am J Public Health.* 2003;93:477–481.

97. McKinney S. Steps to improving WIC usage: office procedures, food package, and nutrition education. *J Am Dietet Assoc.* 2004;93:743–745.

CHAPTER

11

Importance of Public Health Nutrition Programs in Preventing Disease and Promoting Adult Health

JUDITH SHARLIN, PhD, RD

READER OBJECTIVES

After studying this chapter and reflecting on the contents, you should be able to:

1. Identify the primary causes of death and disability in adults in the United States.
2. Describe primary, secondary, and tertiary levels of health prevention and health promotion, and their relationship to nutrition program planning.
3. Identify risk factors for chronic diseases and their implication for nutrition.
4. Describe the dietary risk factors associated with the leading chronic diseases.
5. Discuss the common features of the dietary guidelines issued by the major U.S. health organizations.
6. Compare different dietary interventions a public health nutritionist or dietitian offers to the community, family, or an individual at risk.
7. Recognize the mission and role of public health nutrition in preventing disease and promoting adult health.
8. Name some of the public health nutrition programs that exist today for maintaining adult health.

■ INTRODUCTION

Growing scientific evidence reveals that nutrition or dietary intake in adults contributes significantly to preventing illnesses and premature deaths in the United States.[1] Life expectancy has increased dramatically over the past century, and today the average life expectancy is 77 years.[2] Health and nutrition programs for adults aim at prevention, as well as improving quality of life. However, chronic diseases account for 7 out of every 10 deaths in the United States.[3] The increasing cost of crisis medical care and the growing economic burden provide a cost-effective incentive for individuals and our nation to prevent chronic disease. Chronic diseases cost the United States 75% of the $1 trillion spent on health care annually.[3] Despite this statistic, only 3% of the total annual healthcare expenditures in our nation were spent on prevention.[4] Nutrition interventions and policies target the factors related to adult health, and aim to prevent chronic diseases that are the leading causes of death and disability.

■ CHRONIC DISEASES: THE LEADING CAUSES OF DEATH AND DISABILITY

To successfully create programs to promote health, longevity, and the quality of life, we must examine the leading causes of death and disability. Data from the National Center for Health Statistics (NCHS) show that chronic diseases are the leading causes of death and disability (**Table 11–1**).[5] Cardiovascular diseases and cancer account for half of all deaths in the United States.[3] More than 60% of chronic disease mortality can be attributed to lifestyle factors, such as diet, which can be modified.[6] A recent report on the health status of U.S. adults emphasized that increasing numbers of people still smoke, are physically inactive, and are overweight.[7] Researchers noted in 2000 that about half of the deaths among U.S. adults could have been prevented.[8] These findings revealed that 400,000 deaths occur each year due to poor diet and physical inactivity.[8] This number was found to be 20% less in a 2005 study.[9] It appears that the increasing trend of overweight and obesity will likely overtake tobacco

TABLE 11–1	Deaths and Percentage of Total Deaths for the Ten Leading Causes of Death: United States, 2003–2004					
Cause of Death*	Classification	Rank†	Deaths in 2004 N	Percent of Total Deaths, 2004	Deaths in 2003 N	Percent of Total Deaths, 2003
All Causes			2,397,615	100.0	2,448,288	100.0
Heart diseases	I00–I09, I11, I13, I20–I51	1	652,486	27.2	685,089	28.0
Malignant neoplasms	C00–C97	2	553,888	23.1	556,902	22.7
Cerebrovascular diseases	I60–I69	3	150,074	6.3	157,689	6.4
Chronic lower respiratory diseases	J40–J47	4	121,987	5.1	126,382	5.2
Accidents (unintentional injuries)	V01–X59, Y85–Y86	5	112,012	4.7	109,277	4.5
Diabetes mellitus	E10–E14	6	73,138	3.1	74,219	3.0
Alzheimer's disease	G30	7	65,965	2.8	63,457	2.6
Influenza and pneumonia	J10–J18	8	59,664	2.5	65,163	2.7
Nephritis, nephrotic syndrome and nephrosis	N00–N07, N17–N19, N25–N27	9	42,480	1.8	42,453	1.7
Septicemia	A40–A41	10	33,373	1.4	34,069	1.4

* Based on the *International Classification of Diseases*, Tenth Revision, 1992.
†Rank based on number of deaths
Source: Centers for Disease Control and Prevention, *National Vital Statistics Reports*. Available at http://www.cdc.gov/nchs/products/nvsr.htm. Accessed April 26, 2010.

as the leading preventable cause of mortality in the United States.[8] Although mortality rates from heart disease, stroke, and cancer have declined, behavioral changes have led to an increased prevalence of obesity and diabetes.[10,11] Dietary factors are now associated with 4 of the 10 leading causes of death: coronary heart disease (CHD), some types of cancer, stroke, and type-2 diabetes.[12] The Surgeon General's report confirmed these findings: "For two out of three adult Americans who do not smoke and do not drink excessively, one personal choice seems to influence long-term health prospects more than any other, what we eat."[13]

Risk Factors and Chronic Disease

Chronic diseases, although prevalent and costly, are among the most preventable. Research has identified a Health Promotion and Preventive Action model (HPA) for risk factors.[14] In this model, risk factor identification, reduction, modification, and education are related to human health and developmental stages.[14] Risk factors can be defined as those specific characteristics associated with an increased chance of developing a chronic disease. Risk factors that can be changed or modified, such as diet or physical activity, are under an individual's personal choices.[15] There are four types of risk factors:[2]

1. Biological factors such as an individual's genetic make-up, family history, age, or gender

2. Environmental conditions—social and physical environment
3. Access to quality health care
4. Individual behavior and lifestyle factors such as smoking, exercise, and good eating habits

Healthy People 2010 (HP 2010) provides the most recent guidelines and recommendations for specific health objectives and goals for the nation.[2] HP 2010 reveals that individual biological behaviors and environmental factors are responsible for approximately 70% of all premature deaths.[2] Biological factors such as age or gender are not modifiable. However, the leading causes of death are associated with dietary factors, which are modifiable. The determinants of health illustrate how individual biology and behaviors influence health through the individual's social and physical environments.[2] Finally, health can be improved through policies that provide access to health care and interventions with access to quality health care. Because the leading causes of illness and death in the United States (e.g., CHD, some types of cancer, stroke, type-2 diabetes, and atherosclerosis) are associated with dietary factors, we must address the concern that chronic diseases have resulted from dietary excesses and imbalance.[2] Furthermore, there is evidence that more intensive dietary counseling can lead to reduced intakes of dietary fat and cholesterol, and increased fiber, fruit, and vegetable consumption.[16]

Healthy People 2010 outlines 28 focus areas that include risk factors for chronic diseases and addresses nutrition and overweight, physical activity, tobacco use, cancer, diabetes, cardiovascular disease, and access to quality health care.

■ PREVENTION STRATEGIES

Health promotion and disease prevention provide complementary interventions to change health risk factors. Prevention efforts in public heath, community, and worksite settings are divided into three levels: primary prevention (health promotion), secondary prevention (risk appraisal and reduction), and tertiary prevention (treatment and rehabilitation).[17-19]

Primary Prevention: Health Promotion

Primary prevention strategies, or health promotion, encourage health-enhancing behaviors by giving individuals, families, and communities ways to reduce risk factors associated with disease and injury.[19] Risk factors include environmental, economic, social, and biological aspects. Good examples of primary prevention strategies include nutrition and weight management classes in a community center for adults, environmental changes to provide nutritious choices in a school cafeteria vending machine, and Fruits and Veggies Matter campaigns to increase the availability of fresh fruits and vegetables from farmers' markets.[19] Primary prevention strategies seek to expand the positive potential of health.[20]

A holistic approach, embracing individual lifestyle factors, the environment, and economic, social, and political factors, can help communities and private sector partners achieve health promotion and disease prevention goals. Providing information, available on food labels and through health messages to the public, is one effective method. These messages encourage consumers to apply the U.S. Dietary Guidelines, MyPyramid (formerly called the Food Guide Pyramid), Dietary Reference Intakes, and the Dietary Guidelines Alliance's through the It's All About You campaigns.[21-23] Voluntary community and health organizations, the federal government, worksite programs, and schools can reach consumers daily to promote nutrition interventions.

The media remains an effective means of communicating nutrition issues to the public.[24] Programs to promote physical activity and fitness, good nutrition, and smoking cessation must be broadly accessible. Worksite nutrition-centered health promotion and disease prevention programs provide opportunities to harness social support and influence.[25]

Motivations should be provided for food processors and vendors, restaurant chefs, and school and worksite cafeteria managers to prepare and serve foods lower in fat, calories, and sodium. Finally, legislation and regulations can be ratified to endorse more complete food and nutrition labeling. Food labels that provide short, unequivocal, posi-

tive messages aimed at a single behavior prove beneficial to consumers.[26,27]

Secondary Prevention: Risk Appraisal and Risk Reduction

Secondary prevention includes risk appraisal and screening to emphasize early detection and diagnosis of disease.[14,18,19] Secondary prevention begins at the point where the pathology of a disease may occur. It encompasses diagnostic services that include screening, surveillance, and clinical examinations.[14] Screening strategies include follow-up education, counseling, and health referral. One model for secondary prevention involving screening is a cholesterol screening program for early detection of cardiovascular problems, such as elevated blood pressure, elevated blood cholesterol, and high glucose levels.[28] For people with an elevated blood cholesterol level, this means introducing "therapeutic lifestyle changes" such as reducing total and saturated fat in the diet, increasing physical activity, and reducing or maintaining a healthy weight. If this is not effective, or if low density lipoprotein levels are abnormally high, drug therapy can be recommended by the physician.

Strategies in secondary prevention are aimed at self-care for people with chronic diseases. An example of a secondary prevention program involving self-care would be an educational and awareness program to teach a woman with a history of gestational diabetes how to control her weight through diet and exercise.[18,19]

Tertiary Prevention: Treatment and Rehabilitation

Tertiary prevention involves treatment and rehabilitation, and is defined as the reduction in the amount of disability caused by a disease to achieve the highest level of function.[27] Tertiary factors include diabetes, kidney disease, and angina. The goal of treatment and rehabilitation is the prevention of further disability and any secondary conditions that might result from the initial health problem.

Examples of tertiary prevention programs include medical nutrition therapy (MNT) for people suffering from kidney disease, nutrition education about vitamin and mineral supplementation and feeding strategies to prevent further complications of wasting from HIV/AIDS, and cardiac rehabilitation through diet, exercise, and stress management. The ultimate goal of tertiary prevention is, through rehabilitation, to restore the individual to an "optimal" level of functioning, given the constraints of the disease.[19]

Implications of the Prevention Levels

The prevention levels are useful concepts to help set objectives for public health programs concerned with adult health in communities, worksites, and other settings. Recent findings underscore the need to emphasize population-based prevention programs.[15,29] As discussed earlier, research points to a holistic approach that aims at health, as well as prevention, when using the level concept for public health programs. This approach is embraced in HP 2010 in terms of the nutrition and health objectives.[2] For each goal, the holistic approach involving individual lifestyle factors, environmental factors, social and political issues, and access to quality healthcare is addressed.

Public health endeavors focus on primary or secondary prevention. It is important to choose the appropriate prevention level when planning a public health program. This is illustrated with two different approaches for handling CHD risk factors: one intended to reduce the prevalence of high blood pressure and one to reduce obesity levels.

Almost all Americans have had their blood pressure measured some time in their lives. Ninety percent of Americans had their blood pressure measured in the past two years and could state whether it was normal or abnormally high.[30] Over 90% of Americans are aware of the relationship between hypertension and stroke and hypertension and heart disease.[31] Almost 70% of people with hypertension know about high blood pressure, yet the same percentage (70%) do not have their blood pressure under control (less than 140/90 mm Hg).[32] Recent findings show that systolic (higher number) blood pressure is a more important predictor of heart disease than diastolic blood pressure, especially in the elderly.[33] In addition, ethnic disparities exist for prevalence rates of high blood pressure, and African Americans in the United States have a greater prevalence of high blood pressure than do Caucasians.[32] These data suggest that in order to reduce mortality from hypertension, secondary prevention strategies should be directed toward persons with hypertension (especially those with elevated systolic pressures), African Americans, and the elderly. This would be more effective than primary prevention strategies aimed at increasing public awareness.

In contrast, many Americans are just beginning to be aware of the growing obesity epidemic and the significance of elevated body mass index (BMI) ($\geq$ 30) for the risk of death and illness.[3] Americans understand the viability of lowering this risk factor associated with many chronic diseases. Extensive data exist to substantiate that making lifestyle changes such as engaging in regular physical activity and healthy eating could, at the very least, halt the continued growth of the obesity epidemic.[3] One primary prevention effort is called America on the Move,[34] a national initiative dedicated to helping individuals and communities become more physically active and to eat more healthfully. The program creates and supports an "integrated grassroots network" at the state level to build communities that support individual behavior changes. In addition, America on the Move involves public and private partnerships at the national, state, and local levels. It publicizes small behavioral changes, such as cutting 100 calories a day and taking 2,000 steps daily.

Health promotion and chronic disease prevention programs should focus on coalition building (as previously discussed in Chapter 5) between community-based nutrition and health professionals, government, local businesses,

health agencies, and insurers.[19] In this rapidly changing healthcare environment, continued training and research in public health program development is crucial to provide evidence of the efficacy of health prevention and promotion.

All levels of prevention should be addressed when devising strategies for dietary behavior changes for chronic disease prevention. However, for some diseases, the nutrition strategy may prove similar at each prevention level. Weight reduction, for example, may prevent the onset of hypertension or be part of the treatment for type-2 diabetes. In the case of other diseases, such as cancer, nutrition strategies might vary with the prevention level.

■ DIETARY GUIDELINES FOR DISEASE PREVENTION

Various health organizations and government agencies have issued dietary guidelines and recommendations based on current scientific evidence. In 1989, the National Research Council published its report, *Diet and Health: Implications for Reducing Chronic Disease Risk*, providing evidence for the relationship between all major chronic conditions and diet.[3] More recently, HP 2010 set forth a comprehensive health promotion and disease prevention program for the nation. HP 2010's comprehensive health agenda has two overarching goals: 1) to increase the quality and years of a healthy life, and 2) to eliminate health disparities.[2] These goals embrace the dietary recommendations set forth by several government and health organizations.[35]

In 2001, the U.S. Dietary Guidelines were assessed in terms of surveillance and research needs, especially related to risk for chronic diseases, such as cancer.[36] In the same year, the revised Dietary Guidelines of the American Heart Association (AHA) gave greater emphasis to the diet as a whole and, specifically, to certain protective foods for chronic disease risk prevention.[37] Recent scientifically based dietary

U.S. Dietary Guidelines: http://www.health.gov/dietaryguidelines/

Dietary Guidelines of the American Heart Association: http://www.americanheart.org/presenter.jhtml?identifier=851

American Cancer Society: http://www.cancer.org

American Institute for Cancer Research: http://www.aicr.org

America Dietetic Association: http://www.eatright.org

Alternate Healthy Eating Index: http://www.hsph.harvard.edu/nutritionsource/pyramids.html

American Diabetes Association: http://www.diabetes.org

North American Association for the Study of Obesity: http://www.naaso.org

guidelines from the American Cancer Society and the American Institute for Cancer Research reinforce these guidelines and further emphasize eating foods from plant sources.[38] Dietary recommendations for women issued by the American Dietetic Association reiterated these health-promoting dietary guidelines in 2004.[39] In addition, the Alternate Healthy Eating Index (AHEI) was developed to target food choices and nutrient intake associated with chronic disease risk.[40]

The dietary guidelines from these major health organizations agree in their basic message. The American Institute for Cancer Research stated: "Our research has shown that a diet that prevents cancer can also prevent other chronic diseases...the United States Department of Agriculture (USDA) and other major health organizations are now largely in agreement about specific dietary guidelines that protect overall health."[41]

The American Heart Association, the American Cancer Society, the American Diabetes Association, the American Institute of Cancer Research, and the North American Association for the Study of Obesity concur with the new dietary recommendations.[41] In July 2004, the American Cancer Society, the American Diabetes Association, and the American Heart Association collaborated to work on health promotion and disease prevention.[41] In their collaborative efforts, these organizations are making unified health statements concerning the prevention of heart disease, cancer, diabetes, and related risk factors. Furthermore, all of these organizations agree on the following dietary patterns that may help reduce the risk of chronic diseases[41,42]:

- Consume a diet that emphasizes whole grains and legumes, vegetables, and fruits.
- Decrease saturated fat and dietary cholesterol; limit red meat and full-fat dairy products.
- Limit intake of foods and beverages high in added sugars.
- Limit overall intake of calories and engage in regular physical activity to maintain a healthy body weight.

Despite the evidence of the importance of diet to health, vegetable and fruit consumption among adults continues to be below recommended amounts; fewer than 25% of U.S. adults consume five servings a day.[43] According to the U.S. Department of Agriculture's 1994–1996 Continuing Survey of Food Intakes by Individuals and the Food Guide Pyramid, only 3% of individuals meet four of the five recommendations for the intake of grains, fruits, vegetables, dairy products, and meats.[44]

The 2005 Dietary Guidelines for Americans (6th edition) were released in January 2005 by the Department of Health and Human Services (DHHS) and the USDA. In the past, a diet low in fat was recommended, but in 2000 this recommendation was changed to a diet "moderate" in total fat, and specifically low in saturated fat and cholesterol. The dietary guidelines have consistently encouraged the consumption of complex carbohydrates and fiber by eating more fruits, vegetables, and whole grains. In 2000, the guidelines separated the recommendations for eating fruits and vegetables and eating whole grains. The issue of safe foods was added. The two separate guidelines—"aiming for a healthy weight" and "increasing physical activity"—also were added in 2000.

In revising the Dietary Guidelines and MyPyramid (formerly called the Food Guide Pyramid) for 2010, the following revisions were initiated[45]:

- Balancing calories from foods and beverages according to the amount of calories expended and using MyPyramid to determine appropriate caloric requirements based on age and physical activity levels.
- Select nutritional goals for food intake patterns, such as the USDA Food Guide or DASH eating plan.
- Propose food intake patterns for educating the American public about healthful eating patterns, such as consuming more fruits and vegetables, whole grains, and fat-free or low-fat milk.
- Use "cups" and "ounces" instead of "servings" in educational materials.
- Select appropriate illustrations of food patterns for consumer materials.

See Chapter 2 for more information on these revisions.

In summary, diverse health organizations stress the similarities in the dietary recommendations for reducing disease risk. These recommendations are to eat less saturated fat and cholesterol (limit red meat and full-fat dairy products); increase consumption of fruits, vegetables, whole grains, and legumes; limit added sugar and sodium; drink alcohol in moderation; and increase physical activity. By using clear terms, public health nutrition and dietetic professionals can make the nutrition message easier for the public to understand, value, and implement.

■ DIET AND HEALTH: NUTRITION STRATEGIES AND RISK FACTORS

Nutrition strategies are essential in the prevention and management of several chronic diseases and their risk factors. When developing a public health program, risk factor assessment needs to be addressed. The following criteria can be assessed:

- The risk factor must have a strong association with the development of a chronic disease (e.g., obesity and heart disease).
- The risk factor must affect a significant number of people.
- The risk factor must be modifiable, so it can be reduced or changed.
- The risk factor must have a modification that, when changed or reduced, results in decreased mortality.

Because many risk factors can be modified by healthy lifestyle changes, early recognition of the risk factors for chronic disease prevention is critical.

Obesity

Obesity has reached epidemic proportions in the United States. More than one-third of U.S. adults (over 66%), or 72 million people were obese in 2005–2006.[3,42,46] Rates of excessive weight and obesity are steadily growing in our country. Over 66% of the U.S. adult population was overweight or obese in 2003–2004, compared with 55% in 1988–1994 and 46% in 1976–1980.[43,46] The National Institutes of Health (NIH) Expert Panel uses BMI for defining overweight and obesity.[47] The cut-off point for overweight is a BMI of 25 kg/m². Obesity, defined as having a BMI of $\geq$ 30 kg/m², has doubled among adults since 1980. Extreme obesity (BMI of $\geq$ 40 kg/m²) increased from 4.7% in 1999–2000 to 5.9% in 2003–2004.[48] The age-adjusted prevalence of overweight and obesity (BMI $\geq$ 25 kg/m²) increased from 64.5% in 1999–2000 to 66.3% in 2003–2004. In the same time, obesity (BMI of $\geq$ 30 kg/m²) increased from 30.5% to 34.3%.[46] Many diseases are associated with overweight and obesity, including CHD, stroke, high blood pressure, diabetes, arthritis-related disabilities, sleep apnea, gallbladder disease, and some cancers.[49]

The public health burden of overweight and obesity is overwhelming in terms of premature deaths and disability, lost productivity, and social stigmatization.[50] Medical expenses for obesity accounted for 9.1% of total U.S. medical expenditures in 1998 and may have reached as high as 92.6 billion dollars in 2002.[51] Another estimate places the total cost of obesity at $117 billion.[3] Obesity rates are higher among certain population groups such as Hispanic Americans, African Americans, Native Americans, and Pacific Islander American women.[49] Recent research has reported, however, that overweight has increased in all parts of the U.S. population.[52,53] The recent trend of overweight in the United States has become so severe that if it is not reversed in the next few years, poor diet and lack of physical exercise will likely become the leading preventable cause of mortality among adults.[8]

Many factors contribute to overweight and obesity. For each individual, metabolic and genetic factors, as well as behaviors affecting dietary intake and physical activity, contribute to being overweight. Cultural, environmental, and socioeconomic influences also play a role. Most overweight and obese individuals eat more calories from food than they expend through physical activity. As body weight increases, so does the prevalence of health risks in an individual. For this reason, encouraging obese individuals to adopt new eating and physical activity habits is of vital importance.

Visit http://www.nhlbi.gov for more information about the National Heart, Lung, and Blood Institute's recommendations.

Weight Management

The goals and outcomes of weight management programs should be guided by an assessment of an individual's weight (BMI) and health. The National Heart, Lung, and Blood Institute (NHLBI) guidelines recommend intervention for people who are overweight and have two or more risk factors associated with their weight.[54] Furthermore, according to the position paper of the American Dietetic Association for weight management, assessment should incorporate the following areas[55]:

- *Anthropometrics:* The assessment of height, weight, BMI, and waist circumference (as waist measurement increases, so do health risks)
- *Medical causes:* Identifying potential causes, age of onset, obesity-associated complications, and severity of obesity
- *Psychological causes:* Eating disorders, possible psychological causes, and barriers to treatment
- *Nutritional causes:* Weight history, diet history, current eating patterns, nutritional intake, environmental factors, meals eaten away from home, exercise history, and motivation to change

For an individual, the goal of a weight management program should focus on the prevention of weight gain as well as weight loss. This recommendation encourages individuals to adopt healthier lifestyles, such as increasing physical activity and choosing less calorically dense foods. With this approach, weight loss will lead to reductions of health risks.[56] A weight loss of as little as 10% can improve health risks associated with overweight and obesity.[57]

For effective weight management programs, a multidisciplinary team should be involved, including a physician, a dietitian, an exercise physiologist, and a behavioral therapist. Healthcare professionals ought to be especially dedicated and sensitive to the needs of overweight and obese individuals. It is appropriate to discuss realistic goals of weight loss and maintenance so that shared responsibility for weight management can develop between the provider and individual. Goals might include the following[56]:

- Prevention or cessation of weight gain in an individual who is continuing to see an increase in his or her weight
- Progress in physical and emotional health
- Small, realistic weight losses achieved through sensible eating and exercise
- Improvements in eating, exercise, and any behaviors apart from weight loss

Establishing both short- and long-term treatment goals and documenting measures before implementing the weight management plan and after the individual has started on the plan are an important part of care. Positive behavior changes, other than absolute weight, should be rewarded as these can be very motivating.

Physical activity is highly recommended as an essential part of a weight-management program. It is well established that to maintain weight loss, healthful dietary habits must be coupled with increased physical activity.[47] Physical activity contributes to weight loss not only by changing energy balance, but also by positively changing body composition by increasing lean body mass. Exercise decreases the risk of chronic disease and improves mood and quality of life. Many experts believe that physical inactivity is responsible for the increasing prevalence of overweight and obesity in the United States.[50] Combining weight loss with regular physical activity reduces one's risk for chronic diseases such as heart disease and diabetes by reducing both blood cholesterol and blood glucose levels.

The biggest challenge in weight management is to maintain a healthy weight once it is achieved. It is essential to include physical activity in weight-loss programs because regular physical activity is one of the best predictors of weight maintenance.[58] Unfortunately, studies show that within five years, a majority of people regain the weight they have lost.[59] The NIH recommends that both dietary and physical activity changes need to be continued indefinitely for weight loss to be maintained.[57] A comprehensive lifestyle program that focuses on nutrition, exercise, cognitive behavioral changes, and medical monitoring has been shown to be most effective for long-term success.[60]

Due to the increased prevalence in overweight and obesity in the United States, weight management becomes crucial for primary prevention of many chronic diseases. It is the foundation of secondary and tertiary prevention of hypertension, high blood cholesterol, diabetes, arthritis, and some cancers. It is important for healthcare providers to lobby for public health policies that endorse the treatment and management of weight, as discussed in Chapters 7 and 8. Also, clients must be informed of the known healthy and positive outcomes achieved through weight management programs.

Cardiovascular Disease

Cardiovascular disease is the nation's leading cause of death, accounting for more than 36% of all deaths in the United States. Despite a decline in heart-disease mortality, in 2005, one in three American adults, or more than 864,000 Americans died of cardiovascular disease.[61] Three modifiable health behaviors—poor nutrition, lack of physical activity, and smoking—contribute greatly to the burden of heart disease.

Cardiovascular diseases include diseases of the heart and blood vessels: CHD, stroke, and peripheral vascular diseases. CHD is the most common form of cardiovascular disease, and usually involves atherosclerosis and hypertension. Atherosclerosis is characterized by the build-up of plaques along the inner walls of the arteries, causing inadequate blood flow and leading to serious cardiovascular problems.

The consequences of cardiovascular disease are usually heart disease and stroke; these two diseases combined cause one death every 33 seconds.[3] About 61 million Americans live with the effects of heart disease and stroke. The annual cost of cardiovascular disease and stroke is estimated at $475 billion.[3] The death rate from cardiovascular disease fell by 17% in the last part of the 20th century; however, the number of deaths increased by 2.5% each year due to the growth and size of the population aged 65 years and older.[32] The decrease in the mortality rates due to cardiovascular disease is attributed to primary prevention (e.g., a decrease in dietary intake of saturated fat), secondary prevention (e.g., early detection and treatment of hypertension), and improved medical and surgical treatments.[61] In general, mortality and prevalence rates of cardiovascular disease could be improved by reducing the major risk factors: high blood pressure, high blood cholesterol, tobacco use, physical inactivity, and poor nutrition. Controlling one or more of these risk factors could have a major public health impact in our country.

Hypertension

High blood pressure or hypertension remains a "silent killer" in the United States, affecting about 73.6 million or one in three Americans.[32] High blood pressure is a major independent risk factor for cardiovascular disease. Hypertension increases the risk of heart attack, heart failure, stroke, and kidney disease.[62] This is significant because heart disease and stroke are the first and third leading cause of death in the United States, respectively.[3]

In the latest classification of blood pressure for adults, normal blood pressure is considered to be < 120/80 mm Hg and prehypertension is designated as 120–139 systolic or 80–89 mm Hg diastolic pressure.[62] High blood pressure for adults is defined as a systolic pressure of ≥ 140 mm Hg, or a diastolic pressure of ≥ 90 mm Hg. A recent finding has determined that systolic blood pressure is a more important predictor of CHD in older adults than diastolic blood pressure.[63]

The number of people who were able to control their high blood pressure from lifestyle changes and the use of antihypertensive drugs rose from about 16% in 1971–1972 to about 65% in 1988–1994.[64] The age-adjusted death rate attributed to hypertension rose by about 36.4% over the 1991–2001 decade, with the actual number of deaths increasing by 53%.[42] From 1995 to 2005 the death rate from high blood pressure increased 23% and the actual number of deaths rose to 56.4%.[65] Among people with high blood pressure, 69% are being treated, 45% have it under control, and 54.6% do not have their blood pressure under control.[65] Significant disparities exist among persons diagnosed with hypertension; for example, African Americans have high blood pressure at an earlier age, and in general have higher blood pressures.[66] Twenty-two percent of Americans are unaware that they have hypertension.[65,67]

The latest guidelines for the treatment of hypertension are found in *The Seventh Report of the Joint National Committee on Prevention, Detection, Evaluation, and Treatment*

Visit http://www.nhlbi.nih.gov/guidelines/hypertension/ for more information about the *Seventh Report of the Joint National Committee on Prevention, Detection, Evaluation, and Treatment of High Blood Pressure*.

of High Blood Pressure.[62] This report advocates major lifestyle modifications shown to lower blood pressure, enhance antihypertensive drug efficacy, and decrease cardiovascular risk. General lifestyle modifications include weight reduction for overweight or obese individuals (the goal is for a BMI of 18.5–24.9),[68,69] the adoption of the Dietary Approaches to Stop Hypertension (DASH) eating plan,[66] reducing sodium intake,[70] increasing physical activity,[71] and moderating alcohol consumption.[72,73] The DASH eating plan is a diet rich in calcium and potassium, consisting of fresh fruits, vegetables, and low-fat dairy products.[70,74] The DASH eating plan advocates a low sodium intake; intakes of 1,600 mg have been found to be as effective as single drug therapy in lowering blood pressure.[70] Other specific lifestyle modifications include reducing sodium to 2,400 mg a day, engaging in regular aerobic physical activity at least 30 minutes a day (most days of the week), and limiting alcohol consumption (2 drinks/day for men; 1 drink/day for women).[62] The report's guidelines recommend these lifestyle modifications for all individuals. For those people who have not achieved the goal blood pressure (< 140/90 mm Hg), antihypertensive drugs, such as thiazide-type diuretics, may also be recommended.[75]

A usual food intake in the United States, complete with convenience and fast foods, may provide 10,000–20,000 mg of sodium per day.

Cholesterol

High blood cholesterol is one of the major independent risk factors for heart disease and stroke.[3] Modifying this risk factor is effective in reducing cardiovascular disease mortality. Animal, epidemiologic, and metabolic research show that having elevated blood cholesterol levels is associated with cardiovascular disease. Despite the available recommended dietary guidelines and medications, about 45% of Americans have total blood cholesterol levels of ≥ 200 mg/dL and almost 33% have a low density lipoprotein (LDL) cholesterol of ≥ 130 mg/dL.[3] Recent data show that between 1999–2000 and 2005–2006, mean serum total cholesterol levels in adults aged 20 and older declined from 204 mg/dL to 199 mg/dL.[76]

Research from the 1980s showed that lowering high blood cholesterol significantly reduces the risk for heart attacks and reduces overall mortality rates. As a result, the National Cholesterol Education Program (NCEP) was launched in 1985.[77] Since its inception, the percentage of people who have had their cholesterol checked more than doubled,

from 35% in 1983 to 75% in 1995.[78] Current guidelines recommend that all adults age 20 or older have their blood cholesterol levels checked every five years as a preventive measure.[66] Nevertheless, over 80% of Americans who have high blood cholesterol do not have it under control.

In terms of dietary trends and blood cholesterol levels, as dietary consumption of total fat, saturated fat, and cholesterol declined in the 1980s and 1990s, average blood cholesterol levels in adults declined from 213 mg/dL in 1978 to 203 mg/dL in 1991.[77] Research shows that as little as a 10% decrease in total cholesterol levels can reduce the incidence of CHD by almost 30%.[3]

Statin drugs: These lower blood cholesterol by inhibiting 3-hydroxy-3-methylglutaryl coenzyme A reductase (HMG-CoA reductase), a liver enzyme that is responsible for producing cholesterol.

In 2001, the NCEP released updated clinical guidelines in its report of the Expert Panel on the Detection, Evaluation and Treatment of High Blood Cholesterol in Adults, referred to as the Adult Treatment Panel (ATP) III.[79] This report updated the recommendations made in ATP II and I for people with high blood cholesterol levels, and reinforces findings from studies that confirm elevated LDL cholesterol to be a major cause of CHD. The guidelines in ATP III focus on LDL-lowering cholesterol strategies and on primary prevention in persons with multiple risk factors.[80] In 2004, an update was added to the NCEP guidelines on cholesterol management that advised physicians to consider new, more intensive medical treatments, such as statin drugs for people at high and moderately high risk for a heart attack.[81]

The ATP III report recommends a complete lipoprotein profile that includes total cholesterol, LDL cholesterol, high density lipoprotein (HDL) cholesterol, and triglycerides as the preferred test rather than screening for total cholesterol and HDLs alone. For LDL-lowering therapy, a person's risk status needs to be assessed based on multiple risk factors including cigarette smoking, hypertension, low HDL, family history of premature CHD, and age. Diabetes is considered as a CHD equivalent in assessing a person's risk. In addition, the current guidelines use the Framingham scoring projections of 10-year absolute CHD risk to identify people who need more intensive therapy and those with multiple metabolic risk factors. NCEP[79] defines high-risk patients as those who have CHD, or diabetes, or multiple (≥ 2) risk factors, such as hypertension or smoking, which give them a greater than 20% chance of having a heart attack within 10 years. Very high-risk patients are those who have cardiovascular disease together with either multiple risk factors (especially diabetes), or badly controlled risk factors (e.g., smoking), or metabolic syndrome (a constellation of risk factors associated with obesity). For moderately high-risk and high-risk persons, the ATP III report and update recommend drug therapy in addition to therapeutic lifestyle changes (TLC), which include intensive use of nutrition, weight control, and physical activity.[79,81]

The specific parts of TLC include the following: reducing intakes of saturated fat to < 7% of total calories and decreasing cholesterol to < 200 mg per day. Total fat from calories can be in the 25% to 35% range, as long as saturated and *trans*-fatty acids are kept low. Individuals are encouraged to use plant stanols and sterols in their diet (2 g/day). Small amounts of plant sterols, or phytosterols, occur naturally in pine trees and foods like soybeans, nuts, grains, and oils. Increasing soluble fiber to 10 to 25 g/day is also recommended with weight reduction and increased physical activity. Because overweight and obesity are considered major underlying risk factors for CHD, weight reduction enhances LDL-lowering interventions.

In comparing the recommendations set forth in the ATP III report to the more recent updates, more intensive treatment options are delineated for very high-risk individuals. For high-risk patients, the goal in both reports remains an LDL level of < 100 mg/dL; for very high-risk patients, a therapeutic option is to treat with statins to lower levels to < 70 mg/dL. The update lowers the threshold for drug therapy to an LDL of ≥ 100 mg/dL, and recommends drug therapy for those high-risk people whose LDL is 100 to 129 mg/dL.

According to ATP III, for moderately high-risk persons, the LDL treatment goal is < 130 mg/dL and drug therapy is recommended if LDL levels are ≥ 130 mg/dL. In the update, there is a therapeutic option to set the treatment goal at LDL < 100 mg/dL and to use statin drug therapy if LDL is 100 to 129 mg/dL to reach the goal. In the update, when LDL drug therapy is used, it is advised that enough medication be used to achieve at least a 30% to 40% reduction in LDL levels. In both reports, anyone with LDL above the goal is a candidate for TLC. In the update, any person at high or moderately high risk who has lifestyle-related risk factors should follow TLC, regardless of LDL level.[79,81]

> The decision to go on drug therapy for high LDL levels is dependent on a multitude of risk factors and is decided between the physician and the patient.

As individuals learn about their risk factors and begin TLC, more registered dietitians and nutritionists will be asked to help people make necessary dietary changes. ATP III guidelines recommend that physicians refer individuals to dietitians for medical nutrition therapy.[79] At all stages in the model of TLC, the referral to a dietitian is recommended. This challenges public health providers to provide diet and exercise recommendations that will make a difference to those with elevated blood cholesterol levels. Nutritionists also need to consider prevailing eating and ethnic habits when counseling people to lower blood cholesterol levels.

In terms of adhering to the ATP III protocol guidelines (and the update), patients and healthcare providers are key players in realizing the benefits of cholesterol-lowering and in attaining the highest possible levels of CHD risk reduction. Both screening for risk factors and compliance in adopting the lipid-lowering guidelines are essential; in reality, fewer than 50% of those persons eligible for meeting the criteria actually receive treatment.[79]

Physical Activity

Research demonstrates that virtually all individuals benefit from regular physical activity. Yet, more than 60% of American adults are not regularly physically active.[82] According to recent research, the prevalence of regular leisure-time physical activity among adults is 30.8%.[46] Twenty-five percent of all adults are not active at all. Inactivity increases with age and is more common among women than men. Also, those with lower incomes and less education exercise less than those with higher incomes or education.[82] Physical inactivity thus is a prevalent risk factor in the United States. People who are sedentary are almost twice as likely to develop CHD as people who engage in regular physical activity.[80] The risk imposed by physical inactivity is almost as high as other well-known CHD risk factors, such as high blood cholesterol, high blood pressure, or smoking.[80,82] Even moderate physical activity produces significant health benefits, such as a decreased risk of CHD.[83] Research shows that moderate physical activity, such as walking 30 minutes a day 5 times a week, is more likely to be adopted and maintained than vigorous activity.[84]

There are many health benefits to be gained from regular physical activity. It enhances cardiovascular function, reduces very low density lipoprotein (VLDL) levels, raises HDL cholesterol, and can lower LDL cholesterol levels.[79] Physical activity lowers blood pressure and reduces insulin resistance. Overall, physical activity improves muscle function, cardiovascular function, and physical performance, and aids in weight management.[82] Nutritionists should become aware of the different types of physical activity, especially moderate levels of activity, that can lower an individual's risk for cardiovascular disease.

Smoking

Cigarette smoking is responsible for more than 440,000 deaths each year and is the single largest preventable cause of death and disease among U.S. adults.[85] Public health professionals, concerned about the risk factors for cardiovascular disease, need to discuss smoking with clients because it is a leading risk factor. Of the estimated 12 million deaths from smoking, almost half (5.5 million) are deaths from cardiovascular diseases.[80] In 2003, an estimated 1.1 million Americans had a new or recurrent heart attack. Cigarette smoking results in a two- to threefold risk of dying from coronary heart disease.[85] Smoking-related CHD may also contribute to congestive heart failure, causing 4.6 million to suffer from this disease.[85] Smoking approximately doubles a person's risk of stroke, which is the third leading cause of death in the United States. However, the risk of stroke decreases when an individual stops smoking. Non-smokers exposed to secondary smoke increase their risk of heart disease by 25% to 30%.[86]

Smoking cessation is also effective in preventing heart disease. In fact, after just one year of smoking abstinence, people who quit smoking have a 50% lower risk of death from CHD than those who continue to smoke.[87] Studies have shown that secondhand smoke exposure causes heart disease among adults, with an estimated 35,000 deaths each year.[85,88]

Smoking is a modifiable risk factor, and its modification is effective in preventing cardiovascular disease mortality. Smoking cessation is particularly important in people with other cardiovascular risk factors such as high blood pressure and elevated blood cholesterol, since these risk factors work synergistically. Cigarette smoking is also a risk factor for other leading causes of death and disability, including several kinds of cancer and chronic lung diseases.[85]

Trends

Progress has been made in decreasing mortality and risk factors for cardiovascular diseases. Between 1987 and 1996, the age-adjusted death rate for CHD declined by 22.2%, while deaths caused by stroke declined by 13.2%.[89] However, the HP 2010 objectives on CHD and stroke were not reached. Hypertension rates climbed from 11% to 29%. The prevalence of high blood cholesterol, however, declined from 26% to 19% between 1988 and 1994. There was a slight decline in smoking between 1995 and 1999/2000, yet deaths from smoking, poor diet, and physical inactivity still accounted for almost one-third of all deaths in the United States.[8]

Results from epidemiologic studies suggest that diets rich in fruits, vegetables, whole grains, and low-fat dairy foods are associated with a lower risk of mortality from many chronic diseases, including heart disease.[40] This nutritional pattern is supported by all of the major health organizations. Nevertheless, a large gap remains between recommended dietary patterns and what U.S. adults actually eat. Only about one-fourth of U.S. adults eat the recommended five or more servings of fruits and vegetables each day.[3] Recent research on frequency of fruit and vegetable consump-

tion shows little change from 1994 to 2000.[90] Caloric intake from total fat declined from 36% to 34% from 1976 to 1994, but fell short of the target goal of 30% set by HP 2010.[66] According to data from the National Health and Nutrition Examination Surveys, decreases in calories from dietary fat and dietary cholesterol coincided with decreases in blood cholesterol levels.[91]

From 1950 to 1996, age-adjusted death rates from cardiovascular diseases declined 60%.[89] Although this is a positive trend, other health indicators have not improved significantly. Increasing prevalence rates in obesity and the continued high levels of blood pressure and stroke pose a continued public health challenge.[89]

Cancer

Cancer is an umbrella term used to describe a large group of diseases characterized by uncontrolled growth and spread of abnormal cells.[43] Cancer is the second leading cause of death in the United States, causing one in every four deaths. In 2006, an estimated 560,000 Americans died from this disease.[3] According to the American Cancer Society about one-third of cancer deaths are preventable, and are attributed to dietary factors, physical inactivity, overweight, or obesity.[43] For U.S. adults who don't smoke, dietary choices and physical activity are the most modifiable determinants of cancer risk. All cancers caused by cigarettes and the heavy use of alcohol could be prevented. The National Cancer Institute estimates that about 9.6 million Americans who had been diagnosed with cancer at some point in their life were alive in 2000.[43] This estimate includes people living with cancer and those who were cancer-free.[92] The five-year relative survival rate for all cancers is 63%, or about 6 in 10 persons, which represents people who are living five years after diagnosis of cancer.[43]

Age-standardized death rates from all cancers decreased by 7.2% between 1991 and 2000.[92] Compared to the peak rate of 215.1 deaths per 100,000 in 1991, the cancer death rate decreased 16% in 180.7 to 2006. Despite this decrease in the death rate from cancer, the total number of people who develop or die from cancer each year continues to increase because of our aging population.[93] The overall decrease in death rates from cancer is due to a decline in smoking and more effective detection and screening. The recent decrease in deaths from breast cancer in Caucasian women, for example, is due to a greater use of breast screening in regular medical care. Cancer death rates vary by gender, race, and ethnicity. For example, African Americans are more likely to die from cancer than are Caucasians.[94]

Although inherited genes play a significant role in cancer risk, they only explain part of all cancer incidences.[43] Most of the variation in cancer incidence cannot be explained by inherited factors. The predominant causes of cancer are external factors such as cigarette smoking, diet or nutrition, weight, and physical activity.[43,94] These factors act to modify the risk of cancer at all stages. It is estimated that more than 50% of all cancers could be prevented through dietary improvements, such as reducing total fat and increasing fruit and vegetable consumption, and smoking cessation.[85,95] Doll and Peto[96] estimated that about 10% to 70% of deaths from cancer were attributable to diet. However, recent evidence showing actual causes of death in the United States found that 14% of cancer deaths occurring in 1990 could be attributed to diet.[97] The science of nutrition and cancer is evolving, but still is not as developed as that of diet and cardiovascular disease. Many large-scale studies are currently underway to further elucidate the relationship between various nutrients and cancer.[97] Future research points to the areas of diet and gene interactions, and biomarkers for cancer that will further our understanding in this area.[98]

Current dietary recommendations are based on evidence from the American Cancer Society, the American Institute of Cancer Research/World Cancer Research Fund, and the Harvard Cancer Prevention Study.[43,99,100] In 2001, the American Cancer Society updated its guidelines on nutrition and physical activity after reviewing current scientific evidence.[101] In general, the current dietary guidelines support the existing 2005 and 2010 Dietary Guidelines for Americans, and also encourage the consumption of plant-based diets, without relying on processed foods. The guidelines endorse eating a diet that promotes healthy weight control along with physical activity.[43,100] For cancer prevention, the ACS recommends that individuals eat five or more servings of fruits and vegetables a day. Fruit and vegetable consumption may protect against cancers of the mouth and pharynx, esophagus, lung, stomach, colon, and rectum.[102] In 2007, about one in four adults was eating the recommended amount; however, little improvement in U.S. fruit and vegetable consumption has occurred since the mid-1990s. Specifically, nutrition and food scientists agree on the following recommendations to lower cancer risk[43,102]:

- Eat a plant-based diet that includes a wide variety of fruits, vegetables, whole grains, beans, and legumes. The recommendation is to choose whole grains over refined sources, and eat three to five servings of vegetables and two to four servings of fruits per day.
- Eat less fat from all food sources.
- Limit excess calories and maintain a healthful weight throughout life. Eat a sound diet and incorporate mod-erate or vigorous physical activity five days a week or more to further reduce risks of cancer.
- If you drink alcohol, do so in moderation.

Nutrition supplements are not universally recommended for cancer prevention. Instead, the cancer-prevention benefits of diet are considered among the best due to the interactions of many vitamins, minerals, and other plant-derived substances found naturally occurring in foods.[43,99,102] However, the possible benefits of supplemental folate, calcium, and selenium are noted.[43,101] By eating whole foods and following the cancer-prevention dietary recommendations along with physical activity, the protection of the body's cells may take place during the initiation, promotion, and progression stages of cancer. These food substances may repair damage that has already occurred in cells. Some studies suggest that individuals do not need to be concerned about the pesticide residues on fruits and vegetables, because the benefits of eating fruits and vegetables far outweigh any potential risk.[99] More long-term studies may help to confirm this definitively.

The study of diet and cancer prevention is relatively new. Dietitians and other public healthcare professionals need to stay abreast of these discoveries in order to give appropriate guidance to individuals at risk. The basis of MNT should include those recommendations set forth by the American Cancer Society and the World Cancer Research Fund/American Institute for Cancer Research.[43,99,102]

Diabetes

Diabetes is a serious, costly, and increasingly common chronic disease that poses a significant public health challenge. In 2003–2004, diabetes was the sixth leading cause of death in the United States.[103] About 18 million Americans have diabetes, and over 5 million of these people are unaware that they have the disease.[3] Type-2 diabetes used to be called adult-onset diabetes and may account for about 90% to 95% of all diagnosed cases of diabetes.[104] The total prevalence of diabetes in the United States is expected to more than double from 2005 to 2050: from 5.6% to 12%.[105] By 2050, an estimated 29 million Americans are expected to have been diagnosed with diabetes. The increase in the number of cases has been particularly high within certain ethnic and racial groups in the United States.[106]

Medical complications of type-2 diabetes include heart disease, kidney failure, leg and foot amputations, and blindness. Each year about 12,000 to 24,000 people become blind because of diabetic eye disease.[3] The majority of the deaths caused by diabetes are due to diabetes-associated cardiovascular disease. The presence of diabetes in adults is associated with a two- to fourfold increase in CHD compared to non-diabetic adults. Almost three-quarters of adults with diabetes have hypertension.[3] Diabetes is the cause of 44% of end-stage renal disease cases. Severe forms of nervous system damage occur in 60% to 70% of diabetic adults. Approximately 60% of all non-traumatic amputations in the United States occur in people with diabetes.[107] Periodontal or gum disease is also more common among diabetics. As a result, diabetes is a costly disease, with the total attributable costs (direct and indirect) estimated at $174 billion annually.[107,108]

Type-2 diabetes is associated with the following factors:

- *Age:* Diabetes is most common in people over 60 years of age.[107]
- *Ethnicity:* Deaths from diabetes are twice as high for African Americans than for Caucasians; Native Americans, Hispanic Americans, and certain Pacific Islander American and Asian American populations also have higher rates.[106]
- *Genetics and family history:* Genetic markers that indicate a greater risk for type-2 diabetes have been identified.
- *Obesity:* The increased prevalence of obesity among adults is positively associated with the increased rates of diabetes.[109] Data from clinical trials strongly support the potential of moderate weight loss to reduce the risk of type-2 diabetes.[110]
- *History of gestational diabetes in women:* Gestational diabetes is a form of glucose intolerance that develops in some women during pregnancy. Obesity is associated with gestational diabetes. Women with a family history of gestational diabetes and Hispanic-American and African-American women are at an increased risk.[111]
- *Impaired glucose metabolism:* People with prediabetes, or who are at increased risk of developing diabetes, have impaired fasting blood glucose. Research studies suggest that weight loss and increased physical activity among people with prediabetes may return glucose levels to normal and prevent the onset of diabetes.[106]
- *Physical inactivity:* If you are at higher risk and fairly inactive, or exercise fewer than three times a week, you are more likely to develop type-2 diabetes.

In the United States, recent lifestyle changes such as decreased physical activity and increased energy consumption, which contribute to the increased prevalence rates of obesity, are also strong risk factors for diabetes.[110] On the other hand, positive lifestyle changes such as diet, weight loss of 5% to 7%, and moderate-intensity physical activity (e.g., walking 30 minutes a day) can delay the onset of diabetes. The Diabetes Prevention Program,[110] a major, large-scale study of over 3,000 people at high risk for developing diabetes, confirmed this, and found a 58% reduction in the development of diabetes over a three-year period. The findings from this study, sponsored by the NIH, showed that exercise, a healthy diet, and weight loss can reduce the risk of developing diabetes by as much as 71% in high-risk individuals.[110]

Medical nutrition therapy is an essential part of diabetes management for adults. Its objectives include[111]:

- Attaining and maintaining optimal metabolic outcomes including normalizing blood glucose levels, maintaining a lipid profile that reduces vascular disease risk, and normalizing blood pressure levels
- Preventing, delaying, and treating the onset complications by modifying nutrient intake and lifestyle to prevent and treat obesity, cardiovascular disease, hypertension, and nephropathy
- Optimizing health through sensible food choices and physical activity
- Addressing personal and cultural preferences as well as lifestyle factors, including a person's willingness to change, when determining individual nutritional needs

In terms of specific nutrients and dietary recommendations for type-2 diabetes, studies in healthy subjects and those at risk for type-2 diabetes support the importance of including foods containing complex carbohydrates in the diet, particularly those from whole grains, fruits, vegetables, and low-fat milk.[111] Reduced intake of total fat, especially saturated fat, may reduce the risk of diabetes.

In summary, lifestyle changes such as reduced energy intake, increased physical activity, and nutrition education (with the goal of promoting weight loss) represent essential aspects of type-2 diabetes management for adults. HP 2010[107] discusses the challenges of diabetes and the preventive interventions aimed at them: primary prevention, screening and early diagnosis, access, and quality of care. This includes secondary and tertiary prevention, such as glucose control and decreasing complications from diabetes.[107] As dietitians, public health professionals, and educators, many opportunities exist to contribute to the effective management of diabetes.

Osteoporosis

As one grows, bones develop and become larger, heavier, and denser. At approximately age 30 years peak bone mass is achieved in both men and women. After this time period, adults begin to lose bone mass, and this continues as they get older. Osteoporosis (i.e., porous bone disease) develops when bone loss reaches the point of causing fractures under common, everyday stresses. Due to increased bone fragility, there is a greater susceptibility to fractures of the hip, spine, and wrist. Both men and women suffer from osteoporosis.

Osteoporosis currently affects 44 million Americans, or 55% of people aged 50 and older; 68% of women over 50 have the disease.[112,113] These rates correspond to one in two women and one in four men (aged ≥ 50) who will experience an osteoporosis-related fracture in their lifetime.[112] Osteoporosis causes significant disability with important economic consequences, costing about $19 billion each year in direct expenditures (hospitals and nursing homes).[114] By 2025, experts predict that these costs will rise to about 25.3 billion.[113] Of the 2 million fractures occurring each year due to osteoporosis, over 300,000 are hip fractures, 547,000 are vertebral fractures, and 450,000 are wrist fractures. Of the 300,000 annual hip fractures, 24% result in death following complications from the fracture.[113]

Osteoporosis is often called the "silent disease" because it can occur without any overt symptoms. The technical standard for measuring bone mineral density is dual-energy x-ray absorptiometry (DXA). A low bone mass density is a strong predictor of fracture risk.[113] Bone density tests can detect osteoporosis before a fracture occurs and they can serve as a predictor for future fracture risks.

The chances of developing osteoporosis are greatest in white women beyond menopause. Women have less bone tissue and lose bone more easily than men due to the hormonal changes involved in menopause. Those individuals who have a low dietary intake of calcium and vitamin D over a lifetime, and who are physically inactive, cigarette smokers, excessive alcohol drinkers, thin and small-framed, and who have a family history of osteoporosis are at increased risk.[112,113] White and Asian American women are at highest risk, whereas African-American and Hispanic-American women have lower risks.[113] Excessive intake of protein, sodium, and caffeine also contribute to being at risk for osteoporosis. Anorexia nervosa, the use of certain medications, and low testosterone levels in men are risk factors for osteoporosis.

The five factors that can be modified to prevent osteoporosis are: 1) a diet rich in calcium and vitamin D; 2) weight-bearing exercise; 3) a healthy lifestyle that excludes smoking and excessive alcohol intake; 4) routine bone density measurements; and 5) the use of medication, when appropriate.[113]

Nutrition is an important modifiable risk factor in terms of both bone health and the prevention and treatment of osteoporosis. An adequate amount of calcium and vitamin D contributes significantly to bone health. Low calcium and vitamin D intakes are associated with low bone mass, rapid bone loss, and high fracture rates.[115] Bone is a living, growing tissue, and 99% of the body's calcium is found in bone. Throughout one's lifetime, bone formation and resorption occurs. This process, which is known as *bone turnover*, is responsive to dietary calcium regardless of age. Dietary calcium works to strengthen bone by suppressing bone resorption and parathyroid hormone.[115]

According to the *NIH Consensus Statement on Osteoporosis*,[114] calcium is the most important nutrient for the prevention of osteoporosis. Actual calcium intakes for most of the U.S. population, however, are considerably lower than the current Dietary Reference Intakes (DRI).[116] Many studies have shown that adult skeletal health is improved by increasing dairy foods or calcium intake in the diet.[117] The DASH diet, used to treat hypertension, is a low-fat diet, rich in calcium, that has been shown to reduce bone turnover and reduce the risk of osteoporosis.[70] Calcium requirements can be met with low-fat dairy products; however, low consumption of milk and other dairy products in the U.S. diet is mainly responsible for low calcium intakes among U.S. adults.[117] Other foods contain calcium, such as dark leafy greens, but these usually provide less calcium per serving than milk, and most Americans do not eat these vegetables often. For individuals who do not consume enough calcium in their diets, calcium supplements are recommended.

Vitamin D also plays an important role in calcium absorption and bone health. Vitamin D is a major determinant of intestinal calcium absorption. When skin is exposed to sunlight, the body synthesizes vitamin D. However, studies show decreased production of vitamin D in the elderly and individuals who are housebound, especially in the winter months.[112] Due to inadequate intake of vitamin D in a high proportion of older adults, the most recent DRI have increased the vitamin D requirements for people 50 years and older.[116] Low-fat and nonfat milk, excellent sources of calcium, are fortified with 100 IU of Vitamin D per serving.

In conclusion, osteoporosis is a serious public health disease and is largely preventable. Starting early in life, both females and males should be advised on how to incorporate sources of calcium into their diets. The use of low-fat and nonfat dairy foods should be recommended, and if persons can't consume dairy products, other food sources and calcium supplements are necessary. Adequate vitamin D intake needs to be addressed, as well. Public health nutritionists should encourage individuals to participate regularly in physical activity. Modifiable lifestyle factors should be discussed to promote bone health throughout life.

> For those living in colder climates without much sunshine, vitamin D supplementation is suggested to accompany calcium intake.

Acquired Immune Deficiency Syndrome (AIDS)

In 1981, a new infectious disease, acquired immune deficiency syndrome (AIDS), was first identified in the United States. A few years later, human immunodeficiency virus (HIV) was identified as the viral agent that causes AIDS. HIV/AIDS has affected almost every ethnic, socioeconomic, and age group in the United States.[118]

AIDS, a deadly disease, is the end stage of HIV infection. The infection progresses to overwhelm the immune system and leaves individuals defenseless against numerous other infections and diseases. HIV is spread through direct contact with contaminated body fluids, sexual intercourse, direct blood contact, or from mother to infant. In 1996, death rates from AIDS in the United States declined for the first time.[118] Nevertheless, HIV/AIDS remains a significant cause of illness, disability, and death in the United States. According to the Centers for Disease Control and Prevention (CDC)[118] in 2006, the estimated number of diagnosed AIDS cases was about 1,106,000. Death rates have dropped dramatically in the United States due to the introduction of antiretroviral therapies.[118]

Health complications for people with HIV/AIDS are immune dysfunction and its associated complications, which include malnutrition and wasting. HIV targets the immune system, rendering an individual susceptible to infections and disease. The CDC defines the AIDS-related wasting syndrome as a 10% weight loss in a six-month period accompanied by diarrhea or fever for more than 30 days.[119] Malnutrition and its complications can reduce one's tolerance to medications and other therapies. Malnutrition occurs in the form of tissue wasting, fat accumulation, increased lipid levels, and risk of other chronic disease. The American Dietetic Association's (ADA) *Position Paper*[120] strongly supports nutrition evaluation and medical nutrition therapy as parts of the ongoing health care of HIV-infected individuals. In terms of medical nutrition therapy, this includes early assessment and treatment of nutrient deficiencies, the maintenance and restoration of lean body mass, and continued support for performing daily activities and maintaining quality of life. According to the ADA, nutrition education and guidance should incorporate the following aspects[120]:

- Healthful eating principles
- Water and food safety issues
- Perinatal and breastfeeding issues
- Nutrition management for symptoms such as anorexia, swallowing problems, diarrhea, and so on
- Food–medicine interactions
- Psychosocial and economic issues
- Alternative feeding methods (supplementation, tube feeding, or parenteral nutrition)
- Additional therapies, including physical activity and disease management

- Guidelines for evaluating nutrition information, diet claims, and individual mineral and vitamin supplementation
- Strategies for treatment of altered fat metabolism

In addition, it is important for an HIV-infected individual to have adequate access to food, health care, and other support systems. The maintenance and restoration of nutrition stores are interrelated with recommended medical therapies; therefore, it is essential that a public health nutritionist be an active participant in the healthcare team to provide optimal medical nutrition therapy.

Issues for Discussion

1. What would you propose should be incorporated into public health programs that focus on nutrition as an important preventive factor in illness, disability, and death?

2. What advice would you give to the individual in the community with regard to preventing chronic disease risk factors such as obesity, physical inactivity, and smoking in order to reduce society's financial burden?

3. What proportion of public funds designated for nutrition services should be given for primary, secondary, and tertiary prevention versus acute medical care?

4. Programs such as for-profit weight loss centers proliferate in this country. What are positive and negative aspects of this trend compared with public health weight management programs?

References

1. Frazao E. The high costs of poor eating patterns in the U.S. In: Frazao E., ed. *America's Eating Habits: Changes and Consequences*. Washington, DC: U.S. Department of Agriculture (USDA), Economic Research Service (ERS), AIB-750; 1999.

2. U.S. Department of Health and Human Services. *Healthy People 2010: Understanding and Improving Health*, 2nd ed. Washington, DC: U.S. Government Printing Office; 2000.

3. McRobbie MA, Kolbe LJ. The academy's pivotal role in supporting public-private partnerships to prevent chronic diseases. *Prev Chronic Dis*. 2009;6:A73.

4. Centers for Disease Control and Prevention, National Center for Health Statistics. Effectiveness in disease and injury prevention; estimated national spending on prevention. U.S., 1988. *MMWR Morbid Mortal Wkly Rep*. 1992;41:529–531.

5. Deaths: preliminary data for 2004. *National Vital Statistics Report*. 2006;June 28:54.

6. Krauss RM, Eckel RH, Howard B, et al. AHA dietary guidelines: revision 2000: a statement for healthcare professionals from the Nutrition Committee of the American Heart Association. *Circulation*. 2000;102:2284–2299.

7. National Center for Health Statistics. *Health, U.S., 2003.* Washington, DC: U.S. Government Printing Office; 2003.

8. Mokdad AH, Marks JS, Stroup DF, Gerberding JL. Actual causes of death in the U.S., 2000. *JAMA.* 2004;291:1238–1245.

9. Mokdad AH, Marks JS, Stroup DF, Gerberding JL. Correction: Actual causes of death in the U.S., 2000. *JAMA.* 2005;293:293–294.

10. Department of Health and Human Services, Centers for Disease Control and Prevention. *Health, U.S., 2002.* DHHS Publication No. 1232. Rockville, MD: Department of Health and Human Services, Centers for Disease Control and Prevention; 2002.

11. Koplan JP, Dietz WH. Caloric imbalance and public health policy. *JAMA.* 1999;282:1579–1581.

12. National Center for Health Statistics (NCHS). Report of the final mortality statistics,1995. *Monthly Vital Statistics Report.* 1997;5(suppl. 2).

13. U.S. Department of Health and Human Service (USDHHS), Office of the Surgeon General (OSG) (2006). The health consequences of involuntary exposure to tobacco smoke: A report of the Surgeon General 2006. Available at http://www.surgeongeneral.gov/library/secondhandsmoke/. Accessed June 15, 2009.

14. Elo SL, Caltrop JB. Health promotive action and preventive action model (HPA model) for the classification of healthcare services in public health nursing. *Scand J Public Health.* 2002;30:200–208.

15. Wimbush FB, Peters RM. Identification of cardiovascular risk: use of a cardiovascular-specific genogram. *Public Health Nurs.* 2000;17:148–154.

16. U.S. Preventive Services Task Force. *Guide to Clinical Preventive Services,* 3rd ed. Washington, DC: U.S. Department of Health and Human Services; 2003.

17. Kaufman M, ed. *Nutrition in Public Health: A Handbook for Developing Programs and Services.* Rockville, MD: Aspen Publishers; 1990.

18. Shamansky SL, Clausen C. Levels of prevention: examination of the concept. *Nurs Outlook.* 1980;28:104–108.

19. Position of the American Dietetic Association: the role of nutrition in health promotion and disease prevention programs. *J Am Diet Assoc.* 1998;98:205–208.

20. Brunner E, White I, Thorogood M, Bristow A, Curle D, Marmot M. Can dietary interventions change diet and cardiovascular risk factors? A meta-analysis of randomized controlled trials. *Am J Public Health.* 1997;87:1415–1422.

21. Dietary Guidelines Advisory Committee. *Report of the Dietary Guidelines Advisory Committee on the Dietary Guidelines for Americans, 2000.* Washington, DC: U.S. Department of Agriculture; 2000.

22. U.S. Departments of Agriculture and Health and Human Services. *The Food Guide Pyramid.* Home and Garden Bulletin, No. 249. Washington, DC: U.S. Departments of Agriculture, Health and Human Services; 1992.

23. Dietary Guidelines Alliance. Do it yourself: crafting consumer tips. In: *Reaching Consumers with Meaningful Health Messages.* Washington, DC: Dietary Guidelines Alliance; 1996.

24. Position of the American Dietetic Association: nutrition education for the public. *J Am Diet Assoc.* 1996;96:1183–1187.

25. American Dietetic Association and the Office of Disease Prevention and Health Promotion, Public Health Service, U.S. Department of Health and Human Services. *Worksite Nutrition; A Guide to Planning, Implementation, and Evaluation,* 2nd ed. Chicago, IL: American Dietetic Association; 1993.

26. Goldberg JP. Nutrition and health communication: the message and the media over half a century. *Nutr Rev.* 1992;50:71–77.

27. Pender NJ. *Health Promotion in Nursing Practice,* 3rd ed. Stamford, CT: Appelton-Lange; 1996.

28. Sharlin J, Posner BM, Gershoff S, Zeitlin M, Berger P. Nutrition and behavioral characteristics and determinants of cholesterol levels in men and women. *J Am Diet Assoc.* 1992;92:434–440.

29. Resnicow K, Orlandi M, Vaccaro D, Wynder E. Implementation of a pilot school-site cholesterol reduction intervention. *J School Health.* 1989;59:74–78.

30. U.S. Department of Health and Human Services, Centers for Disease Control and Prevention, National Center for Health Statistics. *National Health Interview Survey (NHIS);* 2003.

31. U.S. Department of Health and Human Services. National Heart, Lung, and Blood Institute (NHLBI). *National High Blood Pressure Education Program.* Available at http://www.nhlbi.nih.gov/about/nhbpep. Accessed April 22, 2010.

32. Centers for Disease Control and Prevention, National Center for Chronic Disease Prevention and Health Promotion, USDHHS. *Preventing Heart Disease and Stroke, Addressing the Nation's Leading Killers.* At-a-Glance Summary Tables. American Heart Association; 2009.

33. Kannel WB, Dawber TR, McGee DL. Perspectives of systolic hypertension, the Framingham Study. *Circulation.* 1980;61:1179–1182.

34. America on the Move. Available at http://www.americaonthemove.org. Accessed April 22, 2010.

35. National Academy of Sciences, National Research Council, Food and Nutrition Board. *Diet and Health: Implications for Reducing Chronic Disease Risk.* Washington, DC: National Academy Press; 1989.

36. The dietary guidelines: Surveillance issues and research needs. *J Nutr* (supplement: AICR 11th Annual Research Conference on Diet, Nutrition and Cancer). 2001;131(suppl 2):3154S–3155S.

37. Kris-Etherton P, Daniels SR, Eckel RH, et al. Summary of the scientific conference on dietary fatty acids and cardiovascular health. Conference summary from the Nutrition Committee of the American Heart Association. *Circulation.* 2001;103:1034–1039.

38. American Institute of Cancer Research. Available at http://www.aicr.org. Accessed on April 22, 2010.

39. Position of The American Dietetic Association and the Dietitians of Canada: nutrition and women's health. *J Am Diet Assoc.* 2004;104:984–1001.

40. McCullough ML, Feskanich D, Stampfer MJ, et al. Diet quality and major chronic disease in men and women: moving toward improved dietary guidance. *Am J Clin Nutr.* 2002;76:1261–1271.

41. American Heart Association. AHA Comment, May 31, 2004. *Health agencies applaud HHS/USDA new dietary guidelines.*

42. Eyre H, Kahn R, Robertson RM. Preventing cancer, cardiovascular disease, and diabetes. *Diabetes Care.* 2004;27:1812–1824.

43. American Cancer Society (ACS). *Cancer Statistics, 2009.* Atlanta, GA: ACS; 2009.

44. U.S. Department of Agriculture. *USDA Continuing Survey of Food Intakes by Individuals (CSFII), 1994–1996.* Washington, DC: USDA; 1998.

45. U.S. Department of Agriculture. *News release: scientific update of food guidance presented to the Dietary Guidelines Committee,* January 28, 2004.

46. U.S. Department of Health and Human Services (USDHHS), Centers for Disease Control and Prevention (CDC), National Center for Health Statistics (2007). Obesity among adults in the US—nonstatistically significant change since 2003–2004. Data brief no. 1, Nov 2007, 8 pp. Available at http://www.cdc.gov/nchs/data/databriefs/db01.pdf. Accessed April 22, 2010.

47. National Institutes of Health, National Heart, Lung, and Blood Institute. *Clinical Guidelines on the Identification, Evaluation, and Treatment of Overweight and Obesity in Adults.* Washington, DC: U.S. DHHS, Public Health Service;1998; xxiii.

48. Ogden CL, Carroll MD, and Flegal KM. High Body mass index for age among US children and adolescents, 2003-2006. *JAMA.* 2008;299:2401–2405.

49. U.S. Department of Health and Human Services. *Healthy People 2010: Understanding and Improving Health*, 2nd ed. Washington, DC: U.S. Government Printing Office; 2000: Chapt 19, Nutrition and Overweight: 19-3-19-9.

50. U.S. Department of Health and Human Services, Public Health Service, Office of the Surgeon General. *Surgeon General's Call to Action to Prevent and Decrease Overweight and Obesity*. Washington, DC: U.S. DHHS; 2001.

51. Finkelstein EA, Flebelkorn IC, Wang G. National medical spending attribuatable to overweight and obesity: how much and who's paying. *Health Aff.* 2003;W3:219–226.

52. Mokdad AH, Bowman BA, Ford ES, Vinicor F, Macks JS, Koplan JC. The continuing epidemics of obesity and diabetes in the U.S. *JAMA.* 2001;286:1195–1200.

53. Flegal KM, Carroll MD, Ogden CL, Johnson CL. Prevalence and trends of obesity among U.S. adults, 1999–2000. *JAMA.* 2002;288:1723–1727.

54. Kuczmarski RJ, Flegal KM. Criteria for definition of overweight in transition: background and recommendations for the U.S. *Am J Clin Nutr.* 2000;72:1074–1081.

55. Position of the American Dietetic Association: weight management. *J Am Diet Assoc.* 2002;102:1145–1155.

56. Kassiger JP, Angell M. Losing weight—an ill-fated New Year's resolution. *N Eng J Med.* 1998;338:52–54.

57. National Institutes of Health and National Heart, Lung, and Blood Institute. Clinical guidelines on the identification, evaluation, and treatment of overweight and obesity in adults—the evidence report. *Obesity Res.* 1998;6:1105–1110.

58. Pavlou KN, Krey S, Stefee WO. Exercise as an adjunct to weight-loss and maintenance in moderately obese subjects. *Am J Clin Nutr.* 1989;49:1115–1123.

59. NIH Technology Assessment Conference Panel. Methods for voluntary weight loss and control. Consensus development conference. March 30–April 1, 1992. *Ann Intern Med.* 1993; 119:764–770.

60. Jeffrey RW, Drewsiowski A, Epstein LH, et al. Long-term maintenance of weight-loss: current status. *Health Psychology.* 2000;1(suppl):5–16.

61. American Heart Association. *Heart Disease and Stroke Statistics: 2009 Update*. Dallas, TX: American Heart Association; 2009.

62. U.S. Department of Health and Human Services, NIH, NHLBI, NHBPEP, JCN 7 Express. *The Seventh Report of the Joint National Committee on Prevention, Detection, Evaluation, and Treatment of High Blood Pressure*. NIH Pub. No. 03-5233. Bethesda MD, National Institutes of Health; 2003.

63. Systolic Hypertension in the Elderly Program (SHEP) Cooperative Research Group. Prevention of stroke by antihypertensive drug treatment in older persons with isolated systolic hypertension. Final results of the SHEP. *JAMA.* 1991;265:3255–3264.

64. National Heart, Lung, and Blood Institute. *Morbidity and Mortality: 1998 Chartbook of Cardiovascular, Lung, and Blood Diseases*. Bethesda, MD: Public Health Service, National Institutes of Health, NHLBI; 1998.

65. American Heart Association. Heart Disease and Stroke Statistics: 2009 Update; 2009. Available at http://www.americanheart.org/presenter.jhtml?identifier=3037327. Accessed April 22, 2010.

66. U.S. Department of Health and Human Services. *Healthy People 2010: Understanding and Improving Health*, 2nd ed. Washington, DC: U.S. DHHS; 2000; Chapter 12-Heart Disease and Stroke: 12-3–12-33.

67. National Heart, Lung, and Blood Institute (NHLBI). *National High Blood Pressure Education Program, Program Description*.

68. The Trials of Hypertension Prevention Collaborative Research Group. Effects of weight-loss and sodium reduction intervention on blood pressure and hypertension incidence in overweight people with high-normal blood pressure. The Trials of Hypertension Prevention, Phase 11. *Arch Intern Med.* 1997;157:657–667.

69. He J, Whelton PK, Appel LJ, Charleston J, Klag MJ. Long-term effects of weight-loss and dietary sodium restriction on incidence of hypertension. *Hypertension.* 2000;35:544–549.

70. Sacks FM, Syerkey LP, Vollmer WM, et al. Effects on blood pressure of reduced dietary sodium and Dietary Approaches to Stop Hypertension (DASH) diet. DASH-Sodium Collaborative Research Group. *N Engl J Med.* 2001;344:3–10.

71. Chobanian AV, Hill M. National Heart, Lung, and Blood Institute Workshop on Sodium and Blood Pressure: a critical review of current scientific evidence. *Hypertension.* 2000;35:858–863.

72. Whelton SP, Chin A, Xin X, He J. Effect of aerobic exercise on blood pressure: a meta-analysis of randomized, controlled trials. *Ann Intern Med.* 2002;136:493–503.

73. Xin X, He J, Frontini MG, et al. Effects of alcohol reduction on blood pressure. A meta-analysis of randomized controlled trials. *Hypertension.* 2001;38:1112–1117.

74. Vollmer WM, Sacks FM, Ard J, et al. Effects of diet and sodium intake on blood pressure. Subgroup analysis of the DASH-sodium trial. *Ann Intern Med.* 2001;135:1019–1028.

75. Psatsy BM, Smith NL, Siscovick DS, et al. Health outcomes associated with antihypertensive therapies used as first-line agents. A systematic review and meta-analysis. *JAMA.* 1997;277:739–745.

76. National Center for Health Statistics (NCHS). High serum total cholesterol—an indicator for monitoring cholesterol-lowering efforts; US adults, 2005-06. NCHS Data brief no. 2; 2007.

77. Cleeman JL, Lenfant C. The National Cholesterol Education Program: progress and prospects. *JAMA.* 1998;280:2099–2104.

78. National Heart, Lung, and Blood Institute. *Consumer Awareness Surveys*. Press conference. Bethesda, MD: NHLBI; December 4, 1995.

79. U.S. Department of Health and Human Services, NHLBI. *National Cholesterol Education Program, Third Report of the Expert Panel on the Detection, Evaluation, and Treatment of High Blood Cholesterol in Adults (Adult Treatment Panel III)*. NIH Pub. No. 01-367. Bethesda, MD: National Institutes of Health; 2001.

80. U.S. Department of Health and Human Services. *Healthy People 2010: Understanding and Improving Health*, 2nd ed. Washington, DC: U.S. DHHS; 2000: 22-Physical activity and fitness. Bethesda, MD; Chapt 22: 22-3–22-36.

81. Grundy SM, Cleeman JI, Barrey Merz CN, et al. For the coordinating committee of the National Cholesterol Education Program. Implications of recent clinical trials for the National Cholesterol Education Program Adult Treatment Panel III Guidelines. *Circulation.* 2004;110:227–239.

82. U.S. Department of Health and Human Services. *Physical activity and health: a report of the Surgeon General, 1996*. Atlanta, GA: Centers for Disease Control and Prevention, National Center for Chronic Disease Prevention and Health Promotion; 1996.

83. NIH Consensus Development Panel on Physical Activity and Cardiovascular Health. Physical activity and cardiovascular health. *JAMA.* 1996;276:241–246.

84. Pate RR, Pratt M, Blair SN, et al. Physical activity and public health: a recommendation from the Centers for Disease Control and Prevention and the American College of Sports Medicine. *JAMA.* 1995;273:402–407.

85. U.S. Department of Health and Human Services. *The Health Consequences of Smoking: A Report of the Surgeon General, 2004*. Atlanta, GA: Centers for Disease Control and Prevention, National Center for Chronic Disease Prevention and Health Promotion, Office on Smoking and Health; 2004.

86. U.S. Department of Health and Human Services. The health consequences of involuntary exposure to tobacco smoke: a report of the Surgeon General; 2006. Available at http://www.surgeongeneral.gov/library/secondhandsmoke/. Accessed April 22, 2010.

87. U.S. Department of Health and Human Services. *The Health Benefits of Smoking Cessation: A Report of the Surgeon General, 1990*. Atlanta, GA: U.S. DHHS, CDC, Center for Chronic Disease Prevention and Health Promotion, Office on Smoking and Health; 1990.

88. Glanz SA, Parmely WW. Passive smoking and heart disease: mechanism and risk. *JAMA*. 1995;272:1047–1053.

89. Centers for Disease Control and Prevention. Decline in deaths from heart disease and stroke—United States, 1990–1999. *MMWR Morbid Mortal Wkly Rep*. 1999;48:649–656.

90. Serdula MK, Gillespie C, Kettel-Khan L, Farris R, Seymour J, Denny C. Trends in fruit and vegetable consumption among adults in the U.S.: Behavioral Risk Factor Surveillance System, 1994–2000. *Am J Public Health*. 2004;94:1014–1018.

91. Ernst ND, Sempos ST, Briefel RR, Clark MB. Consistency between U.S. dietary fat intake and serum total cholesterol concentrations; the National Health and Nutrition Examination Surveys. *Am J Clin Nutr*. 1997;66:965S–972S.

92. Ries L, Eisner M, Kosary C, et al. *SEER: Cancer Statistics Review, 1975–2000*. National Cancer Institute; 2003.

93. Stewart SL, King JB, Thompson TD, Friedman C, Wingo P. Cancer mortality surveillance—U.S., 1990–2000. National Center for Chronic Disease Prevention and Health Promotion. *MMWR Morbid Mortal Wkly Rep*. 2004;53(suppl 503):1–108.

94. Key TJ, Allen NE, Spencer EA, Travis RC. The effect of diet on risk of cancer. *Lancet*. 2002;360:861–868.

95. Willett, W. Diet and nutrition. In: Schottenfield D., Frammeni JF Jr, eds. *Cancer Epidemiology and Prevention*, 2nd ed. New York: Oxford University Press; 1996: 438–461.

96. Doll R, Peto R. The causes of cancer: qualitative estimates of avoidable risks of cancer in the U.S. today. *J Natl Cancer Inst*. 1981;66:1191–1308.

97. McGinnis JM, Forge WH: Actual causes of death in the U.S. *JAMA*. 1993;270:2207–2212.

98. Mandelson MT, Oestreicher N, Porter PL, et al. Breast density as a predictor of mammographic detection: comparison of interval- and screen-detected cancers. *J Natl Canc Inst*. 2000;92:1081–1087.

99. American Institute of Cancer Research. Available at http://www.aicr.org. Accessed April 22, 2010.

100. FANSA. Statement on Diet and Cancer Prevention in the U.S. Available at http://www.eatright.org. Accessed July 7, 2009.

101. Byers T, Nestle M, McTiernan A, et al. American Cancer Society guidelines on nutrition and physical activity for cancer prevention: reducing the risk of cancer with healthy food choices and physical activity. *CA Cancer J Clin*. 2002;52:92–111.

102. American Cancer Society (ACS). Cancer Statistics 2009. Atlanta, GA: ACS;2009.

103. National Vital Statistics Report. *Deaths: Preliminary data for 2004*. November 20, 2007.

104. National Institutes of Health, National Institute of Diabetes and Digestive and Kidney Diseases. Diabetes Prevention Program.

105. Narayan KM, Boyle JP, Geiss MA, et al. Impact of recent increase on incidence on future diabetes burden US, 2005–2050. *Diabetes Care*. 2006;29:2114–2116.

106. Centers for Disease Control and Prevention. *National Diabetes Fact Sheet: General Information and National Estimates on Diabetes in the U.S., 2003*, rvsd ed. Atlanta, GA: U.S. Dept. of Health and Human Services, Centers for Disease Control and Prevention; 2004.

107. U.S. Department of Health and Human Services. *Healthy People 2010: Understanding and Improving Health*. 2nd ed. Washington, DC: U.S. DHHS; 2000;3-34–5-35.

108. National Institute of Diabetes, Digestive and Kidney Diseases (NIDDK). *National Diabetes Statistics, 2007*. Available at http://diabetes.niddk.nih.gov/DM/PUBS/statistics/. Accessed April 22, 2010.

109. Mokdad AH, Ford ES, Bowman BA, et al. Diabetes trends in the U.S.: 1990–1998. *Diabetes Care*. 2000;23:1278–1283.

110. Diabetes Prevention Program Research Group. Reduction in the incidence of type 2 diabetes with lifestyle intervention or metformin. *N Engl J Med*. 2003;346:393–403.

111. Franz MJ, Bantle JP, Beebe CA, et al. Nutrition principles and recommendations in diabetes. *Diabetes Care*. 2004;27:S36.

112. National Institutes of Health. *Osteoporosis and Related Bone Diseases, National Resource Center, 2008*. Available at http://www.niams.nih.gov/Health_Info/Bone/. Accessed April 22, 2010.

113. National Osteoporosis Foundation. *Osteoporosis, Disease Statistics, 2004*. Available at http://www.nof.org/aboutnof/founding.htm. Accessed April 22, 2010.

114. National Institutes of Health. Consensus Development Panel on osteoporosis. *JAMA*. 2001;285:785–795.

115. Heany RP. The importance of calcium intake for lifelong skeletal health. *Calcif Tissue Int*. 2002;70:70–73.

116. Standing Committee on the Scientific Evaluation of Dietary Reference Intakes. Food and Nutrition Board, Institutes of Medicine. *Dietary Reference Intakes for Calcium, Phosphorus, Magnesium, Vitamin D, and Fluoride*. Washington, DC: National Academy Press; 1999.

117. The benefits of dairy foods in health promotion. *Dairy Council Digest*. 2004;75(3):13–18.

118. Centers for Disease Control and Prevention. HIV Prevalence estimate—US, 2006. *MMWR Morbid Mortal Wkly Rep*. 2008; 57(39):1073–1076.

119. U.S. Department of Health and Human Services. *Healthy People 2010: Understanding and Improving Health*. 2nd ed. Washington, DC: U.S. DHHS; 2000. Chapt 13, HIV: 13-3-13-27.

120. Position of the American Dietetic Association and Dietitians of Canada. Nutrition intervention in the care of persons with human immunodeficiency virus infection. *J Am Diet Assoc*. 2000;100:708–717.

CHAPTER 12

Assuring Nutrition for Older Adults

Joseph M. Carlin, MS, RD, LDN, FADA

··

READER OBJECTIVES

After studying this chapter and reflecting on the contents, you should be able to:

1. Describe how the number of older Americans is growing due to improvements in health care, including nutrition.

2. Discuss the degree to which older Americans suffered from food insecurity and hunger prior to the implementation of government-sponsored nutrition intervention programs.

3. Describe the factors that laid the groundwork for federally funded elderly nutrition programs.

4. Outline factors that promoted the success of the Older Americans Nutrition Program.

5. Learn the importance of evaluation as a critical step in planning nutrition interventions.

6. Suggest ideas that might influence better nutrition among the elderly in the future.

··

■ INTRODUCTION

The second half of the 20th century was a time when Americans began to take notice of the growing sea of older people around them. While the total population of the United States grew from 150 million to 302 million from 1950 to 2007 (doubling in size), the population of those 65 and older grew rapidly, as well, representing 6%–7% of the total population.[1] Even more impressive was the growth in the population over 75 years of age, which increased from 4% to 6% of the population.

During the first half of the 20th century, improvements in the prevention and control of infectious diseases had a profound effect on increasing life expectancy. After 1950, improvements in nutrition, housing, hygiene, and medical care contributed to a longer life span. Life expectancy at birth increased for men from 48 years in 1901 to 76 years

of age in 2006; for women, the increases were even more impressive, increasing from 51 to almost 81 years of age.[2] The life expectancy of those in other countries, particularly Japan, holds out hope that longevity can be increased even more in the United States.

One of the major reasons people are living longer is due to decreases in mortality due to heart disease, stroke, and unintentional injuries. Government statistics reveal that although heart disease is still the leading cause of death in the United States, the death rate from heart disease decreased 41% from 1980 to 2007 The death rate from stroke declined during the same period. Both of these diseases are closely associated with high blood pressure, high cholesterol, lack of physical activity, and obesity. Health promotion initiatives, healthier lifestyles, and exercise programs offer the potential of increasing life expectancy.

Joseph M. Carlin, MS, RD, LDN, FADA is a Regional Nutritionist with the U.S. Administration on Aging, Boston, Massachusetts. The views expressed in this paper are the author's and do not necessarily reflect those of the Administration on Aging.

The aging of the population has important consequences to the health and well-being of all Americans. Not only will it put increased demands upon the healthcare system, but at the community level there will be a similar demand for a full range of services, including nutrition services.

Prior to the 1970s, older Americans were more likely to be classified as living in poverty than any other age group. With the availability of inflation-adjusted government social insurance programs—Social Security, Supplemental Security Income, and nutrition intervention programs such as Supplemental Nutrition Assistance Programs and the Elderly Nutrition Program—the poverty rate for older Americans declined rapidly from about 30% in 1970 to about 12% in 2000.

> Search for the different nutrition programs provided by the U.S. government at http://www.nutrition.gov.

One method of assessing food and nutrition problems in the community is the concept of "food insecurity." *Food insecurity* is a term used to convey the idea that the "availability of nutritionally adequate and safe foods or the ability to acquire acceptable foods in socially acceptable ways is limited or uncertain."[3] Among those who experience food insecurity can be people who suffer from true hunger, which is defined as the "uneasy or painful sensation caused by a lack of food."[3] The ideal is to ensure that all older Americans are food secure, meaning that throughout the year they have "access, at all times, to enough food for an active, healthy life."[4] A household food security study conducted by the U.S. Department of Agriculture in 2007 found that the prevalence rate for food insecurity in households with elderly persons was 2.4%. This increased to 2.8% for elderly persons living alone.[5] The idea of food insecurity, and the more precise definition of hunger, are major improvements over the vague and difficult-to-define term malnutrition—both under- and over-malnutrition—that was popular for most of the 20th century.

> Read more about food insecurity in all ages of the U.S. population in Chapter 17.

■ FEEDING AMERICA'S ELDERLY

On March 27, 1972, Congress passed Public Law 92-258, adding a new Title VII to the Older Americans Act (OAA), establishing a permanent program to provide life-saving meals to the elderly. Even though the new Elderly Nutrition Program (ENP) had bi-partisan support in Congress, it was held hostage when the appropriation bill, which provided funding for the new title, was attached to the "Cease Fire in Cambodia Bombing Bill," and was repeatedly vetoed by the President. During the summer of 1973, the funds were finely released to the states. Almost overnight, thousands of community centers opened their doors to the elderly and began the process of delivering meals to older people's homes.

At that time, the law specified that meals were to be served in a congregate setting for socialization purposes and were to be delivered to the homes of those with serious mobility problems. Justification for this new program grew out of the social activism that paralleled America's soul searching during the 1960s, which was at the height of this country's involvement in the Vietnam War and the Civil Rights movement. Providing nutritious meals to America's elderly was viewed as one of the many corrective actions society needed to take to provide for a more just America. Ending the Vietnam War and providing justice for African Americans were similar goals. The elderly were not the only group in society to be singled out for nutrition intervention programs. Both the U.S. Department of Agriculture's Supplemental Nutrition Assistance Program and Commodity Foods Distribution programs were expanded and the Supplemental Nutrition Program for Women, Infants and Children (WIC) were initiated.

> Read more about Public Law 92-258 and Title VII in the Catalog of Federal Domestic Assistance Program Descriptions at: http://www.grantcommunity.com/cfdaprog/p93045.htm.

Following the implementation of these new nutrition intervention programs, the United States became acutely aware of its domestic hunger issues. The Supplemental Nutrition Assistance Program (food stamps) grew from a $288 million program, serving 2.8 million people, to a $6 billion program by 1978. Free or reduced price lunches for poor children grew from a $42 million program for 3 million children to a $1.2 billion program serving 12 million children. Child care and summer food service for children grew from a $3.2 million program serving 140,000 to a $250 million program serving 3 million children.[6]

The idea that would eventually result in the federal government promoting and financing a nutrition program for the elderly started to take shape shortly after World War II. In 1954, a group of women in a Philadelphia neighborhood decided to pack sandwiches in brown paper bags and deliver them to elderly "shut-ins." Newspaper accounts of the efforts of these "angels" delivering "meals on wheels" captured the imagination of America. As the story was repeated across the nation in newspaper accounts, women in other communities began to copy the Philadelphia angels. A survey conducted at the request of the federal government in 1971 counted 311 of these "meals on wheels" programs. Some programs served as few as 10 people a day while others served over 100. No one knows where the women got the original idea for this successful program. We know that in London during World War II, efforts were made by relief groups to deliver meals to older people trapped by the blitz. Some of these Philadelphia women may have heard about these British efforts from their soldier husbands stationed in London during the war.[7]

Before these small efforts to deliver meals to the homebound were created, formal programs to protect the nutritional well-being of the elderly did not exist. It was believed at that time that the needs of older people were being met at home by their families. Forgotten were the tremendous sociological changes that had occurred during the 20th century, particularly after World War II. Children were moving to take jobs a considerable distance away from their parents and grandparents. Furthermore, many older people, particularly women, found themselves living alone after the premature death of a husband. With decreased economic resources to provide for their health and well-being, a large number of older people suffered from food insecurity. When faced with the decision of whether to spend their scarce resources on food, prescription drugs, rent, or utilities, they chose to pay the rent. As their numbers grew, their desperate situation could no longer be ignored. In retrospect, it would not be unreasonable to conclude that prior to the establishment of elderly nutrition programs, many older people suffered from high mortality and morbidity rates because of the lack of proper nutrition.

In the late 1960s, the health and nutrition-related problems of the elderly came to the attention of Congress, particularly the Senate Select Committee on Nutrition and Human Needs chaired by Senator George McGovern. This committee held some of the first hearings ever on the nutritional problems associated with aging in America. These hearings were just one of several defining events during the 1960s that focused attention on the nutritional needs of America's elderly. In 1968, Congress authorized President Johnson to fund several demonstration programs to investigate the extent of the problem and test methods for delivering nutritional resources to the elderly.

The idea for a federally supported nutrition program specifically targeting the elderly began taking root during the 1961 White House Conference on Aging. The deciding event during this turbulent period was the negative findings that came from the USDA's 1965 National Food Study on Food Consumption and Dietary Level. This study produced the shocking finding that as many as 6 to 8 million older persons might have deficient diets. These troubling statistics resulted in the creation of a task force on nutrition to develop both administrative and legislative recommendations for correcting the problem.

This task force decided to spend $2 million yearly for three years on demonstrations and to collect data in a systematic way concerning the nutrition needs of the elderly. These early demonstration programs tested two potential models for providing meals to older people: home-delivered meals and meals provided in-group settings, called *congregate meals*. The home-delivered meals model was clearly modeled after existing community meals-on-wheels programs. The congregate program took as its model programs operated in the Jewish settlement houses located in the lower east side of Manhattan. Two of the original 23 demonstration programs were located in Manhattan at the Henry Street Settlement House and the Hudson Guild-Fulton Senior Association.[8]

By the time the White House Conference on Nutrition and Human Needs was held in 1969, the idea for a federally supported nutrition program for the elderly had the backing of federal policy makers. At the 1971 White House Conference on Aging, solid information from the many Title IV demonstration programs was available. By this time a set of shared principles about the urgent need to respond to the nutritional needs of the elderly existed within the professional nutrition community and among political leaders. These values were incorporated into the Older Americans Act and to this day continue to serve as the basic justification for Congress and the administration to continue to support the program. These fundamental principles, as written into the Older Americans Act, declare that:

> . . . the purpose of the new nutrition program is to meet the acute need for a national policy which: provides older Americans, particularly those with low incomes, with low cost, nutritionally sound meals served in strategically located centers such as schools, churches, community centers, senior citizen centers, and other public or private facilities where they can obtain other social and rehabilitative services. Besides promoting better health among the older segment of the population through improved nutrition, such a program is aimed at reducing the isolation of old age, offering older Americans the opportunity to live their remaining years in dignity.

When the above statement was written, it was not envisioned that home-delivered meals would be a major part of the program. In the beginning, federal regulations required that state plans ensure that nutrition programs "provide home-delivered meals where necessary and feasible to

> More information about the Older Americans Act is available at: http://www.aoa.gov/AOARoot/AoA_Programs/OAA/index.aspx.

meet the needs of target group eligible individuals who are homebound."[9] There was a perception, at least at the federal level, that private meals-on-wheels programs would continue to grow parallel with the OAA home-delivered meals component. Because of this perception, home-delivered meals were capped, and the total number of meals served that way could not exceed 10% of the total meals served in the state. It was assumed that independent meals-on-wheels providers had the capacity to expand and would want to remain independent of the federally funded programs.

This assumption was unfounded, and meals-on-wheels programs soon petitioned the states to be designated as the local service provider. They aggressively pursued federal funding to expand their programs. A few did remain independent, at least for a time, and continued to use the designation meals-on-wheels to distinguish themselves from the rapidly expanding federal home-delivered meals programs.

It soon became clear that the policy restricting home-delivered meals to 10% was unworkable. It was raised incrementally over the first couple of years by the Administration on Aging (AoA) until Congress intervened in 1978 to amend the OAA, eliminating Title VII. The new amendments created the nutrition program anew, providing separate funding for congregate and home-delivered meals.

That separation continues to be in effect, with home-delivered meals representing almost 60% of all meals served. Clearly, the United States' expanding population of very frail elderly homebound is vulnerable and at great nutritional risk. Today, home-delivered meals and meals-on-wheels programs are different names for the same program.

In their yearly budget requests to Congress, the AoA has put the following clear and convincing reasons forward as to why home-delivered meals should continue to exist and even expand.[10] A home-delivered meal:

- "[Is] the first in-home service that an older adult receives . . ."
- "Serves as a primary access point for all other in-home services."
- "Improves participant nutrient intake, decreases food insecurity, increases social interaction and decreases social isolation, contributing to improved quality of life."
- "Play[s] an important role in the treatment, management, and delay of chronic disease and disease-related disability."
- "Provides an essential service to many caregivers by helping them maintain their own health and continued functionality."
- "Assists in decreasing the risk of complications associated with acute and chronic disease and contribute to improvements in quality of life."

In summary, the home-delivered meal program "is a smart, cost-effective investment of public funds."

■ FACTORS THAT PROMOTE PROGRAM SUCCESS

Over the past 30-plus years, the Elderly Nutrition Program, also called the Older Americans Nutrition Program, has been viewed as a resounding success for many reasons. First, it set out to do exactly what it was charged to accomplish and had a positive and lasting nutritional impact on those who participated in the program. Second, states, area agencies on aging, and local service providers did not rely solely upon federal funding to support the program. In addition to participant donations, service providers tapped into their state legislatures for additional funding and received financial support from cities and towns in which the programs operated. To supplement these funds, programs turned to fund-raising and the use of in-kind resources including facilities, and developed one of the most extensive and effective volunteer efforts in the country. In short, this program was made a success by the hundreds of thousands of volunteers who daily perform labor-intensive tasks, such as delivering hot meals to the homes of the isolated elderly.

Another reason for the success of the program, which seldom gets full credit today, is the careful planning that went into its design and implementation. These carefully planned steps ensured the stability and longevity of the program. These steps can serve as a textbook case study of how to implement a complicated nutrition intervention program.

> The Elderly Nutrition Program can be found on the Administration on Aging Web site at http://www.aoa.gov.

AoA put in place an administrative structure, detailed policies and procedures, and a training strategy that effectively ensured that all providers of this new and unproven program had the knowledge and skills to operate a successful program. Even before the first meals were served, AoA had authored a carefully thought-out set of regulations, policies, and a comprehensive training manual. That training manual was so comprehensive and reasoned that after 30 years, it is still in use and is affectionately referred to as the *Green Bible*, because of its green vinyl cover.

Within AoA, a unit was created to oversee this new program, headed up by Donald Watkins, MD, an international authority in the area of nutritional gerontology. He had 3 experienced nutritionists on his immediate staff, plus 10 highly skilled nutritionists, one in each of AoA's 10 regional offices. This team of experienced nutritionists provided technical assistance to the states on issues of nutrition, nutrition education, food service management, and food safety.

AoA funded five training centers strategically located across the country to train state and local service providers. The first directors of these Elderly Nutrition Programs received a minimum of 80 hours of instruction on the nutritional needs of older people, food service operations, sanitation, and basic social gerontology concepts, in addition to accounting and fiscal management basics.

Behind the backbone of this strong administrative structure, training, and technical assistance was the law itself, which provided straightforward guidance to the states on how to implement this program. It was clear from the language in the law that Congress expected the meals to be nutritious. Each meal had to contain one-third of the Recommended Dietary Allowances (RDAs), a reasonable target, given that very little was known about the nutritional needs of older persons at that time. When the program was first created, there was a strong belief that meals should be hot at the time of service, a concession to those older people and professional nutritionists who wanted to set the quality bar as high as possible. Older people, consulted in the 1970s about the design of the program, had vivid memories of the worldwide economic slump lasting from 1929 to 1939, and did not want to participate in a program that would be demeaning or humiliating. They did not want a meal that could in any way be interpreted as "being on the dole." They wanted to sit down to a "hot meal." This program was not to become a soup and sandwich program common during the Great Depression!

Considerable thought was given to the delicate issue of how much participants should contribute to the cost of these meals. Some elderly people clearly had the resources to pay for these meals while others, just as clearly, did not. The solution to this dilemma was to install a donation system; participants could determine for themselves what they considered fair. Furthermore, this donation system was to be implemented in a way that protected the confidentiality and dignity of the participant. The decision not to charge older people for their meals has contributed in large measure to the success of the program. The need for humans to reciprocate in kind with a token of value is a concept that sets our species apart from other animals and has been part of our character throughout our evolutionary progress. In short, human adults feel a sense of anxiety, or at least a state of discomfort, when sharing food with others outside the family. Humans feel a natural tendency to reciprocate with something of equal value when offered food. This something of value can be money. Based upon present data, older people contributed at least $160 million yearly to the support of this program.

The genius of this program lies in part in the simplicity of the legislation and accompanying regulations, which advocate for the needs of the elderly while promoting objectives that respect older people's needs for independence.

Like any law, it was not designed without flaws. As originally written, only hot meals could be served, and each meal had to meet one-third of the RDAs. In 1978, the law was amended to permit other than hot meals to be served, but they still had to meet the strict one-third RDA require-

ment. In 1990, the law was amended again to permit programs to offer a two-meals-a-day program, as long as the two meals combined equaled two-thirds of the RDA. Similarly, if three meals were served, the combined meals had to equal 100% of the RDA. (Note that the RDAs have now been replaced with the Dietary Reference Intakes.) These two changes, although not minor, attest to how well the program was designed in the beginning. These examples also demonstrate three truths: First, it is difficult, if not impossible, to write a flawless law because all variables cannot be anticipated. Second, when writing legislation, extreme care needs to be taken because once something is put in the law, it might take years to make a correction. Third, all programs need to be monitored and periodically evaluated to ensure that the program is doing what it is supposed to do. Changing policy, procedures, or even the law itself may be necessary to put the program back on track. The simplicity of the nutrition provisions in the OAA has afforded both AoA and the states maximum flexibility on administering this program.

Meals are provided in a variety of settings, such as senior centers, senior housing facilities, schools, and church basements. Some meals are cooked on site; others are prepared in central commissaries and delivered to meal sites. In most cases meals are prepared under contract with large food service management companies. A growing number of service providers have turned to frozen pre-plated meals, not only for home-delivered meals but also for congregate participants. Approximately 250 million meals are served yearly, with about 57% home-delivered and 43% congregate.

■ EVALUATION

The question must be asked: Did the Elderly Nutrition Program accomplish what it set out to accomplish? Between 1993 and 1995, AoA funded a nationwide evaluation of the Elderly Nutrition Program (ENP) as required under the Older Americans Act of 1965 when it was amended in

1992.[11] The legislation specified 19 areas for evaluation, with emphasis on the following:

- ENP's effects on participants' nutrition and socialization, compared with a similar population that does not participate in congregate or home-delivered meals programs.
- Is the program targeted to those who need the services most?
- How efficiently and effectively are services administered and delivered?
- What funds are available, and how are they allocated to service providers?

Mathematica Policy Research, Inc. was the contractor for the evaluation. It found that both congregate and home-bound ENP participants, when compared with the overall U.S. population 60 years of age and older, were 1) older by four to six years; 2) more than two-thirds female (69%); 3) lived alone; and 4) were more likely to be impoverished.[12]

For almost all of the nutrients studied, both congregate and home-delivered meals supplied well over a third of participants' daily intake. Many meals provided 40% to 50% of the RDAs. As to how the participants thought about the meals, about two-thirds of both congregate and home-delivered participants described themselves as being "very satisfied" with the taste of the food. The Mathematica team summed up their findings as follows:

> The ENP serves highly vulnerable people with characteristics that tend to put them at increased health and nutritional risk. ENP participants tend to be older, poorer, more likely to be members of racial or ethnic minorities, and more likely to live alone, compared with the overall population in the United States age 60 and older. Participants are also more likely to be in poor health, to have greater difficulty performing everyday tasks, and to have relatively high nutritional risk.[13]

The 1990s evaluation found that the program is serving the target population. This information is critical to the future of the program because it demonstrates that the ENP program is doing exactly what it set out to do. Programs that do what they are designed to do, and do it efficiently and effectively, are more likely to be successful in attracting future funding.

Because comprehensive evaluation research, such as that carried out by Mathematica, is expensive, AoA has used a number of tested performance measurement surveys to get a snapshot of how recipients of services rate the service, whether services are effectively targeted to vulnerable individuals, and whether services help older persons to maintain their independence and avoid premature institutionalization. AoA's 2003 Annual Report[14] shared with the aging network the results on this survey.

AoA found that home-delivered nutrition services "are effectively targeted to vulnerable populations." They found that 59% of respondents lived alone, 69% were 75 years of age or over, and 79% had difficulty with at least one activity of daily living (ADL), such as eating.

One element, critical to the success of the home-delivered meals program, is how well the participants like their meals. If the meals are either not consumed or only half eaten, no benefit is derived. This can be observed directly at congregate sites, but direct observation of eating patterns in the home of participants is difficult. In addition, delivering hot and tasty meals to people's homes has always been a major logistical and quality challenge. Despite the many difficulties in delivering these meals, 94% of respondents surveyed said that they liked the meal; 91% reported that meals almost always arrive when expected.

Since the early 1990s, nutrition programs have been using the *Determine Your Nutritional Health*[15] checklist as a tool to see to what degree participants are at nutritional risk. The survey found that 73% of respondents were at high nutritional risk. This statistic sounds realistic when 62% of respondents are reporting that the typical home-delivered meal provides one-half or more of their daily food intake. Twenty-five percent of respondents said that they did not always have enough money or food stamps to buy food. Clearly, food insecurity is a major problem among this vulnerable population.

> Find the *Determine Your Nutritional Health* checklist at http://www.hospitalmedicine.org/geriresource/toolbox/pdfs/determine.pdf.

When congregate meal participants were surveyed, 64% were 75 years or older and 56% lived alone. As for the quality of the meals, 92% of respondents said they were satisfied with the taste of the food, and 97% were satisfied with the temperature of the food.

When the congregate meals program was designed in the early 1970s, socialization opportunities for participants were one of the primary goals. The importance of socialization as a health factor was highlighted in a major study published in *Science*.[16] After examining the literature on the subject, House et al. found that:

> . . . social relationships, or the relative lack thereof, constitute a major risk factor for health—rivaling the effects of well-established health risk factors such as cigarette smoking, blood pressure, blood lipids, obesity, and physical activity.[16]

AoA's survey found that 96% of respondents like to visit with friends at the site; 73% like to participate in activities at the meal site; and 60% reported that their social opportunities have increased since they started receiving congregate nutrition services.

Over the life of the ENP program, all formal and less formal evaluations have found the same results; the program does exactly what it was designed to do.

■ OTHER NUTRITION INTERVENTIONS

As America's consciousness of the needs of older people grew, old programs were redesigned, others scaled back, and new programs implemented to meet the nutritional needs of the elderly. The government appropriates about $1 billion annually for all food and nutrition intervention programs for older adults.[17] The largest of these is AoA's Older Americans Nutrition Program. Although AoA's program may be the most visible nutrition intervention in the public's mind, it is not the only federal program designed to improve the nutritional well-being of older persons. Other federal interventions include Supplemental Nutrition Assistance Programs, Commodity Supplemental Food Program, Child and Adult Care Food Program, Farmers' Market Nutrition Program, waivers under the Medicaid program, and Medical Nutrition Therapy (MNT) for Medicare beneficiaries. Nutrition education activities carried out in the various states, under the Cooperative Extension Service, can also be added to this list. (Medicare and the other government programs are also discussed in subsequent chapters.)

Supplemental Nutrition Assistance Program

By far the largest of these programs in both numbers of participants and cost is the Supplemental Nutrition Assistance Program administered by the U.S. Department of Agriculture (USDA). The program provides older people with food coupons or electronic benefit transfer cards that can be used to purchase food items at retail stores. The purpose of the program is to assist low-income families, including the elderly, to buy food that is nutritionally adequate.[18]

The Commodity Supplemental Food Program

The Commodity Supplemental Food Program provides packaged food (e.g., juice, powdered milk, canned vegetables, and meat) to low-income participants, including older persons. Older persons must have a household income at or below 130% of the poverty level. In fiscal year 2009, 466,615 persons were served in this program in the United States. In 2009, about 93% (433,951) of those enrolled in this program were older.[19] Only 33 states and 2 Native American reservations participate in the program.[20]

The Child and Adult Care Food Program

The Child and Adult Care Food Program serves any person 60 years of age or older, and any person 18 years of age or older who also has a functional impairment and attends a nonresidential daycare facility. The program provides meal reimbursements to the daycare facility, if licensed or approved by the state. The Food and Nutrition Service, which administers this program, does not maintain statistics on those aged 60 or older.[21]

Seniors Farmers' Market Nutrition Program

In 2000, the USDA created the Seniors Farmers' Market Nutrition Program to improve nutrition and food security among low-income senior citizens by helping them to purchase more fresh fruits and vegetables at farmers' markets.[22] This program is modeled after the Market Coupon Program developed by the Massachusetts Department of Food and Agriculture in 1986, which had as its focus participants in the WIC program. Seniors at nutritional risk were added in 1987.[23]

This program provides coupons to low-income seniors, which can be exchanged for eligible foods at farmers' markets, roadside stands, and community-supported agriculture programs. Besides providing fresh and nutritious foods for the elderly, the program is also designed to increase the domestic consumption of agricultural commodities and to help expand the network of farmers' markets. Fifteen million dollars in direct funding is available to the states each year. About 700,000 older people were served in fiscal year 2003.[24]

■ THE FUTURE

It is impossible to predict how the federally funded nutrition program for the elderly will evolve in the future, but certainly it will change. Those familiar with the program anticipate that issues centered around wellness, lifestyle, health promotion, nutrition education, and exercise will become more important among an aging population as they try to stay healthy and fit as long as possible.

Some nutrition practitioners, disappointed with the poor results of traditional nutrition education strategies whereby older people sit through information-filled lectures, are experimenting with promising new strategies. One model is the Healthy Eating for Successful Living in Older Adults program, an evidence-based healthy eating program developed by an expert advisory panel under the supervision of the Lahey Clinic in Massachusetts. This project is part of the Model Programs Project sponsored by the National Council on the Aging (NCOA) with funding from the John A. Hartford Foundation.[25] It is both an educational and support program designed to help older Americans take control of their nutritional health. The program stresses self-management strategies using behavior modification approaches.

Another opportunity that holds promise for improving the health of seniors is the Internet. Although less than a third (31%) of older Americans have ever gone online, their numbers can be expected to increase dramatically over the next few years. A survey of seniors who use the Internet, released in 2005 by the Kaiser Family Foundation, found that topics related to prescription drugs were the most popular issue, followed by searches for information on nutrition, exercise or weight control, cancer, heart disease, and arthritis. This survey found that seniors say that they consider e-mail and the Internet an important part of their lives that "they wouldn't want to do without."[26]

The future of the Older Americans Nutrition Program, and other federally supported nutrition programs, can be expected to be a valuable part of this nation's "safety net" for ensuring the independence, health, and longevity of America's aging population. To ensure that these programs are efficient and effective, program managers at all levels—federal, state, and community—must continually assess the nutrition needs of the elderly, modify the programs to meet those needs, and periodically evaluate the program to ensure that it is doing what it was designed to do. If these tried and true methods are followed, there is no reason why all Americans can't grow old, knowing that there will be a program to meet their nutrition needs if they ever need it.

Issues for Discussion

1. Compare a nutrition program that is available in another country (research) to the present nutrition program for elders in the United States. What are the similarities and differences?

2. Discuss the ethical implications of a government-funded nutrition program for the elderly.

3. Discuss possible improvements for future nutrition programs for the great number of elders the United States will experience.

References

1. National Center for Health Statistics. *Health, U.S., 2004 with chartbook on trends in the health of Americans.* Hyattsville, MD: U.S. Department of Health and Human Services, Centers for Disease Control and Prevention; 2006. Available at http://www.cdc.gov/nchs/data/hus/hus09.pdf#listtables. Accessed May 13, 2010.

2. National Center for Health Statistics. *Health, U.S., 2004 with chartbook on trends in the health of Americans.* Hyattsville, MD: U.S. Department of Health and Human Services, Centers for Disease Control and Prevention; 2006. Available at http://www.cdc.gov/nchs/data/hus/hus09.pdf#listtables. Accessed May 13, 2010.

3. Frongillo E, Horan CM. Hunger and aging. *Generations.* 2004;3:28–33.

4. Nord M, Andrews M, Carlson S. *Household food security in the U.S., 2007.* Washington, DC: USDA Economic Research Service; 2007:i. Available at http://ers.usda.gov/Publications/ERR66/ERR66.pdf. Accessed on May 13, 2010.

5. Nord M, Andrews M, Carlson S. *Household food security in the U.S., 2007.* Washington, DC: USDA Economic Research Service; 2007:9.

6. Kotz N. *Hunger in America: The federal response.* New York: The Field Foundation; 1979:10–11.

7. Carlin JM. Meals on Wheels. In: *Oxford Encyclopedia of Food and Drink in America.* New York: Oxford University Press; 2004.

8. Bechill WD, Wolgamot I. *Nutrition for the elderly. The program highlights of research and development nutrition projects funded under Title IV of the Older Americans Act of 1965.* Washington, DC: U.S. Department of Health, Education, and Welfare, Administration on Aging; 1973.

9. Administration on Aging. Budget request for fiscal year 2003 by the Administration on Aging. *Federal Register.* August 19, 1972;37(162):16848.

10. Budget request for fiscal year 2003 by the Administration on Aging. Washington, DC: U.S. Department of Health and Human Services; 2003.

11. U.S. House of Representatives. Older Americans Act of 1965 and the Native American Programs Act of 1974 as amended through December 31, 1992. Serial No. 103-E, 22–24. Washington, DC: Committee on Education and Labor of the U.S. House of Representatives; June 15, 1993.

12. Millen BE, Ohls JC, Ponza M, McCool AC. The Elderly Nutrition Program: an effective national framework for preventive nutrition interventions. *J Am Diet Assoc.* 2002:102:234–240.

13. Ponza M, Ohls JC, Millen BE. *Serving Elders at Risk.* Washington, DC: Mathematica Policy Research, Inc. for the U.S. Department of Health and Human Services, Administration on Aging; 1996:12.

14. Administration on Aging. *2003 Annual Report—What we do makes a difference.* Washington, DC: U.S. Department of Health and Human Services; 2004.

15. The Nutrition Screening Initiative. *Nutrition screening manual for professionals caring for older Americans.* Washington, DC: The American Academy of Family Physicians; 1991:4–5.

16. House JS, Landis KR, Umberson D. Social relationships and health. *Science.* 1988;241:541.

17. Wellman NS, Kamp B. Federal food and nutrition assistance programs for older people. *Generations.* 2004;27:78.

18. U.S. General Accounting Office. Food assistance: Options for improving nutrition for older Americans. GAO/RCED-00-238. Washington, DC: U.S. General Accounting Office; 2000:6.

19. U.S. General Accounting Office. Food assistance: Options for improving nutrition for older Americans. GAO/RCED-00-238. Washington, DC: U.S. General Accounting Office. Washington, DC; 2000: 7–8.

20. Wellman NS, Kamp B. Federal food and nutrition assistance programs for older people. *Generations.* 2004;27:85.

21. U.S. General Accounting Office. Food assistance: Options for improving nutrition for older Americans. GAO/RCED-00-238. Washington, DC: U.S. General Accounting Office. 2000:8–9.

22. Older Americans Report. Clinton's food security initiative will help seniors get fresh produce. December 1, 2000:403.

23. Balsam A, Webber D, Oehlke B. The farmers' market coupon program for low-income elders. *J Nutr Elderly.* 1994;13:35–42.

24. Wellman NS, Kamp B. Federal food and nutrition assistance programs for older people. *Generations.* 2004;27:85.

25. *Healthy Eating for Successful Living in Older Adults.* Model Programs Project sponsored by the National Council on the Aging (NCOA) with funding from the John A. Hartford Foundation. Available at http://www.healthyagingprograms.org/resources/EBSummary_HealthyEating_Overview.pdf. Accessed April 26, 2010.

26. e-health and the elderly: How seniors use the Internet for health. Press release. Menlo Park, CA: Kaiser Family Foundation in consultation with Princeton Survey Research Associates (PSRA); January 12, 2005.

CHAPTER

13

Providing Nutrition Services in Public Health Primary Care

ARLENE SPARK, EDD, RD, FADA, FACN

READER OBJECTIVES: After studying this chapter and reflecting on its contents, you should be able to:

1. Define primary health care.
2. Identify primary care providers and its recipients, and the various locations where primary care is practiced.
3. Explain how primary, secondary, and tertiary prevention fit into the primary care model.
4. Summarize how primary care services are financed.
5. Discuss the scope and breadth of nutrition services available in primary care settings, why barriers exist to providing nutrition services in primary health care, and how those barriers may be overcome.

■ INTRODUCTION

There tends to be a lack of clarity and consensus about the term *primary care*. The confusion may be attributed to the numerous meanings of the word *primary*. Among its many meanings are main, chief, most important, key, prime, principal, crucial, fundamental, core, central, essential, basic, and important as well as first, initial, leading, top, and foremost. If *primary* is understood to be first, initial, or leading in time or order, this leads to a relatively narrow concept of primary care as "first contact" or the entry point of healthcare delivery. This narrow definition of primary care connotes only a triage function in which patients are then passed on to a higher level of care. If, on the other hand, *primary* is understood in its sense of chief, principal, or main, then *primary care* is understood as central and fundamental to health care. This latter idea supports the multidimensional view of primary care envisioned in the Institute of Medicine's (IOM) report, *Primary Care: America's Health in a New Era*. That *primary care is fundamental to health care* is also the view envisioned in this chapter.[1]

The IOM defines primary care as "the provision of integrated, accessible health care services by clinicians who are accountable for addressing a large majority of per

sonal health needs, developing a sustained partnership with patients, and practicing in the context of family and community."[1] According to this definition, primary care is a function predicated on relationships and collaboration (rather than boundaries between specialties and disciplines). There is emphasis on the clinician's role as the patient's partner and advocate as the patient navigates his way through the healthcare system. The IOM recommends that primary care should be viewed as a central mission of the health care system (not as a feeder to tertiary care), and that it should be provided by teams that bring "different kinds of expertise...to bear on the patient's needs through collaborative activity, and...permit the delegation of some tasks by broadening the range of professionals involved in primary care.[1]

Primary care is continuing, comprehensive, and preventive personal medical care. The primary care setting includes all public and/or private outpatient clinics and private practices that offer office-based general medical care. (Although not considered here, primary care settings also include emergency rooms, acute care facilities, chronic care facilities, and addiction treatment facilities.) Typically, primary care practice is defined within the categories of pediatrics, adolescent medicine, general internal medicine, family practice, geriatrics, and obstetrics and gynecology.

Providers of primary care include allopathic physicians or medical doctors (MDs) and osteopathic physicians or doctors of osteopathy (DOs). Primary care physicians often work with other healthcare providers, such as physician assistants (PAs), nurse practitioners (NPs), registered nurses (RNs), social workers (MSWs, LMSWs), nutritionists, and behavioral health practitioners.

The concept of primary care is so fundamental to public health that objectives to address primary care appear in the very first chapter of *Healthy People 2010*,[2] the prevention agenda for the nation.

- Increasing the proportion of people who have a specific source of ongoing care.
- Increasing the proportion of persons with a usual primary care provider.
- Reducing the proportion of families that experience difficulties or delays in obtaining health care or do not receive needed care for one or more family members.
- Increasing the proportion of schools training doctors, nurses and other health professionals whose basic curriculum for healthcare providers includes the core competencies in health promotion and disease prevention.
- Increasing the proportion of all health professions, allied and associated health professions, and nursing degrees awarded to members of underrepresented racial and ethnic minorities.
- Reducing hospitalization rates for ambulatory-care–sensitive conditions, such as uncontrolled diabetes. This objective can be accomplished by tighter glycemic control, an aim of diabetes self-management programs, as described in the diabetes sections of this book.

Ten years later, one of the overarching goals of *Healthy People 2020* is to eliminate preventable disease, disability, injury, and premature death. Steps to promote and preserve health and to minimize the occurrence and consequences of disease may or may not save healthcare dollars, but they still improve health and well-being and lead to other positive outcomes. Even people with unpreventable or incurable health conditions can benefit from health promotion and disease prevention efforts that slow functional declines or improve the ability to live independently.[3]

■ ROOM FOR NUTRITION IN PRIMARY CARE

Conducted under the aegis of the National Center for Health Statistics, the National Ambulatory Medical Care Survey (NAMCS) is a national survey that provides information about ambulatory medical care services in the United States. Findings are based on a sample of visits to non-federal employed office-based physicians who are primarily engaged in direct patient care. According to the NAMCS, in 2006 an estimated 902 million visits were made to physicians' of-

fices in the United States. DOs received 60 million of these visits, 6.6% of the total. As indicated in **Table 13–1**, about 58% of the visits were to physicians in the primary care specialties of general family medicine, internal medicine, pediatrics, and obstetrics/gynecology. Tests for blood pressure were the leading diagnostic screening tests, performed during almost one-half of all office visits.

The most common nutrition-related diagnoses were essential hypertension, routine infant or child health check, type-2 diabetes mellitus (formerly known as non-insulin–dependent diabetes), normal pregnancy, and general medical exam–prevention. Almost 12% of the most common diagnoses for office visits are for nutrition-related conditions: essential hypertension (5.9%), diabetes mellitus (4.1%), and hyperlipidemia (1.7%).[4]

In today's healthcare climate, aging Americans are taking a more active role in their health, which translates into increasing numbers of visits to doctors. More than one half of the patients who visited their physicians in 2000 were middle-aged or senior citizens. While the number of people in the United States over 45 years of age rose 11% in the last decade, doctor visits by that age group increased 26% in the same time period. Physicians also are more aggressive in treating chronic disease, which requires more follow-up care.

Nutrition counseling is an appropriate component of treatment for such chronic conditions as diabetes and heart disease. Drugs for nutrition-related conditions of the heart and kidney (Lipitor™, Zocor™, Lasix™) and hormones (Synthroid™, Premarin™) were among the top five types of therapeutic classifications of drugs prescribed during office visits. (Pain, respiratory tract problems, and central nervous system problems were the remaining top conditions for which medicines were prescribed.) Diagnostic and screening tests increased 28% from 1992 to 2001. Visits that included education or counseling increased by a third.

E-mail consultations were not common between doctors and their patients in 2000, when only 6% of physicians

TABLE 13–1	Office Visits to Primary Care Generalists and Specialist Physicians (2006)
Percent of All Office Visits	**Medical Specialty**
22.8	General family medicine
13.9	Internal medicine
13.3	Pediatrics
7.6	Obstetrics/gynecology
42.5	Other (specialty care physicians)

Source: U.S. Department of Health and Human Services, *Health, United States, 2008*. Available at http://www.cdc.gov/nchs/data/hus/hus08.pdf#095/. Accessed February 24, 2010.

made any e-mail consultations. Over the next few decades that number will increase, but as it does, healthcare providers must concern themselves with the quality of consultations, confidentiality, liability, and the challenge of collecting fees. Early e-mail use by healthcare providers has grown without safeguards that adequately address these issues. As e-mail consultations marks a radical shift from the traditional oral modes of communication, patients and healthcare providers alike will need to learn how to use it both safely and effectively.[5]

■ AGENCY FOR HEALTHCARE RESEARCH AND QUALITY

The Agency for Healthcare Research and Quality (AHRQ) is the lead U.S. federal agency for research on healthcare quality, costs, outcomes, and patient safety. It complements the biomedical research mission of its sister agency, the National Institutes of Health (NIH). AHRQ serves as a major source of funding and technical assistance for health services research and research training at leading U.S. universities and other institutions. It is home to research centers that specialize in such major areas of healthcare research as primary care (including preventive services), healthcare organization and delivery systems, and healthcare costs and sources of payment. Goals of AHRQ include supporting improvements in health outcomes by a) supporting research that addresses concerns of very high public priority, such as primary care practice and integrated healthcare delivery systems, b) supporting projects that test and evaluate successful methods that translate research into practice to improve patient care in diverse healthcare settings, and c) translating the recommendations of the U.S. Preventive Services Task Force (USPSTF) into resources for providers, patients, and healthcare systems.

The Task Force produced its first *Guide to Clinical Preventive Services*; individual reports have been released in print and on the AHRQ Web site as they have been completed. The current *Guide* provides recommendations on preventive interventions (screening tests, counseling, immunizations, and chemo prophylactic regimens) for many conditions. It includes assessments of more than 200 services offered in primary care settings for adults, pregnant women, and children. "The patients for whom these services are recommended include asymptomatic individuals of all age groups and risk categories. Thus, the subject matter is relevant to all of the major primary care specialties: family practice, internal medicine, obstetrics-gynecology, and pediatrics. The recommendations in each chapter reflect a standardized review of current scientific evidence and include a summary of published clinical research regarding the clinical effectiveness of each preventive service."[6] Widely used in medical, nursing, and nutrition education as a key reference for teaching preventive care, the 2008 *Guide* is available online and in hard copy.[7]

A variety of clinical preventive services for normal-risk children[8] and adults[9] are recommended by the USPSTF. The recommended nutrition-related screening and counseling services include:

- Screening for phenylketonuria (PKU), sickle cell, hemoglobinopathies, and hypothyroidism at birth
- Measuring head circumference periodically from birth to 2 months
- Measuring height and weight periodically from birth to 18 years
- Screening for anemia and lead at 1 year
- Measuring blood pressure and determining dental health periodically, from 3 to 18 years
- Screening for alcohol use periodically, from 11 to 18 years
- Counseling parents and/or the child regarding development, nutrition, and physical activity, from birth to 18 years
- Screening blood pressure, height, weight, and obesity periodically, starting at age 18 years
- Screening cholesterol every 5 years in men starting at age 35 years and women starting at age 45 years (starting at age 20 in men and women, according to a joint statement issued in 2004 by the American Cancer Society, the American Diabetes Association, and the American Heart Association[10])
- Counseling women for calcium intake periodically, starting at 18 years of age
- Counseling women of childbearing age (18–50 years) on folic acid
- Counseling women 18 to 50 years of age on breast feeding after childbirth

In order to implement these recommendations, in 1994 the Department of Health and Human Service's (DHHS's) Office of Disease Prevention and Health Promotion (ODPHP) launched Put Prevention Into Practice (PPIP).[11] PPIP is a national program to improve delivery of appropriate clinical preventive services, such as the screening tests and counseling recommendations listed above. The purpose of the PPIP initiative is to enable doctors and other healthcare providers to determine which services their patients should receive, facilitate the implementation of the delivery of clinical preventive services, and make it easier for patients to understand and keep track of their preventive care. The PPIP program also works to increase the appropriate use of clinical preventive services through a variety of resources and tools for clinicians, healthcare systems, patients, and the public. For example, growth charts developed by the Centers for Disease Control and Prevention (CDC; available online at http://www.cdc.gov/growthcharts/) are recommended to measure head circumference in infants periodically from birth to 2 months and measure height and weight periodically from birth to 18 years of age. As for adults, diagnostic tests are recommended at prescribed intervals to prevent and treat chronic conditions.

■ BARRIERS TO PROVIDING NUTRITION SERVICES IN PRIMARY CARE AND STRATEGIES FOR INCREASING SERVICES

Despite the myriad opportunities to offer the nutrition services that are described in the previous section of this chapter, multiple factors[12] hamper the fulfillment of this potential. Mitigating factors include characteristics of the physician, the healthcare establishment, financial considerations, and the patient's readiness for change. The physician may be hampered by a lack of confidence and competence in nutrition counseling, and have limited time available to spend with each patient. The organization of the medical office may not be conducive to supporting nutrition services. There may be inadequate third-party reimbursement for nutrition consultation services. Finally, the patient may have a low level of motivation or interest in changing.

Physician Confidence and Skills

Practicing physicians report a lack of confidence and related proficiency in nutrition counseling skills because of inadequate training.[13,14] Despite concerted scientific, educational, and congressional calls to increase nutrition coverage in medicine for more than half a century, most graduating medical students report an inadequate quality and quantity of nutrition training.[15]

Strategies to Improve Confidence and Skills

The Nutrition Academic Award (NAA) Program, developed in 1997 by the National Heart, Lung, and Blood Institute (NHLBI), is an initiative to improve nutrition training across a network of U.S. medical schools. Its purpose is to financially enhance the nutrition curricula for medical students, residents, and practicing physicians to incorporate principles and practice skills of nutrition for their patients. Ten NAA awards were funded for 1998–2003; even more grants were awarded by NHLBI by 2010 and the National Institute of Diabetes and Digestive and Kidney Diseases (NIDDK) funded more as well. While the NHLBI has funded a number of other academic award programs since 1970 to address other topics in medical school curricula, this was the first academic award focusing primarily on nutrition. Products of the NAA program are available online at http://www.nhlbi.nih.gov/funding/training/naa/products.htm.

Of particular interest are the user-friendly tools to make it possible for physicians to quickly determine a patient's diet and exercise habits as well as provide information to aid in the delivery of effective nutrition counseling that were developed at the Albert Einstein College of Medicine.

The Einstein team developed WAVE and REAP, acronyms for tools to help physicians and other healthcare providers conduct nutrition assessments and counseling with their patients in as little as one minute. Weight, Activity, Variety and Excess (WAVE) is designed to encourage provider/patient dialogue about the pros and cons of the patient's status regarding weight, diet, and activity. The Rapid Eating and Activity Assessment for Patients (REAP) is a questionnaire designed to aid providers in performing a quick assessment of diet and physical activity. An accompanying key aids the provider in discussing the patient's answers and provides guidelines for counseling.[16] REAP and WAVE are examples of tools to facilitate nutrition assessment and counseling in the provider office.

Physician's Time Constraints

The frequency, time spent, and factors associated with nutrition counseling in primary care are not well studied, but a few investigations suggest that the amount of time spent on nutrition depends on the reason for the visit and the patient's age. Which patients receive nutrition counseling and how much time do primary care physicians spend discussing diet? Summaries of two surveys answer these questions.

- In 2002, nutrition counseling was measured by direct observation on two days for visits to family physicians. Nutrition counseling occurred in approximately one-fourth (24%) of all office visits, 17% of visits for acute illnesses, 30% of chronic illness visits, and 41% of well-care visits. The average time spent on nutrition counseling was 55 seconds (range < 20 seconds to > 6 min). Nutrition counseling occurred in 45% of visits for diabetes, 33% of visits by obese patients, 31% of visits for hypertension, 26% of prenatal visits, and 25% of visits for cardiovascular disease (CVD). Nutrition counseling was more likely to occur during visits by patients who were older or had diabetes mellitus, during visits for well care or chronic illness, and during longer visits.[17]
- According to a report published in 2004, when trained medical students observed physician, office, and patient characteristics in 4344 patient visits in 38 nonmetropolitan primary care physician offices they found that counseling rates ranged from 0% in some offices to 55% in others. Physicians counseled patients on dietary habits in 25% of visits and exercise in 20% of visits. New patients were counseled 30% more often than established ones. When counseling occurred, physicians (rather than patients) initiated both dietary and exercise counseling 61% of the time. Counseling for dietary habits was associated with counseling for exercise.[18]

Strategies to Reduce Time Constraints

Given the time constraints of primary care practice, nutrition counseling needs to be brief and part of an organized office system that is conducive to supporting nutrition services. When necessary, the physician must be able to refer appropriate patients to qualified nutrition professionals. Strategies targeting both physician and the healthcare system may improve the consistency of physician preventive counseling practices.[13]

AHRQ recommends that primary care physicians utilize the "5 A's" to deliver nutrition counseling.[19] The 5 A's—assess, advise, agree, assist, and arrange—is a mnemonic algorithm that outlines minimal contact interventions that may be provided by a variety of clinical staff in primary care settings.

NAA recipients developed the *Nutrition Curricular Guide for Training Physicians* (available online at: http://www.nhlbi.nih.gov/funding/training/naa/curr_gde/index.htm). Dissemination of this and other NAA materials is facilitated by a national Web site, presentations and publications, and consultants and advisors from the NAA nutrition education programs. The NAA program constitutes a major government-sponsored effort to enhance nutrition knowledge and skills among healthcare providers and to effectively apply the science of human nutrition to clinical medicine.[20]

Cost

In most cases, nutrition counseling is covered by insurance only for adult patients with a diagnosis of hypercholesterolemia, hypertension, or diabetes.[12] Until the mid 1970s most people in the United States had traditional indemnity coverage, which is also referred to as fee-for-service. Indemnity plans are similar to automobile insurance in that one pays a certain amount of one's medical expenses up front in the form of a deductible and afterwards the insurance company pays the majority of the bill. As advances in modern medicine increased the cost of providing health care and made it possible for people to live longer, many insurance companies developed plans to reduce their costs of doing business. This led to the birth of managed care systems. The current health insurance market options include traditional fee-for-service health insurance and managed care plans. Some forms of coverage are highly specialized and others are more comprehensive. The more comprehensive and inclusive the health insurance, the higher the premiums. It is generally in the individual's best interest to purchase group coverage (through an employer) when available. Group coverage is generally more comprehensive and group rates are generally lower because insurance companies can average their costs over many rather than a few people and pass along a portion of those savings to their insurers. Group plans are almost always managed care programs, which contain many restrictions. If group coverage is not available then the individual will need to purchase an individual plan. Individual plans are medically underwritten and there are no guarantees that an insurer will approve the application; premiums for individual policy holders are more in line with their expected healthcare cost than if they

were part of a group coverage. These premiums are also higher for those who are older or less healthy.

■ SYSTEM-WIDE CHANGE STRATEGIES FOR REDUCING THE COST OF MEDICAL CARE

Population-based medicine and chronic disease management are of particular importance to public health nutritionists. Population-based medicine addresses the health care of whole populations rather than that of individual patients. It represents a community-based strategy for disease management and health promotion and places each individual patient within the context of the larger community made up of both sick and healthy people. The community may be as small as an individual physician's private medical practice or as comprehensive as a multi-site HMO. In population-based medicine, disease groups within a given patient population are identified and new levels of disease monitoring and patient education are used to ensure that best practice is systematically applied across the group, accomplished within the traditional relationship of doctor and patient, but with integral support from nurses, nutritionists, pharmacists, health educators, and other members of the healthcare team that are employed by the medical practice.

■ CHRONIC DISEASE MANAGEMENT AND SELF-MANAGEMENT

Disease management is a system of coordinated healthcare interventions and communications for populations with conditions in which patient self-care efforts are significant. Disease management supports the physician or practitioner/patient relationship and plan of care; emphasizes prevention of exacerbations and complications utilizing evidence-based practice guidelines and patient empowerment strategies; and evaluates clinical, humanistic, and economic outcomes on an ongoing basis with the goal of improving overall health. In order to improve health outcomes for the chronically ill, system change interventions that involve primary care and cut across chronic conditions are needed. Chronic disease improvement efforts must create care systems that are designed to meet the needs of patients and their families. The AHRQ and The Robert Wood Johnson Foundation (RJWF) have funded research directed at improving the care of patients with major chronic illnesses. Additionally, valuable experience has been accrued in implementing evidence-based system change ideas in large-scale chronic disease quality improvement programs sponsored by the Bureau of Primary Health Care (BPHC),[21] the CDC, and Improving Chronic Illness Care (ICIC),[22] originally a five-year national demonstration project sponsored by the RWJF and other organizations.

A component of population medicine is chronic disease management (CDM). CDM represents a comprehensive,

Exhibit 13-1 **Summary of Health Insurance Plans**

Indemnity (Fee-for-Service)

Under fee-for-service or indemnity health coverage, the insured has autonomy when it comes to choosing doctors, hospitals, and other healthcare providers. The insured can refer himself to any specialist without getting permission, and the insurance company doesn't get to decide whether the visit was necessary. However, most fee-for-service medicine is managed to a certain extent. Fee-for-service plans usually involve more out-of-pocket expenses, often a deductible amount usually of about $200–$1500, before the insurance company starts paying. Once the deductible is met, the insurer then must pay about 80% of the doctor bills. The insured may have to pay up-front and then submit the bill for reimbursement, or the provider may bill the insurer directly and the insurance company in turn invoices the individual. Under fee-for-service plans, insurers will usually only pay for reasonable and customary medical expenses, taking into account what other practitioners in the area charge for similar services. If the insured's doctor charges more than what the insurance company considers reasonable and customary, the insured probably has to make up the difference. Traditionally, preventive care services like annual check-ups have not been covered under fee-for-service plans, but as evidence mounts that preventive services prevent more costly illnesses, some insurers are including them in the plan. Fee-for-service plans often include a ceiling for out-of-pocket expenses, after which the insurance company will pay 100% of any costs. Traditional fee-for-service coverage offers flexibility in exchange for higher out-of-pocket expenses. Of all visits made to physicians in 2000, approximately 57% were made by patients who listed private insurance as their primary expected source of payment. This may change as health reform begins in 2010.

Managed Care

Preferred Provider Organizations

Preferred Provider Organizations (PPOs) are the least restrictive type of managed care systems. PPOs have made arrangements for lower fees with a network of healthcare providers. PPOs give their policyholders a financial incentive to stay within that network. For example, a visit to an in-network doctor might mean the insured would pay a $10 co-pay. If the insured wanted see an out-of-network doctor, she would have to pay the entire bill up front and then submit the bill to the insurer for an 80% reimbursement. In addition, the insured might have to pay a deductible if she chooses to go outside the network, or pay the difference between what the in-network and out-of-network doctors charge. With a PPO, the insured can self-refer to a specialist without getting approval and, as long as the specialist is an in-network provider, enjoy the same co-pay. Staying within the network means less money coming out of the insured's pocket. Preventive care services may not be covered under a PPO. Exclusive Provider Organizations (EPOs) are PPOs that look like Health Maintenance Organizations (see below). EPOs raise the financial stakes for staying in the network. The insured is responsible for the entire cost of the visit if he chooses a provider outside the network.

Point-of-Service

A Point-of-Service (POS) plan is a little less restrictive type of managed care than the PPO. Like PPOs, POS plans have made arrangements for lower fees with a network of healthcare providers and give their policyholders a financial incentive to stay within that network. However, POS plans introduce the gatekeeper, or primary care physician (PCP). The insured chooses his PCP from among the plan's network of doctors. As with the PPO, the insured can choose to go out of network and still get some kind of coverage. In order to get a referral to a specialist, one usually goes through the PCP. If the insured chooses to self-refer, he will receive less reimbursement. If the PCP refers the insured to a doctor who is out of the network, the plan should pick up most of the cost. Going outside of the network usually also results in paying a deductible. POS plans may cover more preventive care services, and may offer health improvement programs like workshops on nutrition and discounts at health clubs. Rates and coverage vary from state to state.

Health Maintenance Organization

The HMO is the most restrictive type of managed care. Like POS and PPOs, HMOs have made arrangements for lower fees with a network of healthcare providers and give their policyholders a financial incentive to stay within that network. HMO plans also utilize a gatekeeper PCP. The insured selects a PCP from among the HMO's physician network. HMOs require that the insured sees only doctors within their plan. Visits to a specialist occur only after referral from the insured's PCP. In general, the insured must see only HMO-approved physicians and use HMO-approved facilities, or pay the entire cost of the visit oneself. HMO plans generally cover more preventive care services, and may even offer health improvement programs like workshops on nutrition and discounts at health clubs. HMO coverage is a trade-off between premiums paid and plan flexibility. HMOs offer lower premiums but are restrictive when it comes to coverage. Of all office visits to physicians in 2000, approximately 29% were made by patients belonging to HMOs. This may change as health reform begins in 2010.

Government Programs

Medicare

The Health Insurance for the Aged and Disabled Act (title XVIII of the Social Security Act), known as *Medicare*, has made

continues

Exhibit 13-1 *Continued*

available to nearly every American 65 years of age and older a broad program of health insurance designed to assist the nation's elderly to meet hospital, medical, and other health costs. Medicare is administered by the Centers for Medicare & Medicaid Services (CMS). Formerly, Medicare was administered by the Health Care Financing Administrations (HCFA). With approximately 40 million beneficiaries, Medicare is the largest healthcare insurer in the United States. In addition to assisting the elderly, Medicare was also designed to assist persons eligible for Social Security disability payment programs for more than two years, and individuals with end-stage renal disease (ESRD: permanent kidney failure requiring dialysis or kidney transplant), with payments for medical and healthcare services. All payments ultimately come from the federal Medicare Trust Fund, which is financed by Social Security deductions from employee payrolls. Medicare coverage has two parts: A and B. Part A covers inpatient care in hospitals and skilled nursing facilities, home care, and hospital care. Part B covers physician services, outpatient hospital services, durable medical equipment, and other medical services and supplies. There is a monthly premium for Part B coverage for individuals who choose to enroll in the program. Another optional part for drugs was added in 2004.

A list of all the current services covered under Medicaid Part B is available on the CMS Web site at http://www.cms.hhs.gov/. Nutrition-related services that are covered include:
- Rural health clinic services and Federally qualified health center services
- Self-care home dialysis support services
- Diabetes outpatient self-management training services
- Medical nutrition therapy services in the case of a beneficiary with diabetes or a renal disease who 1) has not received diabetes outpatient self-management training services within a time period determined by the Secretary; 2) is not receiving maintenance dialysis for which payment is made under section 1881 of the

Act; and 3) meets such other criteria determined by the Secretary after consideration of protocols established by dietitian or nutrition professional organizations.

The latest information on Medicare enrollment, benefits, and other helpful tools is available at http://www.Medicare.gov, the official U.S. government site for people with Medicare.

Medicaid
Medicaid is the largest source of funding for medical and health-related services for people with limited income. Medicaid, a federally assisted program that became law in 1965, is jointly funded by the federal and state governments (including the District of Columbia and the territories) to assist states in providing medical long-term care assistance to people who meet certain eligibility criteria. Medicaid provides assistance with payment of medical care for eligible low-income persons, the aged, blind, and disabled, and members of families with dependent children in which one parent is absent, incapacitated, or unemployed. The states define eligibility, benefits, and payment schedules. (The program is known as Medi-Cal in California.) CMS provides Medicaid program guidelines at http://www.cms.hhs.gov/home/medicaid.asp.

Currently there are no federal criteria specifically relating to nutrition care services. As of this writing, only some Medicaid programs expressly cover nutrition services, thanks to the efforts of dietitians practicing or residing in those states. States specify the credentials required for dietetic nutrition practitioners, such as whether they must be state licensed or otherwise certified, the designated setting where the service can be provided, and the number of visits allowed, appropriate code numbers to use, and level of reimbursement.

Healthcare reform of 2010 may bring other government santioned health care.

---

ongoing, and coordinated approach to achieving desired outcomes for a population of patients. These outcomes include improving patients' clinical condition, reducing unnecessary healthcare costs and improving patients' quality of life. To achieve these objectives requires rigorous, protocol-based, clinical management in conjunction with intensive patient education, coaching and monitoring: in short, a comprehensive system that incorporates the patient, physician, and health plan into one system with one common goal.

Chronic disease management is now a major component of primary health care. The population is aging, and older adults have many chronic conditions. In addition, some survive for decades with a chronic disease. As indicated in Chapter 9, the leading causes of death in the United States include the chronic diseases CVD and type-2 diabetes. Nutrition is fundamental in the self-management of these conditions. A cost-effective way of delivering nutrition services is through group (or cluster) visits.

Group visits are a cost-effective means of providing self-care guidance and support to chronically ill patients who need more dietary advice than physicians have the resources (skill and time) to deliver. Group (or cluster) visits are designed to help patients manage their health, adhere to their physicians' plans of care, and assure that they seek or obtain medical care they need to reduce their health risks. The term is applied to groups of patients with similar characteristics rather than individual patient-provider appointments. In this model, the healthcare team facilitates an interactive process of care delivery in a periodic group visit program. The group can be conceptualized as an extended doctor's office visit. Invitations are extended by the healthcare team to specific patients on the basis of chronic disease history and utilization patterns. Variations of this group format have been used for disease specific populations, such as diabetes, hypertension, dyslipemia, and weight control. Group visits offer staff a means to interact with patients that makes efficient use of resources, improves access, and uses group process to help motivate behavior change and improve outcomes. Guidelines for planning and implementing group visits have been developed by Improving Chronic Illness Care (ICIC), a national program of the RJW Foundation. The guidelines are available on the ICIC's Web site at http://www.improvingchroniccare. org/tools/criticaltools.html.

An example of an urban, community-based, disease self-management education program is the diabetes program. The diabetes self-management program is led by a nurse and dietitian, who are Certified Diabetes Educators (CDEs). The program consists of a series of six two-hour sessions held in a community location. Participants are recruited through flyers, postings, and newspaper advertisements near the location where the education is to be provided. Group sessions are held with 6 to 18 participants.[23]

Chronic diseases have a long course of illness. They rarely resolve spontaneously and generally are not cured by medication. Today, chronic diseases, such as cardiovascular disease (CVD; primarily heart disease and stroke), cancer, and diabetes, are among the most prevalent, costly, and preventable of all health problems. The prolonged course of illness and disability, from such chronic diseases as diabetes and arthritis, has resulted in extended pain and suffering and decreased quality of life for millions of Americans. These and other chronic, disabling conditions were discussed in Chapter 11.

■ REPRESENTATIVE PROGRAMS THAT DELIVER NUTRITION SERVICES IN PRIMARY CARE SETTINGS

The Indian Health Service

Native Americans are dying at rates up to seven times higher than other Americans of alcoholism, tuberculosis, diabetes, and from accidents, suicide, and homicide. The Indian Health Service (IHS), an agency within the DHHS, is responsible for providing federal health services to American Indians and Alaska Natives (AI/AN). The provision of health services to members of federally recognized tribes grew out of the special government-to-government relationship between the federal government and Indian tribes. This relationship, established in 1787, is based on Article I, Section 8 of the U.S. Constitution, and has been given form

and substance by numerous treaties, laws, Supreme Court decisions, and executive orders. The HIS is charged with upholding the federal government's obligation to promote healthy AI/AN people, communities, and cultures, and to honor and protect the inherent sovereign rights of tribes. As the principal federal healthcare provider and health advocate for indigenous populations, the goal of the IHS is to assure that comprehensive, culturally acceptable personal and public health services are available and accessible. The IHS provides health services to 1.5 to 2 million individuals who belong to more than 557 federally recognized tribes in 35 states, mostly in the western United States and Alaska. For FY 2003, Congress appropriated $2.9 billion to help provide healthcare services to AI/AN.[24]

IHS services are provided directly and through tribally contracted and operated health programs. Health services include health care purchased from more than 9,000 private providers annually. The Federal system consists of hospitals, health centers, health stations, and residential treatment centers. In addition, American Indian tribes and Alaska Native corporations administer hospitals, health centers, residential treatment centers, health stations, and Alaska village clinics. Most of the care supported by the HIS is administered through Community-Oriented Primary Care (COPC), an approach to healthcare delivery that undertakes responsibility for the health of a defined population. COPC is practiced by combining epidemiologic study and social interventions with clinical care of individual patients, so that the primary care practice itself becomes a community medicine program. Both the individual patient and the community in which the patient lives are the foci of diagnosis, treatment and ongoing surveillance.

The IHS employs approximately 15,000 people, including members of virtually every discipline involved in providing health care, social, and environmental health services. All of the IHS senior executive service staff are of AI/AN descent; excluding medical professionals, approximately 88% of IHS staff are of AI/AN descent. Nutritionists and others who have health-related degrees have the option of joining the IHS as civil servants or as commissioned officers in the Public Health Service (PHS). To become familiar with the HIS agency and its programs, visit the Web sites at http:// www.ihs.gov and http://www.info.ihs.gov.

Preventive measures involving environmental, educational, and outreach activities are combined with therapeutic measures into a single national health system. Within these broad categories are special initiatives in traditional medicine, elder care, women's health, children and adolescents, injury prevention, domestic violence and child abuse, health care financing, state health care, sanitation facilities, and oral health.

Most IHS funds are appropriated for American Indians who live on or near reservations. Congress also authorizes programs that provide some access to care for Indians who live in urban areas rather than on reservations or in Alaska Native villages. The National Council of Urban Indian Health was founded in 1998 to meet the unique healthcare needs of the urban Indian population through education, training, and advocacy. Title V of Public Law 94-437, the Indian Health Care Improvement Act, authorizes the appropriation of funds for urban Indian Health Organizations. Title V funds are but one source of funding for urban Indian health organizations. Urban Indian primary care clinics and outreach programs provide culturally acceptable, accessible, affordable, and accountable health services to an underserved off-reservation urban Indian population. These urban health organizations engage in a variety of activities, ranging from the provision of outreach and referral services to the delivery of comprehensive ambulatory health care.

The IHS's *Patient Education Protocols and Codes (PEPC)* were developed to standardize the provision of health services and documentation of patient education encounters from one health professional to another. Among the nutrition-related topics included in the manual are gestational diabetes, type-2 diabetes, obesity, wellness, exercise, medical nutrition therapy. The 14th edition (2008) of the manual is available online at http://www.ihs.gov/NonMedical Programs/HealthEd/index.cfm?module = initiative& option = protocols/.

Type-2 Diabetes

Almost 15% of American Indians and Alaska Natives aged 20 years or older and receiving care from IHS have diabetes. At the regional level, diabetes is least common among Alaska Natives (8.2%) and most common among American Indians in the Southeastern United States (27.8%) and southern Arizona (27.8%). On average, American Indians and Alaska Natives are 2.3 times as likely to have diabetes as non-Hispanic whites of similar age.[25]

Prevention should focus on decreasing the risk, incidence, and consequences of type-2 diabetes mellitus among AI/AN children. Primary prevention efforts by primary healthcare professionals are recommended in two arenas: 1) general community health promotion and health education, and 2) activities in the primary care clinic. Clinically based health promotion activities should not duplicate community-wide health promotion but instead should offer additive benefits. For example, if significant health education is offered at the community level, then motivational interviewing and collaborative problem solving can be offered in the clinical setting. Current evidence suggests that modifiable risks for type-2 diabetes mellitus include obesity and lack of breast feeding.[26] Primary prevention efforts can focus on the prevention of obesity in children and the promotion of breast feeding. Preventing obesity in women of childbearing age is another primary prevention goal, because a diabetic pregnancy places the fetus at increased risk of future onset of diabetes.

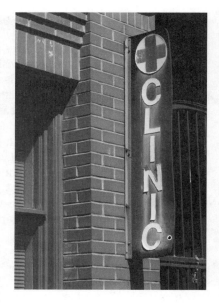

Early diagnosis and optimal medical care are the keys to effective secondary prevention. When type-2 diabetes mellitus is the established diagnosis, secondary prevention efforts by primary healthcare professionals are important for the prevention of complications (e.g., vascular, neural, renal, retinal).

The American Academy of Pediatrics (AAP) Committee on Native American Child Health, in collaboration with the IHS Diabetes Program, the CDC, and the AAP Section on Endocrinology, developed guidelines to improve the medical care for AI/AN children with type-2 diabetes mellitus and those at risk of developing it. The guidelines are consistent with the 2005 American Diabetes Association (ADA) consensus statement on type-2 diabetes mellitus in children and adolescents.[27] The guidelines support the role of the general pediatrician or other primary healthcare professional as the front line for care. Treatment of most AI/AN children with type-2 diabetes mellitus should be managed by primary healthcare professionals with specialty consultation. The guidelines are intended to serve as a framework for the development of diabetes care programs and strategies aimed at decreasing the impact of type-2 diabetes mellitus on AI/AN children and their families and communities.

The IHS Standards of Care for Patients with Type 2 Diabetes (available at http://www.ihs.gov/MedicalPrograms/ Diabetes/HomeDocs/Tools/ClinicalGuidelines/Standards_ Care_508Rev.pdf) was developed and updated by the IHS National Diabetes Program and Area Diabetes Consultants in 2009 to help provide consistent, quality care to AI/AN patients with diabetes. The IHS Diabetes Program supports the American Diabetes Association position that everyone with diabetes should receive regular nutrition counseling and should be seen by an RD every 6 to 12 months. Some people may require more frequent evaluation and counseling.

■ HEALTH RESOURCES AND SERVICES ADMINISTRATION, BUREAU OF PRIMARY HEALTH CARE

The Health Resources and Services Administration (HRSA), an agency of the U.S. DHHS, is the primary federal agency for improving access to healthcare services for people who are uninsured, isolated, or medically vulnerable. HRSA's 6 bureaus and 13 offices provide leadership and financial support to healthcare providers in every state and U.S. territory. HRSA grantees provide health care to uninsured people, people living with HIV/AIDS, and pregnant women, mothers, and children. They train health professionals and improve systems of care in rural communities. HRSA funds almost 1,110 health center grantees that operate more than 7,000 clinics and mobile medical vans. The HSRA budget in FY 2009 was $7 billion. (Note that federal fiscal year, FY, begins October 1st and ends September 30th.)

Four of HRSA's 6 bureaus are discussed in this section: Community Health Centers, Migrant Health Centers, Public Housing Primary Care Program, and Health Care for the Homeless.

Community Health Centers

Community health centers (http://findahealthcenter.hrsa.gov/) offer "one-stop shopping" where primary and preventive healthcare visits, lab services, dental and mental health services, and case management are conveniently located, coordinated, and tailored to meet the patient's needs.[22] Ideally, community health center staff and providers are as diverse as the patients that they serve; many are bilingual and residents of the community. In FY 2009, more than $2.1 billion was appropriated to support the Health Center Program.

Technically known as Federally Qualified Health Centers (FQHCs), community health centers are nonprofit healthcare providers that serve the communities in which they are located. Almost 1,200 health centers serve as the medical home and family physician to 16 million people in the United States, about 5% of the population. Health centers deliver primary and preventive care to over 16 million low-income patients in every state, the District of Columbia, Puerto Rico, the U.S. Virgin Islands, and U.S. possessions in the Pacific.

FQHCs were established in the 1960s as part of the federal government's "War on Poverty." In particular, HRSA's Primary Health Care Programs have their roots in the Migrant Health Act of 1962 and the Economic Opportunity Act of 1964, which established funding for the first community-based clinics. The founders saw quality, personalized medical care as a right of all people and established a policy that no patient would be turned away, regardless of their ability to pay. FQHCs are "by the community, for the community, of the community."[21] Federal law requires that every FQHS have a Board of Directors and that more than half of the Board members must be patients of that center.

Health center patients are among the nation's most vulnerable populations, who are people who even if insured would nonetheless remain isolated from traditional forms of medical care because of where they live, who they are, the language they speak, and their higher levels of complex healthcare needs. About half of health center patients reside in rural areas, while the other half tend to live in economically depressed, inner city communities. Health centers serve one in five low-income children. Two-thirds of health center patients have family incomes at or below the U.S. poverty level ($18,310 annual income for a family of three in 2009). Moreover, nearly one-third of health center patients are uninsured and another one-third depend on Medicaid, much higher than the national rates of 12% and 15%, respectively. Two thirds of health center patients are members of racial and ethnic minorities. All health centers offer a sliding fee scale for the uninsured and low-income patients.

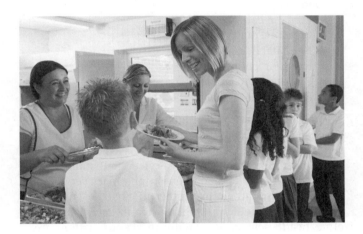

An FQHC is a community health center that has been designated by the federal government as adhering to regulations pertaining to the scope and quality of health services provided to anyone, regardless of ability to pay. Similarly, an *FQHC Look Alike* is a health center that has been identified by the Health Resources and Services Administration (HRSA) and certified by the Centers for Medicare and Medicaid Services as meeting the definition of "health center," although it does not receive grant funding from the federal government. These clinics are reimbursed by Medicaid for their services.

There are benefits of being an FQHC. For FQHCs that are PHS 330 grant recipients, the biggest benefit is the grant funding; for new programs, funding up to $650,000 can be requested. (The funding for new starts is not available to FQHC Look-Alikes.) Other benefits include: enhanced Medicare and Medicaid reimbursement, medical malpractice coverage through the Federal Tort Claims Act, eligibility to purchase prescription and non-prescription medications for outpatients at reduced cost, access to National Health Service Corps (http://nhsc.bhpr.hrsa.gov/index.htm) and eligibility for various other federal grants and programs.

Each FQHC that receives PHS 330 grant funding must meet the requirements of that grant. Community Health

Centers must serve a Medically Underserved Area (MUA) or Medically Underserved Population (MUP). To determine if an area qualifies, search the MUA/MUP database at http://muafind.hrsa.gov/. If an area does not have the MUA/MUP designation, they can apply for it and put in an application for a PHS Section 330 grant while the designation is being processed. Migrant Health Centers, Health Care for the Homeless, and Public Housing Primary Care Programs do not need to meet the MUA/MUP restriction.

FQHCs offer health care to every member of the family throughout the lifespan. Nutrition is a component of many of the comprehensive support services offered by health centers, including:

- Primary care
- Prenatal care
- Breast-feeding classes
- Neonatal home visits
- Nutrition counseling
- Diabetes management
- HIV treatment

Other services provided include: dental services, mental health counseling, immunizations, AIDS family social services, case management, school-based clinics, family planning, homeless support services, substance abuse counseling, treatment and referrals, pharmacy services, lab testing, 12-step programs, domestic violence prevention, senior abuse screening, migrant health care, cancer and other health screenings, childbirth classes, asthma treatment, early education supports, flu clinics transportation, medical interpretation, eye exams, podiatric services, and comprehensive HIV care, including outreach education, prevention and treatment.

The healthcare delivery model used in the community health center has been described is the *patient-centered medical home* (PCMH). This model seeks to 1) strengthen the provider-patient relationship and 2) replace episodic care based on illness with coordinated care based on prevention. The physician-led PCMH team provides all the patient's healthcare needs and, when necessary, arranges for referrals to specialists outside of the practice. The PCMH is being examined as model to be adopted to contain medical costs in the future.[28]

Migrant Health Centers

Since 1962, the Federal Migrant Health Program (MHP) has provided grants to community nonprofit organizations for a broad array of medical and support services to migrant and seasonal farm workers and their families.[29] The MHP was originally authorized by the Migrant Health Act, Public Law 87-692, enacted in September 1962 and is currently authorized under section 330(g) of the Public Health Service Act. The vision of the MHP is the universal accessibility to quality and appropriate health care for the nation's migrant and seasonal farm workers (MSFW) and their families. The MHP provides MSFWs and their families' access to comprehensive, culturally competent, primary care services. The MHP supports the delivery of migrant health services including primary and preventive health care, transportation, outreach, dental, pharmaceutical, occupational health and safety, and environmental health. These programs use bilingual, bicultural lay outreach workers, health personnel, and culturally sensitive appropriate protocols. They also provide prevention-oriented and pediatric services such as immunizations, well baby care, and developmental screenings. Currently the MHP provides grants to 125 public and nonprofit organizations that support the development and operation of 400 migrant clinic sites throughout the United States and Puerto Rico. In 2008, Migrant Health Centers served almost 850,000 migrant and seasonal farm workers and their families. It is estimated that HRSA-funded health center programs serve more than one-quarter of all migrant and seasonal farm workers in the United States MHP funding in FY 2002 was $107 million.

Public Housing Primary Care Program

Across the nation there are over 6.7 million residents living in public housing. The average household size for residents of public housing is 2.2 people, over 21% of who remain in public housing more than five years. Forty percent of the residents are children through 17 years of age. Nearly 15% of residents in public housing are at least 62 years of age, and one-third are disabled. The average annual household income of a household for residents of public housing is $13,306, below the poverty line of $14,570 for a household of two. The primary source of income for a third of public housing resident households is through wages. However, despite the efforts of this working population, more than nearly two-thirds of public housing residents fall into the "Very Low Income" category of the Department of Housing and Urban Development (HUD), with an income of less than 50% of the national median. Social Security payments are the primary source of income for approximately 55% of seniors in public housing.[30,31]

The United States Housing Act of 1937 (P.L. 75-412) created the public housing program. The Act is also known as the Wagner-Steagall Housing Act and the Low-Rent Housing Act. Under the program, the federal government, through the HUD, provides subsidies to local public housing agencies that rent housing to low-income families. Public housing was established to provide decent and safe rental housing for eligible low-income families, the elderly, and persons with disabilities. HUD administers federal aid to local housing agencies that manage the housing for low-income people and also furnishes technical and professional assistance in planning, developing and managing these developments. Approximately 7 million people live in public housing units.

The Public Housing Primary Care (PHPC) Program is a federal grant program created under the Disadvantaged Minority Health Improvement Act of 1990. In 1996, the PHPC Program was reauthorized under the Health Centers Consolidation Act as Section 330(i) of the Public Health Service Act. The PHPC is administered by the Bureau of Primary Health Care (BPHC), a branch of HRSA. The mission of PHPC is to provide accessible comprehensive primary health care and supportive services in order to improve the overall health and well-being of the public housing community, and to eliminate health disparities.

The PHPC Program supports health centers and other health delivery systems in providing services in partnership with other community-based providers of public housing developments or at other locations immediately accessible to residents of public housing. PHPC grantees provide primary healthcare services, including direct medical care, health screening and education, dental, prenatal and perinatal, preventive health, and case management; conduct outreach services to inform residents about health services availability; aid residents in establishing eligibility for assistance under entitlement programs and obtaining government support for health care, mental and oral health, or social services; and train and employ residents of public housing to provide health screenings and health education services.

PHPC health centers have an integrated approach to delivering primary health care, health promotion, and disease prevention. Each PHPC program provides comprehensive primary healthcare services, including internal medicine, pediatrics, OB/GYN care, preventive and restorative dental care, health education, outreach, laboratory services, and case management. Many PHPC health centers also provide behavioral health services, pharmacy, x-ray, optometry, and podiatry, along with nutritional services through the Women, Infants, and Children (WIC) program

In FY 2008, 55 PHPC grantees in 24 states were awarded program funds to provide primary healthcare services. HRSA-funded health centers served nearly 157,000 residents of public housing. At least one-third of the primary diagnoses were nutrition-related (high blood pressure and diabetes), demonstrating the need for nutrition services in this federally sponsored initiative. The PHPC budget in FY 2003 was $18.5 million.

The program publishes quarterly information bulletins that feature updates on the health of residents of public housing, best practices of PHPC health centers, and news about housing authorities' and housing organizations' efforts to promote resident health and self-sufficiency. These are available at online at http://www.healthandpublichousing.org/newsletters.html.

Health Care for the Homeless

An estimated two million are homeless in the United States. Homeless people have the same health problems as people with homes, but get sick with common illnesses much more often than people who are housed. Without a home, there is no place to recuperate from an illness or to treat an injury, and health problems tend to get far worse before they get better. Compared to people with housing, the homeless have higher rates of mental illness (about one-third of people without homes are mentally ill) and current or past drug or alcohol addiction (about one-half), and communicable diseases such as HIV/AIDS and tuberculosis. Infections of every sort are prominent among homeless people, as is trauma resulting from violence and conditions caused by exposure to the elements.

The HRSA-funded Health Care for the Homeless (HCH) Program is a major source of care for homeless persons in the United States, serving patients that live on the street, in shelters, or in transitional housing. In 2008, these health centers served nearly 934,000 persons experiencing homelessness. Programs that deliver primary health care to people without a permanent domicile must be multidisciplinary, as homeless people often have serious, multiple diagnoses. HCH provides primary health care, including diagnosis and treatment for common illnesses. Also provided is behavioral health care, addiction treatment, and mental health services. HCH also offers other services such as access to specialty care, transportation, housing, and medical respite care—services that reflect a wide range of needs. There are HCH programs in every state, the District of Columbia, and Puerto Rico and nearly all major cities in the United States have at least one HCH program. HCH programs are funded primarily by grants from HRSA, but also from state and local governments and donations.

Providers of health care for the homeless need to establish markers of successful outcomes that are unique to the realities of the homeless existence. Seven client-level outcomes have been posited as goals for federally funded HCH projects. Although related, the client-level outcomes can be measured independently of one another. These are improved health status, improved level of functioning, improved quality of life, involvement in treatment, disease self-management, client choice, and client satisfaction.[33]

The National Health Care for the Homeless Council (http://www.nhchc.org/) provides technical assistance to communities trying to obtain HRSA grants or to organize without federal support. Federal grants are only a fraction of the amount required to create a well-rounded program. Not surprisingly, most homeless people are not covered by health insurance, which limits the amount of Medicaid dollars that are billable.

The National Coalition for the Homeless estimates that more than one-half of the homeless population does not receive food stamps. Lack of transportation, lack of knowledge about the program, mental illness, and lack of documentation are some of the common barriers that prevent homeless people from receiving SNAP/Food Stamps. In fact, homeless persons have identical rights under the SNAP/Food Stamp Program as persons who are housed, and they also have some additional rights due to the fact that they are homeless.[33]

Many homeless people rely on shelters and soup kitchens for their food intake. For children, additional sources of food are the National School Lunch Program and the School Breakfast Program as well as the Summer Food Service Program. Referral to the appropriate USDA food assistance program is one of the most important services we can provide to individuals and families who are homeless.

■ RECOMMENDATIONS

Medical caregivers should be able to increase their patients' motivation to improve their diet, just as counseling by medical caregivers has been found to profoundly increase smokers' motivation to stop using tobacco. Unfortunately, physicians may not have the time or the expertise to perform detailed nutrition counseling. The single most important barrier to providing adequate nutrition services in primary care is money. Although there is general consensus regarding the importance of prevention and early detection of the nutrition-related chronic diseases, inadequacies in the structure and organization of healthcare delivery detracts from the adequate delivery of primary and preventive care and recommendations and support of requisite lifestyle changes.

Strategies to improve the delivery of nutrition services in the primary healthcare setting—at a minimum—are three-fold: 1) third party reimbursement for preventive nutrition counseling; 2) training physicians so they feel confident about delivering nutrition advice and are educated on the full armamentarium of nutrition materials that already exist; and 3) reorganizing the primary care office so that self-management is incorporated into disease management.

References

1. Donaldson MS, Yordy KD, Lohr KN, Vanselow NA, eds. *Primary Care: America's Health in a New Era*. Washington, DC: Institute of Medicine National Academy Press; 1996.

2. U.S. Department of Health and Human Services. *Healthy People 2010: Understanding and Improving Health*, 2nd ed. Washington, DC: U.S. Government Printing Office; 2000.

3. U.S. Department of Health and Human Services. *Phase I Report. Recommendations for the Framework and Format of Healthy People 2020*. Available at http://www.healthypeople.gov/hp2020/advisory/PhaseI/summary.htm/. Accessed April 28, 2010.

4. Sloane PD, Slatt LM, Ebell MH, Jacques LB, Smith MA. *Essentials of Family Medicine*, 5th ed. Ch. 8: Introduction to common problems. Philadelphia, PA: Lippincott Williams & Wilkins; 2008.

5. Car J, Sheikh A. Email consultations in health care: 2—acceptability and safe application. *BMJ*. 2004;329:439–442.

6. U.S. Preventive Services Task Force. *Guide to Clinical Preventive Services*, 2nd ed. Washington, DC: U.S. Department of Health and Human Services; 1996. Available at http://odphp.osophs.dhhs.gov/pubs/guidecps/default.htm. Accessed April 28, 2010.

7. Agency for Healthcare Research and Quality (AHRQ). *The Guide to Clinical Preventive Services, 2008*. Publication No. 08-05122., Rockville, MD: AHRQ. 2009 version available at http://www.ahrq.gov/clinic/pocketgd.htm. Accessed April 28, 2010.

8. Agency for Healthcare Research and Quality (AHRQ). *Child and Adolescent Health Resources*. Rockville, MD: AHRQ. Available at http://www.ahrq.gov/ppip/childguide/. Accessed April 28, 2010.

9. Agency for Healthcare Research and Quality (AHRQ). Dissemination and Implementation. Put Prevention into Practice (PPIP). Rockville, MD: AHRQ. Available at http://www.ahrq.gov/clinic/ppipix.htm. Accessed April 28, 2010.

10. Eyre H, Kahn R, Robertson RM, et al. Preventing cancer, cardiovascular disease, and diabetes: a common agenda for the American Cancer Society, the American Diabetes Association, and the American Heart Association. *Circulation*. 2004;109:3244–3255.

11. Agency for Healthcare Research and Quality (AHRQ). *About PPIP. Put Prevention into Practice*. Rockville, MD: AHRQ. Available at http://www.ahrq.gov/ppip/ppipabou.htm. Accessed April 28, 2010.

12. Pollak KI, Krause KM, Yarnall KS, Gradison M, Michener JL, Østbye T. Estimated time spent on preventive services by primary care physicians. *BMC Health Serv Res*. 2008;8:245.

13. Eaton CB, McBride PE, Gans KA, Underbakke GL. Teaching nutrition skills to primary care practitioners. *J Nutr*. 2003;133:563S–566S.

14. Mihalynuk TV, Scott CS, Coombs JB. Self-reported nutrition proficiency is positively correlated with the perceived quality of nutrition training of family physicians in Washington State. *Am J Clin Nutr*. 2003;77:1330–1336.

15. Schulman JA. Nutrition education in medical schools: Trends and implications for health educators. *Med Educ Online*. [serial online] 1999;4,4. Available at http://www.med-ed-online.net/index.php/meo/article/viewFile/4307/4498. Accessed April 28, 2010.

16. Gans KM, Ross E, Barner CW, Wylie-Rosett J, McMurray J, Eaton C. REAP and WAVE: new tools to rapidly assess/discuss nutrition with patients. *J Nutr*. 2003;133:556S–562S.

17. Eaton CB, Goodwin MA, Stange KC. Direct observation of nutrition counseling in community family practice. *Am J Prev Med*. 2002;23:174–179.

18. Anis NA, Lee RE, Ellerbeck EF, Nazir N, Greiner KA, Ahluwalia JS. Direct observation of physician counseling on dietary habits and exercise: patient, physician, and office correlates. *Prev Med*. 2004;38:198–202.

19. Whitlock EP, Orleans T, Pender N, Allan J. Evaluating primary care behavioral counseling interventions: an evidence-based approach. *Am J Prev Med*. 2002;22:267–284.

20. Pearson TA, Stone EJ, Grundy SM, McBride PE, Van Horn L, Tobin BW; NAA Collaborative Group. Translation of nutritional sciences into medical education: the Nutrition Academic Award Program. *Am J Clin Nutr*. 2001;74:164–170.

21. Bureau of Primary Health Care. Primary Health Care: The Health Center Program. Available at http://bphc.hrsa.gov. Accessed April 28, 2010.

22. Improving Chronic Illness Care. Homepage. Available at http://www.improvingchroniccare.org/index.php?p=Home&s=1. Accessed April 28, 2010.

23. Funnell MM, Anderson RM. Working toward the next generation of diabetes self-management education. *Am J Prev Med*. 2002;22(4 Suppl):3–5.

24. Indian Health Service. *Fact Sheet*. Available at http://www.ihs.gov/PublicInfo/PublicAffairs/Welcome_Info/ThisFacts.asp. Accessed April 28, 2010.

25. National Institute of Diabetes and Digestive and Kidney Diseases. *National Diabetes Statistics fact sheet: general information and national estimates on diabetes in the United States, 2007*. Bethesda, MD: U.S. Department of Health and Human Services,

National Institutes of Health. Available at http://diabetes.niddk.nih.gov/dm/pubs/statistics/. Accessed May 14, 2010.

26. Pettitt DJ, Knowler WC. Long-term effects of the intrauterine environment, birth weight, and breast-feeding in Pima Indians. *Diab Care*. 1998;21(suppl 2):B138–B141.

27. American Diabetes Association. Type 2 diabetes in children and adolescents. Available at http://care.diabetesjournals.org/content/30/suppl_1/S91.full. Accessed May 14, 2010.

28. Lipscomb R. Understanding the patient-centered medical home. *J Am Diet Asso*c. 2009;109:1507–1508.

29. Bureau of Primary Health Care. Migrant Health Program. http://bphc.hrsa.gov/programs/MHCProgramInfo.htm. Accessed July 1, 2004.

30. U.S. Department of Housing and Urban Development. Resident Characteristics Report. August 31, 2009.

31. National Center for Health in Public Housing. About NCHPH. Available at http://www.healthinpublichousing.org/about.html. Accessed April 28, 2010.

32. McMurray-Avila M, Gelberg L, Breakey WR. Balancing act: clinical practices that respond to the needs of homeless people. In: Fosburg LB, Dennis DL, eds., for the U.S. Department of Housing and Urban Development. *Practical Lessons: The 1998 National Symposium on Homelessness Research*. Aug 2009. Available at http://aspe.hhs.gov/progsys/homeless/symposium/toc.htm. Accessed April 28, 2010.

33. United States Department of Agriculture (USDA). *SNAP/Food Stamps and Homelessness*. May 2009. Available at http://www.masslegalhelp.org/income-benefits/fshomelessness. Accessed April 28, 2010.

CHAPTER 14

The Baby Boomers: Identification of Wellness Needs

Stacey Chappa, RD

Shirley Chao, MS, RD, LDN

Sari Edelstein, PhD, RD

READER OBJECTIVES

After studying this chapter and reflecting on the contents, you should be able to:

1. Describe the demographic characteristics of the baby boomer population.
2. Discuss the wellness concerns of baby boomers.
3. Identify how public health can best address these wellness concerns.

■ INTRODUCTION

One-third of the United States' population is composed of *baby boomers*, defined as those born between 1946 and 1964. During these decades, the population jumped in number, allowing relative prosperity. This gave individuals opportunities to achieve education levels beyond their prior generations, and to live in a world with major advances in medical science and technology.[1] The initial wave of this cohort has entered the retirement years and is facing the demands of aging. A literature review suggests that these so called "golden boomers" have different characteristics, needs, and demands than most of the elderly population currently served by the public health community.[2] Taking into account the research on education level, family complexity, diversity, income, and health conditions, major needs for these boomers have begun to surface. To sum up current research simply, the baby boomers' needs center on quality of life.

Aging is a multidimensional process influenced by health, desires, family roles, and productivity. Sensitivity to family dynamics and diversity are important considerations when serving baby boomers. The well-being of the boomer generation encompasses screening, assessment, diet, supplement usage, exercise, sexual vitality, pain management, management of health, and

Baby boomers are those persons born between the years 1946 and 1964. There are currently 78.2 million baby boomers in the United States. http://www.census.gov/Press-Release/www/releases/archives/facts_for_features_special_editions/006105.html

living conditions. Boomers acquire health information through education by academia, public health programs, comprehensive health packages offered by the private sector, and personal inquiries. Health packages must integrate alternative and traditional medicine, as long-term care is moving from a traditional medical model towards a holistic approach. To ensure quality of life and overall wellness of boomers, their needs must be addressed and met. This responsibly falls on the community at large, which is comprised of the private, public, government/regulatory, and academic/research sectors. These factors and more are the discussion topics of this chapter.

Growing up after World War II, baby boomers were better educated and better paid than previous American generations. Boomers are becoming our nation's elders; the youngest baby boomer turned 46 years old in 2010 while the oldest was age 64. Between 2011 and 2029, the over-65 population will grow by 77 million people, and that number is expected to increase to 89 million by 2050.[1] In 2010, between 5 and 6 million people were in their 90s.[2]

Boomers have different characteristics, needs, and demands than the elderly population currently served by the community sectors. Boomers' heritage and family structure, formal education, income, employment, and health conditions are different from that of most of today's elders. Assessing the characteristics of boomers' needs and demands provides a portrait of who they are (**Table 14–1**).

As stated previously, the general needs of boomers center on maintaining the quality of their lives. *Health-related quality of life* is a scientific concept that describes a person's perception of their health, well-being, and ability to function. Aging is a multidimensional process characterized by

TABLE 14–1	Characteristics of the Boomer Generation
Characteristic	**Definition**
Heritage and family structure	More ethnically diverse than generations before them. Have fewer children than their parents' generation. Have higher rates of divorce and remarriage than their parents' generation. Grandparents are often raising grandchildren. Formal education. More formal education than today's senior citizens.
Income (median or household)	Higher median family and household incomes than today's senior citizens (although the cost of living is much higher today than it was 20–40 years ago).
Employment	Longer working hours than their parents' generation and more women employed outside of the home.
Health condition	Much more likely to smoke, be overweight, and have a sedentary lifestyle than their parents' generation. Sedentary lifestyle is a risk factor of heart disease, cancer, and diabetes.

biological changes, evolving wants and needs, family roles, and productivity. Another goal of this chapter is to identify boomers' needs so that public health professionals can help to promote a smooth transition into their golden years.[3]

FAMILY STRUCTURE

Boomers have complex family structures and greater diversity than previous generations. Family dynamics are an important consideration when working with boomers. Many are still caring for their elderly parents. Due to the high divorce rate and number of single parents, boomers may also be caring for their grandchildren.[4] Census data from 2000 stated that 5.6 million grandparents nationwide had grandchildren living with them, and 42% of these people reported being the primary caregiver of their grandchildren. Therefore, public health programs must appeal to dynamic families. Public health professionals also need to customize and adjust existing programs, materials, and means of communication to fit the demographic diversity of age, language, and ethnic culture of the boomer population.[4] It is important to have culturally sensitive and knowledgeable workers on staff to best serve this population.

Boomers have more formal education than their elders. According to the 2000 U.S. census summary, about 84% of people between the ages of 35 and 64 graduated high school, compared to only 65% of people over 64 years of age. About 26% of people aged 35 to 64 have a bachelor's degree or higher, whereas only 15% of people over age 64 have a bachelor's degree or higher. The average household income for boomers is $80,000 annually. Boomers are expected to retire later in life and slowly shift from full-time employment to retirement. For them, jobs provide a source of income, add meaning to life, and may prevent social isolation. By creating new identities and roles, boomer women are becoming a strong force in the workplace. Women, as a whole, contribute about 40% of all household income.[5] The health conditions of boomers will directly affect their

quality of life, their wellness needs, and their ability to seek these new roles.

STATE OF HEALTH

The leading causes of death in the United States in the year 2006 were heart disease, cancer, stroke, respiratory disease, accidents, diabetes mellitus, influenza and pneumonia, Alzheimer's disease, and kidney failure.[6-15] Heart disease and cancer accounted for over one-half of all deaths, when combined.[16] Tobacco use, lack of physical activity, and poor nutrition are major contributors to heart disease and cancer.[17] Obesity and lack of physical activity are risk factors for developing type-2 diabetes. According to the third National Health and Nutrition Examination Survey (NHANES III), an estimated 29 million persons (14.4%) aged ≥20 years had either been diagnosed with diabetes, had undiagnosed diabetes, or had an impaired fasting glucose blood level. Diabetes is also the leading cause of kidney failure. More than 193,000 deaths and 60% of all lower-limb amputations occur annually due to diabetes.[17] Behavior modification through diet and exercise, as well as smoking cessation, can decrease the prevalence of heart disease, cancer, and diabetes. One in every five deaths is caused by tobacco.[17] Smokers who die of tobacco-related usage lose about 12 years of expected life.[17] In 2008, Center for Disease Control (CDC) reported that cigarette smoking and exposure to secondhand smoke resulted in an estimated 443,000 deaths and 5.1 million years of potential life lost annually in the United States between 2000 and 2004.[18] About 25% of American adults, or about 47 million, smoke.[17] Elderly smokers who quit can obtain significant health benefits and risk reduction of death, which justifies the need for smoking cessation programs. Arthritis and back pain are other health conditions that affect quality of life and functionality. Some arthritis and back pain may be attributed to carrying excess body weight.

Several factors have contributed to the surge in weight among U.S. adults. Boomers value generous portion sizes and value, as they grew up at the same time the fast food industry was created. Convenience foods were introduced as well as meal replacement drinks and bars to accommodate the busy lifestyles of boomers. Fast food and snacks replaced home-cooked meals. And, boomers adopted a sedentary lifestyle. According to data from NHANES III, approximately one-third of Americans aged 20 to 74 (58 million) are overweight. (These numbers are derived from NHANES III, 1988–1991. NHANES III defines overweight as a BMI value of 27.3% or more for women and 27.8% or more for men.) The Behavioral Risk Factor Surveillance System revealed that 31 states had adult obesity rates between 20% and 24% and four states had obesity rates greater than 25%.[19] If the trends of overweight and obesity continue to rise, it is projected by 2030, 86.3% of adults will be overweight or obese and 51.1% will be obese.[20]

A report in 2010 from the CDC assessed the level of physical activity among adults in the United States. The results indicated that about 60% of adults engaged in some level of physical activity. Forty percent of adults did not achieve the recommended amount of physical activity during leisure time.[17]

Arthritis is one of the most prevalent diseases in the United States and affects 43 billion people. Arthritis limits the boomer's ability to be mobile and perform daily activities without assistance. The ability to function is a component of quality of life. One out of six people have arthritis in the United States, which means that more than 7 million Americans' daily activities are limited by arthritis. Arthritis and other rheumatoid conditions are the leading cause of disability in the United States and will affect an estimated 60 million people by 2020.[17] Low back pain is also prevalent among Americans. According to the American Academy of Orthopedic Surgeons, 80% of Americans will experience back pain at some time in their life.

In the United States, elderly people of all ethnicities are experiencing a proportionately greater rate of new AIDS cases than any other age group. In 2007, there were approximately 8 million persons living with AIDS in the United States. Older adults (50 years and up) accounted for approximately 131,000 cases.[21] Public health educational materials and risk reduction are needed to halt HIV/AIDS infection among the boomers.[21]

■ EDUCATIONAL DEMANDS

Boomers have a need for health education through many sources, as stated previously. The academic sector must continue to conduct research and publish results of trials and studies. Boomers also need more Internet navigation sites to help them sift through the health information online.

More public health programs that promote the health and well-being of boomers through education are needed.

Preventative health measures need to be taken to reduce the prevalence of chronic, preventable diseases in the boomer population. Community and public health classes on diet and exercise should be given that discuss the relationship between lifestyle behaviors and the development of heart disease, cancer, obesity, and diabetes. Smoking cessation programs can be initiated for boomers. Also, sexual health and vitality affect quality of life, and boomers need programs that promote healthy sexual practices. This area, relatively ignored in recent years, has been brought to the forefront with the creation of sexual stimulants marketed to boomers. Americans have already spent over billions on sexual stimulants, and the sales continue to climb.[22] Safe sex education needs to be provided for boomers as they age. With pregnancy no longer a risk, boomers may not practice safe sexual behavior and could be in danger of contracting a sexually transmitted disease (STD), which can include HIV/AIDS.

Public health programs also need to address the accuracy of health information provided by the media. Trained, knowledgeable employees who are familiar with various nutritional supplements and their claims are needed to assist boomers in making informed, smart decisions. Boomers must be careful when purchasing and taking supplements because of possible prescription drug–nutrient interactions and reactions. Independent companies are needed to test health claims for products marketed to the public, which will help consumers and healthcare professionals to evaluate their health, wellness, and nutritional claims more effectively. In 2007, the Food and Drug Administration (FDA) adopted more stringent regulations that require manufacturers of dietary supplements to use Good Manufacturing Practices, which include quality and purity testing. Some companies even provide approval seals on their products to signify passage of laboratory tests for potency, purity, and freedom from harmful contaminants. One is the U.S. Pharmacopeia Dietary Supplement Verification Program, a voluntary testing and auditing program that ensures the safe manufacture of dietary supplements (http://www.usp.org/USPVerified/dietarySupplements/).

In 2003, the FDA launched a grading system for products with health claims, with letters ranging from A to D. Products with health claims now can be supported with various degrees of scientific agreement. For example, grade A indicates the health claim meets the significant scientific agreement standard, whereas a grade D means that very limited and preliminary scientific research has been done, sug-

> Sexually transmitted diseases (STDs) can refer to other diseases besides HIV and AIDS, such as syphilis, gonorrhea, chlamydia, genital herpes, genital warts, hepatitis (A, B, and C), and nonspecific urethritis.

gesting that the FDA concludes that there is little evidence supporting this claim.[23] Of course, because many of these products are not regulated as a drug, many manufacturers do not adhere to those standards to market their products.

Because many boomers seek health information through magazines, newspapers, and the Internet, they need to be educated on which sources are accurate and credible. More than 70% of people who are online access health information.[5] It would be helpful if boomers were knowledgeable about peer-reviewed journal articles and able to distinguish between quality research designs and studies and those with false or misleading claims.

■ HEALTH INSURANCE AND SCREENING

Baby boomers need a comprehensive health package that meets their nutritional and physical needs by integrating medically sound alternative and traditional medicine. Vitamins, supplements, pharmaceuticals, hormone therapies, and other anti-aging substances proliferate in the marketplace and are widely used by this population. For example, supplements and homeopathic remedies are used to manage nutritional status and pain. It is estimated that consumers spend about $14 billion on complementary or integrative medicine in the course of one year.[1]

In 2007, Americans spent more than $23 billion on vitamin, herbal, and other supplements, less than a tenth of the amount spent on prescription drugs.[24] Employers and health maintenance organizations (HMOs) thus should offer comprehensive health programs that include medically recognized homeopathic and complementary services. These services can be included in a health package that should contain screening, education and private consulting, and intervention.

Screening efforts for breast cancer, colorectal cancer, cervical cancer, high blood pressure, arthritis, cholesterol levels, and diabetes mellitus are crucial for the boomer population and need to be continued as a part of traditional medicine as they age. Screening by health professionals must also include nutritional intakes, eating patterns, supplement usage, physical activity patterns, and preferred modes of exercise. During this process, health professionals should also inquire about the boomer's interests or participation in alternative medicine therapies.

Once screening is completed, education through private consultation may be needed. Boomers may want to have several meetings with dietitians or personal trainers to improve their general condition and adopt a healthier lifestyle. Interventions can be developed through these private consultations.

> Homeopathic remedies may include chiropractic, massage, vitamins, yoga, herbals, hypnosis, acupuncture, and many other complementary therapies.

■ HOME ENVIRONMENT

A new concept has emerged, called *aging-in-place*, which describes how a growing number of aging adults prefer to grow old at home.[25,26] Housing trends are shifting toward senior-friendly communities that encourage independent living rather than moving into institutions like nursing homes. Smart home technology assists this population by providing emergency assistance, fall prevention/detection, reminder systems, medication administration, and assistance for those with hearing, visual, or cognitive impairments.[25] Technological advances such as robots that serve as companions and assistants around the house will also likely become more popular for the Boomer generation.[26]

■ INTERVENTIONS

Intervention efforts for boomers include cultivating healthy nutrition behaviors and identifying appealing modes of exercise.

Nutrition

A challenge for the nutritionist is to teach boomers proper, balanced nutrition and motivate them to make changes in their lifestyles. A top trend of Americans is consuming functional foods, that is, nutrient-enhanced, fortified foods as well as nutriceuticals and phytochemicals. People want to manage their health through the foods they eat and make selections based on health benefits. Instead of focusing on components of food, nutritionists may need to focus on the benefits of eating certain foods.

Supplements, as discussed earlier, are another intervention. Supplement use is prevalent among baby boomers. In 2007, 50% of those 55 and older reported using vitamins and supplements.[23] Consumers spent billions on vitamins and on minerals in 2007. The top five vitamins were multivitamin supplements, B vitamins, and vitamins E, C, and A.[27] The top five minerals were calcium, magnesium, iron, chromium, and a zinc/potassium/selenium combination.[27]

Prebiotics and probiotics are also gaining popularity. *Prebiotics* are substances that promote the growth or activity of a limited number of bacterial species in the gut. Prebiotics produce short-chain fatty acids that are critical to gut integrity, immune system functioning, calcium absorption, and cholesterol maintenance.[28] *Probiotics* are live organisms that confer a health effect on the host.[29] Probiotics can be used to fight common female health problems such as urinary tract and vaginal infections. Some studies have shown the lactobacillus GG strain helped manage Crohn's disease and irritable bowel syndrome.[29] Lactobacillus is found in about 80% of the yogurt consumed in the United States.[29] Dairy products are often supplemented with probiotics because they buffer stomach acid and increase the chance the bacteria will survive.

Exercise

Programs, classes, and facilities are needed that will attract boomers to engage in physical fitness. Needs assessment and surveys can articulate where the boomers' interests lie and can help frame programs. In adults, regular physical activity has been associated with decreased risk of coronary heart disease, obesity, type-2 diabetes (formerly known as non-insulin dependent diabetes), osteoporosis, and post-endometrial cancer. Physical activity also has been associated with increased longevity and lower rate of disability.[30]

Both cardiovascular and resistance type of exercise can help maintain the muscle masses of aging adults. Encouraging strength training for both men and women is important. Circuit training that combines cardiovascular fitness and resistance training is popular among boomers. Boomers need to know about how to train prior to exercise, as the most common injuries affecting aging athletes include: ankle and knee sprains; strains in the hamstring, calf, and back muscles; rotator-cuff tendonitis; tennis elbow; stress fractures; and heel spurs.[31] Health professionals also need to encourage regular activity and discourage "weekend warriors." Poor conditioning and stiff bones and muscles in older adults may increase their risk for injuries.

America is a market-driven country, and boomers want to choose which services and products to purchase. Wellness programs need to be affordable and managed by credible, educated professionals. Such programs need to be located near the boomers' homes in order to be accessible, and they must have flexible hours to accommodate boomers' work schedules and family commitments. Finally, programs need to be diverse in order to adapt to each individual's demands. Boomers need a variety of gym options, the choice of meeting with a dietitian or personal trainer, and the option of utilizing medically recognized homeopathic remedies. Dietitians need to package their materials differently to appeal to the boomers and be successful in establishing healthy eating habits. Time is a crucial factor for many boomers, who need an effective workout in a short amount of time. Boomers are seeking not only physical benefits from exercise, but also mind/spirit benefits. This reflects the shift from traditional, Western health care to a more integrative, holistic model.

■ RECOMMENDATIONS FOR THE FUTURE

America's baby boomers have different health needs and demands than the elderly population being served in prior decades. These differences, due to increased longevity, will produce health needs related to a higher incidence of arthritis, obesity, and diabetes. Baby boomers will demand more medical education and intervention than past generations.

A public health needs assessment (as discussed in Chapter 3) should be designed and distributed to boomers across the United States in order to collect information on their wellness needs and wants. California and New York have done preliminary research, and other states need to follow so that appropriate resources may be allocated, desired programs developed, and adequate facilities and staff provided to serve the boomers when they are elderly. In addition to surveying the boomers, existing programs and facilities must be mapped out and inspected so they do not duplicate what is already in place. Once gaps are identified, program planning and development can begin.

Issues for Discussion

1. Given that there are more and more demands made on the public health system, do you think that meeting the baby boomer demands is feasible?

2. Make suggestions as to how the public health system can meet baby boomer demands.

References

1. Bartlett D. The new healthcare consumer. *J Healthcare Finance.* 1999;25:46–51.

2. Mycek S. We're not in Kansas anymore. *Trustee.* 1999;52:22–24.

3. Age power, how the new-old will transform medicine in the 21st century. *Geriatrics.* 1999;54:22–27.

4. *Project 2015, Shaping Public Policy: Preparing for Demographic Change.* The New York State Agencies, Status Report 2005. Available at www.aging.ny.gov/SpecialProjects/Project2015/P2015status05.pdf. Accessed June 1, 2010.

5. Institute for the Future. Fault lines in the shifting landscape: the future of growing older in California 2010. (Published 1999). Available at http://www.archstone.org/publications2292/publications_show.htm?doc_id=33534. Accessed April 29, 2010.

6. Dougherty K, Senelick R. *Baby Boomers' Guide to Women's Health: Living Great the Next 50 Years.* Health South Press; 2003.

7. Naditz A. Coming of age. As the baby boomer ages, long-term care must gear up for its own "boom." *Contemporary, Long-Term Care.* 2003;26:18–19.

8. Hartman-Stein PE, Potkanowicz FS. Behavioral determinants of healthy aging: good news for the baby boomer generation. *Online J Issues Nurs.* 2003;8:6.

9. Rosenbloom AA Jr. New aged and old aged: impact of the baby boomer. *Optometry.* 2003;74:211–213.

10. Bertholf L, Loveless S. Baby boomers and Generation X: strategies to bridge the gap. *Semin Nurse Manag.* 2001;9: 169–172.

11. Mangino M. The aging employee. Impact on occupational health. *AAOHN J.* 2000;48:349–357.

12. Wagner L. Meeting the baby boomer challenge. How will a generation of 70 million elders reshape and redirect long-term care? *Provider.* 2000;26:28–30, 33–34, 36–38.

13. Dunn-Cane KM, Gonzalez JL, Stewart HP. Managing the new generation. *AORN J.* 1999;69:930, 933–936, 939–940.

14. Mangino M. Mid-life is upon us. Preventative care for the baby boomer. *Mich Health Hosp.* 1996;32:22–24.

15. Wilson M. The future of telemedicine. *Stud Health Technol Inform.* 2002;80:129–136.

16. Centers for Disease Control and Prevention. *Natn Vital Stat Rep.* 2002;50(15).

17. Centers for Disease Control and Prevention. The CDC home page. Available at http://www.cdc.gov. Accessed April 29, 2010.

18. Centers for Disease Control. *MMMR Morb Mortal Wkly Rep.* 2009;58:29–33.

19. Yee SL et al. The nutrition and physical activity program to prevent obesity and other chronic diseases: monitoring progress in funded states. *Prev Chronic Dis.* 2006 Jan;3(1):A23.

20. Wang Y, Beydoun MA, Liang L, Caballero B, Kumanyika SK. Will all Americans become overweight or obese? Estimating the progression and cost of the IS obesity epidemic. *Obesity.* 2008;16:2323–2330.

21. Center for Disease Control. Basis Statistics. Available at http://cdc.gov/hiv/topics/surveillance/basic.htm#aidsage. Accessed May 20, 2010.

22. Greenwald J. Drug quest: magic bullets for boomers. *Time Magazine.* 1998;151:54–55.

23. Johnson MA, Sohyun P, Penn D, McClelland, JW, Brown K, AlderA. Nutrition Education Issues for Older Adults. The Forum for Family and Consumer Issues. Available at http://ncsu.edu/ffci/publications/2008/v13-n3-2008-winter/johnson-park-penn-mcclelland-brown-adler.php. Accessed May 20, 2010.

24. Marchione M. Big companies dominate herbal sales. Available at http://www.nctimes.com/lifestyles/health-med-fit/article_8bb3339b-ae67-5c1d-9ae7-09c82d5a1d08.html. Accessed May 2, 2010.

25. Cheek P, Nikpour L, Nowlin HD. Aging well with smart technology. *Nurs Adm Q.* 2005;29:329–338.

26. Robinson KM, Reinhard SC. Looking ahead in long-term care: the next 50 years. *Nurs Clin N Am.* 2009;44:253–262.

27. Madley-Wright R. Vitamins and minerals. *Nutraceuticals World.* 2003:September 1.

28. Douglas L. Prebiotics overview. *Nutraceuticals World.* 2003:September 1.

29. Skovsende A. Probiotics: good for what's bugging you. *Nutraceuticals World.* 2003:September 1.

30. Barnes PM. Physical activity among adults: U.S., 2000. Advance Data, CDC. May 14, 2003: 333.

31. Clark J. A pain in the back for boomers. *Kiplinger's Personal Finance Magazine.* 1997;51:98.

Maintaining Nutrition and Food Service Standards in Group Care

Thelma B. Baker, PhD, RD, LD

READER OBJECTIVES

After studying this chapter and reflecting on the contents, you will be able to:

1. Explain the role of public health nutrition in setting food service standards in acute, long-term, group, and home care facilities.
2. Explain the role of the nutrition professional in providing services for individuals in group care settings.
3. Demonstrate an understanding of the governmental licensing and monitoring agencies that govern nutrition and food service in group care settings.
4. Discuss how nutrition professionals can position themselves as specialists who are responsible for disseminating nutrition and food service information in healthcare facilities.
5. Discuss the information needed by administrators in order to enable the nutrition professional to provide quality nutrition care and food service management.
6. Discuss the difference between licensure, regulations, and accreditation.

■ INTRODUCTION

There has been a marked increase in the need for community group care. This is due to the de-institutionalization of residents in homes for mentally and physically challenged individuals, group homes for persons undergoing alcohol and drug rehabilitation, shelters for battered and abused women, emergency shelters that provide residential and food services to homeless families with children. Also due to the fact that individuals are living longer and the population is aging, there is greater need for assisted living facilities to care for the elderly who are unable to care for themselves. These assisted living communities are the fastest growing type of facility for seniors. As a result, the need for a number of different healthcare service professionals, such as occupational and physical therapists, social services caseworkers, and nutritionists, has increased. Some of these facilities may require the need for food service production; others, where individuals may be reasonably healthy, may not.

Although the provision of nutrition and food service production is guided by federal and state laws, there are organizations in which these laws are not carefully adhered to and it is the responsibility of the nutrition profession to ensure that organizations meet the minimum standards of service. Some of the community institutions that require these services may be denominational, not-for-profit, or for-profit. In providing nutrition and food service systems, therefore, one has to keep in mind the food habits that may need to be altered due to religious, health, or physical reasons that require the nutritional intake to be altered or special provisions improvised for feeding. Nonetheless, the nutritional needs of the individuals must be met and must be demonstrated that they are met in order to satisfy the nutrient needs for a good quality of life.

This chapter proposes to help the reader learn how to apply public health nutrition regulations to traditional and non-traditional healthcare settings, and to interpret guidelines that assist the reader in meeting nutrition needs through the provision of health and nutrition services.

With the expansion of group care to community-based practice, new employment opportunities for nutrition professionals have come into focus. Nutrition professionals can now be found in non-traditional agencies and organizations that provide primary care, promote health, and prevent chronic diseases in the community or in community groups. Nutrition professionals thus are valued and make significant contributions to public health care and service to the community.

■ ROLE OF THE NUTRITIONIST

In some group care organizations, dietitians or nutritionists may be involved only in services such as menu writing, whereas other organizations may need full-time personnel for more complex nutritional services. Listed below are some group care organizations that serve three or more meals each day, and thus require the skills of a nutrition specialist.

Healthcare organizations:
- Hospitals for acute, long-term, or mental health care
- Nursing homes
- Rehabilitation centers
- Assisted living facilities

Community care organizations:
- Group homes for mentally and physically disabled individuals
- Halfway houses for individuals undergoing alcohol and/or drug rehabilitation
- Retirement homes
- Halfway houses for previously incarcerated individuals
- Male and female shelters

Childcare organizations:
- Head Start and preschool programs
- Family daycare homes
- Family foster homes
- Schools

Later in this chapter, we discuss the evolving role of the nutritionist in group care situations.

■ LICENSURE, REGULATION, AND ACCREDITATION

In order to protect the health and safety of consumers, community and healthcare organizations must be licensed by at least one government public health agency. Organizations that provide healthcare services—

including nutrition—and that receive funding from Medicaid and/or Medicare must adhere to specific regulations. These regulations are established by the Healthcare Financing Administration (HCFA) of the U.S. Department of Health and Human Services (DHHS). In addition, these institutions are licensed by states and counties as warranted.

Licensure ensures that the institutions maintain clean and sanitary conditions and staffing patterns that are sufficient to meet the needs, including nutritional needs, of the clients being served. Although hospitals and nursing facilities must be state licensed, in some instances they require additional accreditation by the Joint Commission on Accreditation of Healthcare Organizations (JCAHO). Even though some of the requirements of the various agencies overlap, the goal is to ensure that clients receive appropriate care.

The state health agency, in addition to county government in some instances, is responsible for licensing group care agencies. Licensure laws cover sanitation, safety of facilities, staffing, quality of care, and clients' rights. Regulations cover the safety and sanitation of the food services and the nutritional adequacy of the menu in addition to other requirements. Some of the nutrition requirements specific to hospitals are that clients should be screened by a dietitian/nutritionist or diet technician (RDT) and if warranted, a nutrition assessment must be completed within a specified period of time following admission. The diet recommendation should address the disease state and ultimately should be prescribed by the admitting physician or in some cases by a registered dietitian. Follow-up assessments by the dietitian/nutritionist must also be completed within a specific period of time.

> **JCAHO:** An independent, not-for-profit organization that is a standards-setting and accrediting body in healthcare. Learn more about JCAHO at http://www.jcaho.org.

Evolving Nutrition Standards in Healthcare Organizations

The role of nutrition professionals in healthcare institutions continues to evolve. In earlier decades, nutrition professionals in healthcare settings were responsible for assessing clients' nutritional status based on laboratory parameters and clinical observations, educating clients and family regarding dietary modifications, and making recommendations to physicians for dietary changes. However, in addition to these duties, nutrition professionals, particularly registered dietitians, now serve as active members of the healthcare team and make substantial contributions regarding nutrition and patient care in the area of specialized feedings such as enteral and parenteral nutrition. Registered dietitians teach resident physicians and medical students about nutrition and are responsible for developing and implementing nutrition programs pertaining to lifestyle changes. Nutrition professionals are also responsible for implementing the nutrition care process that addresses the needs of clients specific to nutrition.

Following admission to a healthcare institution, a client's nutrition status must be addressed within a specified period of time and monitored continuously. In situations requiring specialized dietary modifications, continuous quality monitoring is warranted. In addition, nutrition professionals are required to conduct internal audits and patient satisfaction surveys periodically to assure that dietary standards are being maintained.

Bariatric: Refers to the management of morbid obesity by surgery; dietitians assist in educating patients about how to eat properly. Learn more about bariatrics at http://www.asbs.org.

In order to receive funding for health organizations, rules have become more stringent and length of in-hospital stays has decreased. As a consequence, more outpatient treatment centers are being encouraged in order to care for patients and to ensure that health needs are met minimally. Dietitians thus have become an important member of these organizations in order to ensure that dietary needs are being met following discharge. Some of the outpatient programs these dietitians are responsible for are classes in diabetic care, and bariatric and cardiovascular management. In some states and cities, hospital dietitians are required to make house calls to clients in order to provide continuous nutrition care. In these situations, the nutrition professional must take into consideration the client's ability and desire to prepare meals, the living situation, and other conditions that may impact nutrition status.

Evolving Nutrition Standards in Community Organizations

Group Homes for People Who Are Mentally and Physically Disabled

People who are mentally and physically challenged, as a group, are at high nutritional risk for many reasons. This population may have problems with eating and swallowing, limited eating skills, mechanical feeding difficulties or neuromotor dysfunctions, inborn errors of metabolism, problems with underweight and overweight, and malabsorption problems. Fulfilling nutritional needs and malnutrition may be of great concern. If there is neurological impairment, such as stroke or some other forms of trauma, the eating process may be interrupted and the patient may require enteral nutrition. Additionally, there may be a mixture of older and younger clients with developmental disabilities and clients with additional nutritional needs associated with aging. If dementia or poor ambulation is present, this decreases food intake and socialization unless the client is

carefully monitored and encouraged to interact with other clients. Some children who are physically challenged are unable to acquire proper growth and development. The basic goal of nutrition management for all clients therefore is to provide adequate nutrients in order to achieve and maintain optimal health and well-being. Also, in the elderly, the need to ameliorate nutritional health problems related to aging such as diabetes, cardiovascular disease, and diabetes in combination with the mental and physical problems allows the nutrition professional to be creative in addition to engaging the assistance of other health professionals. The need for a multidisciplinary approach to managing such patients is becoming more evident as this population increases and additional problems are identified. In this capacity, the role of the nutrition specialist is very challenging due in part to age range of clients, limited or a lack of communication skills on the part of the individual client, unusual food habits or eating behaviors, multiple medical problems, and physical disabilities that complicate the implementation of nutritional intervention. With neurological disorders, malnutrition can be a serious concern as a result of the inability to fulfill the nutritional needs. The client may be unable to feed himself; therefore, feeders may have to be employed as well as the assistance of families and friends. Depending on the level of the disorder the dysphagia diet may have to be implemented. Also, one has to be very careful in serving liquids, especially liquids of thin consistency such as water or fruit juices, because swallowing liquids of thin consistency can result in aspiration in the lungs and perhaps pneumonia. Liquids can be thickened with cornstarch, dry powered milk, or commercial thickeners.

Determining the client's nutritional status therefore is essential. A comprehensive assessment must include diet information, physical assessment data, laboratory data, and medications affecting nutritional status. Information should be obtained from the direct care staff as well significant persons in the client's life. A nutrition care plan with clearly defined goals for managing each client should be identified in medical charts and adjustments made as necessary. In addition, the nutrition professional should serve as a member of the interdisciplinary healthcare team to address nutrition-related problems, other problems that affect nutrition status, and the client's progress.

Adult Outplacement Homes: Drug and Alcohol Rehabilitation

Adults living in outplacement homes may include otherwise healthy individuals who are undergoing drug or alcohol rehabilitation. These individuals may include adults living with a chronic condition, such as diabetes or hypertension. Homes providing treatment for these recovering individuals are required to be licensed by the state and/or county, and all regulations must be met in order to provide service. In order to ensure that clients receive nutritious meals and meals that are appropriate for their disease condition, a dietitian or nutritionist must be engaged either part-time or as a consultant. With the healthy individual, the dietitian's role is to ensure that the client's diet satisfies the Dietary Reference Intakes (DRIs). The DRIs provide quantitative estimates of nutrient intake that can be used when planning and assessing diets for healthy individuals. Modified diets must be devised for clients requiring them. For example, diets for diabetes, hypertension, obesity, or another condition should be provided by the home. For individuals who are drug and alcohol dependent, the diet must be adequate in energy and other macronutrients, and additional vitamins and minerals may need to be provided in order to correct deficiencies created as a result of drug and alcohol problems. Clients also should be monitored for weight gain due to prescribed medications. Workers should be educated on drug-nutrient interactions, and meals should be timed in order to prevent problems associated with drug-nutrient interactions.

Evolving Nutrition Standards in Retirement Homes

As the older population increases in number, accommodations for individuals not wishing to or unable to care for themselves are increasing. Among these accommodations are assisted living facilities, retirement homes with skilled care services, and nursing homes. Assisted living offers some independence and is a combination of safe housing and supportive social and healthcare services. It is designed to meet the needs of individuals requiring assistance with activities of daily living. Individuals who are unable to care for themselves and require skilled care, or those who have lost the capacity to function independently due to illness, may reside in skilled nursing facilities or skilled care units in retirement communities. These facilities must undergo certification by the Centers for Medicare and Medicaid Services (CMS) and follow established guidelines. In order to receive funding under the federal and state Medicaid program, nursing facilities must have in place a quality care team that assesses patients and establishes measurable clinical goals, outcomes assessments, and approaches to management. This team must include a nutrition professional who assesses clients upon admission and at least 30 days following admission. Clients are reassessed for weight changes, changes in dietary consumption, laboratory parameters affected by nutrition intake, and other clinical incidences. In addition, they must conduct an annual assessment on each resident in order to determine if goals are being met.

Older individuals may suffer from multiple chronic diseases, and data from the third National Health and Nutrition Examination Survey (NHANES) suggest that the older adult is also at risk for malnutrition because of the presence of disease, physical disabilities, poor dental and oral health, many medications (prescribed and over-the-counter), social isolation, financial limitations, or impaired mental health. Physiological changes that accompany aging also place this population at additional risk. Some older adults enter residential homes in order to remove themselves from social isolation and to relieve themselves of the responsibilities associated with their daily care.

In caring for this population, the nutrition professional must take into consideration their unique needs. For example, energy requirements generally decrease with age because of changes in body composition, a reduction in physical activity, and a decrease in the basal energy expenditure. Although the energy requirement is decreased in older adults, the requirements for protein, vitamins, and minerals remain the same or increase in some cases. Adequate sources of carbohydrate-rich foods should be consumed and should be provided in the form of complex carbohydrates, such as whole grains and legumes, in addition to fruits, in order to provide fiber. An adequate supply of water also must be provided in order to prevent dehydration especially if the individual is unable to communicate his/her needs.

As people age and experience a loss of skeletal mass, dietary intake of protein becomes more important. Although the DRI for protein remains the same, in some instances, protein needs may have to be decreased or increased due to some physiological illness; therefore, it is incumbent on the nutrition professional to carefully evaluate the client's nutrition status and any conditions that affect dietary planning. A common marker for nutrition status is the serum albumin level; in acute cases, pre-albumin measures may be required. If depleted albumin stores are exhibited, clients should be evaluated carefully to determine if there are contributing factors, other than diet, that affect albumin levels.

In older adults, intakes of vitamins and minerals should be monitored. It is especially important to provide some sources of calcium other than milk for clients who may have a lactase deficiency, and to offer foods that are low in sodium content especially if the patient is hypertensive or has other medical conditions requiring a low sodium diet.

Individuals requiring skilled care should be serviced meals based on their disease states. Where possible, nutrient-dense foods should be served in situations where a poor appetite exists. Adequate fiber and fluid should be incorporated into the menu in order to prevent dehydration and constipation. Serving attractive and palatable meals in an atmosphere that encourages independent eating helps clients to maintain a sense of self-confidence. Assistance should be provided when necessary to promote the nutritional well-being of the individuals.

Evolving Nutrition Standards for Children in Group Care

School and Head Start Programs

Food service in group settings such as Head Start programs, daycare centers, and preschool programs in elementary schools is regulated by standards established by federal and/or state agencies. These standards, which are administered by regulatory programs, are science-based and are necessary to ensure that childcare food service is of uniformly high quality. Many facilities and some daycare homes participate in the U.S. Department of Agriculture (USDA) Child and Adult Care Food Programs. These programs provide reimbursement on a sliding scale for meals served to children, and each program has nutrient requirements. The programs are designed to assist childcare programs in providing nutritious and healthful meals. Consuming nourishing, wholesome, and attractive food is a foundation for developmentally appropriate learning experiences and contributes to health, well-being, and physical growth. Therefore, in order to provide children with optimal nutrients, a program should offer food that is appealing, wholesome, safely prepared, and age-appropriate.

> See meal patterns for the Child and Adult Care Food Programs at http://riley.nal.usda.gov/nal_display/index.php?info_center=11&tax_level=1&tax_subject=394.

These programs should plan cycle menus, which offer seasonal and cultural foods, and should include foods that are colorful and texture-appropriate. When possible, family-style meals should be encouraged in order to promote independence and self-confidence. Through focus groups, families could be consulted about the inclusion of some food items on menus. Young children do not enjoy mixed dishes and foods that are unidentifiable. Although children usually eat well in group settings, peer influence could have a negative effect on food intake. Refusal of foods by one or more children can affect the entire group. To discourage problem eaters and to strengthen family-style eating, teachers and parents should sit at the table and share the same meal with children. The presence of an adult at the table with children while they are eating also encourages social interactions and conversations about the food.

The nutrition professional can develop nutrition education projects that teachers can incorporate into the lesson plans; mealtime can be an ideal environment for this. Some helpful learning activities include experiencing new foods through identifying and tasting, describing size and shapes, and participating in simple food preparation. Federal guidelines require families who participate in the Head Start program to receive nutrition education, so periodic nutrition classes should be planned for families and teachers. In addition nutrition messages can be sent to families on a weekly or monthly basis in order to keep them abreast of the need for good nutrition and healthy food habits

The latest information on child health has resulted in a shift in emphasis for the child nutrition program from the prevention of dietary deficiencies to the promotion of healthful food practices for prevention of chronic diseases, which are appearing in young children today. (See Chapter 5 on childhood obesity.) In an effort to promote growth and development and good dietary habits that may reduce the incidence of chronic diseases later in life, MyPyramid (formerly called the Food Guide Pyramid) was developed by the USDA. When planning meals, this guide should be utilized in conjunction with the Dietary Guidelines for Americans. Also incorporated into the pyramid is a physical activity regimen, which should be encouraged. (Both are available at http://www.MyPyramid.gov.)

■ THE MISSION OF FOOD SERVICE

In group care organizations, whether healthcare or community care, the mission of the institution guides the food-service delivery system. In healthcare organizations, the mission is to provide food and nutrition that will help to alleviate illnesses and restore health. In community organizations, the mission is to provide meals that meet the nutrient needs of clients; although modified diets may be provided, the emphasis is on maintaining health. In group care for children, the emphasis is on providing food and nutrition that promote growth and development as well as maintain cognitive and emotional health.

If food is not prepared and held in sanitary conditions or if infection control factors are not enforced, the food service delivery system can have a deleterious effect on an individual's nutrition status, causing illness or perhaps death. If incorrect diets are presented to clients, this can also affect nutrition and health status.

In large conventional healthcare organizations such as hospitals and nursing facilities, a multi-layer system for providing meals exists. The first layer is the food service systems staffs, who are responsible for ensuring that foods served to clients are safe and wholesome. In this layer, an administrative dietitian or food service director administers the food service department and may report to an administrative officer of the institution or an officer of a food service company. The next layer of food service is the food production area.

The production area is usually well designed with adequate resources to promote meal preparation and to ensure that acceptable sanitation procedures are adhered to. The recommendations of the Hazard Analysis and Critical Control Point (HACCP) are followed to ensure safety in food handling, cooking, and storage.

Read more about HACCP at http://www.fda.ov/food/foodsafety/hazardanalysis criticalcontrolpointshaccp/default.htm.

The next layer of food service is the menu, which is overseen by a registered dietitian. The cycle menu, designed for a specific period of time, serves as the basis for procurement and food production. All menus must meet the DRIs except for nutrient-modified menus, which the dietitian modifies by altering nutrients where necessary. Diet manuals, authored by nutrition professionals, are available for use by staff.

In privately owned group care facilities for mentally and physically disabled persons, it is mandated that a nutrition specialist be employed for food service oversight. In some states, the professional must be a registered dietitian. Depending on the size of the facility, a full-time, part-time, or consulting dietitian may be employed to ensure that the dietary needs of the clients are met.

The nutrition professional may find problems associated with overseeing a food service operation. There may be limited storage in the production area, resulting in improperly stored foods. Also, the staff may have limited knowledge of meal preparation using a standardized menu. This may result in inconsistencies in taste, appearance, and nutritive value of the meals. Proper measures must be in place to ensure that food is received, stored, and prepared according to acceptable sanitation procedures in order to preserve the nutritive value. Workers should be trained to understand the importance of following menus and recipes as prescribed, the relationship of food storage and sanitation to health, and the reasons for safe food handling and preparation. In addition, a reduction in the use of sodium, total fat, saturated fats, and *trans*-fatty acids should be incorporated into staff training sessions. Alternative methods for the use of seasoning should also be taught. In order to control food costs and decrease waste, recipes for combination dishes should be provided, and detailed shopping lists with quantities for each menu item should be attached.

A daily routine for meal service should be planned into the schedule. Meals should be served at approximately the same time each day. Regulations require that dining space should be adequate to accommodate wheelchairs, and furnishings should be comfortable to serve the number and types of clients for which they are intended. Clients' self-feeding skill can affect their nutritional status; therefore, if necessary, adaptive feeding devices should be provided with comfortable positioning to maximize ingestion. It is also important to ensure that clients are given the correct portions and that all meals including desserts are consumed. Clients who are self-feeders may spill portions of their food, and it is important to replace foods in order to provide adequate nutrition. Although every effort should be made to promote independence, adequate help should be available at mealtime to assist clients who may need to be assisted with feeding when necessary.

■ COUNSELING CLIENTS AND FAMILIES

Clients and family members should be encouraged to participate in nutrition education programs so that they understand the reasons for meals being served to children or relatives in group care facilities. Lessons should be simple, interactive, and fun so that participants do not feel threatened. The provision of basic nutrition information should assist in planning healthy and attractive meals. Good food preparation techniques such as storing, handling, and proper temperature control also should be included in the nutrition education.

One of the requirements of the Head Start Program is that parents receive basic nutrition education so that there can be some continuity in meal planning and preparation. With the increase in obesity, type-2 diabetes, and elevated cholesterol levels in children, parents should be made aware of the link between nutrition and health so that they can become more amenable to practicing healthful nutrition habits for themselves and their families. Where modified diets are served, families should be educated regarding the diets so that they can understand the purpose and, therefore, promote compliance.

■ WHAT ADMINISTRATORS AND STAFF NEED TO KNOW

Although community-based residences are beneficial for many individuals, there can be managerial and staffing issues that are not encountered in formalized institutional settings. One staff training issue unique to community residences is dietary management. In a traditional institution, trained personnel are responsible for menu development, food storage, and meal preparation. In community residences, these responsibilities fall to the direct-care staff, who may have little or no training or experience in institutional food production. Unlike traditional settings (e.g., hospitals), where supervisory personnel are usually present, employees in community-based group homes usually lack continuous on-site supervision for long periods and must make decisions that may affect nutrition status. Therefore, administrators should:

- Be knowledgeable about state and local laws governing nutrition and food service management to ensure appropriate staffing.

- Participate in policy development and implementation that promote and support community nutrition services.
- Take advantage of available resources, such as a local chapter of the American Dietetic Association, registered dietitians at hospitals, and local and state nutritionists in health departments.

Staff in community-based homes:

- Be provided ongoing education, especially in the area of food production, to include receiving, sanitation, storage, and food handling and preparation.
- Who are preparing meals should not be caring for clients simultaneously, to prevent contamination.
- Be knowledgeable about the effects of food preparation on nutrient content.
- Consult with nutrition specialists prior to making menu changes that may affect nutrient intake.

To ensure that safe nutrition and food services standards are maintained in group care, the dietitian/nutritionist should:

- Keep abreast of local and state regulations that affect the clients who are being served. This should include being knowledgeable about public health regulations for group care situations, inclusive of menu patterns.
- Serve as a member of the public health advisory boards that formulate regulations and guidelines for food service in group care, where possible.
- Where possible, should serve as a team member of an organization that conducts inspections and regulates licensure in group care.
- Monitor food guidance systems and public health nutrition education resources to ensure that they are useful and accessible to caregivers at group care facilities.
- Encourage administrators and staff to participate in public health nutrition education training to ensure safe nutrition practices.
- Work in partnership with public health licensing agencies in order to keep abreast of changes in regulations affecting nutrition standards.
- Provide simple references for staff in community sites, such as posters of the appropriate MyPyramid and Dietary Guidelines for Americans.

Issues for Discussion

1. To ensure that nutrition services are being met, should community group organizations be held to the same food and nutrition standards as other healthcare organizations that provide nutrition services? Explain your reasoning.

2. Discuss how and why dietitians/nutritionists should be proactive by ensuring that adequate nutrition services are being provided to clients by means of increasing the ratio of dietitians/nutritionists to clients and increasing the role of the dietitian/nutritionist in these facilities.

3. Discuss ways that dietitians/nutritionists should position themselves politically to better impact the lives of those living in group care situations.

Suggested Reading

American Dietetic Association. Position of The American Dietetic Association: child and adolescent food and nutrition programs. *J Am Diet Assoc.* 2006;106:1467–1475.

Benjamin SE, Copeland KA, Cradock A, Neelon B, Walker E, Slining MM, Gillman MW. *Journal of the American Dietetic Association.* 2009;109:109–115.

Danner KM. Nutritional deficiencies in children on restricted diets. *Pediatric Clinics of North America.* 2009;56:1085–1103.

Gross SM, Cinelli B: Coordinated school health program and dietetics professionals: partners in promoting healthful eating. *J Am Diet Assoc.* 2004;104:793–798.

Horsley JW. Community services and programs. In: Lucas B. Feucht S, Grieger L, eds. *Children with Special Health Care Needs: Nutrition Care Handbook.* Chicago, IL: The American Dietetic Association; 2004.

Humphries K, Traci MA, Seekins T. Nutrition education and support program for community-dwelling adults with intellectual disabilities. *Intellect and Developmental Disabilities.* 2008;46:335–345.

Leydon N, Dahl W. Improving the nutritional status of elderly residents of long-term care. *Journal of Health Services Research and Policy.* 2008;13:Supp 25–29.

Mahan K, Escott-Stump S, eds. *Krause's Food, Nutrition, and Diet Therapy.* Philadelphia: Saunders; 2007.

Rampersaud GC. Breakfast habits, nutritional status, body weight, and academic performance in children and adolescents. *J Am Diet Assoc.* 2005;105:743–760.

Sweitzer SJ, Briley ME, Roberts-Gray C. Do sack lunches provided by parents meet the nutritional needs of young children who attend child care? *J Am Diet Assoc.* 2009;109:141–144.

U.S. Department of Agriculture. *Food Guide Pyramid for Young Children: A Daily Guide for 2 to 6 Year Olds.* Washington, DC: Department of Agriculture, Center for Policy and Promotion; 2010.

▧ USEFUL WEB SITES

Administration on Aging
http://www.aoa.gov

Agency for Healthcare Research and Quality
http://www.ahrq.gov

American Association of Homes and Services for the Aging
http://www.aahs.org

Centers for Medicare and Medicaid Services (CMS)
http://www.cms.hhs.gov

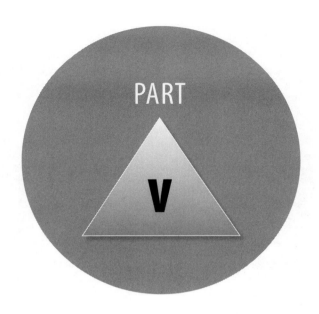

PART

V

Protecting the Public's
Nutritional Health

CHAPTER 16

Safeguarding the Food Supply

Paul N. Taylor, PhD

CHAPTER 17

Food Security and Adequate Food Access for the Public

David H. Holben, PhD, RD, LD

CHAPTER 18

Security of the Food Supply and Bioterrorism Preparedness

Barbara Bruemmer, PhD, RD, CD

Part V includes *Nutrition in Public Health's* newest additions. Although Chapter 16 appeared in the *First Edition*, it has now been greatly enriched. However, Chapters 17 and 18 bring us to a whole new frontier of public health nutrition. Chapter 17 discusses securing adequate food for those who still live in poverty. Despite the present outreach of public health nutrition, a hefty percentage of Americans still live without adequate food and/or live in a constant state of fear of being without food, showing that we have far to go in reaching those at highest risk. Chapter 18 discusses the fact that we must protect ourselves from potential bioterrorism plots directed at our food supply. Our food must be kept secure because it can be a potent avenue for terrorism. Public health nutrition will now have to meet the challenge of keeping food safe from many forms of invasion.

CHAPTER 16

Safeguarding the Food Supply

Paul N. Taylor, PhD

READER OBJECTIVES

After studying this chapter and reflecting on the contents, you should be able to:

1. List and describe the roles of federal, state, and local agencies responsible for the safety of the U.S. food supply.
2. List and describe the hazards to food safety.
3. Identify current national food safety issues.
4. Explain why food safety education should be integrated into public health nutrition programs and describe possible approaches.
5. Understand the importance of keeping informed about food safety.

◼ INTRODUCTION

America's food supply is among the safest in the world. The federal food safety system was recently strengthened in many areas, with new surveillance systems, better prevention programs, faster outbreak responses, enhanced education programs, more focused and coordinated research initiatives, and better risk assessment activities. According to officials, federal food safety agencies are improving their working relationships with each other.[1]

Despite these efforts, every year approximately 76 million Americans contract a foodborne illness, and 5,000 die from it.[2] Causative factors include transportation and refrigeration issues, an increasing volume of imported foods, and more people eating more meals away from home. Among those at greatest risk for foodborne illness are children, the elderly, pregnant women, and immunocompromised persons. Children and the elderly comprised approximately 38% of the population in 1999, and are expected to comprise about 40% of the population by 2021.[3,4]

Americans demand nutritious, wholesome, and safe food that is plentiful, varied, and at reasonable cost. In a rapidly changing world, food producers, processors, vendors, and regulators must constantly adapt to the changing expectations and demands of consumers.

The basic framework of today's federal food safety system was developed early in the 20th century. President Theodore Roosevelt's investigation of Chicago's meat packing industry and Upton Sinclair's exposé of conditions there[5] prompted passage of the Meat Inspection Act of 1906 (concomitant with the Pure Food and Drug Act). Early in this century, terrorist attacks in the United States prompted increased scrutiny of the various food safety regulatory systems and procedures, and passage of antibioterrorism legislation.[6] The Department of Homeland Security absorbed some food safety functions by 2003.[7] Against this backdrop, the full range of food safety issues continues to demand vigilance by industry, government, and consumers.

Public health professionals, nutritionists, and consumers must not become (or remain) complacent about the safety of the nation's food supply. Significant challenges have not been overcome and new challenges emerge frequently (e.g., globalization of food production, manufacturing, and marketing; geographic centralization and consolidation of food processing; some foodborne pathogens' ability to overcome traditional hurdles such as acidity, temperature, or oxygen, employed against them; new foodborne pathogens evolving or being discovered; and bioterrorism directed at food and water supplies). Old paradigms are increasingly irrelevant; yet, as is human nature, powerful forces resist the changes necessary to keep pace with a dynamic system of food production and supply and to ensure safety at all points in the system. The new paradigm for the 21st century should make this chapter's opening line, "America's food supply is among the safest in the world," obsolete by ensuring global food safety.

■ FOOD SAFETY DEFINED

Stier defines *food safety* in terms of hazards and risks:

> A safe food may be defined as a product which contains no physical, chemical or microbial organisms or by-products of those organisms which if consumed by man will result in illness, injury, or death (an unacceptable consumer health risk). The definition purposely does not use the term contaminants because many of the potential hazards in food... are typically found in or on the food. It is their concentration, numbers or size that creates potential safety problems.[8]

Hazard expresses a food's capacity to cause harm (i.e., "Any biological, chemical, or physical property that may cause an unacceptable consumer health risk"[8]). The food does not always cause harm; rather, hazard indicates that the food might cause a specified harm. The probability that the specified harm will occur is the hazard's associated "risk."[9]

To evaluate food safety, scientists must first attempt risk assessment (i.e., to "identify hazards related to foods or food components and then estimate the size of the risk that the hazard will occur"[9]). "When conducting hazard analysis, the [food processor] looks at potential hazards that could realistically cause illness or injury."[8] Risk management involves deciding whether an identified risk is acceptable. "Note that the process outlined... considers all foods to have some degree of risk," that is, "no food is absolutely safe."[9]

Public health nutritionists must understand food safety issues, using critical thinking to evaluate scientific literature and the press, in order to keep consumers informed in today's environment of "junk science" and pseudoscience. Always a dynamic field, food technologies and food safety regulations are changing at an increasingly rapid rate. Food scientists, environmental health specialists, health educators, and other public health colleagues may be consulted to help educate consumers about food safety issues. These professionals can help consumers sort through the many government and scientific Web sites that are available. Lists of these Web sites are maintained by organizations that include The Food Safety Consortium[10] (http://www.uark.edu/depts/fsc/fslinks.htm), the Simmons College Center for Hygiene and Health in Home and Community (http://www.simmons.edu/hygieneand health/links.shtml),[11] and more than 100 Internet sites in the references to this chapter.

■ PROTECTING THE FOOD SUPPLY

Federal Agencies

Several federal agencies, with sometimes overlapping jurisdictions, share responsibility for the safety of the U.S. food supply (**Table 16–1**). The following sections describe the principal federal agencies and their roles.

Food and Drug Administration

The Department of Health and Human Services' (DHHS) Food and Drug Administration (FDA) oversees all domestic and imported food (except meat and poultry) sold in interstate commerce, including seafood, shell eggs, bottled water, and wine beverages containing < 7% alcohol.[12] The FDA enforces food safety laws governing these foods through inspections; food analysis; safety reviews of food and color additives and animal drugs; monitoring of the safety of food-animal feeds; developing model codes, ordinances, guidelines, and interpretations; working with states to implement such models; establishing good food manufacturing practices (GMP); establishing sanitation and packaging requirements; establishing Hazard Analysis and Critical Control Points (HACCP) programs; collaborating with foreign governments to ensure imported foods safety; requesting and monitoring voluntary recalls of unsafe foods; enforcement; research; and industry and consumer food safety education.[12]

Food Safety and Inspection Service

The U.S. Department of Agriculture's (USDA) Food Safety and Inspection Service (FSIS) oversees domestic and imported meat, poultry and related products (e.g., meat- or poultry-containing stews, pizzas, and other frozen foods), and processed egg products (generally liquid, frozen, and dried pasteurized egg products). FSIS enforces food safety laws governing these foods through antemortem and postmortem inspections of food animals, meat and poultry slaughter and processing plant inspections, monitoring and inspecting processed egg products (together with the USDA Agricultural Marketing Service), food analysis, establishing additive and ingredient standards, inspections of foreign meat and poultry processing plants exporting to the United States, requesting and monitoring unsafe meat/poultry products recalls, meat/poultry safety research, and industry and consumer food safety education.[12]

U.S. Environmental Protection Agency

The Environmental Protection Agency (EPA) regulates pesticides and oversees drinking water quality. Its food safety role for foods made from plants, seafood, meat, and poultry includes regulating toxic substances and wastes to prevent entry into the environment or foods, determining new pesticide safety, setting tolerance levels for pesticide residues in foods, and promoting safe use of pesticides (enforcement of these standards is an FDA function).[12] The EPA also establishes safe drinking water standards and assists states in protecting and monitoring drinking water quality.

Customs and Border Protection

In 2003, the Department of Homeland Security (DHS), Customs and Border Protection (CBP) assumed responsibility

TABLE 16–1	**Federal Agencies with Food Safety Responsibilities**		
Agency	**Unit**	**Mission**	**Internet**
Department of Agriculture (USDA)	Animal and Plant Health Inspection Service (APHIS)[a]	Protects and promotes U.S. agricultural health	USDA: http://www.usda.gov APHIS: http://www.aphis.usda.gov FSIS: http://www.fsis.usda.gov
	Food Safety and Inspection Service (FSIS)	Ensures that the nation's commercial supply of meat, poultry, and egg products is safe, wholesome, and correctly labeled and packaged	
	Agricultural Research Service (ARS), National Animal Disease Center (NADC)	Conducts research on animal health and food safety problems	ARS/NADC: http://www.nadc.ars.usda.gov
Department of Commerce (USDC)	National Oceanic and Atmospheric Administration (NOAA)	Administers National Seafood Inspection Program (NSIP) offering seafood inspection, grading, certification, and other services to the seafood industry (voluntary, fee-for-service)	USDC: http://www.commerce.gov NOAA: http://www.noaa.gov NSIP: http://seafood.nmfs.noaa.gov
Department of Health and Human Services (DHHS)	Centers for Disease Control and Prevention (CDC)	Tracks foodborne illness incidents and outbreaks; provides data and information to the other food safety agencies	DHHS: http://www.os.dhhs.gov CDC: http://www.cdc.gov
	Food & Drug Administration (FDA)	Approves food and drugs for widespread use; its Center for Food Safety and Applied Nutrition (CFSAN) ensures that food is safe, nutritious, and wholesome	FDA: http://www.fda.gov CFSAN: http://vm.cfsan.fda.gov/list.html
Department of Homeland Security (DHS)	Customs & Border Protection (CBP)	Inspects agricultural goods arriving in the U.S. at ports and borders	DHS: http://www.dhs.gov/dhspublic/ CBP: http://www.customs.ustreas.gov Introducing the new CBP Agriculture Specialist: http://www.cbp.gov/xp/CustomsToday/2004/May/agSpec.xml
Department of the Treasury	Bureau of Alcohol, Tobacco, Firearms and Explosives (ATF)	Regulates qualification and operations of distilleries, wineries, breweries, importers, and wholesalers	Treasury: http://www.ustreas.gov ATF: http://www.atf.gov
Federal Trade Commission	Bureau of Consumer Protection (BCP); Division of Advertising Practices (DAP); Division of Consumer Protection (DCP); Division of Enforcement (DE)	Protects consumers against unfair, deceptive, or fraudulent practices; protects consumers from deceptive and unsubstantiated advertising (advertising claims for food, particularly those relating to nutritional or health benefits of foods); conducts law enforcement activities to protect consumers	FTC: http://www.ftc.gov BCP: http://www.ftc.gov/bcp/bcp.htm DAP: http://www.ftc.gov/bcp/bcpap.htm DE: http://www.ftc.gov/bcp/bcpenf.htm

[a]Some APHIS functions and personnel transferred to the Department of Homeland Security, Customs and Border Protection, on March 1, 2003.

for inspecting agricultural goods arriving in the United States. Previously, this was a function of the USDA's Animal and Plant Health Inspection Service (APHIS).[13,14] The transfer "linked and integrated the...scientific mission of agriculture border inspection to the expertise and operational capabilities of the primary CBP mission: to prevent terrorists and terrorist weapons from entering the United States."[13] CBP expects to "play an important role in the Department of Homeland Security's multi-layered approach to protect the food supply from the threats of agroterrorism and bioterrorism,"[13] while also detecting and denying entry to animal and plant pests and diseases that could harm U.S. agriculture.

Centers for Disease Control and Prevention

DHHS's Centers for Disease Control and Prevention (CDC) oversees and directs prevention efforts against foodborne and waterborne infections. Collaborating with other domestic and international agencies, the CDC recently expanded its mission to work toward effective global surveillance and control of foodborne and waterborne pathogens. In the United States, the CDC participates in the National Food Safety Initiative (NFSI) with the FDA, USDA, and other agencies to address food safety problems, and collaborates with the EPA and the drinking water industry to improve drinking water safety.[12,15] The CDC also initiated and participates in addressing emerging infectious diseases and preventing future emergent infectious diseases worldwide.[16]

National Oceanic and Atmospheric Administration

The Department of Commerce, National Oceanic and Atmospheric Administration (NOAA) administers a Seafood Inspection Program offering seafood inspection, grading, and certification; vessel and plant sanitation; label review; laboratory analysis; training; and consultative and information services to the seafood industry on a voluntary fee-for-service basis.[17,18] Processors may use official marks on complying products, indicating that they are federally inspected. (Note: All seafood processors must participate in the FDA's seafood HACCP program,[19,20] under which FDA inspects the processors annually. FDA provides guidance on fisheries products hazards and controls while allowing latitude to industry in implementing their HACCP programs.[21])

Bureau of Consumer Protection

The Federal Trade Commission's (FTC) Division of Advertising Practices, Bureau of Consumer Protection protects consumers from deceptive and unsubstantiated advertising. It enforces laws pertaining to advertising claims for food (particularly those claims relating to nutritional or health benefits of foods), television infomercials (to ensure that format and content are non-deceptive), and general advertising.[22]

Alcohol and Tobacco Tax and Trade Bureau

The U.S. Department of the Treasury's Alcohol and Tobacco Tax and Trade Bureau (TTB) regulates distilleries, wineries, breweries, and importers and wholesalers in the industry. TTB tests new alcohol products, determines whether products currently marketed pose a health risk to consumers, and ensures that alcohol beverage labels are not misleading.[23]

State and Local Collaboration

State and local governmental agencies oversee all food products within their jurisdictions, in cooperation with federal agencies. Usually, public health departments and state agriculture departments are the delegated authorities, with responsibilities at the state, county, and city level varying by state. Registered sanitarians, environmental health specialists, and sometimes other classes of employees inspect restaurants, food stores, supermarkets, other retail food establishments, dairy farms, milk processing plants, grain mills, and food manufacturing plants within local jurisdictions. They also may collaborate with federal agencies to develop and implement food safety standards for foods produced within state borders, and seize unsafe food products made or distributed within their jurisdictions.[12] State food sanitation codes usually meet or exceed model federal standards, and for those states maintaining their own commodity inspection programs (e.g., at least 27 states have state meat inspection programs[24]), the state program must be equivalent to the corresponding federal program and operates under federal oversight.

Public health nutritionists should know their jurisdiction's regulatory authorities for sanitation and food safety, and develop working relationships with them to identify and serve the needs of their communities. Inviting these officials to attend or speak at regional, state, and local dietetic or other association meetings is one way to build networking relationships. Nutritionists will find opportunities to assist these officials during natural disasters, in investigating outbreaks of food- and waterborne disease, and during other civil disturbances.[25-27] During the severe acute respiratory syndrome (SARS) crisis in China, for example, "Qualified nutritionists supervised preparations of meals" that were then delivered to quarantined residents in Nanking.[28] Civil emergency preparedness and response organizations should include public health nutritionists and/or registered dietitians on their teams. (Find out who is on your local team—see the American Civil Defense Association's Web site at http://www.tacda.org/defensenow/.[29]) Nutritionists are needed to participate in emergency nutrition and food aid research also.[30,31]

■ FOOD SAFETY LAWS

Major food safety legislation in the United States began in 1906 with the Pure Food and Drug Act (which created the FDA) and the Meat Inspection Act. **Table 16–2** lists several

TABLE 16–2	Selected Federal Regulations Important to Food Safety	

Year	Legislation	Resource
1906	Pure Food and Drug Act	http://www.fda.gov/RegulatoryInformation/Legislation/ucm148690.htm
1906	Federal Meat Inspection Act	http://www.fda.gov/RegulatoryInformation/ Legislation/ucm148693.htm
1967	Wholesome Meat Act	
1968	Wholesome Poultry Products Act	
1938	Federal Food, Drug, and Cosmetic Act	http://www.uvm.edu/nusc/nusc237/ffdcatc.html
1958	Food Additives Amendment	
1960	Color Additives Amendment	
1938	Federal Trade Commission Act (amended for food)	http://www.fda.gov/RegulatoryInformation/Legislation/ucm148712.htm
1957	Federal Poultry Products Inspection Act	http://www.fsis.usda.gov/Regulations/Poultry_Products_ Inspection_Act/index.asp
1966	Fair Packaging and Labeling Act	http://www.ftc.gov/os/statutes/fplajump.shtm
1980	Infant Formula Act	http://vm.cfsan.fda.gov/~dms/inf-guid.html
1990	Nutrition Education and Labeling Act	GuidanceDocuments/FoodLabelingNutrition/FoodLabelingGuide/default.htm
1990	Organic Foods Production Act	http://www.ams.usda.gov/nop/archive/OFPA.html
		http://www.ams.usda.gov/AMSv1.0/nop
		http://www.nal.usda.gov/afsic/pubs/ofp/ofp.shtml
		Olsson F, Weeda PC. *A Primer on the U.S. Department of Agriculture National Organic Program*. Elmwood Park, NJ: Food Institute. Available for purchase at http://www.foodinstitute.com/organic.cfm
		Fishman S. *The Guide to the U.S. Organic Foods Production Act of 1990*. Greenfield, MA: Organic Foods Production Association of North America
1994	Dietary Supplement Health and Education Act	http://vm.cfsan.fda.gov/~dms/dietsupp.html
1996	Food Quality Protection Act	http://www.fda.gov/RegulatoryInformation/Legislation/ FederalFoodDrugandCosmetic ActFDCAct/Significant
1996	Safe Drinking Water Act	http://www4.law.cornell.edu/uscode/42/300f.html
2002	Homeland Security Act	http://www.dhs.gov/xlibrary/assets/hr_5005_enr.pdf
2002	Public Health Security and Bioterrorism Preparedness and Response Act	http://www.fda.gov/Food/FoodDefense/Bioterrorism/ucm111086.htm
2004	Food Allergen Labeling and Consumer Protection Act	http://www.fda.gov/Food/LabelingNutrition/Food AllergensLabeling/GuidanceComplianceRegulatory Information/ucm106187.htm
2008	Food, Conservation and Energy Act	http://www.ers.usda.gov/FarmBill/2008/
		http://frwebgate.access.gpo.gov/cgi-bin/getdoc.cgi?dbname=110_cong_bills&docid= f:h2419enr.txt.pdf

federal laws with applicability to food safety. Some of these laws are discussed in the following sections.

Federal Meat Inspection Act of 1906

The Federal Meat Inspection Act (amended by the Wholesome Meat Act in 1967) requires continuous inspection (an-temortem, during slaughter, and postmortem) by USDA or USDA-sanctioned state meat inspection programs of all cattle, sheep, swine, goats, and horses at slaughter. Additionally, a federal (or state equivalent) inspector must be present for at least part of every shift while meat products are processed for human or animal consumption. Meat and meat products meeting federal standards are stamped "United States Inspected and Passed by Department of Agriculture" (or state equivalent program). Products bearing the federal mark may be shipped and sold in interstate commerce, whereas products bearing state marks may only be shipped and sold in intrastate commerce. State (and city) meat inspection programs must meet federal standards.[32,33]

Federal Food, Drug, and Cosmetic Act of 1938

The Federal Food, Drug, and Cosmetic Act (FDCA) prohibits entry into interstate commerce of any food that is adulterated: containing poisonous or deleterious substances that may make the food unhealthful; containing filth; decomposed; prepared or handled under unsanitary conditions; from a diseased animal; subjected to radiation except as permitted; having a valuable constituent omitted; having an unauthorized ingredient substitution; having a concealed defect; increased in bulk weight or decreased in strength to deceptively improve appearance; or containing an unapproved or uncertified coloring agent or misbranded (not honestly labeled). The FDA establishes guidance and regulatory requirements under the law, codified in Title 21, Code of Federal Regulations. Although the FDA uses inspections to monitor whether food manufacturers adhere to their legal responsibility of producing safe, wholesome foods, the agency's budget and personnel are insufficient and inspections are infrequent. (The USDA, also lacking funding, and the FDA jointly adopted an industry-operated food safety and inspection system, Hazard Analysis and Critical Control Points.)[32,33]

Food Additives Amendment, 1958

The FDA regulates food additives under the 1958 Food Additives Amendment to the FDCA. The FDA must approve an additive before it can be included in food and requires the additive's manufacturer to prove its safety for the ways it will be used in food. Food additives include substances intentionally added for specific purposes, such as carrageenan (a red seaweed gum used to emulsify, stabilize, or thicken foods)[34] or ozone (as an antimicrobial agent in contact with food),[35] and substances unintentionally added to foods, such as acetone (a component of adhesives) or mineral oil (a lubricant, not to exceed 10 ppm in food).[36]

The Food Additives Amendment provided two exemptions:

1. Those additives in use before 1958, which had been determined by the FDA or USDA to be safe for use in specific foods, were given "prior sanctioned" status.[37] For example, sodium nitrite as a preservative in red meats is prior sanctioned and regulated by the USDA, whereas sodium nitrite when added to fish products is an additive regulated by the FDA.[33]
2. Those additives (such as salt and sugar) whose use in foods is Generally Recognized As Safe (GRAS) by

experts,[38-40] based on either an extensive history of common use in food before 1958 or published scientific evidence.[41] Chemicals may be added to or removed from either list as necessary whenever scientific knowledge of the chemical so warrants. The FDA and USDA continuously monitor substances on both lists.[42,43]

Color Additives Amendment, 1960

The Color Additives Amendment to the FDCA brought all colors, natural and synthetic, under federal regulation. The FDA must approve all colors used in foods, drugs, and cosmetics before they can be marketed. Some colors (primarily coal-tar dyes) must be batch-certified (the manufacturer submits samples from each batch produced to the FDA for testing and pays a fee for service); whereas, others (mostly from plant, animal, or mineral sources) are exempt from batch certification.[44,45] Manufacturers and food processors may not use color additives to deceive consumers or to conceal blemishes or inferiorities in food products, and must declare color additives by their common or usual names on labels (e.g., FD&C Yellow 5 or carotene) rather than collectively as "colorings."[46]

The Nutrition Labeling and Education Act of 1990

The Nutrition Labeling and Education Act (NLEA) requires most foods to carry a nutrition label expressing nutrients as a percentage of Daily Values (DVs) for a 2,000-calorie diet rather than the now outdated Recommended Dietary Allowances (RDAs). The Act also 1) mandates more specific definitions for words such as "free," "light," or "reduced"; 2) restricts the use of the terms "sodium free" and "cholesterol free" to products normally containing sodium and/or cholesterol; 3) defines and regulates health claims, such as calcium helping to prevent osteoporosis; and 4) mandates that the total percentage of juice in juice drinks be declared.[47]

Dietary Supplement Health and Education Act of 1994

The Dietary Supplement Health and Education Act (DSHEA) mandates premarket manufacturer responsibility for dietary supplement safety and requires truthful supplement label information. After supplements reach the market, the FDA monitors supplement safety, including voluntary dietary supplement adverse event reporting; monitors product information (e.g., labeling and claims); and takes action against unsafe supplements. The law does not provide for manufacturer registration, nor does it require manufacturers to seek FDA approval before producing or marketing supplements.[48] The law is controversial because, unlike foods or food additives, which must be proven safe by manufacturers before they are marketed, neither the safety nor the efficacy of supplements needs to be proven by producers.[49]

Rather, the FDA must prove that a supplement is unsafe, after marketing, before any action may be taken to remove the product from the market. (For example, it took more than a decade for the FDA to accumulate enough evidence to ban ephedra.[50]) Legislation is pending to address problems with DSHEA and supplement safety.

Food Quality Protection Act of 1996

The Food Quality Protection Act of 1996 (FQPA)[50] amended the FDCA and the Insecticide, Fungicide, and Rodenticide Act (IFRA),[51] changing the way the EPA regulates pesticides (also see the 2003 Pesticide Registration Improvement Act[51]). The zero-tolerance provision of the FDCA's food additives anticancer clause (Delaney Clause[33]) was replaced with a new safety standard, "reasonable certainty of no harm resulting from aggregate exposure," to be applied to all pesticides used on foods. With no provision for phasing in the new requirements, the EPA faced enforcing the new regulations while simultaneously learning to evaluate pesticides under the new rules and developing or approving new, scientifically tested methodologies for evaluating aggregate and cumulative risks.[52–55] Not surprisingly, this led to controversy among the EPA, environmental advocates, and public health organizations.[56,57] In 1993, the EPA was sued by four states and several environmental and public health groups "for allegedly failing to adequately protect children from pesticides used on food...contend[ing] that the EPA set inadequate limits on several organophosphate insecticides."[58]

Public Health Security and Bioterrorism Preparedness and Response Act of 2002

The Bioterrorism Act's Title III specifically addresses food safety, directing:

> ...federal agencies, the food industry, consumer and producer groups, scientific organizations, and the States, [to] develop a crisis communications and education strategy with respect to bioterrorist threats to the food supply. Such strategy shall address threat assessments; technologies and procedures for securing food processing and manufacturing facilities and modes of transportation; response and notification procedures; and risk communications to the public.[59]

Title II covers security strategy, food adulteration, detention, registration, records maintenance, prior notice, and marking.[60] Bioterrorism and food is covered at length in Chapter 18.

Food Allergen Labeling and Consumer Protection Act, 2004

The Food Allergen Labeling and Consumer Protection Act (FALCP, effective 2006) will provide improved food labeling information to consumers who suffer from food allergies. FALCP will require food labels to identify the presence of any of eight major food allergens: milk, eggs, fish, crustaceans, peanuts, tree nuts, wheat, and soybeans. Concomitant with expanding the number of allergens to be identified, the new requirements represent improvements over present labeling standards:

> ...if a product contains the milk-derived protein casein, the product's label would have to use the term "milk" in addition to the term "casein" so that those with milk allergies would clearly understand the presence of an allergen they need to avoid.[61]

Food, Conservation, and Energy Act of 2008

The Food, Conservation, and Energy Act allows federal agricultural programs to continue through fiscal year 2012. Among the 14 titles comprising the Act, two have direct applications to food safety:

1. Title X, "Horticulture and Organic Agriculture," provisions concern:
   - pest and disease management
   - organic agriculture
   - miscellaneous issues
2. Title XI "Livestock," provisions relate to:
   - livestock mandatory reporting;
   - the country of origin labeling;
   - the Agricultural Fair Practices Act of 1967 definitions;
   - an annual report;
   - production contracts;
   - regulations;
   - the sense of Congress regarding pseudorabies eradication program;
   - the sense of Congress regarding the cattle fever tick eradication program;
   - the National Sheep Industry Improvement Center;
   - the trichinae certification program;
   - low pathogenic diseases;
   - animal protection;
   - the National Aquatic Animal Health Plan;
   - the study on bioenergy operations;
   - the interstate shipment of meat and poultry inspected by federal and state agencies for certain small establishments;
   - inspection and grading;
   - food safety improvement.[62,63]

Hazard Analysis and Critical Control Points

The Hazard Analysis and Critical Control Points (HACCP) protocol was developed by the Pillsbury Corporation in 1971 to ensure food safety for astronauts in outer space. Its principles focus on preventing hazards that could cause foodborne illness by identifying and correcting hazards before they develop, following foods from raw materials to finished products.[64,65] HACCP consists of seven principles:

1. Identify hazard(s).
2. Identify critical control point(s) (CCPs) for controlling each hazard identified.
3. Define limits for each CCP.
4. Establish specific procedures for monitoring each CCP.
5. Establish a procedure for taking corrective action whenever a CCP's limits have been exceeded.
6. Implement procedures to verify that the HACCP program is working as intended.
7. Thoroughly document the HACCP program and maintain records of CCP monitoring data. Examples of HACCP plans and flowcharts are easily obtained.[9,66,67]

HACCP programs are used in the seafood industry (since 1995; FDA oversight), meat and poultry processing plants (since 1998; USDA oversight), and the juice industry (since 2001; FDA oversight). Other areas of the food industry, such as food service, also use HACCP programs,[68,69] and the FDA is developing HACCP protocols for use in these segments.[62]

Good Manufacturing Practices

Some regulations published by the FDA are collectively called good manufacturing practices (GMPs), or the Code of GMPs.[70] These specify sanitation, safety, and quality assurance procedures to be followed by food processors.[71] For example, the FDA specifies safe procedures for manufacturing, thermally processing, and packing low-acid canned foods to avoid growth of *Clostridium botulinum* and subsequent toxin formation by the pathogen.[72] The FDA also recognizes that it is impossible to manufacture, process, and package foods that are 100% free of poisonous, deleterious, or aesthetically unpleasant substances, and it has established specific tolerances and rules relating to these substances (e.g., fresh, frozen, and canned clams, mussels, and oysters must not contain > 80 μg paralytic shellfish poisoning toxin/100 g meat;[73] ground nutmeg poses no inherent hazard to health if it contains 100 insect fragments and/or ≤ 1 rodent hair/10 g.[74]

■ HAZARDS TO FOOD SAFETY

Biologic Hazards

Biologic hazards include bacteria, viruses, parasites, and fungi (**Table 16–3**). Although several previously unknown or lesser-known pathogens have emerged in recent years,[75] bacterial pathogens remain the primary cause of foodborne illnesses.[76] These microbes cause either infections or intoxications. In *infections*, pathogens are ingested and multiply in the body, causing illness; in *intoxications*, toxins made by pathogens cause illness. Intoxications result from ingesting live pathogens that go on to multiply and produce toxin in the body, or they can occur without ingesting the live pathogens, if the pathogens are allowed to grow on food and produce heat-stable toxins. Food processing then kills the organisms, but does not damage the toxin.

TABLE 16–3	Some Biologic Hazards Associated with Food[1,2]	
Hazard Type	**Organism**	**Examples of Food Vehicles**
Bacteria	*Bacillus cereus*	Chicken fried rice[3]
	Campylobacter jejuni	Unpasteurized milk and cheese[4]
	Clostridium botulinum	Muktuk (whale meat)[5]
	Clostridium perfringens	Ground turkey and beef casserole[6]
	Escherichia coli	Raw milk and raw colostrum[7]
	Listeria monocytogenes	Jellied pork cold cuts[8]
	Salmonella typhi	Milk (food handler) and water[9]
	Salmonella enteriditis	Dry dog food (unwashed hands)[10]
	Shigella dysenteriae	Sugar snaps (peas)[11]
	Staphylococcus aureus	Precooked packaged ham[12]
	Streptococcus pyogenes	Macaroni and cheese/cook[13]
	Vibrio cholerae	Seafood[14]
	Yersinia enterocolitica	Pork chitterlings[15]
Viruses	Hepatitis A	Green onions/foodhandlers[16]
	Rotavirus	Deli sandwiches[17]
	Noroviruses	Oysters, raspberries, and other berries[18]
	Swine flu (H1N1)	Respiratory transmission[43]
	Avian flu (H5N1)	Direct contact[44]

TABLE 16–3 *(Continued)*

Hazard Type	Organism	Examples of Food Vehicles
Fungi	*Alternaria spp.*	Grain[19]
	Aspergillus spp.	Prob. Kombucha tea[20]
	Byssochlamys spp.	Fruits, vegetables[21]
	Fusarium spp.	Corn; sorghum[22]
	Penicillium spp.	Chestnuts[23]
Parasites	*Clonorchis sinensis*	Fish (frozen, raw, or salted)[24,25]
Flatworms	*Diphyllobothrium latum*	Fish[26]
Protozoans	*Fasciola hepatica*	Watercress[27]
Roundworms	*Fasciolopsis buski*	Raw aquatic plants; untreated water[28]
	Paragonimus spp.	Raw crayfish;[29] undercooked crayfish[30]
	Taenia spp.	Fecal/oral[31]
	Cryptosporidium parvum	Chicken salad[32]
	Cyclospora cayetanensis	Guatemalan raspberries[33]
	Entamoeba histolytica	Prob. ice and ice cream[34]
	Giardia lamblia	Prob. taco ingredients[35]
	Sarcocystis spp.	Raw beef and pork[36]
	Toxoplasma gondii	Raw and undercooked venison[37]
	Anisakis simplex	Raw fish[38]
	Ascaris lumbricoides	Fecal/oral[39]
	Pseudoterranova decipiens	Raw fish[40]
	Trichinella spiralis	Bear, cougar, wild boar meats; pork[41]
Prions	Abnormal prion proteins	Wild game[42] and infected cows[45]
	Bovine spongiform encephalopathy	
	(BSE; also, mad cow disease)	

[1] This is not a complete listing.

[2] For excellent reviews of most of these organisms, see: (a) Hui YH, Pierson MD, Gorham MD, eds. *Foodborne Disease Handbook,* 2nd ed. Vol. 1: Bacterial Pathogens, Vol. 2: Viruses, Parasites, Pathogens, and HACCP, Vol. 3: Plant Toxicants, & Vol. 4: Seafood and Environmental Toxins. New York: Marcel Dekker; 2000. (b) Jay JM. *Modern Food Microbiology,* 6th ed. Gaithersburg, MD: Aspen; 2000. (c) Pommerville JC. *Alcamo's Fundamentals of Microbiology,* 9th ed. Sudbury, MA: Jones and Bartlett Publishers: 2011.

[3] Epidemiologic notes and reports *Bacillus cereus* food poisoning associated with fried rice at two child day care centers—Virginia, 1993. *MMWR Morb Mortal Wkly Rep.* 1994;43:177.

[4] *Campylobacter jejuni* infection associated with unpasteurized milk and cheese—Kansas, 2007. *MMWR Morb Mortal Wkly Rep.* 2009;57:1377.

[5] Outbreak of botulism type E associated with eating a beached whale—Western Alaska, July 2002. *MMWR Morb Mortal Wkly Rep.* 2003;52:24.

[6] *Clostridium perfringens* infection among inmates at a county jail—Wisconsin, August 2008. *MMWR Morb Mortal Wkly Rep.* 2009;58:138.

[7] *Escherichia coli* 0157:H7 infections in children associated with raw milk and raw colostrum from cows—California, 2006. *MMWR Morb Mortal Wkly Rep.* 2008;57:625.

[8] Pichler J, Much P, Kasper S, et al. An outbreak of febrile gastroenteritis associated with jellied pork contaminated with *Listeria monocytogenes. Wiener Klinische Wochenschrift.* 2009;121:149.

[9] Bhunia R, Hutin Y, Ramakrishnan R, Pal N, Sen T, Murhekar M. A typhoid fever outbreak in a slum of South Dumdum municipality, West Bengal, India, 2007: evidence for foodborne and waterborne transmission. *BMC Public Health.* 2009;9:115.

[10] Multistate outbreak of human *Salmonella* infections caused by contaminated dry dog food—United States, 2006–2007. *MMWR Morb Mortal Wkly Rep.* 2008;57:521.

[11] Löfdahl M, Ivarsson S, Andersson S, Långmark J, Plym-Forshell L. An outbreak of Shigella dysenteriae in Sweden, May-June 2009, with sugar snaps as the suspected source. *Eur Surveill.* 2009;14:19268.

[12] Outbreak of staphylococcal food poisoning associated with precooked ham—Florida, 1997. *MMWR Morb Mortal Wkly Rep.* 1997;46:1189.

[13] Farley TA, Wilson SA, Mahoney F, Kelso KY, Johnson DR, Kaplan EL. Direct inoculation of food as the cause of an outbreak of group a streptococcal pharyngitis. *J Infect Dis.* 1993;167:1232.

[14] Crump JA, Bopp CA, Greene KD, et al. Toxigenic *Vibrio cholerae* serogroup O141-associated cholera-like diarrhea and bloodstream infection in the U.S. *J Infect Dis.* 2003;187:866.

[15] *Yersinia enterocolitica* gastroenteritis among infants exposed to chitterlings—Chicago, Illinois, 2002. *MMWR Morb Mortal Wkly Rep.* 2003;52:956.

[16] Hepatitis A outbreak associated with green onions at a restaurant—Monaca, Pennsylvania, 2003. *MMWR Morb Mortal Wkly Rep.* 2003;52:1155.

[17] Foodborne outbreak of group a rotavirus gastroenteritis among college students—District of Columbia, March–April 2000. *MMWR Morb Mortal Wkly Rep.* 2000;49:1131.

[18] Bresee JS, Widdowson M-A, Monroe SS, Glass RI. Foodborne viral gastroenteritis: challenges and opportunities. *Clin Infect Dis.* 2002;35:748.

[19] Liu GT, Qian YZ, Zhang P, et al. Etiological role of Alternaria alternata in human esophageal cancer. *Chinese Med J.* 1992;105:394.

[20] Unexplained severe illness possibly associated with consumption of Kombucha tea—Iowa, 1995. *MMWR Morb Mortal Wkly Rep.* 1995;44:892, 899.

[21] Moss MO. Fungi, quality and safety issues in fresh fruits and vegetables. *J Appl Microbiol.* 2008;104:1239.

[22] Bhat RV, Shetty PH, Amruth RP, Sudershan RV. A foodborne disease outbreak due to the consumption of moldy sorghum and maize containing fumonisin mycotoxins. *J Toxicol Clin Toxicol.* 1997;35:249–255.

continues

> **TABLE 16–3**   *(Continued)*

[23] Overy DP, Seifert KA, Savard ME, Frisvad JC. Spoilage fungi and their mycotoxins in commercially marketed chestnuts. *Int J Food Microbiol.* 2003;88:69.

[24] Fan PC. Viability of metacercariae of Clonorchis sinensis in frozen or salted freshwater fish. *Int J Parasitol.* 1998;28:603.

[25] Choi DW. Clonorchis sinensis: life cycle, intermediate hosts, transmission to man and geographical distribution in Korea. *Arzneimittel-Forschung.* 1984;34:1145.

[26] Arizono N, Yamada M, Nakamura-Uchiyama F, Ohnishi K. Diphyllobothriasis associated with eating raw pacific salmon. *Emerg Infect Dis.* 2009;15:866.

[27] LaPook JD, Magun AM, Nickerson KG, Meltzer JI. Sheep, watercress, and the Internet. *Lancet.* 2000;356:218.

[28] Graczyk TK, Gilman RH, Fried B. Fasciolopsiasis: is it a controllable food-borne disease? *Parasitol Res.* 2001;87:80.

[29] DeFrain M, Hooker R. North American paragonimiasis: case report of a severe clinical infection. *Chest.* 2002;121:1368.

[30] Procop GW, Marty AM, Scheck DN, Mease DR, Maw GM. North American paragonimiasis. A case report. *Acta Cytol.* 2000;44:75.

[31] Locally acquired neurocysticercosis—North Carolina, Massachusetts, and South Carolina, 1989–1991. *MMWR Morb Mortal Wkly Rep.* 1992;41:1.

[32] Foodborne outbreak of diarrheal illness associated with *Cryptosporidium parvum*—Minnesota, 1995. *MMWR Morb Mortal Wkly Rep.* 1995;45:783.

[33] Update: Outbreaks of *Cyclospora cayetanensis* infection—U.S. and Canada, 1996. *MMWR Morb Mortal Wkly Rep.* 1996;45:611.

[34] de Lalla F, Rinaldi E, Santoro D, Nicolin R, Tramarin A. Outbreak of *Entamoeba histolytica* and *Giardia lamblia* infections in travellers returning from the tropics. *Infection.* 1992;20:78.

[35] Epidemiologic notes and reports common-source outbreak of giardiasis—New Mexico. *MMWR Morb Mortal Wkly Rep.* 1989;38:405.

[36] Wilairatana P, Radomyos P, Radomyos B, et al. Intestinal sarcocystosis in Thai laborers. *SE Asian J Trop Med Public Health.* 1996;27:43.

[37] Ross RD, Stec LA, Werner JC, Blumenkranz MS, Glazer L, Williams GA. Presumed acquired ocular toxoplasmosis in deer hunters. *Retina.* 2001;21:226.

[38] Bouree P, Paugam A, Petithory JC. Anisakidosis: report of 25 cases and review of the literature. *Comparative Immunol Microbiol Infect Dis.* 1995;18:75.

[39] Hughes RG, Sharp DS, Hughes MC, et al. Environmental influences on helminthiasis and nutritional status among Pacific schoolchildren. *Int J Environ Health Res.* 2004;14:163.

[40] Adams AM, Murrell KD, Cross JH. Parasites of fish and risks to public health. *Revue Scientifique et Technique.* 1997;16:652.

[41] Trichinellosis surveillance—U.S., 1997–2001. *MMWR Morb Mortal Wkly Rep.* 2002;52(SS06):1.

[42] Fatal degenerative neurologic illnesses in men who participated in wild game feasts—Wisconsin, 2002. *MMWR Morb Mortal Wkly Rep.* 2002;52(7):125.

[43] http://www.cdc.gov/h1n1flu/

[44] http://www.cdc.gov/flu/avian/

[45] http://www.cdc.gov/ncidod/dvrd/prions/index.htm

In 1996, the CDC's Emerging Infections Program's Foodborne Diseases Active Surveillance Network (FoodNet) began collecting data from 10 states for laboratory-diagnosed cases of foodborne illness caused by bacterial pathogens *Campylobacter*, *Shiga* toxin-producing *Escherichia coli* (STEC) O157, *Listeria*, *Salmonella*, *Shigella*, *Vibrio*, and *Yersinia*, and protozoan parasites *Cryptosporidium* and *Cyclospora cayetanensis*. Although the incidence of infections caused by *Campylobacter*, *Cryptosporidium parvum*, *E. coli* O157, *Salmonella*, and *Y. enterocolitica* have varied since 1996, infants and young children continue to suffer a high incidence of infections from several of these nine organisms, and this is a major public health concern.[77] Despite this, seven-year data trends indicate that meeting the

Exhibit Swine Flu: H1N1 Virus

Novel influenza A (H1N1) is a flu virus of swine origin that was first detected in Mexico and the United States in March and April 2009. The first novel H1N1 patient in the United States was confirmed by laboratory testing at CDC on April 15, 2009 and the second was confirmed on April 17, 2009. It was quickly determined that the virus was spreading from person-to-person. On April 22, CDC activated its Emergency Operations Center to better coordinate the public health response. On April 26, 2009, the United States government declared a public health emergency. It's thought that novel influenza A (H1N1) flu spreads in the same way that regular seasonal influenza viruses spread; mainly through the coughs and sneezes of people who are sick with the virus.

CDC has developed a polymerase chain reaction (PCR) diagnostic test kit to detect this novel H1N1 virus and has now distributed test kits to all states in the United States and the District of Columbia and Puerto Rico. The test kits are being shipped internationally as well. This will allow states and other countries to test for this new virus.

The U.S. government is aggressively taking early steps in the process to manufacture a novel H1N1 vaccine, working closely with manufacturing. CDC has isolated the new H1N1 virus, made a candidate vaccine virus that can be used to create vaccine, and has provided this virus to industry so they can begin scaling up for production of a vaccine, if necessary. Making vaccine is a multi-step process requiring several months to complete.

Source: Center for Disease Control and Prevention, 2009 SwineFlu. Available at http://www.cdc.gov/h1n1flu/. Accessed February 24, 2010.

Exhibit Avian Influenza: H5N1 Virus

Avian influenza is an infection caused by avian (bird) influenza (flu) viruses. These influenza viruses occur naturally among birds. Wild birds worldwide carry the viruses in their intestines, but usually do not get sick from them. However, avian influenza is very contagious among birds and can make some domesticated birds, including chickens, ducks, and turkeys, very sick and kill them.

Infected birds shed influenza virus in their saliva, nasal secretions, and feces. Susceptible birds become infected when they have contact with contaminated secretions or excretions or with surfaces that are contaminated with secretions or excretions from infected birds. Domesticated birds may become infected with avian influenza virus through direct contact with infected waterfowl or other infected poultry, or through contact with surfaces (such as dirt or cages) or materials (i.e., water or feed) that have been contaminated with the virus.

Infection with avian influenza viruses in domestic poultry causes two main forms of disease that are distinguished by low and high extremes of virulence. The "low pathogenic" form may go undetected and usually causes only mild symptoms (i.e., ruffled feathers and a drop in egg production). However, the highly pathogenic form spreads more rapidly through flocks of poultry. This form may cause disease that affects multiple internal organs and has a mortality rate that can reach 90% to 100% often within 48 hours.

There are many different subtypes of type A influenza viruses. These subtypes differ because of changes in certain proteins on the surface of the influenza A virus (hemagglutinin [HA] and neuraminidase [NA] proteins). There are 16 known HA subtypes and 9 known NA subtypes of influenza A viruses. Many different combinations of HA and NA proteins are possible. Each combination represents a different subtype. All known subtypes of influenza A viruses can be found in birds.

Usually, "avian influenza virus" refers to influenza A viruses found chiefly in birds, but infections with these viruses can occur in humans. The risk from avian influenza is generally low to most people, because the viruses do not usually infect humans. However, confirmed cases of human infection from several subtypes of avian influenza infection have been reported since 1997. Most cases of avian influenza infection in humans have resulted from contact with infected poultry (e.g., domesticated chicken, ducks, and turkeys) or surfaces contaminated with secretion/excretions from infected birds. The spread of avian influenza viruses from one ill person to another has been reported very rarely, and has been limited, inefficient, and unsustained.

"Human influenza virus" usually refers to those subtypes that spread widely among humans. There are only three known A subtypes of influenza viruses (H1N1, H1N2, and H3N2) currently circulating among humans. It is likely that some genetic parts of current human influenza A viruses came from birds originally. Influenza A viruses are constantly changing, and they might adapt over time to infect and spread among humans.

During an outbreak of avian influenza among poultry, there is a possible risk to people who have contact with infected birds or surfaces that have been contaminated with secretions or excretions from infected birds.

Symptoms of avian influenza in humans have ranged from typical human influenza-like symptoms (e.g., fever, cough, sore throat, and muscle aches) to eye infections, pneumonia, severe respiratory diseases (such as acute respiratory distress), and other severe and life-threatening complications. The symptoms of avian influenza may depend on which virus caused the infection.

Source: Center for Disease Control and Prevention, *Avian Influenza*. Available at http://www.cdc.gov/flu/avian/. Accessed February 24, 2010.

2010 national health objectives of reducing the incidence of foodborne infections is possible.[77,78]

Bacteria

Campylobacter jejuni
Campylobacter jejuni subsp. jejuni, one of about 14 species of *Campylobacter*,[79] is responsible for most cases of foodborne bacterial infection in

the United States.[80] It is found in the intestinal tracts of farm livestock (especially poultry),[79,81] wild birds,[82–84] and rodents,[85,86] and in drinking water[87,88] and unchlorinated water[89,90]; it can also be carried by insects.[91,92] Most cases of campylobacteriosis can be traced to eating undercooked poultry or to other foods contaminated by raw poultry.[93] The next most common route of infection is via unpasteurized milk,[79,93–95] but the largest outbreak, where about 2,000 people were infected, was traced to contaminated water.[79,96] Symptoms include abdominal pain, diarrhea, headache, and fever, and infection rates are higher in immunocompromised individuals (e.g., HIV/AIDS patients, infants, the

---

Exhibit Animal Prion Diseases

Bovine spongiform encephalopathy (BSE)
Chronic wasting disease (CWD)
Scrapie
Transmissible mink encephalopathy
Feline spongiform encephalopathy
Ungulate spongiform encephalopathy

Source: Center for Disease Control and Prevention, *Prion Diseases*. Available at http://www.cdc.gov/ncidod/dvrd/prions/index.htm. Accessed February 24, 2010.

Guillain-Barré syndrome: An inflammatory disorder of the peripheral nerves that is characterized by the rapid onset of weakness and, often, paralysis of the legs, arms, breathing muscles, and face.

Reiter syndrome: A peripheral arthritis lasting longer than one month.

---

elderly)[93,97–99] In severe cases of campylobacteriosis there may be bloody diarrhea.[79,99] Among the sequelae to infection are Guillain-Barré syndrome[100,101] and Reiter syndrome.[102]

Escherichia coli *Escherichia coli* (*E. coli*), a known human pathogen since the 18th century,[103] gained widespread recognition in 1971 after an enteritis outbreak was traced to contaminated imported cheeses.[104] *E. coli* is one of four genera of coliform bacteria used as indicators of food safety (microbiological coliform test), and *E. coli* is often specifically assayed because it is more indicative of fecal contamination than are the other three genera.[105] Within the genus *Escherichia* there are some 200 O and 30 H serotypes.[104] *E. coli* O157 inhabit the intestinal tracts of cattle; other *E. coli* are normal inhabitants of human intestinal tracts. When people become ill from *E. coli*, the usual transmission vehicles are raw or undercooked ground beef and other red meats, and occasionally prepared foods such as mashed potatoes and cream pies. Untreated water, raw milk, cheeses, and fish have also been implicated. Shiga toxin-producing *E. coli* (STEC) O157:H7 (a toxin similar to that of *Shigella dysenteriae*) was first recognized in 1982.[106–110] Causing either infection or intoxication, symptoms of illness resemble those of shigellosis, including, for infection, bloody diarrhea and colitis, and for intoxication, severe abdominal pain, nausea, vomiting, diarrhea, and sometimes fever.[111,112] Hemolytic uremic syndrome (HUS) and hemorrhagic colitis are especially severe and are particularly serious for children; several fatalities have occurred in the last 20 years. Although STEC is the organism monitored by the CDC, other strains of *E. coli* cause diarrhea (e.g., enteroaggregative *E. coli*[113]).

E. coli is among the leading causes of travelers' diarrhea (others include Noroviruses, *Campylobacter jejuni/coli*, and *Giardia lamblia*[105]). To prevent foodborne illness caused by *E. coli* (and other pathogens), nutritionists should advise that foods be cooked thoroughly and that a thermometer be used to ensure that proper temperatures are reached. Avoiding cross-contamination, proper handling/reheating of leftovers, and handwashing/personal hygiene are also appropriate control measures against *E. coli*.

Listeria The genus *Listeria* has six recognized species. *Listeria monocytogenes*, the primary pathogen, has 13 serovars.[114] For many years listeriosis was recognized as an animal disease, but *Listeria*'s association with foodborne illness in humans is a recent phenomenon. The organisms are widespread in nature, in wild and domestic animals and birds, in water and soil, and in vegetation. Found in raw milk, soft cheeses, raw meats, and poultry, it can also contaminate raw soil-grown vegetables such as lettuce. Symptoms of listeriosis include nausea, vomiting, and headache, but the health of the host determines the course and severity of the disease—many healthy people never develop clinical manifestations.[114] However, infants may be congenitally infected, and infected pregnant women (often with no or mild symptoms) may spontaneously abort, deliver prematurely, or deliver a stillborn infant.[114] Immunocompromised individuals, such as those with HIV/AIDS, are particularly susceptible, and neoplasms, alcoholism, diabetes (especially type 1), cardiovascular disease, renal transplant, and corticosteroid therapy predispose individuals to clinical listeriosis, characterized by meningitis, meningoencephalitis, or encephalitis.[114] *Listeria* can grow at cold temperatures, so refrigeration is inadequate as a control. Thorough cooking, using pasteurized milk and dairy products, avoiding cross-contamination, handwashing/personal hygiene, and maintaining clean, dry food storage and preparation areas are all effective against *Listeria*.

Salmonella The salmonellae are a large group of bacteria, but there are only two species, *Salmonella enterica* and *S. Bongori*. These species are further classified into four subspecies and one subspecies, respectively, and further into 2,324 serovars—these are commonly treated as separate species.[115] *Salmonella spp.* (*spp.* is defined as all individual species within a genus) are found in animal intestinal tracts, including birds, livestock, humans, reptiles, and some insects. Shed in feces, they may then be spread by insects and other vermin.[115] Animal feeds may serve as routes of infection for livestock,[116] and animal carcasses may be contaminated with gastrointestinal salmonellae during slaughter and processing. People who eat undercooked *Salmonella*-contaminated meats, poultry, or eggs, or drink *Salmonella*-contaminated water develop nausea, vomiting, abdominal pain, diarrhea, headache, and fever. The strains most com-

Exhibit **Bovine Spongiform Encephalopathy**

Bovine spongiform encephalopathy (BSE) is a progressive neurological disorder of cattle that results from infection by an unusual transmissible agent called a prion. The nature of the transmissible agent is not well understood. Currently, the most accepted theory is that the agent is a modified form of a normal protein known as prion protein. For reasons that are not yet understood, the normal prion protein changes into a pathogenic (harmful) form that then damages the central nervous system of cattle.

Research indicates that the first probable infections of BSE in cows occurred during the 1970s, with two cases of BSE being identified in 1986. BSE possibly originated as a result of feeding cattle meat-and-bone meal that contained BSE-infected products from a spontaneously occurring case of BSE or scrapie-infected sheep products. Scrapie is a prion disease of sheep. There is strong evidence and general agreement that the outbreak was then amplified and spread throughout the United Kingdom cattle industry by feeding rendered, prion-infected, bovine meat-and-bone meal to young calves.

The BSE epidemic in the United Kingdom peaked in January 1993 at almost 1,000 new cases per week. Through the end of 2007, more than 184,500 cases of BSE had been confirmed in the United Kingdom alone in more than 35,000 herds.

Strong epidemiologic and laboratory evidence exists for a causal association between a new human prion disease called variant Creutzfeldt-Jakob disease (vCJD), which was first reported from the United Kingdom in 1996 and the BSE outbreak in cattle. The interval between the most likely period for the initial extended exposure of the population to potentially BSE-contaminated food (1984–1986) and the onset of initial vCJD cases (1994–1996) is consistent with known incubation periods for the human forms of prion disease.

Source: Center for Disease Control and Prevention, *Prion Diseases*. Available at http://www.cdc.gov/ncidod/dvrd/prions/index.htm. Accessed February 24, 2010.

monly responsible for human illness are *S. Typhimurium* and *S. Enteritidis*. (The incidence of cases of non-typhoid *Salmonella* infections has increased substantially since about 1950.[75]) *S. enteritidis* infections have been increasing since the 1970s and are often associated with eggs, egg products, or egg-containing foods.[115,117–119] Because *S. enteritidis* may be present in fresh, uncracked shell eggs,[120–122] eating undercooked or raw eggs is ill-advised unless the eggs have been pasteurized in the shell.[123,124]

Shigella   The genus *Shigella* has four species: *S. dysenteriae*, *S. flexneri*, *S. boydii*, and *S. sonnei*. Although *S. dysenteriae* causes bacillary dysentery and can be carried in food or water, it is not considered a food-poisoning organism.[115] The other three species cause shigellosis infection, characterized by diarrhea, abdominal pain, fever, and chills. *Shigella* is unique among the bacteria discussed thus far, because there are no known non-human reservoirs.[115] Poor personal hygiene therefore is usually behind outbreaks, with shellfish, raw produce, chicken, and salads the usual vehicles.[115] People may carry *Shigella* for several weeks, excreting the bacteria in their stool. Flies and other vermin also may transmit the bacteria to foods. Control measures include fastidious handwashing/personal hygiene, rapid cooling of foods, vermin control, and use of potable water.

Vibrio   The genus *Vibrio* includes about 28 species, 5 being of public health significance: *V. parahaemolyticus*, *V. vul-*

nificus, *V. hollisae*, *V. alginolyticus*, and *V. cholerae*.[79] These are marine organisms, so the usual vehicle for foodborne illness is seafood, especially shellfish and dried fish, or other foods cross-contaminated by seafood.[79] *V. parahaemolyticus* is the leading cause of foodborne illness in Japan, and in the United States it has been responsible for many outbreaks, usually associated with eating raw oysters or clams. *V. vulnificus* causes soft-tissue infections and primary septicemia, particularly affecting immunocompromised individuals and those with liver cirrhosis. The organism consumed via raw oysters is responsible for about 95% of seafood-associated mortality in the United States.[79] *V. hollisae* causes gastroenteritis via shellfish consumption, and *V. alginolyticus* can cause gastroenteritis, but is more often implicated in soft-tissue and ear infections among swimmers.[79] *V. cholerae* is well known as the causative agent of cholera. Several foodborne gastroenteritis infections have been recorded in the United States, all in patients who had eaten raw oysters. Other foods implicated in small outbreaks (1–6 individuals) were raw seaweed, palm fruit, and coconut milk.[79] Control measures against vibriosis include avoiding raw shellfish and seafood, purchasing shellfish/seafood from approved sources, avoiding cross-contamination, and good handwashing/personal hygiene habits.

Yersinia   The genus *Yersinia* includes 11 species, among them the plague-causing *Y. pestis*. *Y. enterocolitica* is the primary organism of importance to food safety.[79] Swine are the usual reservoirs, but *Yersinia* is also associated with milk, seafood, and vegetables.[79] Foodborne yersiniosis manifestations include gastroenteritis, pseudoappendicitis, lymphadenitis, and many others.[79] The gastroenteritis is characterized by abdominal pain and diarrhea, and the illness may progress to a variety of systemic syndromes.[79] Children and the elderly are more susceptible than middle-aged adults.

Viruses

Viruses differ from bacteria in that they require a vector (i.e., virus-contaminated food or hands) in order to enter the body and cause disease. Pathogenic viruses have always been associated with foods, but some such as the Norwalk viruses,[125] newly renamed "Noroviruses,"[126] have been known as food-associated pathogens only since the 1970s.[127–129] Before then, causative agents for most gastroenteritis cases could not be identified. Noroviruses are responsible for most of the cases of acute gastroenteritis in the United States.[130] Norwalk virus is "the prototype strain of genetically and antigenically diverse single stranded RNA (ribonucleic acid) viruses,"[125] formerly known as small, round structural viruses. It was first identified as the causative agent for a school outbreak of gastroenteritis in 1968, in Norwalk, Ohio.[130] Norovirus outbreaks have been associated with contaminated water, fruits, raw oysters, and scallops,[130–132] and are notorious for their association with acute gastroenteritis outbreaks on cruise ships.[133]

In the United States, food- and waterborne hepatitis A outbreaks are relatively uncommon. However, transmission via the fecal-oral route is possible; food handler carriers of hepatitis A are often identified, and raw or undercooked shellfish may carry the virus, so prevention and control measures (see Vibrio previously) are necessary.[134,135]

Parasites

Parasites include flatworms, roundworms, tapeworms, protozoans, and other organisms that use the body as a host in order to live and multiply. Some familiar parasites are listed in Table 16–3. These are usually ingested in raw or undercooked foods or water in which the parasites live; for example, *Trichinella spiralis* (roundworm of pork, also found in game, like bear and walrus) causes trichinellosis,[116] and *Giardia lamblia*, a waterborne protozoan, causes giardiasis ("beaver fever").[136] Parasites emerging recently as significant to food safety include Cryptosporidium and Cyclospora, and liver flukes (e.g., *Fasciola hepatica* and *F. gigantica*).[137]

Cryptosporidium parvum, a protozoan found in mammals, reptiles, and birds, causes diarrhea in humans (it is particularly severe in immunocompromised individuals). Abdominal pain, nausea, vomiting, and fever are often reported.[138] Cryptosporidiosis is "acquired by at least one of five known transmission routes: zoonotic, person to person,

water, nosocomial, or food."[138] People are infected by ingesting oocysts of the parasite, which are shed in the feces of the host.[138] Major outbreaks of cryptosporidiosis have occurred in Maine (1993, unpasteurized apple cider),[139] Minnesota (1995, chicken salad),[140] New York (1996, unpasteurized apple cider),[141] and Washington (1997, raw green onions).[142]

Cyclospora cayetanensis, a protozoan similar to *Cryptosporidium*, causes symptoms similar to cryptosporidiosis in infected humans. Like cryptosporidiosis, cyclosporiasis is much more serious in immunocompromised individuals.[143] The most notorious foodborne cyclosporiasis outbreak "occurred in 1996 in 20 U.S. states and two Canadian provinces, infecting 1,465 people who had eaten imported Guatemalan raspberries."[138]

Prions

Problems in the British beef industry in the 1980s brought prion diseases under increased scientific scrutiny and public curiosity.[130,144–146] Prions, the etiologic agents of, among others, Creutzfeldt-Jakob disease (CJD) and kuru in humans[147,148] and chronic wasting disease and sheep scrapie in animals, are physiological cellular glycoproteins. The bovine spongiform encephalopathy (BSE; "mad cow disease") prion (PrPSc) is an infectious variant of a normal copper-binding prion (PrPC) on cell surfaces.[149] BSE is one of several transmissible spongiform encephalopathies (the human form of BSE is variant Creutzfeldt-Jakob disease, vCJD[150]) that are emerging, serious public health concerns.[151,152] Critics of U.S. regulatory policies regarding BSE cite half-hearted efforts to monitor for the disease, lack of research funding, and undue meat industry pressure.[153] After two BSE-infected cows were detected in the United States, one each in 2003 and 2004, public, professional, and Congressional lobbying for changes in regulatory oversight ensued. The FDA and USDA have strengthened safeguards protecting consumers from PrPSc, prohibiting "the use of certain cattle-derived materials in human food (including dietary supplements) and cosmetics."[154–156]

Chemical Hazards

Nutritionists understand that foods consist of chemicals, but the public grossly misunderstands the word *chemicals*. Several chemical hazards are associated with foods, some naturally occurring (e.g., aflatoxin, alkaloids, histamine), some indirectly added (e.g., pesticides, compounds that migrate from packaging materials, lubricants from food processing machinery), and others directly added (e.g., colors, preservatives).[9]

Naturally Occurring Toxicants Many foods contain natural toxins that may be harmful when consumed at certain levels, such as aflatoxin and mushroom toxins, whereas others contain toxins that are harmful over time, such as mercury. Mycotoxins, potato glycoalkaloids, shellfish toxins, and methylmercury are illustrative of this group, but there are many others, including oxalic acid, goitrogens, hemagglutinens, and protease inhibitors.

Mycotoxins are mold-produced toxins, many of which are of public health importance. The aflatoxins (*Aspergillus flavus* toxin), highly substituted coumarins, are the most studied.[157] Usually associated with corn, cottonseed, peanuts, and products made from them, aflatoxins are also found in milk, cheese,[158] meats, and other foods. Aflatoxins produce liver cancer in animals.[159] Developing countries in Africa and Asia have the greatest incidence of aflatoxin-related cancers.[160] The FDA specifies limits for aflatoxins in animal feeds and foods for human consumption, currently 20 ppb for food, feeds, Brazil nuts, peanuts, peanut products, and pistachios, and 0.5 ppb for milk.[160,161] At the international level, the Codex Alimentarius Commission[162] recommends maximums of 15 µg/kg of aflatoxin in peanuts for further processing and 0.05 µg/kg of aflatoxin in milk.[163]

Other molds, such as *Aspergillus*, *Alternaria*, *Fusarium*, and *Penicillium*, produce toxins in foods. *Aspergillus spp.* produce ochratoxins, found in corn, nuts, grains, meats, and other foods.[157] These heat-stable toxins are hepatotoxic and nephrotoxic in rats.[157] Alternariol and other *Alternaria*-produced toxins have been found in grains and fruits.[164,165] Fumonisins are *Fusarium*-produced toxins found in corn and other grains. These are associated with high rates of esophageal cancer in Africa and Asia.[166,167] Citrinin and patulin are toxins produced by *Penicillium spp.* Citrinin is found in many foods, including bread, rice, other cereal grains, and country-cured hams, and patulin has been found in bread, sausage, fruits, and juices.[157] The Codex Alimentarius Commission recommends maximums of 50 µg/kg of patulin in apple juice and apple juice as an ingredient in other beverages, and 5 µg/kg ochratoxin A in cereals and cereal products.[163]

Mycotoxins survive food-processing methods,[168] but continuous monitoring for them ensures safety of the foods affected. Although mycotoxins are not formed (or are formed in very small quantities) at refrigerator temperatures (generally, 36°–41°F),[169] consumers should be advised to throw out foods that develop molds. Preformed toxins are not affected by refrigeration, freezing, or cooking. Consumers also should be advised to store foods to minimize mold growth, by storing foods in small quantities, under refrigeration, and dry.

Alkaloids are found in many food products. Various glycoalkaloids are present in potatoes and potato products[170–176] and can increase with exposure to light,[177–179] heat,[180,181] and insect damage during the growing season.[182] Toxic effects of glycoalkaloids include abdominal pain, diarrhea, and vomiting at low doses; fever, hypotension, neurological disorders, tachycardia, tachypnea,[183] and death[184] at higher doses. Glycoalkaloid poisoning is uncommon, however, and individual responses to glycoalkaloids vary. For many years, nutritionists and other health professionals merely cautioned people to avoid eating the green parts of potatoes. The generally accepted safe limit for potato glycoalkaloids is 200 mg/kg.[185] Recently, as scientists have broadened their understanding of the biochemistry of glycoalkaloids, warnings about chronic versus acute effects of ingested glycoalkaloids have become more strident.[186] Glycoalkaloids increase risk for some cancers[187]; are teratogenic, embryotoxic, and genotoxic[188,189]; and may interfere with or interact with commonly prescribed pharmaceuticals.[190] With the food industry's interest in developing value-added products from potato peels[191,192] (and in reducing the glycoalkaloid content[193]) and the increasing likelihood that nutritionists will encounter clients (such as Bangladeshis[172]) for whom potato leaves and potato peels are acceptable food choices, regular monitoring of the scientific literature pertaining to potato glycoalkaloids is warranted.

Toxins causing amnesic shellfish poisoning (ASP), ciguatera poisoning, and paralytic shellfish poisoning (PSP) are not produced by shellfish or fish. Rather, they are produced by microscopic phytoplankton (diatoms and dinoflagellates) consumed by the shellfish and fish. The diatom *Pseudonitzschia pungens* produces domoic acid, which acts as a glutamic acid antagonist in the human central nervous system,[130] producing sometimes fatal ASP.[194] Several outbreaks have occurred since 1988.[195–198]

Ciguatoxin is produced by the dinoflagellate *Gambierdiscus toxicus*. Humans ingest the toxin in predatory fish, such as barracuda, groupers, and sea bass, which in turn have ingested herbivorous fish in which the toxin is concentrated in organs and muscles. Symptoms of ciguatoxin poisoning are similar to those of PSP (nausea, oral paresthesia, and respiratory paralysis), but the onset of symptoms is somewhat longer (3–6 hours vs. 2 hours for PSP). Long considered an illness of the tropics,[199,200] modern food transportation systems can deliver ciguatoxic fish to locations far removed from their home waters.[201–204]

PSP is caused by ingesting toxins (decarbamoyl saxitoxin, neosaxitoxin, gonyautoxins, and others[205,206]) in bivalve mollusks that have eaten dinoflagellates such as *Gonyaulax catenella* and *G. acatenella* (Pacific Coast), and *G. tamarensis* (Atlantic Coast), among others. The toxins are heat-stable and can cause cardiovascular collapse and respiratory failure.[130] PSP mortality can reach 22%.[207]

The National Shellfish Sanitation Program (NSSP),

...a voluntary, tripartite program composed of state officials, the shellfish industry, and Federal agencies...is designed to prevent human illness associated with the consumption of fresh and frozen shellfish (oysters, clams, and mussels) through the establishment of sanitary controls over all phases of the growing, harvesting, shucking, packing and distribution of fresh and frozen shellfish.[208]

The FDA oversees the NSSP and, together with state agencies, manages the sanitation programs at the state level. Foreign countries (e.g., Canada, Chile, Korea, Mexico, New Zealand) may import shellfish into the United States by agreeing to abide by the provisions of the NSSP as set forth in a Memorandum of Understanding between countries. Public health nutritionists should consult the Interstate Certified Shellfish Shippers List (ICSSL),[209] published monthly by the FDA, because under the NSSP all states require that shellfish be from a certified source, proof of which is dealer listing in the ICSSL.

Metals such as mercury are persistent environmental pollutants and can cause foodborne illness. Foods usually implicated are fish, shellfish, and marine mammals. These animals ingest and accumulate methylmercury from their foods. Mercury enters the environment and food chains from both human activities (coal-fired power plant emissions, medical and electronics wastes, etc.) and natural processes.[210] Methylmercury is neurotoxic[210] and possibly immunomodulating[211] in humans, usually over time with chronic exposure. The human fetus is particularly susceptible to methylmercury poisoning. The FDA's seafood Web site (http://vm.cfsan.fda.gov/seafood1.html) has links to population-specific seafood advisories[212,213] and data on mercury levels in commonly consumed fish and shellfish.[214,215] One example is the irreversible neurologic damage from the chemical methylmercury found in fish and shellfish living in polluted waters that may be tempered by nutrition.[216-218] Until more is known, some authorities question current recommendations to eat more fish to improve cardiovascular health.[219]

Directly Added Chemicals

Food Additives   Humans have added chemicals to food since before recorded history. Primitive food preservation methods included salting, smoking, and fermentation, all still in use today, and herbs and spices were used to retard spoilage and to mask flavors caused by spoilage. Today, with fewer people cooking meals "from scratch" and with fewer meals eaten in the home, consumers are increasingly leaving decisions about which chemicals are added to foods to the food industry and its government regulators. Nutritionists are likely to encounter ignorance of the purposes of food additives in foods consumed by their clients as well as fear of the chemical names listed on ingredient labels. At least, this may be true for those who actually read the labels; some nutritionists believe that many do not read food labels,[220,221] and among those who do, comprehension is not what it should be.[222,223] Many people are influenced by the popular press and news media, where innuendo, half-truths, and patently false statements compete with sound

science on issues surrounding chemical use in foods. The food and chemical industries and government regulatory agencies often exacerbate the confusion by offering platitudes in response to accusations. Steps have been taken to restore public confidence in food safety and in the industries themselves.[224-229] This constant interchange between science and pseudo-science is one of the most daunting obstacles a nutritionist is likely to face. We must regularly evaluate the scientific literature and government policy to better inform clients and to provide guidance in critically evaluating claims made about food additives.

Chemicals are added to foods for many reasons: to increase nutritional quality; to aid in food processing; to increase, decrease, or neutralize certain sensory characteristics of foods; to prolong storage stability; and to inhibit microbial growth. Within broad categories of additives (**Table 16–4**) there are usually several alternatives available to gain the same desired effect. For some applications, combinations of additives are applied to meet specific requirements (e.g., a manufacturer may use a blend of acesulfame-K and aspartame to obtain an optimum low-calorie sweetener for hot coffee and tea beverages[230]). Development, testing, and approval of new chemical food additives continue at a rapid pace.

Antioxidants   Foods containing fats are subject to oxidative rancidity during storage. To enable foods such as crackers, nuts, and potato chips to be packaged and stored while retaining freshness, antioxidant chemicals such as ascorbic acid (vitamin C), butylated hydroxyanisole (BHA), butylated hydroxytoluene (BHT), sulfur dioxide, and tocopherols (vitamin E), among others, are used, singly or in combinations.[9]

Alternative Sweeteners   Sweeteners may be classified as nutritive (or caloric; e.g., sucrose, honey, corn syrups) or non-nutritive (or noncaloric; e.g., acesulfame-K, saccharin). Some nutritive alternative sweeteners are so much sweeter than sucrose that they are essentially reduced-calorie sweeteners (e.g., aspartame at 4 kcal/g is approximately 200 times sweeter than sucrose[231] and thus is calorically negligible in foods to which it has been added). Reduced-calorie or noncaloric alternatively sweetened foods are popularly used in weight-reducing diets and weight-maintenance plans to reduce the incidence of dental caries or to manage diabetes. Food scientists and food technologists continue to research

TABLE 16–4	Examples of Chemical Food Additives[1]	
Class	**Representative Chemicals**	**Purposes**
Antioxidants	Ascorbic acid (vitamin C) butylated hydroxyanisole, butylated hydroxytoluene, sulfur dioxide, tocopherols (vitamin E)	Retard deterioration, rancidity, discoloration from oxidation; free radical scavengers
Flour bleaching agents, flour maturing agents, starch bleaching agents, starch modifiers	Acetone peroxides, calcium bromate, sodium hypochlorite, adipic anhydride (esterifier), propylene oxide (etherifier)	Enhance whiteness of flour or starch; enhance baking qualities of flour; modify starch functional characteristics to applications desired
Buffers, acids, alkalis	Acetic acid, ammonium hydroxide, citric acid, fumaric acid, malic acid, oxalic acid, sodium carbonate, succinic acid, tartaric acid	Lower or raise pH; buffer pH against change
Colors (exempt from batch certification)[2]	Annatto extract, caramel, carmine, grape skin extract, turmeric	Impart, enhance, or preserve food color or shading
Colors (must be batch certified)[3]	FD&C Blue No. 1, FD&C Green No. 3, Orange B, Citrus Red No. 2, FD&C Yellow No. 5	Impart, enhance, or preserve food color or shading
Flavors, chemical	2-acetyl thiazole, 3-heptanone, benzaldehyde, cresyl acetate, decanal, eugenol, quinine sulfate	Impart or enhance a flavor or flavor "note" in food
Nutritional additives	Amino acids (e.g., DL-leucine), β-carotene, kelp, minerals (e.g., ferrous sulfate), vitamins (e.g., biotin)	Necessary for the body's nutritional and metabolic processes
Preservatives	Benzoic acid, butyl P-hydroxybenzoate, calcium benzoate, calcium disodium EDTA, calcium sorbate, cupric sulfate, heptylparaben	Retard microbial spoilage; block ripening and enzymatic processes; antioxidation
Sequestrants	Calcium acetate, calcium disodium EDTA, citric acid, disodium EDTA, glucono δ-lactone	Combine with polyvalent metal ions to form a soluble metal complex; improve product quality and stability
Stabilizers and thickeners	Carrageenan, carob bean gum, dammar gum, dextrin, edible gelatin, modified starches, tara gum	Increase viscosity of solutions; produce/improve dispersions; impart body, improve consistency, or stabilize emulsions
Surface-active agents: detergents; dispersants; defoaming agents; foaming agents; solubilizing agents; wetting agents; whipping agents	TERG-A-ZYME™[4] microcrystalline cellulose decanoic acid	Modify surface properties of liquid food components
Miscellaneous additives: alternative sweeteners; anti-caking agents; anti-sticking agents; clarifying agents; fat replacers[5]; firming agents; growth promoters; lubricants; solvents	acacia 1,3-butylene glycol dioctyl sodium sulfosuccinate calcium polyphosphates aspartame, sucralose, tagatose aluminum silicate castor oil polyvinylpolypyrrolidone dextrins, whey protein, olestra aluminum sulfate calcium lactate (yeast food) mineral oil ethylene dichloride	For specific applications

[1]Not a complete list. For extensive lists, see the *NutritionData Food Additive Identifier*, http://www.nutritiondata.com/food-additives.html; "Food Additives Permitted for Direct Addition to Food for Human Consumption," Code of Federal Regulations, Title 21, Vol. 3, (U.S. Government Printing Office, April 1, 2003), Ch. 1, Part 172; "Secondary Direct Food Additives Permitted in Food for Human Consumption," Code of Federal Regulations, Title 21, Vol. 3, (U.S. Government Printing Office, April 1, 2003), Ch. 1, Part 173; "Indirect Food Additives," Code of Federal Regulations, Title 21, Vol. 3, (U.S. Government Printing Office, April 1, 2003), Ch. 1, Parts 174–178.

[2]See "Color Additives Approved for Use in Human Food. Part 73, Subpart A: Color Additives Exempt from Batch Certification," http://www.cfsan.fda.gov/~dms/opa-col2.html#table1A. Accessed July 1, 2009.

[3]See "Color Additives Approved for Use in Human Food. Part 74, Subpart A: Color Additives Subject to Batch Certification," http://www.cfsan.fda.gov/~dms/opa-col2.html#table1A. Accessed July 1, 2009.

[4]TERG-A-ZYME consists of sodium linear alkylaryl sulfonate, phosphates, carbonates, and protease enzyme (*Bacillus licheniformis subtilisin Carlsberg*). See Document #123, "TERG-A-ZYME Technical Bulletin" (White Plains NY: Alconox, http://www.alconox.com/downloads/pdf/techbull_tergazyme.pdf. Accessed July 1, 2009).

[5]For a current list of fat replacers, see the Calorie Control Council's Web site at http://www.caloriecontrol.org/frgloss.html. Accessed July 1, 2009.

and develop alternative sweeteners; the most recently approved sweetener is tagatose, a natural sugar.[232]

Nutritionists can help consumers recognize the various sugars (e.g., corn syrup, dextrose, fructose, high fructose corn syrup [HFCS], honey, lactose, sucrose) and alternative sweeteners[233] listed on food labels, and to choose foods sweetened with additives that are suited to their individual health profiles, diets, and lifestyles. Nutritionists may also be asked about alternative sweeteners that, although legally used abroad, are not approved for additive use in the United States, such as stevia (powdered extract of the plant *Stevia rebaudiana Bertoni*),[234] currently regulated and sold as a food supplement. (Stevia is purported to have antihyperglycemic[235] and antihypertensive properties.[236-238]) Finally, nutritionists must thoroughly understand the controversial aspects of some additive sweeteners (e.g., the alleged association of HFCS with the increasing worldwide prevalence of obesity;[239] the purported carcinogenicity of sodium saccharin;[240,241] and the alleged adverse health effects of dietary aspartame[242-247] and sucralose[248-251]) and critically evaluate the evidence available to make the best possible recommendations to consumers. The Dietary Guidelines for Americans,[252] the Dietary Reference Intakes,[253] and the position statement on sweeteners of the American Dietetic Association[254] are useful guidelines.

Bleaching Agents, Maturing Agents, and Starch Modifiers   Oxidizing agents such as benzoyl peroxide and chlorine dioxide are used to bleach flour color and to mature flour to improve baking properties. Modified food starches are used to improve the appearance, stability, texture, and quality of food products.[9] Starches may be cross-linked with phosphates or adipates, stabilized by etherification or esterification (acetate- or hydroxypropyl-modified), or thinned by dextrinization or acid hydrolysis.[255]

Buffers, Acids, and Alkalis   Buffers (e.g., acetic acid/sodium acetate), acids (e.g., acetic, malic, tartaric acids), and alkalis (e.g., ammonium hydroxide, carbonates) are used in foods to control or adjust pH. They may be from natural sources, fermentation-derived, or chemically synthesized.[9,256]

Colors   Natural and synthetic colors are added to foods to enhance visual appeal. Natural colors may be obtained from plant (e.g., beets, grapes, saffron), mineral (e.g., iron oxide, titanium dioxide), and animal (e.g., cochineal extract or carmine from female scale insects, Coccus cacti) sources.[9]

Flavors   Flavoring agents constitute the largest group of food additives. Natural flavor substances include spices (e.g., anise, paprika, vanilla), herbs (e.g., basil, parsley, thyme), essential oils (e.g., clove, lime, rose), and plant extracts (e.g., almond, garlic, rosemary). Some natural flavor substances may appear in multiple categories; for example, chervil may be added to foods as a spice, an oil, or an extract, among other designations.[257] Synthetic flavoring agents are also used (e.g., allyl disulfide, isopropyl alcohol, thymol). Flavoring agents may be listed on food labels as "flavorings," "natural flavors," "artificial flavors," and "spices." Monosodium glutamate (MSG), a flavor enhancer, is associated with adverse reaction symptoms (chest pain, edema, facial or oral numbness, headache, perspiration, and cranial or facial pressure such as "Chinese Restaurant Syndrome"[258-264] and MSG-induced asthma[265,266]) in some people, but is listed GRAS by the FDA and is reported safe by the Joint Food and Agriculture Organization/World Health Organization (FAO/WHO) Expert Committee on Food Additives,[267] in the absence of conclusive proof that it is harmful. Many health professionals do recognize, however, a subpopulation of MSG-sensitive individuals. Nutritionists should be prepared to help these consumers identify MSG-containing foods (MSG may be hidden in general ingredient label statements, such as "hydrolyzed vegetable protein," "natural flavorings," "seasonings") and to suggest alternatives.

Nutritional Additives   Vitamins and minerals are added as enrichments and fortifiers to several foods. Although there is no legal distinction between *enrichment* and *fortification* in the United States—the FDA uses the terms interchangeably[268])—enrichment usually signifies replacement of nutrients lost in flour and cereal processing. Enriched flour has had B vitamins and iron added, most breakfast cereals are vitamin and mineral enriched, and polished rice is usually enriched. Fortification also signifies the replacement of lost nutrients, usually in foods other than flour and cereals, as well as the addition of nutrients to commonly used foods to redress deficiency of the nutrient(s) in most diets. Milk thus may be fortified with vitamin D because the diet of children and older adults is often deficient in vitamin D[269]; no-fat and low-fat milks have vitamins A (by law) and D (optional) added because these vitamins are lost when fat is removed; salt may be fortified with iodine to prevent goiter; and cereal and grain products are fortified with folic acid to prevent neural tube defects.[270]

Food fortification is one of the leading research areas in food technology today.[271-273] For example, consumers can buy calcium-fortified and vitamin D–fortified orange juice[274] and vitamin-and-herb-fortified spring water (e.g., Kraft Foods' Fruit2O Plus™). Unfortunately, most people purchase fortified foods with little or no knowledge of bioavailability or potential toxicities of the substances used to fortify the foods.[275,276]

Preservatives   Preservatives (e.g., butylated hydroxyanisole [BHA], butylated hydroxytoluene [BHT], sodium propionate, sulfur dioxide) are used as antimicrobial agents to retard microbial spoilage of foods, as metal chelators to block ripening and enzymatic processes that continue in foods after harvest, and as antioxidants to retard rancidity and browning, allowing consumers to enjoy a variety of foods, from global sources, year-round.[277,278] Nutritionists may receive questions from consumers concerning the safety of BHA,[279–282] BHT,[279,280,282] sulfites,[283,284] nitrites,[285–287] and food irradiation ("cold pasteurization," considered a food additive by the FDA).[288–297] Currently, several classes of foods may be irradiated at doses between 4.5 and 7.0 kGy[298] in the United States, including some fresh fruits and vegetables, spices and seasonings, meats, poultry, and prepackaged foods.

Sequestrants Chelating agents (e.g., EDTA, citric acid) are used to sequester metal ions in foods. Left alone, metals such as iron and copper contribute to off colors and catalyze oxidation reactions in foods.[9]

Stabilizers and Thickeners Processed foods, such as gravies, puddings, and salad dressings, are stabilized and thickened by substances such as carboxymethyl cellulose, gums, and pectin.[9] Foods containing little or no fat, such as low-fat salad dressings, are formulated using stabilizers and thickeners to resemble their full-fat counterparts.

Surface-Active Agents Emulsifiers, defoaming agents, and detergents are all active at molecular surfaces. Emulsifiers (e.g., lecithin, mono- and diglycerides, and fatty acids) are used to keep food mixtures, such as oil in water and water in oil, stable.[9]

Miscellaneous Additives Many other additives (e.g., anticaking and anti-sticking agents, clarifying agents, firming agents, growth promoters, lubricants, solvents) are used for very specific applications.[9] Macrocomponents, such as fat replacers, are added to foods to replace some or all of a food component. Substances such as bean pastes, fruit pastes, or microparticulated whey protein concentrates (e.g., Simplesse®) and emulsifiers may be used to replace some or all of the fat in baked goods.[299,300]

Agricultural Chemicals Agricultural chemicals include antibiotics, growth hormones, herbicides, fertilizers, fungicides, insecticides, and rodenticides, all of which may enter the food supply. Antibiotics at subtherapeutic doses are used to promote animal growth (in the United States) and to prevent disease. Evidence that antibiotic-resistant strains of bacteria develop in food animals and might be passed on to humans, and that consuming antibiotic residues in food might inhibit the efficacy of therapeutic antibiotic use in humans, is controversial.[301,302] Growth hormones, such as recombinant bovine growth hormone (rbGH or BGH) or recombinant bovine somatotropin (rbST or BST), are considered safe when used as directed.[303,304] However, prod-

uct labeling is controversial, particularly the use of label statements such as "BST-free."[305–308] Herbicides, fertilizers, fungicides, insecticides, and other pesticides are regulated by the EPA. Residues of these chemicals in food[309–312] are under FDA jurisdiction.

Physical Hazards

Physical hazards include extraneous objects or foreign materials in food that may cause illness or injury if consumed. The most common physical hazards found in foods are:

- Metal (from fields, equipment, premises), bullets and BB shot (from animals shot in the field), and hypodermic needles (broken off when treating animals)
- Jewelry (buttons, earrings, rings, etc.)
- Stones and rocks (from fields, ceilings, walls), wood (from fields, ceilings, walls, boxes, pallets), and insulation (from buildings)
- Glass (from bottles, jars, light fixtures, utensils, equipment)
- Insects, insect parts, and other filth (from fields, premises, entry after processing)
- Bone (from improper processing; also from fields and premises)
- Plastic (from fields, packaging and packing, employees)
- Personal effects (bandages, pens, pencils, thermometers, etc.)[8]

Less common physical hazards include capsules, crystals (e.g., struvite), paper, pits, scum, shells, and slime.[313] Food processors must identify potential physical hazards and determine procedures to control each hazard; if warranted, control points should be implemented as part of the facility HACCP plan.[314]

Agroterrorism and Bioterrorism

For centuries, humans have targeted agricultural crops and employed biological agents in adversarial confrontations with each other,[315] but for most of the 20th century, these methods were thought unlikely to be employed. In the 1990s, government and public health professionals began to assess vulnerabilities and to prepare countermeasures against acts of warfare or terrorism directed against the agricultural, food, and water systems of the national infrastructure.[316–318] The CDC identified many biological and chemical agents that could be used for these purposes.[319,320] The effects of several of these, such as mercury, could be insidious, whereas others, such as Salmonella, would make it difficult to distinguish disease outbreaks due to bioterrorism from those due to mundane incidents.

In 1984, a bioterrorist act was perpetrated by a religious cult attempting to gain political control of Wasco County, Oregon. More than 700 people were sickened after *Salmonella* was sprinkled over salad bars in 10 restaurants. What was most frightening about this incident was that it went unrecognized as bioterrorism until disgruntled members of the cult told their stories.[321,322]

Public health nutritionists will most likely be involved with bioterrorism directed at food and water systems. A consensus is forming that preventing and detecting these incidents will require more than the usual precautions taken by government and the food and water industries, and that improvements made or contemplated by these entities will be inadequate. Rather, the focus should be on improving surveillance systems with the aim of detecting outbreaks early enough to intervene.[323–325] Consumers are an integral part of this plan but currently do not seek medical care for gastrointestinal illnesses.[325] This is one area where nutritionists can help. Public health nutritionists are routinely involved in educating consumers and should actively seek ways to expand their roles to encompass antibioterrorism. (As noted earlier, nutritionists should be involved in investigating and monitoring outbreaks of foodborne disease and in emergency preparedness planning and response.)[326,327] Bioterrorism and the food supply are discussed at length in the Chapter 18.

■ FOOD SAFETY IN THE 21ST CENTURY

Among the many food safety issues that will occupy our nation in the 21st century, expect these five to be prominent in the early years:

1. *Federal regulation/oversight by a single agency.* Government and some industry groups contend that the current array of federal (see Table 16–1), state, and local agencies results in overlapping jurisdictions and in duplicated efforts that often impede the progress of new food safety initiatives and slow responses to emerging food safety issues.[328–332] Limited resources end up being divided among the many federal agencies, reducing the effectiveness of each tax dollar. Others in government and industry contend that creating a single food safety agency is unnecessary, pointing out that the United States sets the international standard for food safety.[333–335] Proponents favor increasing cooperation and collaboration among agencies, increasing funding for the agencies, and adopting a single national food safety policy.

2. *Safety of bioengineered foods.* Genetically engineered food crops and animals are controversial.[336–338] Whereas most scientists agree that bioengineered foods are safe,[339,340] some make persuasive opposing arguments,[341,342] and consumers hold strong views at either extreme.[342–346] There are also those who question labeling of foods with respect to consumers' right to know what they are buying.[347]

3. *Chronic health effects of natural and synthetic chemicals ingested in foods.* As synthesis of new food additives, pesticides, and antibiotics continues, and as new uses for these chemicals and combinations of them continue to be found, the need for research on chronic effects of low-level exposure to these chemicals will be needed. Studies of interactions among additives, naturally occurring chemicals and toxicants, and environmental chemicals and toxicants as well as their acute and chronic effects on humans are needed also. Research addressing these issues in specific subpopulations, such as children, pregnant and lactating women, the elderly, and the immunocompromised, must be accomplished.[348–353]

4. *Prions as infective agents of foodborne disease.* The experience with BSE and vCJD in the United Kingdom initiated intense research efforts into prions as infective agents.[145] When a cow with BSE was thought to have entered the food supply in the United States, a series of reforms in regulating the meat industry were undertaken.[150,354] As research on prions and prion diseases[146,355]—as well as other issues concerning emerging microbial pathogens—continues, public health nutritionists should be prepared to assist consumers in understanding this issue within the context of hazards and risks.

5. *Home food safety.* Today, more meals than ever before are eaten outside the home. Ready-prepared meals for home consumption have never been more popular. Despite these trends, a significant number of foodborne illnesses result from hygiene errors committed at home.[356–362] In the area of home hygiene alone, the public health nutritionist can make a difference in consumer habits affecting individual and community health. For example, workshops and individual training could be offered to reinforce the food safety messages that should have been received in elementary and high school health classes. Occasional focused articles can be submitted to newspapers to reach a broader audience. Through partnerships with other professionals, such as sanitarians and school health teachers, consumers can be apprised of the many resources available to them in their communities. For all of the various federal, state, and local food safety initiatives, present and future, to succeed, food safety must begin at home.

Issues for Discussion

1. How can nutritionists help consumers understand food safety hazards and risks?

2. How should nutritionists approach other health agency staff to offer expertise on food safety issues? How is the nutritionist's perspective likely to differ from other health professionals' perspectives?

3. What possible roles exist for nutritionists to identify and combat bioterrorism directed against the food supply system?

4. Considering risks versus benefits, what specific recommendations should be made to clients concerned about bovine growth hormones in milk?

5. How can nutritionists help to instill a sense of individual responsibility for food safety?

References

1. Schwetz BA. Statement before the Committee on Governmental Affairs, Subcommittee on Oversight of Government Management, Restructuring and the District of Columbia. (October 10, 2001). Available at http://www.fda.gov/NewsEvents/Testimony/ucm114861.htm. Accessed July 1, 2009.

2. Mead PS, Slutsker L, Dietz V, McCaig LF, Bresee JS, Shapiro C, et al. Food-related illness and death in the United States. *Emerg Infect Dis.* 1999;5:607.

3. Interagency Forum on Child and Family Statistics. *America's Children: Key National Indicators of Well-Being, 2009.* Available at http://www.childstats.gov/americaschildren/index.asp. Accessed July 1, 2009.

4. Anderson GF, Hussey PS. *Health and Population Aging: A Multinational Comparison.* Baltimore MD: Johns Hopkins University; October 1999:6.

5. Sinclair U. *The Jungle.* New York: Doubleday; 1906. Available at http://sunsite.berkeley.edu/Literature/Sinclair/TheJungle/. Accessed July 1, 2009.

6. Dingell JD. *Food safety and the bioterrorism legislation.* Remarks before the Consumer Federation of America's 26th Annual National Food Policy Conference 2002. (April 23, 2002). Available at http://archives.energycommerce.house.gov/press/107rm4.shtml. Accessed July 1, 2009.

7. Veneman AM. *Testimony before the Subcommittee on Agriculture, Rural Development, Food and Drug Administration, and Related Agencies Committee on Appropriations*, U.S. House of Representatives. (February 27, 2003). Available at http://www.usda.gov/news/special/ctc33.htm. Accessed July 1, 2009.

8. Stier RF. The dirty dozen: Ways to reduce the 12 biggest foreign materials problems. *FoodSafety Magazine.* 2003;9:44.

9. Potter NN, Hotchkiss JH. *Food Science,* 5th ed. Gaithersburg, MD: Aspen Publishers; 1998:533.

10. University of Arkansas. *The Food Safety Consortium.* Available at http://www.uark.edu/depts/fsc/fslinks.htm. Accessed July 1, 2009.

11. Simmons College. *Simmons Center for Hygiene and Health.* Available at http://www.simmons.edu/hygieneandhealth. Accessed July 1, 2009.

12. U.S. Food and Drug Administration. *Food Safety: A Team Approach. FDA Backgrounder.* (September 24, 1998). Available at http://vm.cfsan.fda.gov/~lrd/foodteam.html. Accessed July 1, 2009.

13. Remarks of Commissioner Robert C. Bonner, Customs and Border Protection National Plant Board Annual Meeting. (August 12, 2003). Available at http://www.cbp.gov/xp/cgov/newsroom/commissioner/speeches_statements/archives/2003/aug122003.xml. Accessed July 1, 2009.

14. Applebaum RS. Protecting the nation's food supply from bioterrorism. *FoodSafety Magazine.* 2004;10:30.

15. Centers for Disease Control and Prevention (CDC). *Drinking water.* Available at http://www.cdc.gov/healthywater/drinking/. Accessed July 1, 2009.

16. Preventing emerging infectious diseases: a strategy for the 21st century. Overview of the updated CDC plan. *MMWR Morb Mortal Wkly Rep.* 1998;47(15):1.

17. U.S. Department of Commerce, NOAA. Seafood Inspection Program. (undated). *NOAA Handbook 25.* Available at http://www.seafood.nmfs.noaa.gov/NOAA Handbook25/NOAA Handbook.pdf. Accessed July 1, 2009.

18. Title 50, U.S. Code of Federal Regulations, Part 260-261. Subpart A: Inspection and certification of establishments and fishery products for human consumption. Available at http://www.seafood.nmfs.noaa.gov/50CFR260-261.PDF. Accessed July 1, 2009.

19. Becker GS, Upton HF. Seafood safety: background and issues. (2009). Congressional Research Service 7-5700. Available at http://www.nationalaglawcenter.org/assets/crs/RS22797.pdf. Accessed July 1, 2009.

20. Foulke J. Seafood safety regulations announced. HHS News, P95-9. (December 5, 1995). Available at http://www.scienceblog.com/community/older/archives/A/hhs1286.html. Accessed July 1, 2009.

21. U.S. Food & Drug Administration (USDA). *Fish and Fisheries Products Hazards and Controls Guidance,* 3rd ed. (2001) Available at http://www.fda.gov/Food/GuidanceCompliance RegulatoryInformation/GuidanceDocuments/Seafood/Fish andFisheriesProductsHazardsandControlsGuide/default.htm. Accessed July 1, 2009.

22. Federal Trade Commission (FTC). *For Consumers: Division of Advertising Practices.* Available at http://www.ftc.gov/bcp/bcpap.htm. Accessed July 1, 2009.

23. Goldammer T. *The Brewer's Handbook. The Complete Book to Brewing Beer,* 2nd ed. Clifton VA: Apex Publishers; 2008:411.

24. United States Department of Agriculture (USDA), Food Safety and Inspection Service (FSIS). State Inspection Programs. (2009). Available at http://www.fsis.usda.gov/Regulations_&_Policies/state_inspection_programs/index.asp. Accessed July 1, 2009.

25. Landman J. Food aid in emergencies: a case for wheat? *Proc Nutr Soc.* 1999;58:355.

26. Stevens S. Just a matter of time. *Food Manage.* 1990;25:116–119.

27. Gemperlein J. When the earth moved. *Food Manage.* 1990;25:130–134.

28. *The China Post.* "Over 200 Taipei citizens quarantined over SARS." (March 23, 2003). Available at http://www.chinapost.com.tw/taiwan/detail.asp?ID=36279&GRP=B. Accessed July 1, 2009.

29. The American Civil Defense Association. *Local & State Resources.* (2009). Available at http://www.tacda.org/resources/local/local.htm. Accessed July 1, 2009.

30. Marchione TJ. Foods provided through U.S. government emergency food aid programs: policies and customs governing their formulation, selection and distribution. *J Nutr.* 2002;132:2104S.

31. Reed BA, Habicht J-P, Garza C. Translating nutrition research into action in humanitarian emergencies. *J Nutr.* 2002;132:2112S.

32. HR 875: *Food Safety Modernization Act of 2009.* (2009). Available at http://www.govtrack.us/congress/bill.xpd?bill=h111-875. Accessed July 1, 2009.

33. Potter NN, Hotchkiss JH. *Food Science,* 5th ed. Gaithersburg, MD: Aspen; 1998:562.

34. Food additives permitted for direct addition to food for human consumption. Code of Federal Regulations (Title 21, Vol. 3, April 1, 2003), Ch. 1, Part 172.

35. Secondary direct food additives permitted in food for human consumption. Code of Federal Regulations (Title 21, Vol. 3, April 1, 2003), Ch. 1, Part 173.

36. Indirect food additives. Code of Federal Regulations (Title 21, Vol. 3, April 1, 2003), Ch. 1, Parts 174–178.

37. Prior-sanctioned food ingredients. Code of Federal Regulations (Title 21, Vol. 3, April 1, 2003), Ch. 1, Part 181.

38. Substances generally recognized as safe. Code of Federal Regulations (Title 21, Vol. 3, April 1, 2003), Ch. 1, Part 182.

39. Direct food substances affirmed as generally recognized as safe. Code of Federal Regulations (Title 21, Vol. 3, April 1, 2003), Ch. 1, Part 184.

40. Indirect food substances affirmed as generally recognized as safe. Code of Federal Regulations (Title 21, Vol. 3, April 1, 2003), Ch. 1, Part 186.

41. Burdock GA, Carabin IG. Generally recognized as safe (GRAS): history and description. *Toxicol Lett.* 2004;150:3.

42. Rados C. GRAS: time-tested, and trusted, food ingredients. *FDA Consumer.* 2004;38:20.

43. Folkenberg J. A primer on food additives. *FDA Consumer.* 1988;Nov:44.

44. Henkel J. From shampoo to cereal. Seeing to the safety of color additives. *FDA Consumer.* 1993;Dec:1.

45. Food and Drug Administration (FDA). (2007). *Summary of Color Additives for Use in United States in Foods, Drugs, Cosmetics, and Medical Devices.* Available at http://www.fda. gov/ForIndustry/ColorAdditives/ColorAdditiveInventories/ ucm115641.htm. Accessed July 1, 2009.

46. United States Department of Agriculture (USDA), FSIS. *Additives in Meat and Poultry Products.* (2008). Available at http://www.fsis.usda.gov/Fact_Sheets/Additives_in_Meat_&_ Poultry_Products/index.asp. Accessed July 1, 2009.

47. *How to Understand and Use the Nutrition Facts Label.* (2004). Available at http://www.fda.gov/Food/LabelingNutrition/ ConsumerInformation/ucm078889.htm. Accessed July 1, 2009.

48. Food and Drug Administration (FDA). Dietary supplements. (2009). Available at http://www.fda.gov/Food/Dietary Supplements/default.htm. Accessed July 1, 2009.

49. Hileman B. Reining in dietary supplements. Food additives critics demand changes in the law governing supplement. *Chem Eng News.* 2004;82:21.

50. Food and Drug Administration (FDA). *Food Quality Protection Act of 1996.* (2009). Available at http://www.fda.gov/Regulatory Information/Legislation/FederalFoodDrugandCosmeticActFDC Act/SignificantAmendmentstotheFDCAct/ucm148008.htm. Accessed July 1, 2009.

51. Environmental Protection Agency (EPA). (2009). *Laws and Regulations.* Available at http://www.epa.gov/pesticides/ regulating/laws.htm. Accessed July 1, 2009.

52. Environmental Protection Agency (EPA). *Food Quality Protection Act (FQPA).* Available at http://www.epa.gov/agriculture/lqpa. html. Accessed July 1, 2009.

53. Tomerlin JR. The U.S. Food Quality Protection Act–Policy implications of variability and consumer risk. *Food Additives and Contaminants.* 2000;17(7):641.

54. Sumner D. The Food Quality Protection Act: A public health perspective. *Neurotoxicology.* 2000;21:183.

55. DiFonzo C. Food Quality Protection Act. In: *Pesticide Policy and Michigan Specialty Crops Food Quality Protection Act.* (1997). East Lansing, MI: Michigan State University. Available at http:// ipmworld.umn.edu/chapters/fqpa96.htm. Accessed July 1, 2009.

56. Measure continues ban on human tests. *Chem Eng News.* 2003;81:21.

57. Wagner JM. Food Quality Protection Act: Its impact on the pesticide industry. *Qual Assur.* 1997;5:279.

58. EPA sued over pesticide standards. *Chem Eng News.* 2003;81:25.

59. Food and Drug Administration (FDA). *Public Health Security and Bioterrorism Preparedness and Response Act of 2002 (PL107-188).* Letter from Center Director, 2002. Available at http:// www.fda.gov/Food/FoodDefense/Bioterrorism/ucm111086.htm. Accessed July 1, 2009.

60. Food and Drug Administration (FDA). *Bioterrorism Act of 2002.* Available at http://www.fda.gov/RegulatoryInformation/ Legislation/ucm148797.htm. Accessed July 1, 2009.

61. Food and Drug Administration (FDA). FDA commends passage by the House of Representatives of S. 741, a bill providing improved consumer protection and incentives for animal drug development. *FDA News* P04-72. (July 20, 2004). Available at http://www.fda.gov/NewsEvents/Newsroom/ PressAnnouncements/2004/ucm108329.htm. Accessed July 1, 2009.

62. Weber JA. More than a farm bill: food, conservation, and energy act of 2008. *J Am Diet Assoc.* 2008;108:1428.

63. Global Legal Information Network, U.S. Library of Congress. *Food, Conservation, and Energy Act of 2008.* Available at http://www.glin.gov/view.action?glinID=210274. Accessed July 1, 2009.

64. Food and Drug Administration (FDA). *Hazard analysis & critical control points (HACCP).* (2009). Available at http:// www.fda.gov/Food/FoodSafety/HazardAnalysisCritical ControlPointsHACCP/default.htm. Accessed July 1, 2009.

65. National Restaurant Association. *Applied Foodservice Sanitation: A Certification Coursebook,* 4th ed. Chicago, IL: The Educational Foundation of the National Restaurant Association; 1995:80.

66. Food and Drug Administration (FDA). *HACCP guidelines.* (2000). Available at http://vm.cfsan.fda.gov/ ~ dms/fc99-a5. html. Accessed July 1, 2009.

67. Food and Drug Administration (FDA). *Hazard analysis and critical control point principles and application guidelines.* (1997). Available at http://www.fda.gov/Food/FoodSafety/ HazardAnalysisCriticalControlPointsHACCP/ucm114868.htm. Accessed July 1, 2009.

68. Arvanitoyannis IS. *HACCP and ISO 22000: Application to foods of animal origin.* Ames, IO: Wiley-Blackwell; 2009:1–549.

69. Arduser L, Brown DR. *HACCP & sanitation in restaurants and food service operations: A practical guide based on the FDA food code.* Ocala, FL: Atlantic Publishing Group; 2005:1–541.

70. Code of Federal Regulations, Title 21, Vol. 2, Part 110 (2009). *Food and drugs. Current good manufacturing practice in manufacturing, packing, or holding human food.* eCFR document. Available at http://ecfr.gpoaccess.gov/cgi/t/text/ text-idx?c = ecfr;sid = 03c0f0ea8b688b533744ae63a89f6aa4;rgn = div5;view = text;node = 21%3A2.0.1.1.10;idno = 21;cc = ecfr#21:2 .0.1.1.10.1.1.2. Accessed July 1, 2009.

71. Gould WA. *Current Good Manufacturing Practices/Food Plant Sanitation,* 2nd ed. Cockeysville, MD: CTI Publications; 1994: Ch. 2.

72. Potter NN, Hotchkiss JS. *Food Science,* 5th ed. Gaithersburg, MD: Aspen; 1998:161.

73. Food and Drug Administration (FDA). *Guidance for Industry: Action Levels for Poisonous or Deleterious Substances in Human Food and Animal Feed.* (2000). Available at http://www. fda.gov/Food/GuidanceComplianceRegulatoryInformation/ GuidanceDocuments/ChemicalContaminantsandPesticides/ ucm077969.htm. Accessed July 1, 2009.

74. Food and Drug Administration (FDA). (2009). *Defect levels handbook.* The food defect action levels. Levels of natural or unavoidable defects in foods that present no health hazards for humans. Available at http://www.fda.gov/Food/Guidance ComplianceRegulatoryInformation/GuidanceDocuments/ Sanitation/ucm056174.htm. Accessed July 1, 2009.

75. Tauxe RV. Emerging foodborne diseases: An evolving public health challenge. *Emerg Infect Dis.* 1997;3:425.

76. Altekruse SF, Swerdlow DL. The changing epidemiology of foodborne diseases. *Am J Med Sci.* 1996;311:23.

77. Preliminary FoodNet data on the incidence of infection with pathogens transmitted commonly through food—10 states, 2008. *MMWR Morb Mortal Wkly Rep.* 2008;58(13):333.

78. U.S. Department of Health and Human Services. *Healthy People 2010: Understanding and Improving Health*, 2nd ed., Objective 10, Washington, DC: Government Printing Office; November 2000.

79. Jay JM. *Modern Food Microbiology*, 6th ed. Gaithersburg, MD: Aspen; 2000:560.

80. Tauxe RV. Epidemiology of *Campylobacter jejuni* infections in the United States and other industrialized nations. In: Nachamkin I, Blaser MJ, Tompkins LS, eds. *Campylobacter jejuni: Current Status and Future Trends*. Washington, DC: American Society of Microbiology; 1992:9–19.

81. Blaser MJ. *Campylobacter jejuni* and food. *Food Technol.* 1982; 36:89.

82. Moore JE, Gilpin D, Crothers E, Canney A, Kaneko A, Matsuda M. Occurrence of *Campylobacter spp.* and *Cryptosporidium spp.* in seagulls (*Larus spp.*). *Vector Borne Zoon Dis.* 2002;2:111.

83. Yogasundram K, Shane SM, Harrington KS. Prevalence of *Campylobacter jejuni* in selected domestic and wild birds in Louisiana. *Avian Dis.* 1989;33:664.

84. Stelzer W, Mochmann H, Richter U, Dobberkau HJ. A study of *Campylobacter jejuni* and *Campylobacter coli* in a river system. *Zentralblatt für Hygiene und Umweltmedizin.* 1989;189:20.

85. Pacha RE, Clark GW, Williams EA, Carter AM, Scheffelmaier JJ, Debusschere P. Small rodents and other mammals associated with mountain meadows as reservoirs of *Giardia spp.* and *Campylobacter spp. Appl Environ Microbiol.* 1987;53:1574.

86. Rosef O, Gondrosen B, Kapperud G, Underdal B. Isolation and characterization of *Campylobacter jejuni* and *Campylobacter coli* from domestic and wild mammals in Norway. *Appl Environ Microbiol.* 1983;46:855.

87. Cools I, Uyttendaele M, Caro C, D'Haese E, Nelis HJ, Debevere J. Survival of *Campylobacter jejuni* strains of different origin in drinking water. *J Appl Microbiol.* 2003;94:886.

88. Moore J, Caldwell P, Millar B. Molecular detection of *Campylobacter spp.* in drinking, recreational and environmental water supplies. *Int J Hygiene Environ Health.* 2001;204:185.

89. Skirrow MB. Epidemiology of *Campylobacter enteritis. Int J Food Microbiol.* 1991;12:9.

90. Palmer SR, Gully PR, White JM, et al. Water-borne outbreak of *Campylobacter* gastroenteritis. *Lancet.* 1983;1:287.

91. Bates C, Hiett KL, Stern NJ. Relationship of *Campylobacter* isolated from poultry and from darkling beetles in New Zealand. *Avian Dis* 2004;48:138.

92. Gregory E, Barnhart H, Dreesen DW, Stern NJ, Corn JL. Epidemiological study of *Campylobacter spp.* in broilers: source, time of colonization, and prevalence. *Avian Dis.* 1997;41:890.

93. Altekruse SF, Stern NJ, Fields PI, Swerdlow DL. *Campylobacter jejuni*—an emerging foodborne pathogen. *Emerg Infect Dis.* 1999;5:28.

94. Birkhead G, Vogt RL, Heun E, Evelti CM, Patton CM. A multiple-strain outbreak of *Campylobacter* enteritis due to consumption of inadequately pasteurized milk. *J Infect Dis.* 1988;157:1095.

95. Hudson PJ, Vogt RL, Brondum J, Patton CM. Isolation of *Campylobacter jejuni* from milk during an outbreak of campylobacteriosis. *J Infect Dis.* 1984;150:789.

96. Vogt RL, Sours HE, Barret T, Feldman TA, Dickinson RJ, Witherell L. *Campylobacter* enteritis associated with contaminated water. *Ann Intern Med.* 1982;96:292.

97. Manfredi R, Nanetti A, Ferri M, Chiodo F. Fatal *Campylobacter jejuni* bacteraemia in patients with AIDS. *J Med Microbiol.* 1999;48:601.

98. Meier PA, Dooley DP, Jorgensen JH, Sanders CC, Huang WM, Patterson JE. Development of quinolone-resistant *Campylobacter* fetus bacteremia in human immunodeficiency virus-infected patients. *J Infect Dis.* 1998;177:951.

99. Tauxe RV, Pegues DA, Hargrett-Bean N. *Campylobacter* infections: the emerging national pattern. *Am J Public Health.* 1987;77:1219.

100. Bereswill S, Kist M. Recent developments in *Campylobacter* pathogenesis. *Curr Opin Infect Dis.* 2003;16:487.

101. Tsang RS. The relationship of *Campylobacter jejuni* infection and the development of Guillain-Barré syndrome. *Curr Opin Infect Dis.* 2002;15:221.

102. Locht H, Krogfelt KA. Comparison of rheumatological and gastrointestinal symptoms after infection with *Campylobacter jejuni/coli* and enterotoxigenic *Escherichia coli. Ann Rheum Dis.* 2002;61:448.

103. Neill MA, Tarr PI, Taylor DN, Wolf M. *Escherichia coli.* In: YH Hui, MD Pierson, JR Gorham, eds. *Foodborne Disease Handbook*, 2nd ed., vol. 1: Bacterial pathogens. New York: Marcel Dekker; 2000:196.

104. Jay J M. *Modern Food Microbiology*, 6th ed. Gaithersburg, MD: Aspen; 2000:531.

105. Jay JM. *Modern Food Microbiology*, 6th ed. Gaithersburg, MD: Aspen; 2000:387–406.

106. Besser RE, Griffin PM, Slutsker L. *Escherichia coli* O157:H7 gastroenteritis and the hemolytic uremic syndrome: an emerging infectious disease. *Ann Rev Med.* 1999;50:355.

107. Nauschuetz W. Emerging foodborne pathogens: enterohemorrhagic *Escherichia coli. Clin Lab Sci.* 1998;11:298.

108. Qadri SM, Kayali S. Enterohemorrhagic *Escherichia coli.* A dangerous food-borne pathogen. *Postgrad Med.* 1998;103:179.

109. Isolation of *E. coli* O157:H7 from sporadic cases of hemorrhagic colitis—U.S. 1982. *MMWR Morb Mortal Wkly Rep.* 1997; 46:700.

110. Doyle MP. *Escherichia coli* O157:H7 and its significance in foods. *Int J Food Microbiol.* 1991;12:289.

111. Griffin PM, Ostroff SM, Tauxe RV, et al. Illnesses associated with *Escherichia coli* O157:H7 infections. A broad clinical spectrum. *Ann Intern Med.* 1988;109:705.

112. Riley LW, Remis RS, Helgerson SD, et al. Hemorrhagic colitis associated with a rare *Escherichia coli* serotype. *N Engl J Med.* 1983;308:681.

113. Nataro JP, Steiner T, Guerrant RL. Enteroaggregative *Escherichia coli. Emerg Infect Dis.* 1998;4:251.

114. Jay JM. *Modern Food Microbiology*, 6th ed. Gaithersburg, MD: Aspen; 2000:488.

115. Jay JM. *Modern Food Microbiology*, 6th ed. Gaithersburg, MD: Aspen; 2000:511–513.

116. Orriss GD. Animal diseases of public health importance. *Emerg Infect Dis.* 1997;3:497.

117. Hogue A, White P, Guard-Petter J, et al. Epidemiology and control of egg-associated *salmonella enteritidis* in the United States of America. *Rev Sci Tech.* 1997;16:542–553.

118. Barnhart HM, Dreesen DW, Bastien R, Pancorbo OC. Prevalence of *Salmonella enteritidis* and other serovars in ovaries of layer hens at time of slaughter. *J Food Protect.* 1991;54:488.

119. St. Louis ME, Morse DL, Potter ME, et al. The emergence of grade A eggs as major source of *Salmonella enteritis* infections: New implications for the control of salmonellosis. *JAMA.* 1988; 259:2103.

120. Guard-Petter J. The chicken, the egg and *Salmonella enteritidis*: minireview. *Environ Microbiol.* 2001;3:421.

121. Humphrey TJ. Contamination of egg shell and contents with *Salmonella enteritidis*: a review. *Int J Food Microbiol.* 1994;21:31.

122. Perales I, Audicana A. *Salmonella enteritidis* and eggs. *Lancet* 1988;2:1133.

123. United States Department of Agriculture (USDA), FSIS. *Shell eggs from farm to table. Fact sheets.* (2008). Available at http://www.fsis.usda.gov/Fact_Sheets/Focus_On_Shell_Eggs/index.asp. Accessed July 1, 2009.

124. Mermelstein NH. Pasteurization of shell eggs. *Food Technol.* 2001;55:72.

125. Parashar U, Quiroz ES, Mounts AW, et al. "Norwalk-like viruses": public health consequences and outbreak management. Recommendations and Reports. *MMWR Morb Mortal Wkly Rep.* 2001;50(RR-9):1.

126. Centers for Disease Control and Prevention (CDC), National Center for Infectious Diseases, Division of Viral and Rickettsial Diseases, Respiratory and Enteric Viruses Branch. *Norovirus: Q&A.* (2006). Available at http://www.cdc.gov/ncidod/dvrd/revb/gastro/norovirus-qa.htm. Accessed July 1, 2009.

127. Goldrick BA. Foodborne diseases: more efforts needed to meet the Healthy People 2010 objectives. *Am J Nurs.* 2003;103:105–106.

128. Mao Y, Zhu C, Boedeker EC. Foodborne enteric infections. *Curr Opin Gastroenterol.* 2003;19:11–22.

129. Lasky T. Foodborne illness—old problem, new relevance. *Epidemiology.* 2002;13:593–598.

130. Jay JM. *Modern Food Microbiology*, 6th ed. Gaithersburg, MD: Aspen; 2000:614–615.

131. Norovirus activity—United States, 2006–2007. *MMWR Morb Mortal Wkly Rep.* 2007;56(33):842.

132. Bresee JS, Widdowson MA, Monroe SS, Glass RI. Foodborne viral gastroenteritis. *Clin Infect Dis.* 2002;35:748.

133. Outbreaks of gastroenteritis associated with noroviruses on cruise ships—U.S. *MMWR Morb Mortal Wkly Rep.* 2002;51:1112.

134. Centers for Disease Control and Prevention (CDC). *Viral Hepatitis.* (2008). Available at http://www.cdc.gov/hepatitis/index.htm. Accessed July 1, 2009.

135. Fiore AE. Hepatitis A transmitted by food. *Clin Infect Dis.* 2004;38:705.

136. Yoder JS, Beach MJ. Giardiasis surveillance—United States, 2003–2005. *MMWR Morb Mortal Wkly Rep.* 2007;56(SS07):11.

137. Slifko TR, Smith HV, Rose JB. Emerging parasite zoonoses associated with water and food. *Int J Parasitol.* 2000;30:1379.

138. Jay JM. *Modern Food Microbiology*, 6th ed. Gaithersburg, MD: Aspen; 2000:576–578.

139. Millard PS, Gensheimer KF, Addiss DG, Sosin DM, Beckett GA, Houck-Jankoski A, Hudson A. An outbreak of cryptosporidiosis from fresh-pressed apple cider. *JAMA.* 1994;272:1592.

140. Foodborne outbreak of diarrheal illness associated with *Cryptosporidium parvum*—Minnesota, 1995. *MMWR Morb Mortal Wkly Rep.* 1996;45:783.

141. Outbreaks of *Escherichia coli* O157:H7 infection and cryptosporidiosis associated with drinking unpasteurized apple cider—Connecticut and New York, October 1996. *MMWR Morb Mortal Wkly Rep.* 1997;46(1):4.

142. Foodborne outbreak of cryptosporidiosis—Spokane, Washington, 1997. *MMWR Morb Mortal Wkly Rep.* 1998;47(27):565.

143. Soave R. Cyclospora: an overview. *Clin Infect Dis.* 1996;23:429.

144. Harris DA, ed. *Mad Cow Disease and Related Spongiform Encephalopathies.* New York: Springer-Verlag.

145. Yam P. *The Pathological Protein: Mad Cow, Chronic Wasting, and Other Deadly Prion Diseases.* New York: Copernicus Books; 2003:1–284.

146. Brown P, Will RG, Bradley R, Asher DM, Detwiler L. Bovine spongiform encephalopathy and variant Creutzfeldt-Jakob disease: background, evolution, and current concerns. *Emerg Infect Dis.* 2001;7:6.

147. Pedersen NS, Smith E. Prion diseases: epidemiology in man. *Acta Pathol Microbiol Immunol Scand.* 2002;110:14.

148. Ironside JW. Prion diseases in man. *J Pathol.* 1998;186:227.

149. Kretzschmar HA. Molecular pathogenesis of prion diseases. *Eur Arch Psychiatry Clin Neurosci.* 1999;249(suppl 3):56.

150. Scott MR, Will R, Ironside J, et al. Compelling transgenetic evidence for transmission of bovine spongiform encephalopathy prions to humans. *Proc Natl Acad Sci USA.* 1999;96:15137–15142.

151. Food and Drug Administration (FDA). *Bovine Spongiform Encephalopathy.* Available at http://www.fda.gov/AnimalVeterinary/GuidanceComplianceEnforcement/ComplianceEnforcement/BovineSpongiformEncephalopathy/default.htm. Accessed July 1, 2009.

152. Brown P. The risk of bovine spongiform encephalopathy ("mad cow disease") to human health. *JAMA.* 1997;278:1008.

153. Hileman B. Mad cow disease. Regulatory changes stemming from discovery of one diseased cow create new conflicts spawned in part by gaps in scientific understanding. *Chem Eng News.* 2004;82:21.

154. United States Department of Agriculture (USDA), FDA. *USDA and HHS Strengthen Safeguards Against Bovine Spongiform Encephalopathy.* (2004). Available at http://www.fda.gov/NewsEvents/Newsroom/PressAnnouncements/2004/ucm108319.htm. Accessed July 1, 2009.

155. Food and Drug Administration (FDA). *BSE Rules–FDA Prohibits Some Cattle Material in Foods, Cosmetics.* (2004). Available at http://www.fda.gov/AnimalVeterinary/NewsEvents/FDAVeterinarianNewsletter/ucm093808.htm. Accessed July 1, 2009.

156. Food and Drug Administration (FDA). USDA proposes mad cow regulations. *Chem Eng News.* 2004;82:15.

157. Jay JM. *Modern Food Microbiology*, 6th ed. Gaithersburg, MD: Aspen; 2000:595–600.

158. Lie JL, Marth EH. Formation of aflatoxin in cheddar cheese by *Aspergillus flavus* and *Aspergillus parasiticus*. *J Dairy Sci.* 1967;50:1708.

159. Van Rensburg SJ. Primary liver cancer rate and aflatoxin intake in a high cancer area. *S African Med J.* 1974;48:2508a.

160. Park DL. Controlling aflatoxin in food and feed. *Food Technol.* 1993;47:92.

161. Labuza TP. Regulation of mycotoxins in food. *J Food Protect.* 1983;46:260.

162. Food and Agriculture Organization/World Health Organization (FAO/WHO). *FAO/WHO Food Standards.* Codex Alimentarius. Available at http://www.codexalimentarius.net/web/index_en.jsp. Accessed July 1, 2009.

163. Newsome R. Issues in international trade: looking to the Codex Alimentarius Commission. *Food Technol.* 1999;53:26.

164. Stinson EE, Osman SF, Heisler EG, Siciliano J, Bills DD. Mycotoxin production in whole tomatoes, apples, oranges, and lemons. *J Agric Food Chem.* 1981;29:790.

165. Stinson EE, Bills DD, Osman SF, Siciliano J, Ceponis MJ, Heisler EG. Mycotoxin production by *Alternaria* species grown on apples, tomatoes, and blueberries. *J Agric Food Chem.* 1980;28:960.

166. Marasas WFO, Jaskiewicz K, Venter FS, Van Schalkwyk DJ. *Fusarium moniliforme* contamination of maize in oesophageal cancer areas in Transkei. *S African Med J.* 1988;74:110.

167. Yoshizawa T, Yamashita A, Luo Y. *Fumonisin* occurrence in corn from high- and low-risk areas for human esophageal cancer in China. *Applied Environ Microbiol.* 1994;60:1626.

168. Bennett GA, Richard JL. Influence of processing on Fusarium mycotoxins in contaminated grains. *Food Technol.* 1996;50:235.

169. Mycotoxins and food safety. *Food Technol.* 1986;40:59.

170. Friedman M, Roitman JN, Kozukue N. Glycoalkaloid and calystegine contents of eight potato cultivars. *J Agric Food Chem.* 2003;51:2964.

171. Friedman M, McDonald GM. Glycoalkaloids in fresh and processed potatoes. In: Lee T-C, Kim H-J, eds. *Chemical Markers for Processed and Stored Foods.* Washington, DC: American Chemical Society; 1996:189.

172. Phillips BJ, Hughes JA, Phillips JC, Walters DG, Anderson D, Tahourdin CSM. A study of the toxic hazard that might be associated with the consumption of green potato tops. *Food Chem Toxicol.* 1996;34:439.

173. Hellenas KE, Branzell C, Johnsson H, Slanina P. Glycoalkaloid content of early potato varieties. *J Sci Food Agric.* 1995;67:125.

174. Zhao J, Camire ME, Bushway RJ, Bushway AA. Glycoalkaloid content and in vitro glycoalkaloid solubility of extruded potato peels. *J Agric Food Chem.* 1994;42:2570.

175. Friedman M. Composition and safety evaluation of potato berries, potato and tomato seeds, potatoes, and potato alkaloids. *ACS Symposium Series.* 1992;484:429.

176. Friedman M, Dao L. Distribution of glycoalkaloids in potato plants and commercial potato products. *J Agric Food Chem.* 1992;40:419.

177. Edwards EJ, Cobb AH. The effect of prior storage on the potential of potato tubers (*Solanum tuberosum L*) to accumulate glycoalkaloids and chlorophylls during light exposure, including artificial neural network modelling. *J Sci Food Agric.* 1999;79:1289.

178. Griffiths DW, Bain H, Dale MFB. Effect of storage temperature on potato (*Solanum tuberosum L.*) tuber glycoalkaloid content and the subsequent accumulation of glycoalkaloids and chlorophyll in response to light exposure. *J Agric Food Chem.* 1998;46:5262.

179. Percival G, Dixon GR, Sword A. Glycoalkaloid concentration of potato tubers following exposure to daylight. *J Sci Food Agric.* 1996;71:59.

180. Coria NA, Sarquis JI, Penalosa I, Urzua M. Heat-induced damage in potato (*Solanum tuberosum*) tubers: membrane stability, tissue viability, and accumulation of glycoalkaloids. *J Agric Food Chem.* 1998;46:4524.

181. Griffiths DW, Bain H, Dale MFB. The effect of low-temperature storage on the glycoalkaloid content of potato (*Solanum tuberosum*) tubers. *J Sci Food Agric.* 1997;74:301.

182. Hlywka JJ, Stephenson GR, Sears MK, Yada RY. Effects of insect damage on glycoalkaloid content in potatoes (*Solanum tuberosum*). *J Agric Food Chem.* 1994;42:2545.

183. Rayburn JR, Bantle JA, Friedman M. Role of carbohydrate side chains of potato glycoalkaloids in developmental toxicity. *J Agric Food Chem.* 1994;42:1511.

184. Friedman M, McDonald GM. Potato glycoalkaloids chemistry analysis, safety and plant physiology. *Crit Rev Plant Sci.* 1997;16:55.

185. New safeguards against glycoalkaloids. *Agricultural Research Magazine.* 1997;45:14.

186. Korpan YI, Nazarenko EA, Skryshevskaya LV, Martelet C, Jaffrezic-Renault N, El'skaya AV. Potato glycoalkaloids: true safety or false sense of security. *Trend Biotechnol.* 2004;22:147.

187. Friedman M, Henika PR, Mackey BE. Effect of feeding solanidine, solasodine, and tomatidine to non-pregnant and pregnant mice. *Food Chem Toxicol.* 2003;41:61.

188. Smith DB, Roddick JG, Jones JL. Potato glycoalkaloids: some unanswered questions. *Trend Food Sci Technol.* 1996;7:126.

189. Nigg HH, Beier RC. Evaluation of food for potential toxicants. In: *Phytochemicals and Health: Proceedings, Tenth Annual Penn State Symposium in Plant Physiology*; 1995 (May 18–20): 192–201.

190. Tanne JH. Foods and drugs alter response to anaesthesia. *BMJ.* 1998;317:1102.

191. Arora A, Camire ME. Performance of potato peels in muffins and cookies. *Food Res Int.* 1994;27:15.

192. Camire ME, Flint SI. Thermal processing effects on dietary fiber composition and hydration capacity in corn meal, oat meal, and potato peels. *Cereal Chem.* 1991;68:645.

193. Surjawan I, Dougherty MP, Bushway RJ, Bushway AA, Briggs JL, Camire ME. Sulfur compounds reduce potato toxins during extrusion cooking. *J Agric Food Chem.* 2001;49:2835.

194. Teitelbaum JS, Zatorre RJ, Carpenter S, et al. Neurologic sequelae of domoic acid intoxication due to the ingestion of contaminated mussels. *N Engl J Med.* 1990;322:1781.

195. Perl TM, Bédard L, Kotsatsky T, Hockin JC, Todd EC, Remis RS. An outbreak of toxic encephalopathy caused by eating mussels contaminated with domoic acid. *N Engl J Med.* 1990;322:1775.

196. Stewart GR, Zorumski CF, Price MT, Olney JW. Domoic acid: a dementia-inducing excitotoxic food poison with kainic acid receptor specificity. *Exp Neurol.* 1990;110:127.

197. Zatorre RJ. Memory loss following domoic acid intoxication from ingestion of toxic mussels. *Can Dis Wkly Rep.* 1990; 16(suppl 1E):101.

198. Iverson F, Truelove J, Nera E, Tryphonas L, Campbell J, Lok E. Domoic acid poisoning and mussel-associated intoxication: preliminary investigations into the response of mice and rats to toxic mussel extract. *Food Chem Toxicol.* 1989;27:377.

199. Pottier I, Vernoux JP, Lewis RJ. Ciguatera fish poisoning in the Caribbean islands and Western Atlantic. *Rev Environ Contam Toxicol.* 2001;168:99.

200. Ting JY, Brown AF, Pearn JH. Ciguatera poisoning: an example of a public health challenge. *Austr N Zealand J Public Health.* 1998;22:140.

201. Pearn J. Neurology of ciguatera. *J Neurol Neurosurg Psychiatry.* 2001;70:4.

202. Bruneau A, Mahanty S, al-Azraqui T, MacLean J, Bourque M, Desroches F. Ciguatera fish poisoning linked to the ingestion of barracuda in a Montreal restaurant—Quebec. *Can Commun Dis Rep.* 1997;23:153.

203. Klemme TM, Lösch RR. Ciguatera-Eine Tückische Fischvergiftung. Durch Fischimporte ist das Risiko Potentiell auch Hierzulande Gegeben. *Fortschritte der Medizin.* 1997;115:39. (in German)

204. Sanders WE Jr. Intoxications from the seas: Ciguatera, scombroid, and paralytic shellfish poisoning. *Infect Dis Clin N Am.* 1987;1:665.

205. Lawrence JF, Niedzwiadek B, Menard C. Quantitative determination of paralytic shellfish poisoning toxins in shellfish using prechromatographic oxidation and liquid chromatography with fluorescence detection: Interlaboratory study. *J AOAC Int.* 2004;87:83.

206. Biré R, Krys S, Frémy JM, Dragacci S. Improved solid-phase extraction procedure in the analysis of paralytic shellfish poisoning toxins by liquid chromatography with fluorescence detection. *J Agric Food Chem.* 2003;51:6386.

207. Lehane L. Paralytic shellfish poisoning: a potential public health problem. *Med J Aust.* 2001;175:29.

208. Food and Drug Administration (FDA), CFSAN. *The National Shellfish Sanitation Program. A Protocol for International Participation.* (2001). Available at http://vm.cfsan.fda.gov/~ear/nsspprot.html. Accessed July 1, 2009.

209. Food and Drug Administration (FDA). *Interstate Certified Shellfish Shippers List (ICSSL).* Available at http://www.fda.gov/Food/FoodSafety/Product-SpecificInformation/Seafood/FederalStatePrograms/InterstateShellfishShippersList/default.htm. Accessed July 1, 2009.

210. Castoldi AF, Coccini T, Manzo L. Neurotoxic and molecular effects of methylmercury in humans. *Rev Environ Health.* 2003;18:19.

211. Sweet LI, Zelikoff JT. Toxicology and immunotoxicology of mercury: a comparative review in fish and humans. *J Toxicol Environ Health. Part B, Crit Rev.* 2001;4:161.

212. Food and Drug Administration (FDA). *What you need to know about mercury in fish and shellfish–March 2004.* 2004 EPA and FDA advice for: Women who might become pregnant, women who are pregnant, nursing mothers, young children. (2004). Available at http://www.fda.gov/Food/FoodSafety/Product-SpecificInformation/Seafood/FoodbornePathogensContaminants/Methylmercury/ucm115662.htm. Accessed July 1, 2009.

213. Environmental Protection Agency (EPA). *Consumption advice. Joint federal advisory for mercury in fish.* Backgrounder for the 2004 FDA/EPA consumer advisory: What you need to know about mercury in fish and shellfish. (2004). Available at http://www.epa.gov/waterscience/fish/advice/factsheet.html. Accessed July 1, 2009.

214. Food and Drug Administration (FDA). *Mercury levels in commercial fish and shellfish.* (2009). Available at http://www.fda.gov/Food/FoodSafety/Product-SpecificInformation/Seafood/FoodbornePathogensContaminants/Methylmercury/ucm115644.htm. Accessed July 1, 2009.

215. Food and Drug Administration (FDA). *Mercury level data in commercial fish (1990–2004).* Mercury concentrations in fish: FDA monitoring program (1990–2004). (2009). Available at http://www.fda.gov/Food/FoodSafety/Product-Specific Information/Seafood/FoodbornePathogensContaminants/Methylmercury/ucm115658.htm. Accessed July 1, 2009.

216. Clarkson TW, Strain JJ. Nutritional factors may modify the toxic action of methyl mercury in fish-eating populations. *J Nutr.* 2003; 133(suppl 1):1539S.

217. Shipp AM, Gentry PR, Lawrence G, Van Landingham C, et al. Determination of a site-specific reference dose for methylmercury for fish-eating populations. *Toxicol Indust Health.* 2000;16:335.

218. Chapman L, Chan HM. The influence of nutrition on methyl mercury intoxication. *Environ Health Perspec.* 2000;108 (suppl 1):29.

219. Chan HM, Egeland GM. Fish consumption, mercury exposure, and heart diseases. *Nutr Rev.* 2004;62:68.

220. Smith SC, Taylor JG, Stephen AM. Use of food labels and beliefs about diet-disease relationships among university students. *Public Health Nutr.* 2000;3:175.

221. Elbon SM, Johnson MA, Fischer JG, Searcy CA. Demographic factors, nutrition knowledge, and health-seeking behaviors influence nutrition label reading behaviors among older American adults. *J Nutr Elderly.* 2000;19:31.

222. Joshi P, Mofidi S, Sicherer SH. Interpretation of commercial food ingredient labels by parents of food-allergic children. *J Allergy Clin Immunol.* 2002;109:1019–1021.

223. Levy L, Patterson RE, Kristal AR, Li SS. How well do consumers understand percentage daily value on food labels? *Am J Health Promot.* 2000;14:157.

224. Verbeke W, Frewer LJ, Scholderer J, De Brabander HF. Why consumers behave as they do with respect to food safety and risk information. *Anal Chim Acta.* 2007;586:2.

225. Henson S, Annou M, Cranfield J, Ryks J. Understanding consumer attitudes toward food technologies in Canada. *Risk Anal.* 2008;28:1601.

226. McLellan MR. IFT's strategic plan: changing direction. *Food Technol.* 2002;56:62.

227. Reisch MS. Track us, trust us. American Chemistry Council says will supply the facts to earn the public's trust. *Chem Eng News.* 2004;82:24.

228. Thayer A. ACC convenes amid upheaval. Industry group wrestles with issues of money, resignations, and image. *Chem Eng News.* 2003;81:10.

229. Storck W. ACC tests new ad image program. By stressing "chemistry" not "chemicals," group hopes to change public's view of industry. *Chem Eng News.* 2001;79:13.

230. Pszczola DE. Sweetener + sweetener enhances the equation. *Food Technol.* 2003;57:48.

231. Homler BE. Properties and stability of aspartame. *Food Technol.* 1984;38:50.

232. Levin GV. Tagatose, the new GRAS sweetener and health product. *J Med Food.* 2002;5:23.

233. Gilman V. Artificial sweeteners. No-calorie sugar substitutes provide options for enjoying the sweet life. *Chem Eng News.* 2004;82:43.

234. Geuns JM. Stevioside. *Phytochemistry.* 2003;64:913.

235. Gregersen S, Jeppesen PB, Holst JJ, Hermansen K. Antihyperglycemic effects of stevioside in type 2 diabetic subjects. *Metabol Clin Exp.* 2003;53:73.

236. Hsieh MH, Chan P, Sue YM, et al. Efficacy and tolerability of oral stevioside in patients with mild essential hypertension: a two-year, randomized, placebo-controlled study. *Clin Ther.* 2003;25:2797.

237. Jeppesen PB, Gregersen S, Rolfsen SE, et al. Antihyperglycemic and blood pressure-reducing effects of stevioside in the diabetic Goto-Kakizaki rat. *Metabol Clin Exp.* 2003;52:372.

238. Chan P, Tomlinson B, Chen YJ, Liu JC, Hsieh MH, Cheng JT. A double-blind placebo-controlled study of the effectiveness and tolerability of oral stevioside in human hypertension. *Br J Clin Pharmacol.* 2000;50:215.

239. Bray GA, Nielsen SJ, Popkin BM. Consumption of high-fructose corn syrup in beverages may play a role in the epidemic of obesity. *Am J Clin Nutr.* 2004;79:537.

240. Chappel CI. A review and biological risk assessment of sodium saccharin. *Reg Toxicol Pharmacol.* 1992;15:253.

241. Ellwein LB, Cohen SM. The health risks of saccharin revisited. *Crit Rev Toxicol.* 1990;20:311.

242. Butchko HH, Stargel WW, Comer CP, et al. Aspartame: review of safety. *Reg Toxicol Pharmacol.* 2002;35:S1.

243. Potenza DP, el-Mallakh RS. Aspartame: clinical update. *Connecticut Med.* 1989;53:395.

244. Yost DA. Clinical safety of aspartame. *Am Fam Physician.* 1989; 39:201.

245. Garriga MM, Metcalfe DD. Aspartame intolerance. *Ann Allergy.* 1988;61:63.

246. Janssen PJ, van der Heijden CA. Aspartame: review of recent experimental and observational data. *Toxicology.* 1988;50:1.

247. SteBink LD. The aspartame story: a model for the clinical testing of a food additive. *Am J Clin Nutr.* 1987;46(suppl 1):204.

248. Finn JP, Lord GH. Neurotoxicity studies on sucralose and its hydrolysis products with special reference to histopathologic and ultrastructural changes. *Food Chem Toxicol.* 2000;38 (suppl 2):S7.

249. Goldsmith LA. Acute and subchronic toxicity of sucralose. *Food Chem Toxicol.* 2000;38(suppl 2):S53.

250. Grice HC, Goldsmith LA. Sucralose–an overview of the toxicity data. *Food Chem Toxicol.* 2000;38(suppl 2):S1.

251. Knight I. The development and applications of sucralose, a new high-intensity sweetener. *Can J Physiol Pharmacol.* 1994;72:435.

252. Department of Health and Human Services (DHHS) and USDA. *Dietary Guidelines for Americans*, 6th ed. (2005). Available at http://www.health.gov/dietaryguidelines/dga2005/document/default.htm. Accessed July 1, 2009.

253. United States Department of Agriculture (USDA), National Agricultural Library, Food and Nutrition Information Center. In: *Dietary Guidance.* (2009). Available at http://fnic.nal.usda.gov/nal_display/index.php?info_center=4&tax_level=2&tax_subject=256&level3_id=0&level4_id=0&level5_id=0&topic_id=1342&&placement_default=0. Accessed July 1, 2009.

254. American Dietetic Association. Position of the American Dietetic Association: use of nutritive and nonnutritive sweeteners. *J Am Diet Assoc.* 2004;104:255.

255. Tate & Lyle. *About Food Starches.* Available at http://www.amylum.com/TateAndLyle/products_applications/_products/food_starches/default.htm. Accessed July 1, 2009.

256. Wittrig B. *Preservative analysis by liquid and gas chromatography.* State College, PA: Restek Corp; 2003. Available at http://www.restek.com/restek/images/external/pres-2003-preserv.pdf. Accessed July 1, 2009.

257. Duke J. *Module 19. Botanicals generally recognized as safe.* Available at http://www.ars-grin.gov/duke/syllabus/gras.htm. Accessed July 1, 2009.

258. Geha RS, Beiser A, Ren C, et al. Review of alleged reaction to monosodium glutamate and outcome of a multicenter double-blind placebo-controlled study. *J Nutr.* 2000;130(suppl 4S):1058S.

259. Yang WH, Drouin MA, Herbert M, Mao Y, Karsh J. The monosodium glutamate symptom complex: Assessment in a double-blind, placebo-controlled, randomized study. *J Allergy Clin Immunol.* 1997;99:757.

260. Tarasoff L, Kelly MF. Monosodium L-glutamate: a double-blind study and review. *Food Chem Toxicol.* 1993;31:1019.

261. Scher W, Scher BM. A possible role for nitric oxide in glutamate (MSG)-induced Chinese restaurant syndrome, glutamate-induced asthma, "hot-dog headache," pugilistic Alzheimer's disease, and other disorders. *Med Hypotheses.* 1992;38:185.

262. Pulce C, Vial T, Verdier F, Testud F, Nicolas B, Descotes J. The Chinese restaurant syndrome: a reappraisal of monosodium glutamate's causative role. *Adverse Drug React Toxicol Rev.* 1992;11:19.

263. Sands GH, Newman L, Lipton R. Cough, exertional, and other miscellaneous headaches. *Med Clin N Am.* 1991;75:733.

264. Scopp AL. MSG and hydrolyzed vegetable protein induced headache: review and case studies. *Headache.* 1991;31:107.

265. Stevenson DD. Monosodium glutamate and asthma. *J Nutr.* 2000;130(suppl 4S):1067S.

266. Woods RK, Weiner JM, Thien F, Abramson M, Walters EH. The effects of monosodium glutamate in adults with asthma who perceive themselves to be monosodium glutamate-intolerant. *J Allergy Clin Immunol.* 1998;101:762.

267. Walker R, Lupien JR. The safety evaluation of monosodium glutamate. *J Nutr.* 2000;130(suppl 4S):1049S.

268. Junod SW. *Folic acid fortification: fact and folly.* (2001). Available at http://www.fda.gov/AboutFDA/WhatWeDo/History/ProductRegulation/SelectionsFromFDLIUpdate SeriesonFDAHistory/ucm091883.htm. Accessed July 1, 2009.

269. Food and Drug Administration (FDA). PMO 2007: Appendix O. Vitamin fortification of fluid milk products. Grade "A" pasteurized milk ordinance (2007 Revision). Available at http://www.fda.gov/Food/FoodSafety/Product-Specific Information/MilkSafety/NationalConferenceonInterstate MilkShipmentsNCIMSModelDocuments/PasteurizedMilk Ordinance2007/ucm089032.htm. Accessed July 1, 2009.

270. Kurtzweil P. How folate can help prevent birth defects. *FDA Consumer.* (1999). Available at http://vm.cfsan.fda.gov/~dms/fdafolic.html. Accessed July 1, 2009.

271. Global trends. (Market trends): Fortified beverages. *Prepared Foods.* 2002;171:9.

272. Health sells!!! Refrigerators, etc. *Business World.* 2002; May 27: 38.

273. Fortifying sales: lifestyle choices support demand for fortified foods. *Gourmet Retailer.* 2002;23:42.

274. Food additives permitted for direct addition to food for human consumption; vitamin D3. *Federal Register.* February 27, 2003; 68:9000.

275. Penniston KL, Tanumihardjo SA. Vitamin A in dietary supplements and fortified foods: too much of a good thing? *J Am Diet Assoc.* 2003;103:1185.

276. Greger JL. Food, supplements, and fortified foods: scientific evaluations in regard to toxicology and nutrient bioavailability. *J Am Diet Assoc.* 1987;87:1369.

277. Dalton L. What's that stuff? Food preservatives. *Chem Eng News.* 2002;80:40.

278. Foulke JE. A Fresh Look at Food Preservatives. *FDA Consumer.* (1993; updated 2003). Available at http://vm.cfsan.fda.gov/~dms/fdpreser.html. Accessed July 1, 2009.

279. Williams GM, Iatropoulos MJ, Whysner J. Safety assessment of butylated hydroxyanisole and butylated hydroxytoluene as antioxidant food additives. *Food Chem Toxicol.* 1999;37:1027.

280. Whysner J, Williams GM. Butylated hydroxyanisole mechanistic data and risk assessment: conditional species-specific cytotoxicity, enhanced cell proliferation, and tumor promotion. *Pharmacol Ther.* 1996;71:137.

281. Iverson F. Phenolic antioxidants: Health protection branch studies on butylated hydroxyanisole. *Cancer Lett.* 1995;93:49.

282. Huang MT, Ferraro T. Phenolic compounds in food and cancer prevention. *ACS Symp Series.* 1992;507:8.

283. Lester MR. Sulfite sensitivity: significance in human health. *J Am Coll Nutr.* 1995;14:229.

284. Lecos C. Reacting to sulfites. *FDA Consumer.* 1995;19:17.

285. Skovgaard N. Microbiological aspects and technological need: technological needs for nitrates and nitrites. *Food AdditContam.* 1992;9:391.

286. Mirvish SS. The significance for human health of nitrate, nitrite and n-nitroso compounds. *NATO ASI Series: Series G: Ecological Sciences.* 1991;30:253.

287. Nitrate, nitrite, and nitroso compounds in foods. *Food Technol.* 1987;41:127.

288. Food and Drug Administration (FDA). *Packaging Materials Listed in 21 CFR 179.45 for Use during Irradiation of Prepackaged Foods.* (2007). Available at http://www.fda.gov/Food/FoodIngredientsPackaging/IrradiatedFoodPackaging/ucm074764.htm. Accessed July 1, 2009.

289. United States Department of Agriculture (USDA), FSIS. *Irradiation and Food Safety. Answers to Frequently Asked Questions.* (2005). Available at http://www.fsis.usda.gov/Fact_Sheets/Irradiation_and_Food_Safety/index.asp. Accessed July 1, 2009.

290. American Dietetic Association. Position of the American Dietetic Association: Food irradiation. *J Am Diet Assoc.* 2000;100:246.

291. Tritsch GL. Food irradiation. *Nutrition.* 2000;16:698.

292. Pauli GH. *U.S. regulatory requirements for irradiating foods.* (1999). Available at http://www.fda.gov/Food/FoodIngredients Packaging/IrradiatedFoodPackaging/ucm110730.htm. Accessed July 1, 2009.

293. Farkas J. Irradiation as a method for decontaminating food. A review. *Int J Food Microbiol.* 1998;44:189.

294. Morehouse KM. Food irradiation: the treatment of foods with ionizing radiation. *Food Test Anal.* 1998;4:9.

295. Loaharanu P. Irradiation as a cold pasteurization process of food. *Vet Parasitol.* 1996;64:71.

296. Dodd NJ. Free radicals and food irradiation. *Biochem Soc Symp.* 1995;61:247.

297. Lagunas-Solar MC. Radiation processing of foods: an overview of scientific principles and current status. *J Food Protect.* 1995;58:186.

298. Irradiation in the production, processing and handling of food. *Federal Register.* December 3, 1997;62(232):64107.

299. Swanson RB, Munsayac LJ. Acceptability of fruit purees in peanut butter, oatmeal, and chocolate chip reduced-fat cookies. *J Am Diet Assoc.* 1999;99:343.

300. Pszczola DE. Blends reduce fat in bakery products. *Food Technol.* 1994;48:168.

301. Phillips I, Casewell M, Cox T, et al. Does the use of antibiotics in food animals pose a risk to human health? A critical review of published data. *J Antimicrob Chemother.* 2004;53:28.

302. Wegener HC. Antibiotics in animal feed and their role in resistance development. *Curr Opin Microbiol.* 2003;6:439.

303. Bauman DE. Bovine somatotropin: review of an emerging animal technology. *J Dairy Sci.* 1992;75:3432.

304. Juskevich JC, Guyer CG. Bovine growth hormone: human food safety evaluation. *Science.* 1990;249:875.

305. Bradley T. "Monsanto's victory in Maine rBGH lawsuit a setback for consumers." *Portland Press Herald.* December 30, 2003:10A.

306. Mohl B. "Got growth hormone? Dairies play on fear in marketing milk without the additive." *The Boston Globe.* September 28, 2003:J1.

307. Mills LN. *Science and Social Context: The Regulation of Recombinant Bovine Growth Hormone in North America.* Montreal: McGill-Queen's University Press; 2002:1–207.

308. Centner TJ, Lathrop KW. Legislative and legal restrictions on labeling information regarding the use of recombinant bovine somatotropin. *J Dairy Sci.* 1997;80:215.

309. Hamilton D, Ambrus A, Dieterle R, et al. Pesticide residues in food–acute dietary exposure. *Pest Manag Sci.* 2004;60:311.

310. Potter TL, Marti L, Belflower S, Truman CC. Multiresidue analysis of cotton defoliant, herbicide, and insecticide residues in water by solid-phase extraction and GC-NPD, GC-MS, and HPLC-diode array detection. *J Agric Food Chem.* 2000;48:4103.

311. Cabras P, Angioni A. Pesticide residues in grapes, wine, and their processing products. *J Agric Food Chem.* 2000;48:967.

312. Mukherjee I, Gopal M. Insecticide residues in baby food, animal feed, and vegetables by gas liquid chromatography. *Bull Environ Contam Toxicol.* 1996;56:381.

313. Hyman FN, Klontz KC, Tollefson L. Food and Drug Administration surveillance of the role of foreign objects in foodborne injuries. *Public Health Rep.* 1993;108:54.

314. University of Nebraska Cooperative Extension. *Physical Hazards.* (2005). Available at http://foodsafety.unl.edu/haccp/start/physical.html. Accessed July 1, 2009.

315. Jacobs MK. The history of biologic warfare and bioterrorism. *Dermatol Clinics.* 2004;22:231.

316. Martin W. Legal and public policy responses of states to bioterrorism. *Am J Public Health.* 2004;94:1093.

317. Hassler KE. *Agricultural Bioterrorism: Why It Is a Concern and What We Must Do.* Carlisle Barracks, PA: U.S. Army War College; 2003:1–44.

318. Pellerin C. The next target of bioterrorism: your food. *Environ Health Perspect.* 2000;108:A126–A129.

319. Centers for Disease Control and Prevention (CDC). *Emergency preparedness and response. Bioterrorism agents/diseases.* Available at http://www.bt.cdc.gov/agent/agentlist.asp. Accessed July 1, 2009.

320. Centers for Disease Control and Prevention (CDC). *Emergency Preparedness and Response. Chemical agents.* Available at http://www.bt.cdc.gov/agent/agentlistchem.asp. Accessed July 1, 2009.

321. Grossman LK. The story of a truly contaminated election. *Columbia Journalism Review.* 2001;39:65.

322. Török TJ, Tauxe RV, Wise RP, et al. A large community outbreak of salmonellosis caused by intentional contamination of restaurant salad bars. *JAMA.* 1997;278:389.

323. American Dietetic Association. Position of the American Dietetic Association: food and water safety. *J Am Diet Assoc.* 2003;103:1203.

324. Sobel J, Khan AS, Swerdlow DL. Threat of a biological terrorist attack on the U.S. food supply: the CDC perspective. *Lancet.* 2002;359:874.

325. Khan AS, Swerdlow DL, Juranek DD. Precautions against biological and chemical terrorism directed at food and water supplies. *Public Health Rep.* 2001;116:3.

326. Bruemmer B. Food biosecurity. *J Am Diet Assoc.* 2003;103:687.

327. Peregrin T. Bioterrorism and food safety: what nutrition professionals need to know to educate the American public. *J Am Diet Assoc.* 2002;102:14.

328. Abbott C. "USDA's Vilsack favors single food safety agency." Washington, DC: Reuters; 2009. Available at http://www.reuters.com/article/politicsNews/idUSTRE5156DQ20090206. Accessed July 1, 2009.

329. Stevens S. "Recent industry poll favors single food safety agency." Milwaukee, WI: Gass Weber Mullins LLC; 2009. Available at http://www.defendingfoodsafety.com/2009/02/articles/food-safety-news/recent-industry-poll-favors-single-food-safety-agency/. Accessed July 1, 2009.

330. Center for Science in the Public Interest (CSPI). Congressional leaders call for single food safety agency. CSPI supports effort to modernize food safety laws. (2007). Available at http://cspinet.org/new/200702143.html. Accessed July 1, 2009.

331. Committee to Ensure Safe Food from Production to Consumption (Institute of Medicine and National Research Council). *Ensuring Safe Food: From Production to Consumption.* Washington, DC: National Academies Press; 2003:1–206.

332. Mermelstein NH. Terrorism spurs renewed call for single food safety agency. *Food Technol.* 2001;55:32.

333. Anon. Vilsack backs away from single food safety agency commitment. *The Food & Fiber Letter.* (2009). Available at http://www.entrepreneur.com/tradejournals/article/200117471.html. Accessed July 1, 2009.

334. Pray L, Yaktine A. *Managing Food Safety Practices from Farm to Table: Workshop Summary.* Washington, DC: National Academies Press; 2009:Ch. 4.

335. Toops D. A conversation with food safety czar David W. K. Acheson. FoodProcessing.com. (2008). Available at http://www.foodprocessing.com/articles/2008/367.html. Accessed July 1, 2009.

336. Polkinghorne JC. Ethical issues in biotechnology. *Trend Biotechnol.* 2000;18:8.

337. Serageldin I. Biotechnology and food security in the 21st century. *Science.* 1999;285:387.

338. Burke D. Why all the fuss about genetically modified food? Much depends on who benefits. *BMJ.* 1998;316:1845.

339. Kuiper HA, König A, Kleter GA, Hammes WP, Knudsen I. Safety assessment, detection and traceability, and societal aspects of genetically modified foods. European Network on Safety Assessment of Genetically Modified Food Crops (ENTRANSFOOD). Concluding remarks. *Food Chem Toxicol.* 2004;42:1195.

340. Perr HA. Children and genetically engineered food: Potentials and problems. *J Pediatr Gastroenterol Nutr.* 2002;35:475.

341. Leeder SR. Genetically modified foods—food for thought. *Med J Aust.* 2000;172:173.

342. Macilwain C. U.S. food-safety body hears protests over genetically modified food. *Nature.* 1999;402:571.

343. Finucane ML. Mad cows, mad corn and mad communities: the role of socio-cultural factors in the perceived risk of genetically modified food. *Proc Nutr Soc.* 2002;61:31.

344. Hino A. Safety assessment and public concerns for genetically modified food products: the Japanese experience. *Toxicol Pathol.* 2002;30:126.

345. Moseley BE. Safety assessment and public concern for genetically modified food products: the European view. *Toxicol Pathol.* 2002;30:129.

346. Harlander SK. Safety assessments and public concern for genetically modified food products: the American view. *Toxicol Pathol.* 2002;30:132.

347. Consumer protection from an EU regulation on the mandatory labelling of genetically modified food. *Clin Lab.* 2004;50:380.

348. Breakey J. Is food intolerance due to an inborn error of metabolism? *Asia Pac J Clin Nutr.* 2004;13(suppl):S175.

349. Schafer KS, Kegley SE. Persistent toxic chemicals in the U.S. food supply. *J Epidemiol Comm Health.* 2002;56:813.

350. Goldman LR, Koduru S. Chemicals in the environment and developmental toxicity to children: a public health and policy perspective. *Environ Health Persp.* 2000;108:443.

351. Käferstein F, Abdussalam M. Food safety in the 21st century. Bull WHO. 1999;77:347.

352. Bro-Rasmussen F. Contamination by persistent chemicals in food chain and human health. *Science Total Environ.* 1996;188(suppl 1):S45.

353. Abbott PJ. Carcinogenic chemicals in food: evaluating the health risk. *Food Chem Toxicol.* 1992;30:327.

354. United States Department of Agriculture (USDA), FSIS and APHIS, and DHHS, FDA. *USDA and HHS Strengthen Safeguards against Bovine Spongiform Encephalopathy.* (2004). Available at http://www.fda.gov/NewsEvents/Newsroom/PressAnnouncements/2004/ucm108319.htm. Accessed July 1, 2009.

355. Legname G, Baskakov IV, Nguyen HO, et al. Synthetic mammalian prions. *Science.* 2004;305:673.

356. Anderson JB, Shuster TA, Hansen KE, Levy AS, Volk A. A camera's view of consumer food-handling behaviors. *J Am Diet Assoc.* 2004;104:186.

357. Sharp K, Walker H. A microbiological survey of communal kitchens used by undergraduate students. *International Journal of Consumer Studies.* 2003;27:11.

358. Scott E. Relationship between cross-contamination and the transmission of foodborne pathogens in the home. *Pediatr Infect Dis J.* 2000;19(10 suppl):S111.

359. Sattar SA, Tetro J, Springthorpe VS. Impact of changing societal trends on the spread of infections in American and Canadian homes. *Am J Infect Control.* 1999;27:S4.

360. Scott E. Hygiene issues in the home. *Am J Infect Control.* 1999; 27:S22.

361. Bloomfield SF, Scott E. Mini review: cross-contamination and infection in the domestic environment and the role of chemical disinfectants. *J Appl Microbiol.* 1997;83:1.

362. Scott E. A review of foodborne disease and other hygiene issues in the home. *J Appl Bacteriol.* 1996;80:5.

CHAPTER 17

Food Security and Adequate Food Access for the Public

DAVID H. HOLBEN, PHD, RD, LD

READER OBJECTIVES

After studying this chapter and reflecting on the contents, you should be able to:

1. Define food security and hunger.
2. Discuss and carry out food security measurement.
3. Interpret food security data from nutrition monitoring and research studies.
4. Understand the consequences of food security and its relationship to selected health issues.
5. Apply food security knowledge to program and client assessment strategies.
6. Discuss programs that assist the public in securing adequate food.

■ INTRODUCTION

Healthy People 2010 goals relate to increasing the quality and years of healthy life and eliminating health disparities among Americans.[1] Securing adequate food for the public is paramount to achieving and maintaining health; therefore, Healthy People 2010 objectives include increasing food security among U.S. households to 94%.[1] Food insecurity persists at an unacceptable rate in the United States, with the most recent estimates indicating that about 85% of households were food secure throughout the entire year in 2008.[2]

Food security exists when all people, at all times, have access to sufficient food for an active and healthy life without resorting to emergency food supplies or socially unacceptable ways of obtaining food, including begging, stealing, or scavenging.[3] On the other hand, food insecure families or individuals have limited resources and ability to acquire food, which often leads them to resort to socially unacceptable means of food acquisition.[3,4] A possible consequence of food insecurity is hunger, the uneasy or painful sensation caused by a lack of food or the recurrent and involuntary lack of access to food.[3] Common definitions of food security and related terms are summarized in **Table 17–1**.

Securing adequate food for the public is paramount. Public health nutrition professionals must not only be aware of programs that can assist the public in securing adequate food, but also know how to assess:

- The proportion of the public that is food secure
- The consequences of food insecurity
- If a particular program designed to improve food security is actually doing so

This chapter therefore was designed to:

- Review the definitions of food security and hunger
- Outline food security measurement strategies
- Summarize the food security status of the United States
- Highlight the consequences of food security and its relationship to selected health issues
- Review how food security measurement can be used for program and client assessment strategies
- Discuss public health programs designed to improve food access by the public

■ MEASURING THE FOOD SECURITY STATUS OF THE PUBLIC

Although food insecurity is broad in scope, its primary dimension is food insufficiency, which can be measured along a continuum of successive stages. These stages, as noted by Bickel and others,[4] each have specific characteristics, that is, conditions and experiences related to being unable to fully meet the basic needs of household members followed

TABLE 17–1	Definitions of Food Security and Related Terms
Term	**Definition**
Community food security	"The state in which all persons obtain a nutritionally adequate, culturally acceptable diet at all times through local non-emergency sources."[a]
Food security	"Access by all people, at all times to sufficient food for an active and healthy life...[and] includes at a minimum: the ready availability of nutritionally adequate and safe foods, and an assured ability to acquire acceptable foods in socially acceptable ways."[b]
Food insecurity	"Limited or uncertain availability of nutritionally adequate and safe foods or limited or uncertain ability to acquire acceptable foods in socially acceptable ways."[b]
Food insufficiency	"An inadequate amount of food intake due to a lack of resources."[c]
Hunger	"The uneasy or painful sensation caused by a lack of food. The recurrent and involuntary lack of access to food...[which] may produce malnutrition over time."[b]
Nutrition security	"The provision of an environment that encourages and motivates society to make food choices consistent with short- and long-term good health."[d]

[a]Gottlieb R, Fisher A. Community food security and environmental justice: searching for a common discourse. *Agriculture Hum Values*. 1996;3:23–32.
[b]Life Science Research Office. Federation of American Societies for Experimental Biology. Core indicator of nutritional state for difficult to sample populations. *J Nutr.* 1990;102:1599–1600.
[c]Briefel R, Woteki C. Development of the food sufficiency questions for the Third National Health and Nutrition Examination Survey. *J Nutr Educ.* 1992;24:24S–28S.
[d]*Nutrition Action Themes for the United States: A Report in Response to the International Conference on Nutrition.* Washington, DC: U.S. Department of Agriculture Center for Nutrition Policy and Promotion; 1996. CNPP-2 Occasional Paper.

by the behavioral responses to those conditions and experiences. Public health nutrition professionals must be able to understand the federal, state, and local reports related to food security and their implications on public health issues. In addition, they need to be able to develop strategies in order to measure the effectiveness of interventions intended to improve food security.

Household food security status is one outcome measure that provides insight into the public's ability to secure adequate food. Bickel and colleagues have summarized food security measurement for U.S. households in *Guide to Measuring Household Food Security, Revised 2000*.[4]

The National Nutrition Monitoring and Related Research Act of 1990 (**Table 17–2**) prompted the development of the Food Security Measurement Project.[5] This project is an ongoing collaboration among federal agencies, academic researchers, and private commercial and nonprofit organizations. Standardized questionnaires for measuring household food security status and methods for editing and scoring those instruments have been one outcome of the project.[5]

The foundation for measuring the public's food security was laid through work conducted by Radimer and colleagues[6,7] and Wehler and others[8]; their work led to the development of an instrument capable of measuring the food security status of U.S. households. This instrument[4] is called the Food Security Survey Module (**Table 17–3**). Federal estimates of household food security status are measured using this instrument as part of the Census Bureau's Current Population Survey (http://www.bls.gov/cps/home.htm).[9] Other national surveys that contain the Food Security Survey Module include:

- Early Childhood Longitudinal Study[10]
- National Health and Nutrition Examination Survey[11]
- Panel Study of Income Dynamics[12]
- Survey of Program Dynamics[13]

Table 17–4 provides a brief summary of each of these national surveys. In addition to these, states, academic and private researchers, and public health nutrition professionals use the Food Security Survey Module to measure household food security status.

TABLE 17–2	The National Nutrition Monitoring and Related Research Act of 1990

Facts about This Legislation

- Public Law 101-445.
- Enacted October 22, 1990.
- Leadership/Responsibility: U.S. Department of Health and Human Services and U.S. Department of Agriculture.
- Reports are filed at least every 5 years on the dietary, nutritional, and health-related status of people in the United States.
- Purposes of the Act

  1. "Make more effective use of Federal and State expenditures for nutrition monitoring, and enhance the performance and benefits of current Federal nutrition monitoring and related research activities."

  2. "Establish and facilitate the timely implementation of a coordinated National Nutrition Monitoring and Related Program, and thereby provide a scientific basis for the maintenance and improvement of the nutritional status of the people of the United States and the nutritional quality…of food consumed in the United States."

  3. "Establish and implement a comprehensive plan for the National Nutrition Monitoring and Related Research Program to assess, on a continuing basis, the dietary and nutritional status of the people of the United States and the trends with respect to such status, the state of the art with respect to nutrition monitoring and related research, future monitoring and related research priorities, and the relevant policy implications."

  4. "Establish and improve the quality of national nutritional health status data related data bases and networks, and stimulate research necessary to develop uniform indicators, standards, methodologies, technologies, and procedures for nutrition monitoring."

  5. "Establish a central Federal focus for the coordination, management, and direction of Federal nutrition monitoring activities."

  6. "Establish mechanisms for addressing the nutrition monitoring needs of Federal, State, and local governments, the private sector, scientific and engineering communities, healthcare professionals, and the public in support of the foregoing purposes."

  7. "Provide for the conduct of such scientific research and development as may be necessary or appropriate in support of such purposes."

Sources: Office of the Law Revision Counsel. Available at http://uscode.house.gov/download/pls/07C84.txt. Accessed May 11, 2010.
National Nutrition Monitoring and Related Research Act of 1990. Available at http://uscode.house.gov/download/pls/07C84.txt. Accessed May 11, 2010.

The Food Security Survey Module poses questions to respondents about:

- Anxiety related to food budget or supply and whether the budget is able to meet basic needs;
- Experiences relating to running out of food without being able to obtain more due to financial constraints;
- Perceptions of intake adequacy by themselves or other household members; and
- Food use.[4]

This instrument measures only the "sufficiency" dimension of food security, and does not measure other aspects of food security, including the nutritional adequacy or safety of diets.[4] Other instruments therefore must be used to capture this information in a research project or programmatic evaluation. As seen in Table 17–3, all of the questions in the Food Security Survey Module specify financial limitations as the reason for the reported behaviors or conditions and ask about circumstances that occurred within the past 12 months; however, shorter time periods can be utilized.[4] For example, if a public health nutrition intervention (e.g., community gardening project) was initiated in the spring and concluded in the fall, the food security status of participating households could be measured in the spring and re-measured after four months when the program ends.

Responses to the Food Security Survey Module questions are tabulated, as summarized by Bickel and colleagues[4] and the United States Department of Agriculture (USDA),[14] resulting in a scale that measures the degree of the severity of food insecurity and hunger experienced by a household. In addition to being assigned a score ranging from 0 to 10, with larger numbers corresponding to a greater level of food insecurity, households can be categorized into three groupings of food security status, each representing a range of severity on the food security scale (**Table 17–5**).[1]

As summarized by the USDA,[14] food-secure households can be classified into those with high food security or marginal food security. Households classified as having high food security report no indications of food-access problems or limitations. Households classified as having marginal food security have little or no indication of changes in diet or food intake and only report one or two indications of food security, which is typically anxiety over food sufficiency or shortage of food in the house. Essentially, for high or marginally food secure households, there is no or minimal evidence of food insecurity; that is, they are able to secure nutritionally adequate, safe foods in socially acceptable ways.[14]

TABLE 17–3 Food Security Survey Module

- "(I/We) worried whether (my/our) food would run out before (I/we) got money to buy more." Was that often true, sometimes true, or never true for (you/your household) in the last 12 months?

- "The food that (I/we) bought just didn't last, and (I/we) didn't have money to get more." Was that often, sometimes, or never true for (you/your household) in the last 12 months?

- "(I/We) couldn't afford to eat balanced meals." Was that often, sometimes, or never true for (you/your household) in the last 12 months?

- "(I/We) relied on only a few kinds of low-cost food to feed (my/our) (child/children) because (I was/we were) running out of money to buy food." Was that often, sometimes, or never true for (you/your household) in the last 12 months?

- "(I/We) couldn't feed (my/our) (child/children) a balanced meal, because (I/we) couldn't afford that." Was that often, sometimes, or never true for (you/your household) in the last 12 months?

- "(My/our) (child was/children were) not eating enough because (I/we) just couldn't afford enough food." Was that often, sometimes, or never true for (you/your household) in the last 12 months?

- In the last 12 months, since last (name of current month), did (you/you or other adults in your household) ever cut the size of your meals or skip meals because there wasn't enough money for food? Yes No

- If yes, how often did this happen—almost every month, some months but not every month, or in only 1 or 2 months?

- In the last 12 months, did you ever eat less than you felt you should because there wasn't enough money to buy food? Yes No

- In the last 12 months, were you ever hungry but didn't eat because you couldn't afford enough food? Yes No

- In the last 12 months, did you lose weight because you didn't have enough money for food? Yes No

- In the last 12 months, did (you/you or other adults in your household) ever not eat for a whole day because there wasn't enough money for food? Yes No

- If yes, how often did this happen—almost every month, some months but not every month, or in only 1 or 2 months?

- In the last 12 months, since (current month) of last year, did you ever cut the size of (your child's/any of the children's) meals because there wasn't enough money for food? Yes No

- In the last 12 months, did (CHILD'S NAME/any of the children) ever skip meals because there wasn't enough money for food? Yes No

- If yes, how often did this happen—almost every month, some months but not every month, or in only 1 or 2 months?

- In the last 12 months, (was your child/were the children) ever hungry but you just couldn't afford more food? Yes No

- In the last 12 months, did (your child/any of the children) ever not eat for a whole day because there wasn't enough money for food? Yes No

Note: Questions relating to children are only asked if there are children under 18 in the household. Specific guidelines for using the Core Module, including screening techniques, can be found in the source below.

Source: Bickel G, Nord M, Price C, Hamilton W, Cook J. *Guide to Measuring Household Food Security, Revised 2000.* Alexandria, VA: U.S. Department of Agriculture, Food and Nutrition Service; 2000.

TABLE 17–4 National Surveys That Include Food Security Measurement

Survey	Web Site	Brief Summary
Current Population Survey	http://www.bls.gov/cps/home.htm	A nationally representative study of employment and unemployment experiences. Used to provide U.S. food security estimates.
Early Childhood Longitudinal Study	http://nces.ed.gov/ecls/	National data with two overlapping cohorts, birth (birth through first grade) and kindergarten (kindergarten through fifth grade), on children's status at birth and thereafter. Includes family, school, community, and individual variables on development, early learning, and early performance in school.
National Health and Nutrition Examination Survey	http://www.cdc.gov/nchs/nhanes.htm	A nationally representative health and dietary study of the non-institutionalized civilian population.
Panel Study of Income Dynamics	http://psidonline.isr.umich.edu	A nationally representative longitudinal study of U.S. families on economic, health, and social behavior.
Survey of Program Dynamics	http://www.sipp.census.gov/spd/	A nationally representative longitudinal, demographic survey on the economic, household, and social characteristics of the United States.

TABLE 17–5	Food Security Survey Module Categories of Food Security Status	
Food Secure		
High Food Security	No reported indications of food-access problems or limitations	
Marginal Food Security	One or two reported indications—typically of anxiety over food sufficiency or shortage of food in the house. Little or no indication of changes in diets or food intake	
Food Insecure		
Low Food Security	Reports of reduced quality, variety, or desirability of diet. Little or no indication of reduced food intake	
Very Low Food Security	Reports of multiple indications of disrupted eating patterns and reduced food intake	

Source: Economic Research Service, *Food Security in the United States: Definitions of Hunger and Food Security.* Available at http://www.ers.usda.gov/Briefing/FoodSecurity/labels.htm. Accessed May 11, 2010.

On the other hand, households that are food-insecure can be classified into those with low food security or very low food security. Households with low food security have members concerned about the adequacy of the household food supply and management. This may include reduced quality, variety, or desirability of the diet and increased use of unusual coping patterns. However, in this category, little or no reduction in members' food intake is reported. Households at the most severe level, those with very low food security, report multiple indications of disrupted eating patterns and reduced food intake. In fact, some have members who may go one or more entire days with no food due to lack of resources, or food intake may be reduced to an extent that members have repeatedly experienced the physical sensation of hunger. In households with children, typically at the early stages, food reductions are not observed for children. However, at the most severe level, even children have reduced food intake to an extent that physical sensations of hunger have been experienced; however, children are often protected from hunger by other family members.[15] Finally, at the most severe stages of food insecurity, adults in households with and without children have repeatedly experienced extensive reductions in food intake.[14]

Generally, the Food Security Survey Module takes less than four minutes to administer, unless screening is performed, which would decrease the time needed to administer the survey instrument to approximately two minutes.[4] Less time is needed because when screening is performed, all questions may not be asked if responses inconsistent with food insecurity are provided for the initial survey questions.

Some public health nutrition professionals may find it difficult to administer the 18-question module for a variety of reasons, but are still interested in food security status as an outcome or factor impacting public health program development and delivery. Therefore, if utilizing the entire Food Security Survey Module (all 18 questions) is not possible due to time constraints, an agency can use an abbreviated 6-item subset that is available at http://www.ers.usda.gov/briefing/foodsecurity/surveytools.[16] This tool also provides food security scale scores for classifying households by level of food security status.[4] However, use of this 6-item subset does have limitations. Overall, researchers[16] were able to demonstrate that the abbreviated instrument correctly classified 98% of households correctly, but the abbreviated food security instrument was not able to differentiate the more severe range of food insecurity where child hunger had been experienced. This is because the abbreviated version does not include questions about these more extreme experiences and behaviors. Consequently, if a public health nutrition professional intends to utilize this tool, it is important for him or her to have a preliminary idea of what levels of food insecurity are likely to exist in the target population before choosing the abbreviated subset.

When the entire Food Security Survey Module is used, a subset of the questions can be employed to assess the extent to which children were hungry in the household.[17] **Table 17–6** highlights these questions.

■ FOOD SECURITY IN THE UNITED STATES

The agricultural bounty of the United States has not completely overcome the problem of hunger. In 2008, almost 85% of U.S. households were food secure. However, 14.6% were food insecure at some time during the year,[2] as shown in **Figure 17–1**. Trends in food insecurity and prevalence in the United States are shown in **Figure 17–2**.

Figure 17–3 summarizes the 2007–2008 food security data. **Figure 17–4** summarizes the prevalence of very low food insecurity for 2007–2008. Overall, food insecurity was greater in 2008 than in 2007 among 1) households with incomes below the official poverty line; 2) households with children headed by a single woman or man; 3) African-American or Hispanic households; and 4) households located in central cities or non-metropolitan areas. Overall, all households with food insecurity fared worse in 2008 than in 2007.[2] Hunger patterns were similar.[2]

TABLE 17–6	**Child-Related Food Security Survey Module Questions**[a]

- "(I/We) relied on only a few kinds of low-cost food to feed (my/our) (child/children) because (I was/we were) running out of money to buy food." Was that often, sometimes, or never true for (you/your household) in the last 12 months?

- "(I/We) couldn't feed (my/our) (child/children) a balanced meal, because (I/we) couldn't afford that." Was that often, sometimes, or never true for (you/your household) in the last 12 months?

- "(My/our) (child was/children were) not eating enough because (I/we) just couldn't afford enough food." Was that often, sometimes, or never true for (you/your household) in the last 12 months?

- In the last 12 months, since (current month) of last year, did you ever cut the size of (your child's/any of the children's) meals because there wasn't enough money for food? Yes No

- In the last 12 months, did (CHILD'S NAME/any of the children) ever skip meals because there wasn't enough money for food? Yes No

- If yes, how often did this happen—almost every month, some months but not every month, or in only 1 or 2 months?

- In the last 12 months, (was your child/were the children) ever hungry but you just couldn't afford more food? Yes No

- In the last 12 months, did (your child/any of the children) ever not eat for a whole day because there wasn't enough money for food? Yes No

[a]A self-administered food security survey module is also available for youth age 12 and older. Available at http://www.ers.usda.gov/Briefing/FoodSecurity/surveytools.htm#youth. Accessed May 11, 2010.

Source: Bickel G, Nord M, Price C, Hamilton W, Cook J. *Guide to Measuring Household Food Security, Revised 2000*. Alexandria, VA: U.S. Department of Agriculture, Food and Nutrition Service; 2000.

Although these national estimates paint a picture of the United States as a whole, regions within the United States and particular states may vary with regard to food security status. The prevalence of food security and hunger by state is summarized in **Table 17–7**. Again, although a particular state may experience food insecurity and hunger below the national average, a community within a state may exceed the state and national averages, necessitating the need for programmatic intervention.

In the United States, food insecurity is evident when families have limited resources, lack access to food (due to limited resources, lack of transportation, living in remote areas, or limited access to food stores), depend on food assistance programs, skip meals, substitute nutritious foods with less expensive alternatives, and seek assistance from soup kitchens and food pantries.[18,19] A low income, coupled

with high housing and healthcare costs, can result in hunger and food insecurity,[20] possibly leading to malnutrition and various health problems.[21]

Coping Strategies Used by the Public to Avoid Food Insecurity

People often use coping strategies to minimize household food security. Food management practices used by people with limited resources have been identified by Kempson and colleagues[22] including:

- Strategizing food preparation (e.g., making low-cost dishes; removing mold, insects, and slime from cheese, grain, and meats)
- Rationing the household food supply
- Conserving food
- Inadequately preserving food

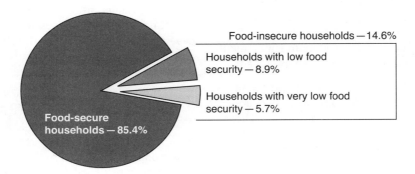

FIGURE 17–1 U.S. Households by Food Security Status, 2008

Source: Calculated by ERS using data from December 2008 Current Population Survey Food Security Supplement.

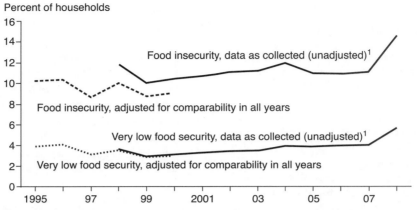

Percent of households

¹Data as collected in 1995–1997 are not directly comparable with data collected in 1998–2008.

FIGURE 17-2 Trends in the Prevalence of Food Insecurity in U.S. Households, 1995–2008
Source: Calculated by ERS using data from December 2008 Current Population Survey Food Security Supplement. Available at http://www.ers.usda.gov/Briefing/FoodSecurity/Stats_Graphs.htm#trends. Accessed August 30, 2010.

- Restricting personal food intake
- Overeating when food is available
- Obtaining food opportunistically
- Cycling monthly eating patterns
- Eating low-cost foods

Supporting some of these ideas, Greder and Brotherson[23] and other researchers[24] have identified coping strategies used in households with low incomes. These tactics included depending upon others (family, friends, community resources),[23,24] adjusting resources and making trade-offs (securing multiple jobs, not paying bills or only paying a portion of them in order to have enough money to buy food and other basic needs),[23] adjusting food consumption,[23] decreasing budgets to pay rent and utilities,[23] and obtaining nutrition and shopping knowledge and skills through nutrition education programs like the Expanded Food and Nutrition Education Program and the Special Supplemental Nutrition Program for Women, Infants and Children (WIC).[23]

As noted by Nord, Andrews, and Carlson,[2] households with limited resources employ a variety of methods to help meet their food needs, including participating in one or more federal food assistance programs or obtaining food from community emergency food providers to supplement the household food purchased. Nord and others[2] noted:

> Households that turn to federal and community food assistance programs typically do so because they are having difficulty in meeting their food needs. The use of such programs by low-income households and the relationship between the food security status and use of food assistance programs by these households provide insight into the extent of their difficulties in obtaining enough food and the ways they cope with those difficulties.

Food assistance programs in the United States, that is, the *nutrition safety net*, have been key in helping the U.S. public secure adequate food. In fact, federally funded and community-based programs are vital in helping households make ends meet. Several program summaries follow.

Child and Adult Care Food Program

This program provides nutritious meals and snacks to children and adults who receive day care or after-school care away from home. It also provides these provisions to children residing in homeless shelters. This program is usually administered by the state education agency.

> More information about the Child and Adult Care Food Program can be found at http://www.fns.usda.gov/cnd/CARE/CACFP/cacfphome.htm.[25]

Expanded Food and Nutrition Education Program

This program helps families with limited incomes acquire knowledge, skills, attitudes, and behavior changes necessary to maintain nutritionally sound diets and enhance personal development, including basic nutrition, food preparation, and resource management skills. There are several food distribution programs, including:

- Child Nutrition Commodity Support
- Nutrition Services Incentive Program
- Commodity Supplemental Food Program
- Food Distribution Disaster Assistance
- Food Distribution Program on Indian Reservations
- Emergency Food Assistance Program

Overall, these programs support the nutrition safety net through commodity distribution and other nutrition

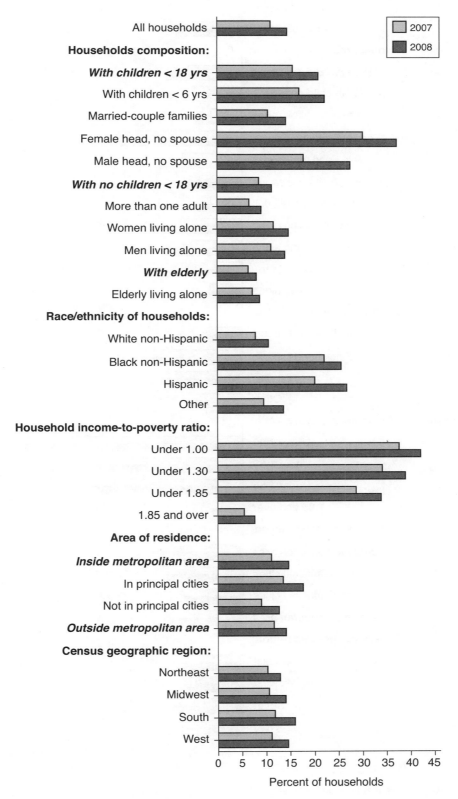

FIGURE 17–3 Prevalence of Food Insecurity, 2007 and 2008

Source: Calculated by ERS based on Current Population Survey Food Security Supplement data, December 2007 and December 2008.

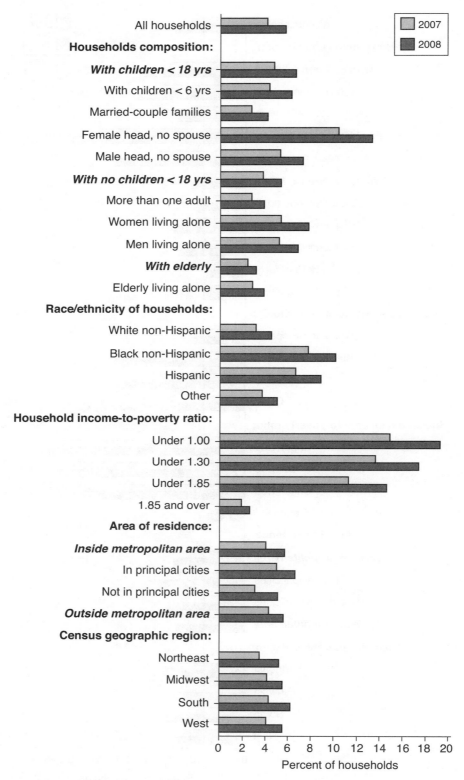

FIGURE 17–4 Prevalence of Very Low Food Security, 2007 and 2008

Source: Calculated by ERS based on Current Population Survey Food Security Supplement data, December 2007 and December 2008.

TABLE 17–7	Prevalence of Household-Level Food Insecurity and Very Low Food Security by State, Average 2004–2006[1]				

	Number of Households		Food Insecurity (low or very low food security)		Very Low Food Security	
State	Average 2004–06[2]	Interviewed	Prevalence	Margin of Error[3]	Prevalence	Margin of Error[3]
	Number	Number	Percent	Percentage points	Percent	Percentage points
U.S.	114,338,000	141,683	11.3	0.26	3.9	0.14
AK	243,000	1,785	12.6	1.36	5.1*	0.71
AL	1,831,000	1,685	12.1	1.55	3.3	1.10
AR	1,125,000	1,687	14.3*	1.17	5.8*	1.04
AZ	2,216,000	1,868	13.1*	1.55	4.3	0.72
CA	12,807,000	10,155	10.9	0.73	3.7	0.45
CO	1,874,000	2,988	12.0	1.31	4.4	0.65
CT	1,386,000	2,758	8.6*	0.95	2.7*	0.46
DC	266,000	1,970	12.5*	0.90	3.8	0.84
DE	328,000	2,118	7.8*	1.43	2.6*	0.61
FL	7,242,000	5,893	8.9*	0.56	3.1*	0.24
GA	3,523,000	2,844	12.6	1.65	5.0*	0.89
HI	448,000	1,843	7.8*	0.59	2.8*	0.62
IA	1,210,000	2,857	11.4	1.33	3.9	0.58
ID	526,000	1,696	12.7*	0.88	3.5	0.59
IL	4,937,000	4,373	9.8*	0.85	3.5*	0.34
IN	2,480,000	2,453	10.8	1.44	4.0	0.57
KS	1,098,000	2,303	12.5*	0.80	4.5*	0.34
KY	1,690,000	2,064	13.6*	1.66	4.6*	0.66
LA	1,585,000	1,251	14.4*	1.41	5.0	1.24
MA	2,492,000	2,246	8.1*	0.83	3.0	0.47
MD	2,125,000	3,119	9.5*	1.13	3.9	0.45
ME	545,000	2,945	12.9*	1.04	5.3*	0.79
MI	3,985,000	3,529	12.2	1.19	4.6	0.80
MN	2,043,000	3,415	8.2*	0.94	3.2*	0.48
MO	2,383,000	2,598	12.3	1.12	4.4*	0.46
MS	1,103,000	1,312	18.1*	1.87	6.4*	0.80
MT	412,000	1,697	9.9	1.44	4.3	0.59
NC	3,426,000	2,939	12.9*	1.24	4.4	0.64
ND	262,000	2,048	6.4*	0.94	2.2*	0.53
NE	709,000	2,323	9.5*	1.68	3.8	0.71
NH	509,000	2,889	7.4*	0.94	2.2*	0.38
NJ	3,172,000	2,660	7.7*	0.87	2.1*	0.41
NM	770,000	1,453	16.1	2.00	5.8*	1.16
NV	923,000	2,232	8.8*	0.66	3.2*	0.41
NY	7,468,000	5,726	9.8*	0.47	3.2*	0.26
OH	4,617,000	4,180	12.7*	0.89	4.1	0.40
OK	1,401,000	1,884	14.6*	1.36	5.3*	0.68
OR	1,434,000	1,997	11.9	1.32	4.4	0.82
PA	4,916,000	4,604	10.0*	0.78	3.3*	0.33
RI	429,000	2,407	11.3	1.26	3.7	0.65
SC	1,703,000	1,991	14.7*	1.58	5.9*	0.69
SD	324,000	2,392	9.5*	0.69	3.3*	0.51
TN	2,418,000	1,967	12.5	1.72	4.3	0.83
TX	8,371,000	6,567	15.9*	0.50	5.3*	0.30
UT	806,000	1,629	14.5*	1.69	5.1	1.65
VA	2,827,000	2,939	7.9*	0.86	2.8*	0.49
VT	261,000	2,116	9.6*	1.29	4.3	0.88
WA	2,492,000	2,523	10.3	1.51	3.6	0.80
WI	2,253,000	2,925	8.9*	0.99	2.7*	0.44
WV	733,000	1,808	9.3*	0.68	3.2	0.77
WY	209,000	2,032	10.6	0.98	3.7	0.87

*Difference from U.S. average was statistically significant with 90 percent confidence (t > 1.645).

[1]Prevalence rates for1996–96 reported in *Prevalence of Food Insecurity and Hunger, by State, 1996–1998* (Nord et al, 1999) are not directly comparable with the rates reported here because of differences in screening procedures in the CPS Food Security Supplements from 1995 to1998. Comparable statistics for the earlier periods are presented in Appendix D of this document.

[2]Totals exclude households whose food security status is unknown because they did not give a valid response to any of the questions in the food security scale. These represented about 0.3 percent of all households in each year.

[3]Margin of error with 90 percent confidence (1.645 times the standard error of the estimated prevalence rate).

Source: Nord M, Andrews M, Carlson S. *Household Food Security in the United States, 2007* (ERR66). Alexandria, VA: Food and Rural Economics Division, Economic Research Service, U.S. Department of Agriculture; 2008.

More information about the Expanded Food and Nutrition Education Program can be found at http://www.csrees.usda.gov/nea/food/efnep/about.html.[26]

More information about Feeding America can be found at http://www.feedingamerica.org, http://www.fns.usda.gov/fdd/.[27–29]

assistance to families with low incomes, emergency feeding programs, Native American reservations, and older adults. Local food banks and pantries or other agencies or organizations, including faith-based groups, typically receive supplemental foods. Local food banks can be accessed through Feeding America. (See more about this program later in this section.)

Supplemental Nutrition Assistance Program

More information about Supplemental Nutrition Assistance Program (food stamps) can be found at http://www.fns.usda.gov/fsp/.[30]

This program enables families with low incomes to buy nutritious food with coupons and electronic benefits transfer cards. Food stamp recipients spend their benefits to buy eligible food in authorized retail food stores.

National Meals on Wheels Foundation

More information about the National Meals on Wheels Foundation can be found at http://www.nationalmealsonwheels.org.[31]

This program delivers meals to homebound older adults and those at congregate meal sites. A variety of organizations, including local communities, churches, charitable organizations, and concerned citizens administer this program.

National School Lunch and School Breakfast Programs

More information about the National School Lunch and School Breakfast Programs can be found at http://www.fns.usda.gov/cnd/lunch/default.htm and http://www.fns.usda.gov/cnd/breakfast/default.htm.[32,33]

These programs provide nutritionally balanced, low-cost or free breakfasts and lunches to children enrolled in public and nonprofit private schools and residential childcare institutions. They also provide snacks served in after-school educational and enrichment programs for children through 18 years of age.

Senior Farmers' Market Nutrition Program

This program provides older adults, with low incomes, coupons that can be exchanged for fresh, nutritious, unprocessed fruits, vegetables, and fresh-cut herbs at farmers' markets, roadside stands, and community-supported agriculture programs during the harvest season.

More information about the Senior Farmers' Market Nutrition Program can be found at http://www.fns.usda.gov/wic/seniorFMNP/SFMNPmenu.htm.[34]

WIC and the WIC Farmers' Market Nutrition Program

Both of these programs provide supplemental foods, nutrition education and counseling, and access to health services to low-income pregnant, breast-feeding, and non–breast-feeding postpartum women, and to infants and children up to five years of age who are found to be at nutritional risk. As part of the WIC Farmers' Market Nutrition Program, as in the Senior Farmers' Market Nutrition Program, a variety of fresh, nutritious, unprepared, locally grown fruits, vegetables, and herbs may be purchased with coupons.

More information about WIC and the WIC Farmers' Market Nutrition Program can be found at http://www.fns.usda.gov/wic and http://www.fns.usda.gov/wic/FMNP/FMNPfaqs.htm.[35,36]

Summer Food Service Program

This program provides nutritious breakfasts, lunches, and snacks to ensure that children in areas with lower incomes continue to receive nutritious meals during long school vacations, when they typically would not have access to the school breakfast and lunch programs. Programs vary by area and may be accessed through local summer programs or through schools.

More information about the Summer Food Service Program can be found at http://www.summerfood.usda.gov.[37]

Feeding America

This is the largest domestic hunger-relief organization in the United States.[1] Emergency food providers include food pantries, soup kitchens, shelters, and other charitable agencies that feed hungry people. Feeding America is a national network of 200 member food banks. Annually, it distributes 2 billion pounds of food to hungry Americans in the fifty states, District of Columbia, and Puerto Rico through more than 94,000 programs, including food pantries, soup kitchens, emergency shelters, after-school programs, and Kids Cafes operated by private nonprofit organizations, government-affiliated agencies, or faith-based agencies affiliated with churches, mosques, synagogues, and other organizations.[27]

IMPACT OF FOOD INSECURITY ON THE PUBLIC

Food insecurity can have grave consequences on health, including physical impairments such as illness and fatigue; psychological suffering such as feelings of constraint to go against norms and values, and stress at home; and sociofamilial disturbances such as modifications of eating patterns and ritual, disruption of household dynamics, and distortion of the means of food acquisition and management.[38] Dietary quality also can be negatively impacted by food insecurity or insufficiency, including lower dietary intakes of fruits and vegetables[40] and other foods containing essential nutrients.[39-40] Over time these suboptimal intakes could increase the public's risk of developing diet-related, chronic diseases.[41] In fact, overweight/obesity has been associated with food insecurity.[42-44] It has been asserted that the relationship between obesity and food insecurity may be mediated by the low cost of energy-dense foods and reinforced by the pleasing taste of sugar and fat.[45] Poorer functional health status has also been associated with food insecurity.[46] Regarding children, evidence links food insecurity with grave consequences, including poor health status,[47] psychosocial problems,[48,49] lower cognitive and academic performance,[50] and poor nutritional status.[51,52]

STRATEGIES TO ASSIST THE PUBLIC IN SECURING ADEQUATE FOOD

Public health nutrition professionals, registered dietitians, dietetic technicians, registered nurses, and physicians, along with other members of the healthcare team, can assist the public in improving food security. This is paramount, because noncompliance with dietary suggestions may simply be due to poor access to food rather than a lack of understanding of the regimen. Practical suggestions have been published for incorporating food security principles into practice.[53,54] During an interview, health professionals should inquire about issues similar to those assessed in the

food security survey module: 1) anxiety related to food budget or supply and whether the budget is able to meet basic needs; 2) experiences relating to running out of food without being able to obtain more due to financial constraints; 3) perceptions of intake adequacy; and 4) food use.[4]

For example, in the context of having inadequate resources, questions could be posed about eating balanced meals, cutting meal size or skipping meals, and experiencing unintentional weight loss. In addition, questions to include should be related to:

- Available resources, including household income, that the individual has for food to implement dietary and nutrition interventions
- Storage facilities for food, including having a refrigerator and/or freezer in the household
- Availability of utilities, including gas, electric, and water, to the household
- Participation in federal and non-federal food assistance programs in their community, including food pantries, soup kitchens, and community gardens
- How the household acquires food, including gardening practices, hunting for game or fish, and related food safety issues related to dressing fish and game
- Meal planning and purchasing tips related to preserving food resources and reducing food waste[53,54]

Although the educational needs of clients vary, such as in meal planning and purchasing tips, in the face of scarce resources, training may be necessary. In addition, being prepared to discuss the rationale for federal and non-federal food assistance programs and their benefits as well as being able to assist clients in accessing these programs or referring them to another professional should be considered; in fact, an educational resource could be developed and updated periodically.[53] Other educational strategies may include an explanation of manufacturers' expiration codes and other information found on packages, such as "use-by" and "sell-by" dates, to help clients preserve scarce resources. Food safety education related to food preservation methods, including canning and freezing, and food storage processes should be included,[53] as should those related to some of the unsafe practices discussed previously.[22]

CONCLUSIONS

Securing adequate food for the public is paramount to achieving and maintaining health. Food security exists when all people, at all times, have access to sufficient food for an active and healthy life without resorting to emergency food supplies or socially unacceptable ways of obtaining food, including begging, stealing, or scavenging.[3] Understanding food security measurement strategies for programmatic evaluation and inclusion in community needs assessments, as well as the consequences of food insecurity and programs designed to assist the public in securing adequate food, is vital for public health professionals. Several resources will assist public nutrition professionals in staying abreast of food security-related issues, including the Food Security Briefing Room of the Economic Research Service (http://www.ers.usda.gov/briefing/foodsecurity)[5] and the Food Research and Action Center (http://www.frac.org).[55]

Issues for Discussion

1. You are developing a nutrition intervention that you think will impact the food security status of households in the community. The intervention is planned to be 12 months in length. Develop an assessment/evaluation strategy to assess the impact of the program on food security status.

2. Individuals in the local community have had trouble securing adequate food for their households, and your agency's public health nutrition team is working with these individuals. During a meeting you plan to discuss how some of the clients are coping to minimize household food insecurity. Develop a list of strategies that you believe would be generated from such a discussion and the risks associated with those strategies.

3. Select a life-span group—for example, older adults—and discuss food assistance programs that may be accessed in the community, noting what resources each program provides.

4. Develop an interviewing strategy that will assist you in identifying clients at risk for food insecurity.

References

1. Office of Disease Prevention and Health Promotion, U.S. Department of Health and Human Services. *Healthy People 2010.* Available at http://www.healthypeople.gov. Accessed May 12, 2010.

2. Nord M, Andrews M, Carlson S. *Household Food Security in the United States, 2008 (ERR66).* Alexandria, VA: Food and Rural Economics Division, Economic Research Service, U.S. Department of Agriculture; 2010.

3. Life Science Research Office. Federation of American Societies for Experimental Biology. Core indicator of nutritional state for difficult to sample populations. *J Nutr.* 1990;102:1599–1600.

4. Bickel G, Nord M, Price C, Hamilton W, Cook J. *Guide to Measuring Household Food Security, Revised 2000.* Alexandria, VA: U.S. Department of Agriculture, Food and Nutrition Service; 2000.

5. Economic Research Service, U.S. Department of Agriculture. *Briefing Room—Food Security in the United States.* Available at http://www.ers.usda.gov/briefing/foodsecurity/. Accessed September 1, 2009.

6. Radimer KL, Olson CM, Campbell CC. Development of indicators to assess hunger. *J Nutr.* 1990;120:1544–1548.

7. Radimer KL, Olson CM, Greene JC, Campbell CC, Habicht J-P. Understanding hunger and developing indicators to assess it in women and children. *J Nutr.* 1992;24:36S–45S.

8. Wehler CA, Scott RI, Anderson JJ. The Community Childhood Hunger Identification Project: a model of domestic hunger—demonstration project in Seattle, Washington. *J Nurs Educ.* 1992;24:29S–35S.

9. Bureau of Labor Statistics, U.S. Department of Labor. *Labor Force Statistics from the Current Population Survey.* Available at http://www.bls.gov/cps/home.htm. Accessed May 12, 2010.

10. National Center for Education Statistics. Early Childhood Longitudinal Study. Available at http://nces.ed.gov/ecls. Accessed May 12, 2010.

11. National Center for Health Statistics, Centers for Disease Control and Prevention. *National Health and Nutrition Examination Survey.* Available at http://www.cdc.gov/nchs/nhanes.htm. Accessed May 12, 2010.

12. Institute for Social Research, University of Michigan. *Panel Study of Income Dynamics.* Available at http://psidonline.isr.umich.edu. Accessed May 12, 2010.

13. U.S. Census Bureau. *Survey of Program Dynamics.* Available at http://www.sipp.census.gov/spd/. Accessed May 12, 2010.

14. USDA. *Food Security in the United States: Definitions of Hunger and Food Security.* Available at http://www.ers.usda.gov/Briefing/FoodSecurity/labels.htm. Accessed on May 12, 2010.

15. McIntyre L, Glanvill NT, Raine KD, Dayle JB, Anerson B, Battaglia N. Do low-income lone mothers compromise their nutrition to feed their children? *Can Med Assoc J.* 2003;168:686–691.

16. Blumberg SJ, Bialososky K, Hamilton WL, Briefel RR. The effectiveness of a short form of the household food security scale. *Am J Public Health.* 1999;89:1231–1234.

17. Nord M, Bickel G. *Measuring Children's Food Security in the United States, 1995–1999 (FANRR-25).* Alexandria, VA: Food and Rural Economics Division, Economic Research Service, U.S. Department of Agriculture; 2002.

18. Andrews M, Nord M, Bickel G, Carlson S. *Household Food Security in the United States, 1999 (FANRR-8).* Alexandria, VA: Food and Rural Economics Division, Economic Research Service, U.S. Department of Agriculture; 2000.

19. Holben DH, McClincy MC, Holcomb JP, Dean KL, Walker CE. Food security status of households in Appalachian Ohio with children in Head Start. *J Am Diet Assoc.* 2004;104:238–241.

20. LeBlanc C, McMurry K. Discussion paper on food security. *Fam Econ Nutr Rev.* 1998;2:49–78.

21. Olivera V. *The Food Stamp Program and Food Insufficiency.* Washington, DC: Economic Research Service; 1998.

22. Kempson KM, Keenan DP, Sadani PS, Ridlen S, Rosato NS. Food management practices used by people with limited resources to maintain food sufficiency as reported by nutrition educators. *J Am Diet Assoc.* 2002;102:1795–1799.

23. Greder K, Brotherson MJ. Food security and low-income families: Research to inform policy and programs. *J Fam Cons Sci.* 2002;94:40–47.

24. Holben DH, Shih K-P, Manoogian MM. Relationship of food insecurity to physical and mental health of women from rural, low-income households in West Virginia. *FASEB J.* 2004;18:A109.

25. Food and Nutrition Service, U.S. Department of Agriculture. *Child and Adult Care Food Program.* Available at http://www.fns.usda.gov/cnd/CARE/CACFP/cacfphome.htm. Accessed May 12, 2010.

26. Cooperative State Research, Education, and Extension Service. *Expanded Food and Nutrition Education Program.* Available at http://www.csrees.usda.gov/nea/food/efnep/about.html. Accessed April 15, 2009.

27. *Feeding America.* Available at http://www.feedingamerica.org. Accessed May 12, 2010.

28. Food and Nutrition Service, U.S. Department of Agriculture. *Food Distribution Programs.* Available at http://www.fns.usda.gov/fdd/. Accessed May 12, 2010.

29. Food and Nutrition Service, U.S. Department of Agriculture. *Nutrition Assistance Programs.* Available at http://www.fns.usda.gov/fns/. Accessed May 12, 2010.

30. Food and Nutrition Service, U.S. Department of Agriculture. *Food Stamp Program.* Available at http://www.fns.usda.gov/fsp/. Accessed April 15, 2009.

31. National Meals on Wheels Foundation. Available at http://www.nationalmealsonwheels.org. Accessed May 12, 2010.

32. Food and Nutrition Service, U.S. Department of Agriculture. *National School Lunch Program.* Available at http://www.fns.usda.gov/cnd/lunch/. Accessed April 15, 2009.

33. Food and Nutrition Service, U.S. Department of Agriculture. *School Breakfast Program.* Available at http://www.fns.usda.gov/cnd/breakfast/. Accessed May 12, 2010.

34. Food and Nutrition Service, U.S. Department of Agriculture. *Senior Farmers' Market Nutrition Program.* Available at http://www.fns.usda.gov/wic/SeniorFMNP/SFMNPmenu.htm. Accessed May 12, 2010.

35. Food and Nutrition Service, U.S. Department of Agriculture. *Special Supplemental Nutrition Program for Women, Infants and Children (WIC).* Available at http://www.fns.usda.gov/wic/. Accessed May 12, 2010.

36. Food and Nutrition Service, U.S. Department of Agriculture. *WIC Farmers' Market Nutrition Program.* Available at http://www.fns.usda.gov/wic/FMNP/FMNPfaqs.htm. Accessed May 12, 2010.

37. Food and Nutrition Service, U.S. Department of Agriculture. *Summer Food Service Program.* Available at http://www.fns.usda.gov/cnd/summer/. Accessed May 12, 2010.

38. Hamelin A-M, Habicht J-P, Beaudry M. Food insecurity: consequences for the household and broader social implications. *J Nutr.* 1999;129:525S–528S.

39. Rose D, Oliveira V. Nutrient intakes of individuals from food insufficient households in the United States. *Am J Public Health.* 1997;87:1956–1961.

40. Kendell A, Olson CM, Frongillo EA Jr. Relationship of hunger and food insecurity to food availability and consumption. *J Am Diet Assoc.* 1996;96:1019–1024.

41. Dixon LB, Winkleby M, Radimer K. Dietary intakes and serum nutrients differ between adults from food-insufficient and food-sufficient families: Third National Health and Nutrition Examination Survey, 1988–1994. *J Nutr.* 2001;131:1232–1246.

42. Frongillo EA Jr, Olson CM, Raschenbach BS, Kendall A. *Nutritional Consequences of Food Insecurity in a Rural New York County.* Discussion Paper no. 1120-97. Madison, WI: Institute for Research on Poverty, University of Wisconsin-Madison; 1997.

43. Olson CM. Nutrition and health outcomes associated with food insecurity and hunger. *J Nutr.* 1999;129:521S–524S.

44. Holben DH, Pheley AM. Obesity, diabetes, and BMI are greater in food insecure households in rural Appalachian Ohio. *J Am Diet Assoc.* 2001;101:A-78.

45. Drewnowski A, Specter SE. Poverty and obesity: the role of energy density and energy costs. *Am J Clin Nutr.* 2004;79:6–16.

46. Pheley AM, Holben DH, Graham AS, Simpson C. Food security and perceptions of health status: a preliminary study in rural Appalachia. *J Rural Health.* 2002;18:447–454.

47. Alaimo K, Olson CM, Frongillo EA, Jr. Food insufficiency, family income, and health in U.S. preschool and school-aged children. *Am J Public Health.* 2001;91:781–786.

48. Kleinman RE, Murphy JM, Little M, Pagano J, Wehler CA, Regal K, Jellinek MS. Hunger in children in the United States: potential behavioral and emotional correlates. *Pediatrics.* 1998;101:1–6.

49. Murphy JM, Wehler CA, Pagano ME, Little M, Kleinman RE, Jellinek MS. Relationship between hunger and psychosocial functioning in low-income American children. *J Am Acad Child Adolesc Psychiatry.* 1998;37:163–170.

50. Alaimo K, Olson CM, Frongillo EA, Jr. Food insufficiency and American school-aged children's cognitive, academic and psychosocial development. *Pediatrics.* 2001;108:44–53.

51. Casey PH, Szeto K, Lensing S, Bogle M, Weber J. Children in food-insufficient, low-income families. Prevalence, health and nutrition status. *Arch Pediatr Adolesc Med.* 2001;155:508–514.

52. Kaiser LL, Melgar-Quinonez H, Lamp CL, Johns MC, Sutherlin JM, Harwood JO. Food insecurity and nutritional outcomes of preschool-age Mexican-American children. *J Am Diet Assoc.* 2002;102:924–929.

53. Boeing KL, Holben DH. Self-identified food security knowledge and practices of licensed dietitians in Ohio: Implications for dietetics and clinical nutrition practice. *Top Clin Nutr.* 2003;18:185–191.

54. Holben DH, Myles W. Food insecurity in the United States: how it affects our patients. *Am Fam Physician.* 2004;69:1058–1063.

55. Food Research and Action Center. Available at http://www.frac.org. Accessed May 12, 2010.

CHAPTER 18

Security of the Food Supply and Bioterrorism Preparedness

Barbara Bruemmer, PhD, RD, CD

READER OBJECTIVES

After studying this chapter and reflecting on the contents, you should be able to:

1. Describe the scope of the bioterrorist threat to the food supply.
2. Identify organisms that may be disseminated by ingestion.
3. Describe the foods most at risk of intentional contamination.
4. Compare and contrast the challenges in distinguishing an intentional food contamination from an unintentional food contamination.
5. Summarize the strengths and weaknesses of our current food biosecurity efforts.
6. Recommend actions public health nutritionists can take to promote preparedness for the community and the consumer.

■ INTRODUCTION

The safety and security of our food supply is essential for physical survival as well as social stability and economic prosperity. In a developed country such as the United States, individuals may live a life quite removed from the acts that produce, process, and transport food for various levels of home, retail, and restaurant preparation and presentation. This chapter examines the complex risks from bioterrorism that are inherent in a stratified food economy.

There are many historical precedents for biological warfare as far back as 184 BC, when Hannibal had pots filled with serpents placed on the decks of enemy ships.[1] In modern history, the Biological and Toxin Weapons Convention was signed by over 140 countries in the early 1970s. This agreement addressed research on offensive biological weapons and destruction of existing weapons. Although such international agreement on the development of biological weapons is necessary, certain rogue states and terrorist groups have declared their intent to fight an economic and political war with the United States. During the Persian Gulf War in 1995, Iraq not only had stocks of botulinum toxin, the deadliest know substance to humans, but also had loaded 11,200 liters into Scud missile warheads.[2]

Historically, food has been a vehicle for terrorist attacks both nationally and internationally. In 1984, a religious cult contaminated salad bars at 10 restaurants with *Salmonella typhimurium*, sickening 751 people in The Dalles, Oregon.[3] Chemical agents, as well as biologic agents, have also been added to food. In 2003, 200 pounds of ground beef were contaminated with nicotine by a supermarket employee. This attack resulted in illness in 111 people, 40 of whom were children.[4] Mark Wheelis noted, "Every major state biological weapons program we know of has included an anti-agricultural component."[5]

The potential for causing sickness in larger populations has been demonstrated with unintentional foodborne illness. The largest reported incident of unintentional foodborne illness occurred in China in 1991, where 300,000 reported victims suffered from an outbreak of hepatitis A that was linked to tainted clams.[6] When contamination occurs at a central food processing or distribution point, food thus may be a vehicle for wide dissemination of a biologic or chemical agent.

Assessment and quantification of this risk has been considered by numerous government agencies, including the Center for Food Safety and Applied Nutrition of the FDA. Its report of October 2003 noted:

> Though the likelihood of a biological or chemical attack on the U.S. food supply is uncertain, significant scientific evidence documents the risk to public health of food that has been inadvertently contaminated. Notwithstanding the uncertainties described in this risk assessment, and given the broad range of agents that may contaminate the food supply that FDA regulates, the agency concludes that there is a high likelihood, over the course of a year, that a significant number of people will be affected by an act of food terrorism or by an incident of unintentional food contamination that results in serious foodborne illness.[4]

In light of the terrorism threat to the United States, how can we defend and protect public health and these vital resources? In the event of an attack, how can we assure an adequate supply of safe food for victims and minimize short- and long-term impacts?

Terrorism: The unlawful use of force or violence against persons or property to intimidate or coerce a government, the civilian population, or any segment thereof, in furtherance of political or social objectives.

■ FOOD AS A TARGET

Food is vulnerable not only because of the physical need for survival, but also because of the complex layers of societal involvement. As illustrated in **Figure 18–1**, both individual and societal factors may be profoundly impacted by an attack on the food supply. The individual components are both physical and psychological; societal components can be economic and political.

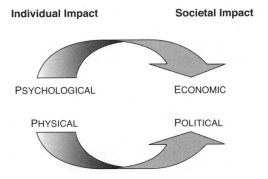

Individual Impact   **Societal Impact**

PSYCHOLOGICAL   ECONOMIC

PHYSICAL   POLITICAL

FIGURE 18–1 Potential Consequences of a Major Food Bioterrorism Event

Physical

The physical consequences start with our dependence on food for survival. Although this simple statement appears as a *prima fascia* tenet, so obvious that it should not need acknowledgment, it is our assumption that food is always available that contributes to our vulnerability. Our population does not regard food insufficiency as a risk that all may face; however, it is certainly recognized as a vulnerability of select groups, such as the homeless and poor. But the concept that a food shortage could occur is generally not considered a threat. The lack of food in the short term could cause physical discomfort, could be associated with mild malnutrition, or in an extreme situation could threaten life. Certain segments of the population could be more vulnerable to shortages, such as groups who may be isolated and unable to obtain emergency supplies, or those who by their physical limitations may have less reserves or increased needs, such as pregnant women, infants, small children, and older adults.

Another potential physical consequence is the destruction or contamination of food that has been exposed to a biological weapon. This could potentially remove needed food supplies from circulation and cause disruption in the transportation and distribution of replacement food supplies to the public, retail outlets, restaurants, and institutional feeding sites.

Psychological

The terrorist attacks on the United States in 2001, where millions of people experienced anxiety and distress, demonstrated the widespread psychological impact of terrorist events. Individuals would understandably respond to attacks on the food supply in a similar fashion, but the degree of psychological harm may be very difficult to assess and control. Factors that may influence the magnitude of emotional response include the weapon (severity of the attack, type of weapon used, and duration of the attack or multiple attacks), emergency communication (perceived accuracy and timeliness of information, level of detail on individual victims, extent and duration of media coverage), perception of personal risk (uncertainty regarding personal defense strategies), and the coexistence of deprivation or discomfort. Factors that may contribute to public alarm and panic include rumors and misinformation that establish public mistrust, the appearance of favoritism for some individuals over others, a perception that there is a small chance of escape, requests for isolation, declarations of quarantine, social disruption, and civil discord and violence.[7] The psychological response to an attack on food would certainly be magnified for individuals who have inadequate food, suffer from hunger pains, or would be responsible for others, such as hungry children. Also, the majority of Americans are not accustomed to eating spoiled food, which might be a necessity in the situation of a shortage.

Response: Those activities and programs designed to address the immediate and short-term effects of the onset of an emergency or disaster.

The National Academy of Sciences (NAS) has published a report, *Preparing for the Psychological Consequences of Terrorism: A Public Health Strategy*,[8] that describes three spheres of psychological consequence: distress response, psychiatric illness, and behavioral change. The authors note the level of psychological response to terrorism may include "insomnia, fear, anxiety, vulnerability, anger, increased alcohol consumption or smoking; and, a minority will develop psychiatric illnesses, such as posttraumatic stress disorder or depression." Several elements related to food and psychological distress should be considered in public health preparedness. During an attack, availability of basic supplies including food is the responsibility of the public health infrastructure. The first of the 10 recommendations from the NAS report is the "Provision of basic resources including food, shelter, communication, transportation, information, guidance, and medical services." During a recovery phase, we must recognize that attitudes toward a food or a food group may be altered as a psychological response, particularly if a food has been the vehicle to deliver a terrorist weapon. Such responses may result in short-term or long-term maladaptive behaviors, such as food aversions. Research on this area of behavioral change not only would help us to assure the return to psychological health, but also may help us avoid severe economic and/or nutritional consequences of long-term shifts in consumption patterns.

Recovery: As defined here, includes all types of emergency actions dedicated to the continued protection of the public or to promoting the resumption of normal activities in the affected area.

The final element to consider regarding psychological consequences is the amount of damage that potentially may result from small, sporadic terrorist attacks on food, where the main target is psychological health itself. Although few individuals were actually exposed to the anthrax bacterium in 2001, the uncertainty of the exposure and resulting perception created additional "victims" of this attack.

Economic

An attack on our food supply has the potential to cause tremendous economic damage both for domestic consumption and for our export markets and balance of trade. As described by Chalk,[9] an agroterrorist attack would generate costs on three levels:

1. *Direct losses:* From containment measures and the destruction of disease-ridden livestock

2. *Indirect multiplier effects:* From compensation costs paid to farmers

3. *International costs:* From protective trade embargoes imposed by major external trading partners

Following the events of September 2001, the food industry experienced:

...a dramatic decline in some travel-dependent sectors of food service, a temporary slowdown in new grocery product introductions, impacts on transportation in small segments of the industry and increased security costs.[10]

Increased economic costs are continuing for agriculture and industry as preparedness plans are developed, implemented, evaluated, and revised. The consequences to our economy are difficult to estimate but could potentially be profound with an agent delivered at a central distribution point with widespread contamination. Even random attacks on the food supply could have major economic impacts if consumers alter eating patterns, shopping habits, and food storage inventory. Also, a stigma with economic consequences may be associated with an industry or a food product. In 1993, after the outbreak of *E. coli* O157:H7 was traced to Jack in the Box® restaurants in the Pacific Northwest, the parent company, Foodmakers, saw its stock value drop by 30%.[11]

Treatment costs following an outbreak also may be substantial. Trevejo and others reported that the median cost of hospitalization of patients with salmonellosis from 1990 to 1999 ranged from $160 to $3.2 million dollars (median 9.054).[12]

Political

How would these factors then impact the political situation? The outbreak of bovine spongiform encephalopathy (BSE; also known as "mad cow disease") led to a loss of confidence in the political system and political destabilization in Great Britain. Much of this fallout was due to communication missteps where the public was given assurances of safety that later proved to be unsubstantiated.[4] Certainly the election in Spain in the winter of 2004 was influenced by the March 11 train bombings in Madrid. In the United States, the events of September 2001 and subsequent activities unmistakably influenced the political arena.

■ PUBLIC HEALTH PREPAREDNESS FOR FOOD BIOSECURITY

In the face of these consequences of an attack on the food supply, federal agencies, state and local public health jurisdictions, emergency responders, academic institutions, researchers, and community groups have taken specific steps to safeguard the food supply and upgrade the public health infrastructure to lessen risk. The Centers for Disease Control and Prevention (CDC) uses a paradigm for preparedness that includes planning, surveillance, detection, and response. The Department of Health and Human Services also highlights the element of awareness in preparedness efforts.[13] Each of these components has unique challenges in regard to food biosecurity. The issue of awareness is particularly appropriate regarding food security. Although the events of September 2001 certainly maximized awareness of the potential for terrorist attacks, the risk to the food supply is still obscured by complacency that exists at various levels among institutions and individuals.

> Live agents cannot be detected by the human senses. The first indication of a biologic attack therefore is usually the first observed casualty, most often detected by local physicians who then report it to local public health officials.

The elements of effective planning include the identification of appropriate regulatory agencies, which are then responsible for the assessment of areas of risk; development of preparedness priorities, strategies, and plans to diminish risk; communication; training; and evaluation. Planning activities also depend on interagency cooperation. The FBI has prepared a Concepts of Operations Plan (CONPLAN), which provides overall guidance on response to a potential or actual terrorist threat.[14]

To plan a strong defense system, it is important to assess those elements of our food environment that may be involved in a terrorist attack. There are two main approaches to our defense systems. First, we must recognize that food may be a vehicle to deliver a terrorist weapon; second, other types of terrorist activities may compromise the availability of safe food in adequate amounts. In both situations, we must provide defense, but also plan and empower local communities and individuals to be prepared with knowledge, skills, and reserves of necessary water and food.

Potential Agents

Food, as a vehicle for the delivery of a bioterrorist weapon, may be contaminated with either biological or chemical weapons that may be viable through the gastrointestinal tract. The CDC has created a list of agents that have been assigned to categories based on a number of criteria including:

> ...need for hospitalization, mortality rates for exposed untreated persons, potential for initial dissemination to a large population, potential for continued propagation by person-to-person transmission, potential for overall dissemination, capability for mass production,

potential for rapid, large-scale dissemination including most effective route of infection and general environmental stability, source of the agent, i.e., soil, animal/insect, or plant source versus laboratory or clinical sources, and main routes of infection, i.e., respiratory versus gastrointestinal.[15]

This report noted several important aspects of this classification process. First, these agents are not ranked on their likelihood of use, but on their potential impact. Second, historically the presumed target for biological weapons was military personnel and military capability. The virulence of these agents would be quite different in young, physically fit individuals in the military service compared to a cross-section of the population with varying levels of immune function and comorbidities.

> **Virulence:** The relative severity of the disease produced by a pathogen.

Ingestion of biological agents may occur by:

- Contaminated food or drinking water (non-aerosols can contaminate food supplies or drinking water over long distances)
- Hand-to-mouth contact after touching contaminated surfaces
- Swallowing mucus that contains particles lodged in the nose and throat[16]

Potential targets include food crops, livestock (using aerosols, sprays, and crop dusters), food processing plants, imported foods and food additives, point of sale (i.e., grocery stores), restaurants, institutional feeding sites, and congregate meals.[16] Because the contaminants may be spread from hand to food, packaging may be a target also. Individual packages, such as milk cartons or other sealed containers, may be penetrated with a syringe.

Table 18–1 provides information on the category A and category B agents that may be viable through the gastrointestinal tract. Of these agents, botulism is certainly one that potentially could lead to substantial loss of life. It is considered the most toxic agent known. Knobler and colleagues stated that, "one hundred grams of botulinum toxin evenly distributed in a food or beverage and ingested, could kill over one million people."[17] However, many of the traditional foodborne agents, such as *Salmonella*, that do not have a high fatality rate may still cause significant morbidity, social disruption, and psychological damage, particularly in vulnerable populations.

TABLE 18–1	CDC Information on Bioterrorism Agents and Diseases[36,37,42,43]				
Category A	**Characteristics of Agent**	**Dissemination**	**Incubation Period**	**Symptoms**	**Case Fatality Ratio (CFR) or Lethality**
Anthrax[36,44] *Bacillus anthracis*	Encapsulated, aerobic, gram-positive, spore-forming, rod-shaped bacterium	Aerosol Cutaneous Ingestion	1–7 days	GI: Nausea, anorexia, vomiting, and fever progressing to severe abdominal pain, hematemesis, and diarrhea that is almost always bloody	Gastrointestinal has mortality rate of 50–100% despite treatment.
Botulism[45,46] Toxin of *Clostridium botulinum*	Most lethal agent known to man. Spore-forming, rod-shaped organisms that grow in anaerobic environments. The toxin interferes with the presynaptic release of acetylcholine at the neuromuscular junction. Seven types of toxin; A–F are toxic in humans. Victims with respiratory symptoms may require ventilatory support. No person-to-person transmission. No natural occurrence of inhalation botulism.	Ingestion Aerosol	18–36 hours (may range from 6 hours to 10 days, dose dependent)	Acute abdomen picture with rebound tenderness may develop. Initial: Blurred vision, double vision, drooping eyelids, slurred speech, difficulty swallowing, dry mouth, muscle weakness. Later: Descending neurologic impairment. GI: nausea, vomiting, abdominal cramps or abdominal pain, diarrhea.[47]	High mortality, 60% if untreated. Hospitalization rate 80%. Lethal dose 1ng/kg.
Plague[42,48] *Yersinia pestis*	Pneumonic plague refers to respiratory infection. Person-to-person transmission from respiratory droplets.	Aerosols	2–6 days	Swollen and tender lymph gland accompanied by pain.	Untreated bubonic plague. CFR 50%
Smallpox[42] *Variola major*	High transmissibility. Quarantine may be necessary for containment.	Aerosol	10–12 days	Fever, hypotension, rash.	Death occurs in 30% of cases.
Tularemia[49] *Francisella tularensis*	Bacterium found in animals. Highly infectious (10-50 organisms can cause disease). May remain alive for weeks in water.	Aerosol (most likely method for bioterrorism) Ingestion	3–5 days (may range 1–14 days)	Depends on site of exposure. Skin ulcers, swollen and painful lymph glands, sore throat, mouth sores, diarrhea, or pneumonia	CFR for Jellison type A: 5–10%
Viral hemorrhagic[36,42] **fevers**	Causes increased capillary permeability, leucopenia, and thrombocytopenia	Contact Aerosol	4–16 days	Fever, easy bleeding, edema, malaise, headache, vomiting, diarrhea, jaundice, shock, sore throat, rash	Lethality is moderate to high

TABLE 18–1	*(Continued)*

Category B (Those that may be ingested)	Characteristics of Agent	Dissemination	Incubation Period	Symptoms	Case Fatality Ratio (CFR) or Lethality
Brucellosis[50] *Brucella species*	Natural *Brucella* species affect sheep, goats, cattle, deer, elk, pigs, dogs, and several other animals.	Ingestion Aerosol Cutaneous through skin wounds	5–60 days	Acute form: Non-specific flu-like symptoms Undulant form: Undulant fevers, arthritis, and epididymo-orchitis in males. Chronic form: Chronic-fatigue syndrome, depression, and arthritis. Nausea, abdominal cramps, watery diarrhea.	CFR: 5%. Hospitalization rate: 55%.
Epsilon toxin of *Clostridium Perfringens*[47]	An anaerobic, gram-positive, spore-forming rod commonly found in the intestines of humans, domestic and feral animals [FDA]. The toxins bind to enterocytes and form protein complexes that alter cell permeability [Smedley].*	Ingestion	8–16 hours	Nausea, abdominal cramps, watery diarrhea.	CFR: 0.005% Hospitalization rate: 0.3%

Food Safety Threats	Characteristics of Agent	Dissemination	Incubation Period	Symptoms	Case Fatality Ratio (CFR) or Lethality
Salmonella **species**	Generally resolves in 5–7 days and does not usually require hospitalization. Victim may require rehydration. Estimated cases per year in U.S.: 400,000; mortality: 600. Person-to-person contact likely with fecal-oral transmission. Good hygiene and sanitation essential.	Ingestion	12–72 hours	Diarrhea, fever, abdominal cramps. 3–8 days with a median of 3–4 days.	Non-typhoidal. CFR: 0.8%. Hospitalization rate: 22%. Typhoid. CFR: 0.4%. Hospitalization rate: 75%. Severe bloody diarrhea and abdominal cramps.
Escherichia coli **O:157:H7**[52]	Gram-negative rod-shaped bacterium. Estimated cases per year in U.S.: 73,000; mortality: 61. Person-to-person contact likely with fecal-oral transmission. Good hygiene and sanitation essential. Children under 5 and the elderly are at risk of the complication of hemolytic uremia syndrome.	Ingestion	3–8 days	Severe bloody diarrhea and abdominal cramps.	CFR: 0.83%. Hospitalization rate: 29.5%.
Dysentery *Shigella*[53]	Estimated cases per year in U.S.: 18,000. Person-to-person contact likely with fecal-oral transmission. Good hygiene and sanitation essential.	Ingestion	3 days**	Diarrhea (often bloody), fever, stomach cramps.	CFR: 0.16%. Hospitalization rate: 0.14%.

continues

TABLE 18–1	*(Continued)*				

Food Safety Threats	Characteristics of Agent	Dissemination	Incubation Period	Symptoms	Case Fatality Ratio (CFR) or Lethality
Cholera[36,42,50–53] ***Vibrio cholerae***	The disease is rare in industrialized nations. Person-to-person contact likely with fecal-oral transmission. Good hygiene and sanitation essential.	Aerosol Ingestion	12–72 hours	Sudden onset of profuse, watery diarrhea, cramps, vomiting, headache	CFR: 0.6%. Hospitalization rate: 34%.
Cryptosporidium Parvum[43,47]	Parasitic infection of the intestinal epithelium. Person-to-person contact likely with fecal-oral transmission. Good hygiene and sanitation essential.	Ingestion	7 days (range, 2–28 days)	Watery diarrhea, abdominal cramps, low-grade fever, malaise, fatigue, anorexia, occasionally nausea and vomiting.	CFR: 0.5%. Hospitalization rate: 0.05%
Q Fever[36] ***Coxiella burnetii***	Acute rickettsial disease.	Aerosol Ingestion	14–16 days	Fever, chills, malaise, headache, myaldia, eye pain, hyperaesthesias, pulmonary syndrome, cough, chest pain.	Untreated CFR < 1%.
Ricin toxin[36] From *Ricinus communis* (castor bean)	Causes damage to the liver and bone marrow.	Aerosol Ingestion	1–12 hours	Vomiting, nausea, diarrhea, cramps, bloody nose, fever, pulmonary edema 18–24 hours after inhalation, severe respiratory distress and death in 36–72 hours.	High lethality.
Staphylococcal Enterotoxin B[36]	Causes damage to the gastrointestinal and respiratory systems.	Aerosol Ingestion	1 hour (range may be 3–12 hours)	Sudden onset of fever, chills, headache, nausea, muscle aches, pulmonary syndrome, vomiting, and diarrhea if ingested.	Fatality < 1%

Agents that may be disseminated through ingestion are shown in bold type.

*Food and Drug Administration. Bad Bug Book. Available at http://www.cfsan.fda.gov/~mow/chap11.html. Accessed April 25, 2005.

**Jojosky RA, Groseclose SL. Evaluation of reporting timeliness of public health surveillance systems for infectious diseases. *BMC Public Health*. 2004;4: 29. Available at http://www.biomedcentral.com/1471-2458/4/29. Accessed April 24, 2005.

Healthcare providers and public health professionals should be familiar with the latency periods and presenting symptoms of these agents to assist in communication for early detection and to provide informed responses to the public if one of these agents be suspected in an attack.

Foods at Risk

Two factors influence the magnitude of the impact of a foodborne bioweapon: 1) the range of distribution of the vehicle (food) and 2) the rate of introduction of the vehicle combined with the rate of clearance. Many of our current foods, including dietary staples, are centrally processed and widely distributed. These foods therefore would present a more attractive profile with which to deliver a bioweapon. A National Academy of Sciences (NAS) report has noted that food and water supply networks have a ready-made distribution system for the rapid and widespread introduction of biological and chemical weapons.[18] The rate of introduction of the vehicle into the food supply and the rate of clearance, however, limits the effectiveness of many distribution systems. Foods that have a long shelf life would be less desirable, because the source of contamination may be identified and isolated before the food reaches many of the intended victims. Highly perishable foods with a large distribution range would be most vulnerable to contamination. This category includes dairy products, fresh fruits and vegetables, and certain baked goods. These foods are staples for many of the most vulnerable in our population, such as children. The consequences of an attack on these foods would include a high level of publicity and the associated psychological impact, even though the actual human losses may be limited.

> **Perishable food:** Food that is not heat-treated, frozen, or otherwise preserved in a manner so as to prevent the quality of the food from being adversely affected if held longer than seven days under normal shipping and storage conditions.

■ FOOD BIOSECURITY TRIAD: FOOD SYSTEMS SECURITY, PUBLIC HEALTH VANGUARD, AND CONSUMER ENGAGEMENT

Our efforts to address the risks are focused on three areas, which are described as a triad: 1) the security of the food supply; 2) mobilizing public health and federal agencies as vanguards in preparedness; and 3) the engagement of individual consumers in this process (**Figure 18–2**).

Food System Security

In this first area, actions have been taken to increase the security of the food supply with increased agency funding, expanded regulations, and revised guidelines for food producers and food importers. Title III of the Public Health Security and Bioterrorism Preparedness and Response Act of 2002 contained specific information related to protecting the food supply. The Food and Drug Administration (FDA), through the Center for Food Safety and Applied Nutrition (CFSAN), has implemented provisions for registration of food facilities and prior notice of imported food, as noted in **Table 18–2**. These actions will assist in communication regarding food that may have been contaminated, as well as serving as a deterrent.

The U.S. Department of Agriculture (USDA), through the Food Safety and Inspection Service (FSIS), also has taken action regarding meat, poultry, and egg products with guidelines for food processors and for the transportation and distribution of these foods. Many of these actions are based on directives from the Public Health Security and Bioterrorism Preparedness and Response Act of 2002. Additional procedures have been added during times of heightened threat levels (orange or red) to enhance inspection activity; enhance surveillance of transportation, storage, retail sites, and import facilities; conduct random laboratory sampling for threat agents in high-risk commodities; and increase surveillance of human illness.[19] These actions should improve security at sites that could potentially serve as distribution points for an attack. The key to the success of these actions is consistent high standards for compliance and ongoing evaluations. Vigilance in this regard is essential.

Another tool that has been promoted in the food industry is the Hazard Analysis and Critical Control Point (HACCP) approach to food safety. The FSIS has reported a reduction in Salmonella prevalence on raw meat and poultry products with the enforcement of the Pathogen Reduction/HACCP rule.[20] Guidelines for HACCP procedures to diminish the risk of a bioterrorist attack include:

1. Evaluate significant food security hazards and evaluate the likelihood of these risks.
2. Develop and institute preventive or risk control measures to reduce hazards.
3. Determine the points in your operation that are critical for managing a specific risk. These could be locations, processes, functions, or times when your operation is at greatest risk.
4. Develop monitoring procedures for each critical point.

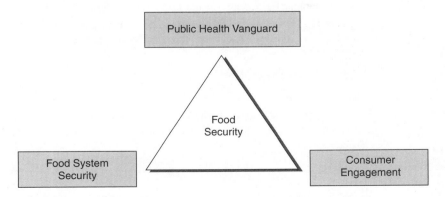

FIGURE 18–2 Triad of Food Security

TABLE 18–2	Food Biosecurity Triad: Food Systems Security

Food and Drug Administration (FDA)	

Center for Food Safety and Applied Nutrition

Legislation: Public Health Security and Bioterrorism Preparedness and Response Act of 2002

Title III: Protecting Safety and Security of Food and Drug Supply

Implementation: December 12, 2003

Activities related to Bioterrorism Act

Title III, Section 305

• Registration of Food Facilities

"Domestic and foreign facilities that manufacture, process, pack or hold food, as defined in the regulation, for human or animal consumption in the US must register with FDA."

The purpose is to allow the FDA to: "determine the location and source of a potential bioterrorism incident or an outbreak of food-borne illness and to quickly notify facilities that may be affected."

Examples provided by FDA:

Included food:
• Dietary supplements and dietary ingredients
• Infant formulas
• Beverages (including alcoholic beverages and bottled water)
• Fruits and vegetables
• Fish and seafood
• Dairy products and shell eggs
• Raw agricultural commodities for use as food or components of food
• Bakery goods, snack food, and candy (including chewing gum)
• Live food animals
• Animal feeds and pet food

Excluded food:
• Food contact substances
• Pesticides

Facilities that do NOT need to register:
• Private residences of individuals
• Non-bottled water, such as municipal water systems
• Transport vehicles that hold food only in the usual course of their business as carriers
• Farms
• Restaurants
• Nonprofit food facilities [501(c)(3)]
• Fishing vessels that harvest and transport fish
• Facilities regulated exclusively and throughout the entire facility by the USDA—facilities that handle only meat, poultry, or egg products.

For additional information and instructions on registration see http://www.cfsan.fda.gov/~dms/fsbtact.html.

Title III, Section 307

• Prior Notice of Imported Food

"Act requires that FDA receive prior notice for food imported or offered for import into the U.S.

The Act also provides that if an article of food arrives at the port of arrival with inadequate prior notice (i.e., no prior notice, inaccurate prior notice, or untimely prior notice), the food is subject to refusal of admission."

http:www.cfsan.fda.gov/~pn/cpgpn.html

Issued Guidelines:

CFSAN Guidance for Industry: Retail Food Stores and Food Service Establishments: Food Security Preventive Measures Guidance. http://www.cfsan.fda.gov/~dms/secgui11.html.

TABLE 18–2 *(Continued)*	

U.S. Department of Agriculture (USDA)

Food Safety and Inspection Service (FSIS) Public Health Security and Bioterrorism Preparedness and Response Act of 2002. Responsible for the regulation of meat, poultry, and egg products.	**Actions authorized under the legislation:** • "Enhance the ability of the Service to inspect and ensure the safety and wholesomeness of meat and poultry products. • Improve the capacity of the Service to inspect international products at points of origin and ports of entry. • Strengthen the ability of the Service to collaborate with relevant agencies within USDA and other entities within the Federal Government, States and Indian Tribes. • Otherwise expand the capacity to protect against the threat of bioterrorism."[19] **Issued Guidelines:** FSIS Security Guidelines for Food Processors Elements include: 1. Food security plan management: establish a team with a food security manager; develop and implement a plan; identify potential corrective action and recommendations for recall of adultered products; link to analytical labs; develop a procedure for notification of law enforcement; identify facility entry points; determine local emergency and public health contacts; provide for training, inspections, communication, and response to threats; and liaison with Homeland Security officials. 2. Checklists for: outside security, general inside security, slaughter and processing security, storage security, shipping and receiving security, water and ice security, mail handling security, and personnel security. See http://www.fsis.usda.gov. **FSIS Safety and Security Guidelines for the Transportation and Distribution of Meat, Poultry, and Egg Products:** Elements include: 1. Assess vulnerabilities 2. Emergency operations 3. Train and test 4. Screen and educate employees 5. Secure the facility

Industry Actions

National Food Processors Association	Alliance for Food Security Includes government agencies, agricultural and food industry organizations. Actions: Food Security Checklist, regarding food plant operations. www.nfpa-food.org
Dietary Managers Association	Articles for Dietary Managers and Food Protection Publications. www.dmaonline.org

5. Develop a procedure to fix security problems or failures that occur if a critical control has been breached or compromised, similar to a corrective-action program in HACCP.
6. Verify or test your security program periodically.[21]

While these agencies are in a transition period to a higher state of preparedness, however, there are still many areas that have not been addressed and that result in serious weaknesses in protecting the food supply. In November 2003, the General Accounting Office (GAO) provided testimony to Congress on the bioterrorist threat to agriculture. The GAO found gaps in federal controls for protecting agriculture and the food supply, which it concludes renders the United States vulnerable to bioterrorism.[22] Four specific areas had been studied and found deficient: prevention of foot and mouth disease, improvements in the composition of animal feed to prevent mad cow disease, food-processing security, and the Plum Island Animal Disease Center. Each of these areas represents opportunities for the introduction of a weapon into the food biosystem.

Another report from the GAO focused on the overlapping and inefficient partitioning of food service regulation among multiple agencies. As noted by Robin Strongin,[23] 12 different federal agencies administer 35 different laws on food safety, with an additional 28 House and Senate subcommittees having food safety oversight. The GAO review recommended fundamental changes with: 1) comprehensive, uniform, and risk-based food safety legislation; and 2) establishment of a single, independent food safety agency.[24] Its assessment of the hazards for attack is that terrorists would attack livestock and crops to cause severe economic harm, but would contaminate finished food products to cause harm to humans. As an example of the lapses in oversight, the report noted that neither the FDA nor the USDA considers itself to have the authority to require processors to adopt physical facility security measures. Taken together, these omissions and inefficiencies contribute to food system vulnerability.

Public Health Vanguard

In this second area, progress has been made to create bridge organizations that address interagency coordination, communication, and harmonization activities and to integrate technology into surveillance systems (**Table 18–3**).

The Food Emergency Response Network (FERN; the lead agency of the FDA) coordinates activities among federal, state, regional, and university laboratories to identify bioterrorist agents in food. The FERN Steering Committee has included representatives of the FDA, Office of Regulatory Affairs, CFSAN, CDC, USDA, FSIS, Animal and Plant Health Inspection Service, Agriculture Marketing Service, Grain Inspection Packers and Stockyards Administration, Customs, Department of Defense, FBI, Environmental Protection Agency, Association of Public Health Laboratories, the agriculture community, and public health.[25] Surveillance activities include federal and state sampling programs for domestic and imported food. The agency also examines response and recovery capabilities. Surge capacity has previously been identified as a critical weakness in public health efforts. The potential large number of casualties, as

well as the number of worried well, may indeed overwhelm current health facilities. Response issues specific to a foodborne attack include the rapid dissemination of information on the affected food; the tracking, isolation, and recall of tainted food; and the ability to maintain adequate food in circulation.

OFSEP was created in 2002 and assumed the function of the Food Biosecurity Action Team (F-BAT).

While these agencies function to enhance planning, response, and recovery, the function of surveillance is divided among many groups (Table 18–3). The challenge of surveillance of foodborne agents is unique because many of the potential agents (Table 18–1) are common in unintentional foodborne illness. Surveillance thus must distinguish between the background "noise" of seasonal incidents and sentinel events from a bioweapon. The CDC and other agencies have drawn on efforts to enhance food safety to link state and local laboratories with national databases. As noted by Sobel et al.,[2] "The adequacy of response will depend on the capacity of public-health officials to respond to all foodborne disease outbreaks." Technology has greatly enhanced the ability to conduct passive, automated surveillance. Syndromic surveillance is an approach that is being tested to examine trends in various syndromic criteria that may be suggestive of a bioterrorist attack. In theory, this method would provide a more rapid alert system than conventional reporting systems.[26] Ashford et al.[27] reviewed CDC outbreak investigations, including those outside of the United States, for agents with a high potential for bioterrorism. Of the 1,099 investigations, healthcare providers and infection control practitioners reported 36.3% and health departments reported 30.5%. The lag time for reporting had a range of up to 26 days.[27] The CONPLAN highlights specific differences between an attack with weapons of mass destruction and other incidents, noting that the

> The Department of Homeland Security and the USDA coordinate food security activities through the USDA Homeland Security Council. The Office of Food Security and Emergency Preparedness (OFSEP; the lead agency of FSIS) functions with the FDA and CDC. It is the lead office for: emergency preparedness and response; federal/state/industry relations; continuity of operations; scientific expertise in biological, chemical, physical, and radiological terrorism; and security clearance and safeguarding classified information.[2]

> **Lead agency:** The federal department or agency assigned lead responsibility under U.S. law to manage and coordinate the federal response in a specific functional area. For the purposes of the CONPLAN, there are two lead agencies: the FBI for crisis management and FEMA for consequence management.

TABLE 18–3	Food Biosecurity Triad: Public Health Vanguard

Agency	Information
Department of Homeland Security	State Homeland Security and Emergency Services. http://www.dhs.gov/dhspublic/
Federal Emergency Management Agency (FEMA)	Antiterrorism hazard mitigation information. http://www.fema.gov/fima/antiterrorism/
	NEMB-CAP: National Emergency Management Baseline Capability Assessment Program. A program to assess, analyze, evaluate, and collectively review state capabilities against a national standard. http://www.fema.gov
Department of Health and Human Services (DHHS)	
Centers for Disease Control and Prevention (CDC)	Epi-X: The Epidemic Information Exchange System A secure Web-based communication network for public health professionals. http://www.cdc.gov/mmwr/epix/epix.html
	PHLIS: Public Health Laboratory Information System An electronic reporting system.
	PHIN: Public Health Information Network. A framework to support communication and data exchange. http://www.cdc.gov/phin/
	CDC Surveillance Systems: BioNet Combines PulseNet and the Laboratory Response Network (LRN) to detect links between disease agents during terrorist attacks. http://www.bt.cdc.gov/surveillance/bionet.asp
	EARS, Early Aberration Reporting System A syndromic surveillance tool. http://www.bt.cdc.gov/surveillance/ears/
	FoodNet: Foodborne Diseases Active Surveillance Network A laboratory-based surveillance for foodborne illness. http://www.cdc.gov/foodnet/
	NEDSS: National Electronic Disease Surveillance System A component of PHIN. This system promotes standards for data and information systems. http://www.cdc.gov/nedss/index.htm
	NETSS: National Electronic Telecommunications System for Surveillance A computerized public health system that provides the CDC with weekly data on notifiable diseases. http://www.cdc.gov/epo/dphsi/netss.htm
	PulseNet National Molecular Subtyping Network for Foodborne Disease Surveillance is a network of public health laboratories that provides an early warning system for foodborne illness. http://www.cdc.gov/pulsenet/
	CDC Response Systems: HAN: Health Alert Network A system to link local health departments and other organizations for preparedness and response. Other partners for HAN include the National Association of County and City Health Officials (NACCHO) and the Association of State and Territorial Health Officials (ASTHO). http://www.bt.cdc.gov/documentsapp/HAN/han.asp
Food and Drug Administration (FDA)	CBER, Center for Biologics Evaluation and Research "Responsible for the development of products to diagnose, treat or prevent outbreaks from exposure to the pathogens that have been identified as bioterrorist agents." http://www.fda.gov/cber/cntrbio/cntrbio.htm

continues

TABLE 18–3 *(Continued)*	
	eLEXNET: Electronic Laboratory Exchange Network An Internet-based data exchange system for federal, state, and local government food safety laboratories.
U.S. Department of Agriculture (USDA)	
Food Safety and Inspection Service (FSIS)	OFSEP, Office of Food Security and Emergency Preparedness Manages homeland security activities with FSIS. http://www.fsis.usda.gov/About_FSIS/OFSEP/index.asp
Multi-agency: FDA, CDC, USDA	FERN, Food Emergency Response Network Coordinates activities among federal, state, regional, and university laboratories to identify bioterrorist agents in food.
Industry	
Food Marketing Institute, Grocery Manufacturers of America	FoodElert Food Safety and Security Rapid Alert Database may be used in emergencies to obtain contact information and access a listserv to send e-mail messages. http://www.fmi.org/foodelert/

situation may not initially be recognizable until there are multiple casualties, and there may be multiple events with the intent to influence another event's outcome.[14] Time to detection thus is critical for tainted food to be identified and the threat neutralized.

To combat these challenges, our vanguard of public health agencies must have the resources and structure to respond. However, as noted by a report of the Trust for America's Health, there are many concerns regarding public health preparedness, including insufficient funds; unspent federal aid; agencies unprepared for stockpiling; the exclusion of local agencies, which are unprepared for natural as well as bioterrorist threats; and a workforce crisis.[29] A GAO report notes that state and local jurisdictions have requested additional guidance from the federal government on preparedness standards, and specifically cited the example of a state that had ceased testing for foodborne or waterborne diseases until more guidance was provided.[30]

Syndromic surveillance: Surveillance activities that enable early detection of epidemics with data analysis for patterns of prodromal illnesses including the use of medications, illness syndromes, or events.[28]

Consumer Engagement

The third element of the triad is the engagement of individuals/consumers. **Table 18–4** outlines some of the recommendations to consumers to raise awareness and direct action for food reserves and disaster plans in the event of a bioterrorism attack. For example, the Federal Emergency Management Agency (FEMA) has prepared both educational brochures describing personal preparation for emergencies and recommendations for specific items that should be stored in the event of an emergency. This material needs to be reviewed and revised based on simulations and surveys. Recommendations should be founded on the best in evidence-based medicine and practice.

However, should we consider individuals as active or passive partners in preparedness? Government agencies and food industries engage in preparedness activities (e.g., awareness, planning, surveillance, response, and recovery), but do individuals? As Figure 18–1 illustrates earlier in this chapter, physical and psychological consequences to the individual are antecedents to economic and political outcomes. So how well prepared are our citizens?

Most families have some stockpile of food on hand, although the suitability for use during a crisis may be limited. An ironic resource is our high prevalence of overweight and obesity, certainly a reserve of energy stores. With over 50% of our population overweight, we may analytically recognize that these individuals may be able to tolerate short-term food deprivation with the provision of water and vitamin and mineral supplements. However, although discomfort may be acceptable during intentional dieting, we know that the perception of risk is altered when the situation is not voluntary. The estimates of the amount of calories that may be necessary to sustain individuals during food shortages varies from the estimates for refugees of 2,100 calories per day[31] to the levels that were available in Biosphere 2, which was 1,780 calories per day.[32] FEMA currently recommends that shelters plan on providing 2,400 to 3,000 calories per person/per day Table 18–4. Certainly, the estimated needs will vary with energy expenditure. Are we prepared to convey messages to individuals to assist them in distinguishing discomfort from true risk?

TABLE 18–4   **Food Biosecurity Triad: Consumer Engagement**

Agency	Activity/Message	Recommendations Regarding Food for Consumers' Preparedness
Department of Homeland Security	• "Preparing makes sense" • "Make a Kit • Make a Plan • Be Informed" Web information: http://www.ready.gov[a]	Make a Kit: Supply Checklists: "Emergency supplies of water, food and clean air Recommendations include: • Water—One gallon of water per person per day, for drinking and sanitation • Food—At least a 3-day supply of non-perishable food • Can opener for food • Infant formula, if you have an infant"
Federal Emergency Management Agency (FEMA) Shelters	"Toolkit for managing the emergency consequences of terrorist incidents" Guidelines for stocking shelters following a terrorist incident.[b]	Water: Quantity required: • 1–2 gallons per person per day for drinking (infants may need more) • 1–2 gallons per person per day for sanitation needs Possible source: • Bottled water companies • Soft-drink companies • National Guard Food: Quantity required: • Three 800- to 1000-calorie meals per person per day (prepackaged or hot) • A 4- to 7-day supply should be readily accessible. Possible source: • Red Cross suppliers • Salvation Army suppliers • Local fast food vendors • Existing supplies in school and church kitchens • Local food growers, farmers, and co-ops
Individuals and families	"Food and Water in an Emergency"[c]	• Short-term (2 weeks) food supply Comments: • "Eat at least one well-balanced meal each day. • Drink enough liquid to enable your body to function properly (2 quarts per day) • Take in enough calories to enable you to do any necessary work • Include vitamin, mineral and protein supplements in your stockpile to assure adequate nutrition." Other comments and recommendations: • "If activity is reduced, healthy people can survive on half their usual food intake for an extended period and without any food for many days. Food, unlike water, may be rationed safely, except for children and pregnant women."

continues

TABLE 18–4	*(Continued)*	
Agency	**Activity/Message**	**Recommendations Regarding Food for Consumers' Preparedness**
	"Your Family Disaster Supplies Kit"[d]	Recommendations: • Food: "Include a selection of the following foods in your Disaster Supplies Kit: • Ready-to-eat canned meats, fruits and vegetables • Canned juices, milk, soup (if powdered, store extra water) • Staples—sugar, salt, pepper • High-energy foods—peanut butter, jelly, crackers, granola bars, trail mix • Vitamins • Foods for infants, elderly persons or persons on special diets • Comfort/stress foods—cookies, hard candy, sweetened cereals, lollipops, instant coffee, tea bags." Other recommendations: • Practice and maintain your plan. Long-term (greater than 2 weeks) Food: "Store large amounts of staples along with a variety of canned and dried foods Stock the following amounts per person per month: • Wheat—20 pounds • Powdered milk (for babies and infants)—20 pounds* • Corn—20 pounds • Iodized salt—1 pound • Soybeans—10 pounds • Vitamin C—15 gms" Supplies: A hand-cranked grain mill to grind the corn and wheat
Department of Health and Human Services (DHHS) Food and Drug Administration (FDA) Center for Food Safety and Applied Nutrition (CFSAN)	"Food Tampering: An Extra Ounce of Caution"[e]	Recommendations: • Examine food packaging. • Check anti-tampering devices. • Do not eat food from a package that appears damaged
U.S. Department of Agriculture (USDA)	"Food Safety and Food Security: What Consumers Need to Know"[f]	Recommendations: • Examine all food product packaging. • Be aware of the normal appearance of food containers. • Contact local health department or law enforcement agency if tampering is suspected and preserve the evidence. "Most of the food safety practices already in place apply equally to intentional contamination." To report unusual characteristics of meat, poultry, and egg products: USDA Meat and Poultry Hotline: 1-888-674-6854

[a]U.S. Department of Homeland Security. *Ready.gov*. Available at http://www.ready.gov. Accessed May 13, 2010.

[b]Federal Emergency Management Agency. *Toolkit for Managing the Emergency Consequences of Terrorist Incidents. Appendix A—Biological Weapons*. July 2002. Available at http://www.oregon.gov/OMD/OEM/docs/dom_prep/01-_table_of_contents.pdf. Accessed May 14, 2010.

[c]Federal Emergency Management Agency. *Food and Water in an Emergency*. Available at www.fema.gov/pdf/library/f&web.pdf. Accessed June 21, 2010.

[d]Federal Emergency Management Agency. *Your Family Disaster Supplies Kit*. Available at www.fdem-mediacenter.org/PDF/Family_Disaster_Supplies.pdf. Accessed June 21, 2010.

[e]Center for Food Safety and Applied Nutrition, Food and Drug Administration. *Food Tampering: An Extra Ounce of Caution*. Available at www.fda.gov/downloads/Food/ResourcesForYou/.../ucm079231.pdf. Accessed June 21, 2010.

[f]Food Safety and Inspection Service, U.S. Department of Agriculture. *Food Safety and Food Security: What Consumers Need to Know*. Available at www.fsis.usda.gov/oa/topics/foodsec_cons.pdf. Accessed May 13, 2010.

*Families with infants should stock infant formula as opposed to powdered milk.

Our current food culture has substantially lessened the need for food preparation skills and familiarity with raw foods. Yet, the foods recommended by FEMA for long-term food supply (greater than 2 weeks) includes grinding corn and wheat. What data should be gathered to provide insight into the utility of these recommendations? Food preparation skills are rapidly diminishing in our population. Do we have a mechanism for disseminating information in a time of crisis? The actual endpoint may be more related to psychological well-being than actual food intake.

There is a lack of survey and observational data on consumer reaction to a bioterrorist attack. One observational study examined a simulated attack and found that 50% of residents said they would compete for vaccine for themselves and their families, and 75% said they would comply with a rumor of quarantine and not try to leave.[33] Overall, the sample indicated that before the bioterrorism agent was identified and implications were known, they would put more trust in local sources of information; after the bioterrorism was confirmed, no single source of information was preferred. The sample size for this exercise was small ($N = 39$), but the issues raised are very important, and additional scenarios involving contaminated food are necessary.

Should we challenge ourselves and our neighbors to engage in food preparedness by conducting drills? We recognize the need for first responders and public health officials to be familiar with response processes, yet consumers do not have specific events to increase food biosecurity awareness. It may be beneficial to have a "vanguard" exercise periodically, such as the last week of June leading up to the Fourth of July. This exercise might serve to raise awareness, build skills, and engage in the preparedness process. Such an exercise may have specific goals such as:

- Review food and water supplies, including dating and circulating food stocks.
- Stockpile the appropriate amount of water and food for short-term needs.
- Include the preparation of one raw food during the vanguard period.
- Do a food safety check of the home.

These activities could be integrated with other measures to improve preparedness. Families may then be better prepared, both physically and psychologically, for a disruption in food availability that may actually have the most benefit during natural disasters. It would be an opportunity to raise awareness and support of food banks also.

Currently, our citizens are not prepared to make reasonable decisions on food biosecurity. Can these limitations be overcome with central planning and resources? How much physical and psychological damage can be diminished with preparedness, and, therefore, how much can we safeguard against economic and political consequences?

■ FROM AWARENESS TO SECURITY

The events of September 2001 have reshaped our national awareness of food safety related to the potential of a bioterrorism attack. Accomplishments to date have focused on critically vulnerable areas but, given the scope of the challenge, significant risks remain. As previously noted, the FDA has summarized our current situation by concluding that there is a high likelihood of an attack on the food supply.[4] Of additional concern is the potential for engineered bioweapons, which may increase the ability of a virus to kill infected cells, overcome vaccine-induced immunity, increase the agent's ability to survive environmental stress, and increase the potential for dissemination.[34] The technology required to produce such weapons is not obscure, and Smith and others[34] noted that, "The distinction between good biology and its 'dark side' lies only in intent and application."

Public health nutritionists possess skills and competencies to support preparedness at all levels, including community interventions and consumer outreach. Consider their didactic and experiential training in food safety, nutritional requirements, nutrition education, and food service management. Professional associations may play a pivotal role in raising awareness among these individuals that they may serve as responders should a foodborne bioweapon or chemical weapon be suspected or confirmed. Such resources are vital to preserve and sustain food security.

Issues for Discussion

1. How well-prepared are our communities to provide food to individuals in the event of an intentional attack on the food supply? In the event of an attack that compromises access to food? In the event of a quarantine?

2. What research is necessary to identify community and consumer capacity to use food on hand in the event of food shortages?

3. What priority should food security receive in public health preparedness efforts?

4. What level of investment is appropriate for security of the food supply, and who should provide the funding?

5. Are public health nutritionists involved in preparedness activities?

6. What role should nutrition professionals assume for risk assessment, surveillance, planning, response, and recovery in the event of an attack?

■ TERMS RELEVANT TO PUBLIC HEALTH PREPAREDNESS

Agroterrorism: The deliberate introduction of a disease agent, either against livestock or into the food chain, for purposes of undermining the socioeconomic stability and/or generating fear.[9]

Biologic toxin: The toxic material of plants, animals, microorganisms, viruses, fungi, or infectious substances of a recombinant molecule, whatever its origin or method of production, including 1) any poisonous substance or biological product engineered as a result of biotechnology produced by a living organism; or 2) any poisonous isomer of biologic products, homolog, or derivative of such a substance.[35]

Carriers: Infected humans who can transmit contagious diseases to other humans.[36]

CDC: Bioterrorism Agents/Diseases
  Category A
  - Can be easily disseminated or transmitted from person to person
  - Result in high mortality rates and have the potential for major public health impact
  - Might cause public panic and social disruption
  - Require special action for public health preparedness
  Category B
  - Are moderately easy to disseminate
  - Result in moderate morbidity rates and low mortality rates
  - Require specific enhancements of the CDC's diagnostic capacity and enhanced disease surveillance
  Category C
    Emerging pathogens that could be engineered for mass dissemination in the future because of availability, ease of production and dissemination, and potential for high morbidity and mortality rates and major health impact.[37]

Consequence management: Includes measures to protect public health and safety; restore essential government services; and provide emergency relief to governments, businesses, and individuals affected by the consequences of terrorism. A consequence management response will be managed by FEMA using structures and resources of the Federal Response Plan (FRP).[14]

Crisis management: Crisis management is predominantly a law enforcement function and includes measures to identify, acquire, and plan the use of resources needed to anticipate, prevent, and/or resolve a threat or act of terrorism.

Debarment: Authorizes the FDA to debar (prohibit from importing food) persons who have been convicted of a felony relating to the importation of any food or who have engaged in a pattern of importing adulterated food that presents a threat of serious adverse health consequences or death to humans or animals.[38]

Disaster field office (DFO): An office established in or near the designated area to support federal and state response and recovery operations. The disaster field office houses the federal coordinating officer (FCO), the emergency response team, and, where possible, the state coordinating officer and support staff.

Emergency operations center (EOC): Site from which civil government officials (municipal, county, state, and federal) exercise direction and control in an emergency.

Emergency public information: Information that is disseminated primarily in anticipation of an emergency or at the actual time of an emergency; in addition to providing information, it frequently directs actions, instructs, and transmits direct orders.

Emergency response team: A team composed of federal program and support personnel, which FEMA activates and deploys into an area affected by a major disaster or emergency.

Emergency support function: A functional area of response activity established to facilitate coordinated federal delivery of assistance required during the response phase to save lives, protect property and health, and maintain public safety.

Evacuation: Organized, phased, and supervised dispersal of civilians from dangerous or potentially dangerous areas, and their reception and care in safe areas.

Federal coordinating officer (FCO): Person appointed by the FEMA director, following a declaration of a major disaster or of an emergency by the president, to coordinate federal assistance.

Federal Response Plan (FRP): Plan designed to address the consequences of any disaster or emergency situation in which there is a need for federal assistance.

First responder: Local police, fire, and emergency medical personnel who first arrive on the scene of an incident and take action to save lives, protect property, and meet basic human needs.

Incubation period: Time between exposure and appearance of symptoms of a disease, syndrome, or illness.

Infectivity: Ease with which a microorganism establishes itself in a host species.

Joint information center (JIC): A center established to coordinate the federal public information activity on-scene.

Lead federal agency (LFA): Agency designated by the President to lead and coordinate the overall federal response; it is determined by the type of emergency.

Local government: Any county, city, village, town, district, or political subdivision of any state, Indian tribe or authorized tribal organization, or Alaska Native village or organization, including any rural community or unincorporated town or village or any other public entity.

Mitigate: To cause to become less harsh or hostile; to make less severe or painful.[39]

Public information officer: Official at headquarters or in the field responsible for preparing and coordinating the dissemination of public information in cooperation with other responding federal, state, and local agencies.

Recovery plan: A plan developed by each state, with assistance from the responding federal agencies, to restore the affected area.

Regional director: The director of one of FEMA's 10 regional offices and principal representative for working with other federal regions, state and local governments, and the private sector in that jurisdiction.

Regional operations center (ROC): Temporary operations facility for the coordination of federal response and recovery activities, located at the FEMA regional office.

State coordinating officer: An official designated by the governor of the affected state, upon a declaration of a major disaster or emergency, to coordinate state and local disaster assistance efforts with those of the federal government, and to act in cooperation with the FCO to administer disaster recovery efforts.

Toxicity: Relative severity of the illness or incapacitation produced by a toxin.

Trace backward: Retailers, wholesalers, carriers, and others who have received products from federally inspected meat, poultry, or egg processing establishments should be able to identify the source of the products quickly and efficiently.[40]

Trace forward: Shippers (including operators of federally inspected meat, poultry, and egg processing establishments) and carriers should have systems in place for quickly and effectively locating products that have been distributed to wholesalers and retailers.[40]

Transmissibility: Ease with which disease is transmitted by victims. Methods may be direct (personal contact), indirect (through material contaminated by the infected person), or secondary (through particles spread by coughing or sneezing).

Vectors: Infected animals or insects that serve as hosts to the organism.

Weaponization for aerosol: As it pertains to the use of anthrax as a bioterrorist weapon, this generally involves use of a small particle size, a high concentration of spores, treatment to reduce clumping, neutralization of the electrical charge, and use of antimicrobial-resistant strains or genetic modification of the organism to increase virulence or escape vaccine protection.[41]

Weapon of mass destruction (WMD): Any device, material, or substance used in a manner, in a quantity or type, or under circumstances evidencing an intent to cause death or serious injury to persons or significant damage to property.

References

1. Osterholm MT, Schwartz J. *Living Terrors: What America Needs to Know to Survive the Coming Bioterrorist Catastrophe.* New York: Dalacort Press; 2000.
2. Sobel J, Khan AS, Swerdlow DL. Threat of a biological terrorist attack on the U.S. food supply: the CDC perspective. *Lancet.* 2002;359:874–880.
3. Torok TJ, Tauxe RV, Wise RB, et al. A large community outbreak of salmonellosis caused by intentional contamination of restaurant salad bars. *JAMA.* 1997;278:389–395.
4. Center for Food Safety and Applied Nutrition, Food and Drug Administration. *Risk Assessment for Food Terrorism and Other Food Safety Concerns.* October 7, 2003. Available at http://www.fda.gov/OHRMS/DOCKETS/98fr/03-25850. Accessed March 13, 2010.
5. Wheelis M. Agricultural biowarfare & bioterrorism: an analytical framework & recommendations for the fifth BTWC review conference. *Bioscience,* 2002.
6. Halliday ML, Kang L-Y, Zhou T-K, et al. An epidemic of hepatitis A attributable to the ingestion of raw clams in Shanghai China. *J Infect Dis.* 1991;164:852–859.
7. Hall MJ, Norwood AE, Ursao RJ, Fullerton CS. The psychological impacts of bioterrorism. *Biosecur Bioterror.* 2003;1:139–144.
8. Committee on Responding to the Psychological Consequences of Terrorism, National Research Council. *Preparing for the Psychological Consequences of Terrorism: A Public Health Strategy.* Washington, DC: National Academy Press; 2003.
9. Chalk P. *Hitting America's Soft Underbelly: The Potential Threat of Deliberate Biological Attacks Against the U.S. Agricultural and Food Industry.* Santa Monica, CA: RAND Publications; 2004.
10. Neff J. Food industry deals with crisis: from disruptions to previously unimaginable threats, the food industry braces for a new reality post-Sept. 11. *Food Processing.* 2001;Nov 2.
11. Nestle M. *Safe Food: Bacteria, Biotechnology, and Bioterrorism.* Berkeley, CA: University of California Press; 2003.
12. Trevejo RT, Courtney JG, Starr M, Vugia DJ. Epidemiology of salmonellosis in California, 1990–1999: Morbidity, mortality, and hospitalization costs. *Am J Epidemiol.* 2003;157:48–57.
13. Meadows M. The FDA and the fight against terrorism. *FDA Consumer Mag.* 2004: January–February.
14. Federal Bureau of Investigation. *U.S. Government Interagency Domestic Terrorism Concept of Operations Plan.* January 2001. Available at http://www.fbi.gov/publications/conplan/conplan.pdf. Accessed May 12, 2010.
15. Rotz LD, Khan AS, Lillibridge SR, Ostroff SM, Hughes JM. Public health assessment of potential biological terrorism agents. *CDC Emerging Infect Dis.* 2002;8(2):225–230. Available at http://www.cdc.gov/ncidod/EID/vol8no2/01-0164.htm. Accessed May 12, 2010.
16. Federal Emergency Management Agency. *Managing the Emergency Consequences of Terrorist Incidents.* Available at www.fema.gov/pdf/plan/managingemerconseq.pdf. Accessed June 14, 2010.
17. Knobler SL, Mahmoud AAF, Pray LA. *Biological Threats and Terrorism: Assessing the Science and Response Capabilities: Workshop Summary.* Washington, DC: Institute of Medicine, National Academy Press; 2002. Available at http://www.nap.edu/openbook/0309082536/html/43.html. Accessed May 12, 2010.
18. Committee on Science and Technology for Countering Terrorism, National Research Council. *Making the Nation Safer, the Role of Science and Technology in Countering Terrorism.* Washington, DC: National Academy Press; 2002.
19. U.S. Department of Agriculture, Food Safety and Inspection Service. *Protecting America's Meat, Poultry, and Egg Products: A Report to the Secretary on the Food Security Accomplishments of the Food Safety and Inspection Service.* Available at www.

meatami.com/ht/a/GetDocumentAction/i/1455. Accessed July 21, 2010.

20. U.S. Department of Agriculture, Food Safety Inspection Service. *Keynote Address, Taking Food Safety and HACCP to a New Level.* May 17, 2002. Available at http://www.fsis.usda.gov/OA/speeches/2002/mp_haccp.htm. Accessed May 12, 2010.

21. Bledsoe GE, Rasco BA. Addressing the risk of bioterrorism in food production. *Food Technol.* 2002;56:43–47.

22. Government Accounting Office. *Bioterrorism: A Threat to Agriculture and the Food Supply.* Testimony Before the Committee on Governmental Affairs, U.S. Senate. November 19, 2003. Washington, DC: GAO. GAO-04-259T.

23. Strongin RJ. How vulnerable is the nation's food supply? Linking food safety and food security. *Nat Health Policy Forum.* 2002; 773:2–22.

24. Dyckman LJ. *Federal Food Safety and Security System: Fundamental Restructuring Is Needed to Address Fragmentation and Overlap.* Testimony Before the Subcommittee on Civil Service and Agency Organization, Committee on Government Reform, House of Representatives. Washington, DC: Government Accounting Office; March 30, 2004. GAO-04-588T.

25. Food and Drug Administration. *FDA Science Board Advisory Committee.* November 6, 2003. Available at http://www.fda.gov/ohrms/dockets/ac/03/transcripts/4001t1.txt. Accessed May 12, 2010.

26. Buehler JW, Berkelman RL, Hartley DM, Peters CJ. Syndromic surveillance and bioterrorism-related epidemics. *Emerging Infect Dis.* 2003;9(10). Available at http://www.cdc.gov/ncidod/EID/vol9no10/03-0231.htm. Accessed May 12, 2010.

27. Ashford DA, Kaiser RM, Bales ME, et al. Planning against biological terrorism: Lessons from outbreak investigations. *Emerging Infect Dis.* 2003;9:515–519.

28. Buehler JW, Berkelman RL, Hartley DM, Peters CJ. Syndromic surveillance and bioterrorism-related epidemics. *Emerg Infect Dis.* 2003;9:1197–1204. Available at http://www.cdc.gov/ncidod/EID/vol9no10/03-0231.htm. Accessed May 12, 2010.

29. *Trust for America's Health. Ready or Not? Protecting the Public's Health from Disease, Disaster, and Bioterrorism.* December 2009. Available at http://www.healthyamericans.org. Accessed March 14, 2010.

30. General Accounting Office. *Bioterrorism: Preparedness Varied across State and Local Jurisdictions.* Report to Congressional Committees. Washington, DC: GAO; April 2003. GAO-03-373.

31. United Nations News Service, Relief Web. UN Appeals for $10 Million to Feed Refugees in Ethiopia This Year. February 24, 2004. Available at http://www.reliefweb.int/w/rwb.nsf/s/42DD226AEE3B209285256E440069149D. Accessed May 12, 2010.

32. Walford RL, Harris SB, Gunion MW. The calorically restricted low-fat nutrient-dense diet in Biosphere 2 significantly lowers blood glucose, total leukocyte count, cholesterol, and blood pressure in humans. *Proc Natl Acad Sci.* 1992;89:11533–11537.

33. DiGiovanni C, Reynolds B, Harwell R, Stonecipher EB, Burkle FM. Community reaction to bioterrorism: prospective study of simulated outbreak. *Emerging Infect Dis.* 2003;9:708–712.

34. Smith BT, Inglesby TV, O'Toole T. Biodefense R&D: anticipating future threats, establishing a strategic environment. *Biosecur Bioterror.* 2003;1:193–202.

35. Food and Drug Administration. *Chemical and Biological Emergency Response Plan.* Available at http://www.cdc.gov/mmwr/preview/mmwrhtml/rr4904a1.htm. Accessed May 7, 2010.

36. Federal Emergency Management Agency. *Toolkit for Managing the Emergency Consequences of Terrorist Incidents. Appendix A—Biological Weapons.* July 2002. Available at http://www.oregon.gov/OMD/OEM/docs/dom_prep/01-_table_of_contents.pdf. Accessed May 14, 2010.

37. Centers for Disease Control and Prevention. *Emergency Preparedness & Response.* Available at http://www.bt.cdc.gov/agent/agentlist-category.asp. Accessed May 12, 2010.

38. Food and Drug Administration. *The Bioterrorism Act of 2002: Title III. Protecting safety and security of food and drug supply.* Available at http://www.fda.gov/RegulatoryInformation/Legislation/ucm155769.htm Accessed April 19, 2010.

39. U.S. Department of Homeland Security. *Ready. Prepare. Plan. Stay Informed.* Available at http://www.ready.gov. Accessed May 12, 2010.

40. U.S. Department of Agriculture, Food Safety and Inspection Service. *FSIS Safety and Security Guidelines for the Transportation and Distribution of Meat, Poultry, and Egg Products.* Available at http://www.fsis.usda.gov/oa/topics/transportguide_text_aug.pdf. Accessed May 12, 2010.

41. Center for Infectious Disease Research and Policy (CIDRAP) and the Infectious Diseases Society of America. *Anthrax Medical Summary.* Available at http://www.swcphp.ouhsc.edu/CD06/CERT04/Bioterrorism%20Manual/B.%20%20Anthrax/4a_Anthrax%20-%20Comprehensive%20Information.htm. Accessed April 23, 2010.

42. National Library of Medicine, Specialized Information Services. Biological Warfare. Available at http://sis.nlm.nih.gov/enviro/biologicalwarfare.htm. Accessed July 21, 2010.

43. Mead PS, Slutsker L, Dietz V, et al. Food-related illness and death in the United States. *CDC Emerg Infect Dis.* 2000;5. Available at http://www.cdc.gov/ncidod/eid/vol5no5/mead.htm. Accessed April 12, 2009.

44. Centers for Disease Control and Prevention. Fact Sheet: Anthrax Information for Healthcare Providers. Available at http://www.bt.cdc.gov/agent/anthrax/anthrax-hcp-factsheet.asp. Accessed April 23, 2009.

45. Centers for Disease Control and Prevention. Botulism, General Information. Available at http://www.cdc.gov/nczved/divisions/dfbmd/diseases/botulism. Accessed July 21, 2010.

46. Centers for Disease Control and Prevention. Anthrax: Diagnosis/Evaluation (Signs and Symptoms). Available at http://www.bt.cdc.gov/agent/anthrax/diagnosis/index.asp. Accessed April 2, 2009.

47. Center for Infectious Disease Research and Policy. Initial Assessment of Food System Biosecurity Threats. Available at http://www.cidrap.umn.edu/cidrap/content/biosecurity/food-biosec/threats/assess.html. Accessed March 22, 2009.

48. Centers for Disease Control and Prevention. Questions and Answers About Plague. Available at http://www.cdc.gov/ncidod/dvbid/plague/qa.htm. Accessed April 2, 2009.

49. Centers for Disease Control and Prevention. Tularemia, Frequently Asked Questions About Tularemia. Available at http://www.bt.cdc.gov/agent/tularemia/faq.asp. Accessed April 23, 2009.

50. Centers for Disease Control and Prevention. Brucellosis, Technical Information. Available at http://www.cdc.gov/ncidod/dbmd/diseaseinfo/brucellosis_t.htm. Accessed April 2, 2009.

51. Centers for Disease Control and Prevention. Salmonellosis, General Information. Available at http://www.cdc.gov/nczved/divisions/dfbmd/diseases/salmonellosis/. Accessed April 2, 2009.

52. Centers for Disease Control and Prevention. Escherichia Coli O157:H7, General Information. Available at http://www.cdc.gov/nczved/divisions/dfbmd/diseases/ecoli_o157h7/. Accessed April 2, 2009.

53. Centers for Disease Control and Prevention. Shigellosis, General Information. Available at http://www.cdc.gov/nczved/divisions/dfbmd/diseases/shigellosis/. Accessed April 2, 2009.

PART

VI

Managing the System

Part VI provides fundamental information about public health nutrition funding. Chapter 19 details how nutrition services are planned and evaluated so that effective programs can be implemented that will result in positive performance and financial outcomes. To evaluate the effectiveness and cost of a program, data must be collected and managed appropriately, as discussed in Chapter 20. Finally, Chapter 21 examines how money is managed, which will help take public health nutrition through the stages from funding to appropriations.

CHAPTER 19

JULIE M. MORESCHI, MS, RD, LDN

Planning and Evaluating Nutrition Services for the Community

READER OBJECTIVES

After studying this chapter and reflecting on the contents, you should be able to:

1. Define planning.
2. List the types of planning.
3. Discuss the need for and advantages of planning.
4. Discuss the history of health education planning models.
5. Become familiar with a variety of planning models that could be applied when the reader is responsible for program management.
6. Understand the elements of program implementation.
7. List the value of a planning group and identify the potential membership.
8. Describe why program evaluation is essential.
9. Discuss program impact evaluation.
10. Discuss cost-effectiveness evaluation.

■ INTRODUCTION

What is planning? Why is planning of tremendous relevance to a public health nutritionist's success? This chapter will help expand your ability to answer these questions, and you will be able to use the concepts presented here to enhance your work performance in this essential management area.

Planning refers to the management function that involves setting goals and deciding the best route for achieving them. In essence, planning deals with the what, where, when, and how of management. It focuses on solving problems and planning for events in the future. Planning is continuous. It involves following certain steps, and proceeding with these steps in a logical, preset manner, as listed in these the steps[1]:

1. Understanding and engaging
2. Assessing needs
3. Setting goals and objectives
4. Developing an intervention
5. Implementing the intervention
6. Evaluating the results

Types of Planning

There are three main types of planning in public health: strategic, long-term (planning that addresses an organization's overall goals and usually encompasses 3–5 years), and operational (short-term, and deals with the activities required to meet the organization's goals).

A public health nutritionist is involved in all three of these types of planning. Of the three, the nutrition professional in public health is most often involved in program/project management. Program/project management can occur in any of the three types of planning listed above. The majority of this chapter thus focuses on the planning, implementation, and evaluation aspects of this form of management.

A great deal of data are available regarding the health status of the U.S. population. Many of the health issues affecting this population can be significantly improved by nutrition and lifestyle changes. It follows that the public health nutritionist may find him- or herself creating and implementing programs to impact these relevant and profound health concerns.

For example, in 2006–2010 the three leading causes of death in the United States, as reported by the Center for Disease Control's (CDC) National Vital Statistics System,[2] were diseases of the heart, malignant neoplasm, and cerebrovascular diseases, as discussed in previous chapters. The top three risk factors that contribute to the leading causes of death in the United States are smoking, alcohol consumption, and poor nutrition/diet.[3] Health promotion and disease prevention activities focused on these risk factors could substantially impact on unnecessary illness and death. In addition, a public health nutritionist could be involved in implementing programs relevant to achieving the objectives of *Healthy People 2020*[4] Planning is essential in the implementation of programs that answer the call to reduce or eliminate these particular healthcare problems.

As discussed in Chapter 3, when conducting a needs assessment in the community, a public health nutritionist may discover certain nutritional issues that trigger the need for program planning. The following are some program planning tasks:

- Assess the needs of the target population
- Identify the problem(s)
- Develop appropriate goals and objectives
- Create an intervention that is likely to achieve desired results
- Implement the intervention
- Evaluate the results

The process of program planning can provide several advantages to an organization. Some of them include:

- Consensus and prioritization regarding organizational goals
- Identification of key membership relative to the project
- Development of specific, measurable objectives
- Identification of steps necessary to reach the established goals
- Sharing task completion among all project members
- Setting specific target dates for task completion
- Focusing on outcomes that will impact the population being served

In summary, planning focuses on approaching work in an organized and defined manner. This results in positive outcomes for employees, managers, and the members of the community that are served.

■ HISTORY OF HEALTH EDUCATION PLANNING

When approaching public health planning, organizations have no shortage of available models to consider as resources and for potential adoption into their facilities. This fact is illustrated in a 1995 review by Carol Campbell of the Mississippi Cooperative Extension Service. Her article, "Health Education Planning Models—A Review of the Literature, Part II," presented models that since then have been used in a variety of settings and resulted in some degree of success. Campbell also suggested a generic set of tasks that are necessary to planning, regardless of the model selected or designed (**Table 19–1**).[5]

■ PLANNING MODELS

Most public health nutritionists find it helpful to have a variety of planning models to choose from when organizing and implementing public health programs. A variety of models may be needed due to the nature of the project, or a nutritionist and/or the project team may embrace the concepts of one model over another. When choosing a model, the project team should keep in mind that any chosen model serves as a frame from which to build, and provides structure and organization for the planning process. No model is perfect. The public health nutritionist can decide to use a model in its entirety, in parts, or by combining elements from a variety of models. Doing so assures a good fit to meet the demands of the individual project's mission and goals.

The following section acquaints the reader with a variety of program planning models, and serves as a reference when selecting models to use in tackling their organization or community public health issues. We begin by discussing two historic models used in large governmental project applications.

Logic Model

During the 1960s a planning approach called the Logic Model was developed. Logic Models are often used for managing projects for the U.S. government, and a public health nutritionist most likely will be exposed to an application of it when working on large collaborative projects. A *Logic Model* is a framework for building a common language for accountability and evaluation across the organization. Logic Models are often referred to as a "roadmap," and they serve to display the sequence of actions that describe what the program is and what it will do. It is a simple linear model that includes elements related to inputs, outputs, and outcomes. An example of a Logic Model is given in **Figure 19–1**, where the CDC charts a sequence of gathering information about a youth campaign.

Several organizations—such as the W.K. Kellogg Foundation, CDC, United Way of America, Harvard Family Research Project, and several State Cooperative Extension Services—currently use the Logic Model as their planning framework. Logic models have a variety of advantages to a project team. They keep everyone moving in the same direction, provide a common language and common points of reference for the project team, and create a map of action.

TABLE 19–1	Health Education Planning Models	
Planning Model	**Author**	**Year Developed**
Comprehensive Health Education Model	Sullivan	1973
Model of Health Education Planning	Ross and Mico	1980
The PRECEDE Framework	Green et al.	1980
Model for Health Education Planning and Resource Development	Bates and Winder	1984
Generic Health/Fitness Delivery System	Patton, Corry, Gettman and Graf	1986
Community Wellness Model	Jenkins	1991
The PRECEDE-PROCEED Model	Green and Keuter	1991
The PEN-3 MODEL	Airhihenbuwa	1992
APEXPH and PATCH	Centers for Disease Control and Prevention	1993
Formative Evaluation, Consultation, and Systems Technique	Goodman and Wandersman	1994
The PRECEDE-PROCEED Model for for public health education	Ottoson and Green	2001
The PRECEDE-PROCEED Model for patient counseling	Chiang and Lu	2003
The PRECEDE-PROCEED Model for educational and ecological approach	Green and Kreuter	2005

Sources: Adapted from Campbell C. *Health Education Planning Models—A Review of the Literature, Part II*. Mississippi Cooperative Extension Service; 1995. Green LW, Kreuter MW. *Health Program Planning: An Educational and Ecological Approach*. 4th ed. New York: McGraw-Hill Higher Education, 2005. Kreuter MW, Lezin N, Kreuter M, Green LW. *Community Health Promotion Ideas That Work*, 2nd ed. Sudbury, MA: Jones & Bartlett Publishers, 2003. Ottoson JM, Green LW. Public health education and health promotion. In Novick LF, Mays GP, eds. *Public Health Administration: Principles for Population-Based Management*. 2nd ed. Sudbury, MA: Jones & Bartlett Publichers. 2006:300–323. Chiang L, Huang J, Lu C. Educational diagnosis of self-management behaviors of parents with asthmatic children by triagulation based on PRECEDE-PROCEED model in Taiwan. *Patient Education and Counseling* 2003:49:19–25.

APEXPH and PATCH

Assessment Protocol for Excellence in Public Health (APEXPH) and Planned Approach To Community Health (PATCH) are two planning processes developed by the CDC. APEXPH was designed for use by local public health departments, and a workbook is available to assist in implementing the program. The program consists of three major parts:

Part I: Organizational capacity assessment

Part II: The community process

Part III: Completing the cycle

In Part I, the public health department conducts a self-assessment and determines the strengths and weaknesses of the organization in meeting the community's health needs. In Part II, the community health needs are assessed and health status goals and program objectives are defined. Part III establishes the basic monitoring and evaluation tools.

PATCH is a model intended for use in implementing chronic disease prevention and health promotion programs.

PATCH was originally established in the mid-1980s with good results; APEXPH was introduced in 1993 to enhance the existing PATCH model. Similar to PRECEDE, the model begins with the individual in mind. PATCH incorporates five phases:

Phase I: Mobilize the community. A group is formed to define the community, address health issues, and create working groups.

Phase II: Collect and analyze data. Data are collected and used to determine health priorities and program planning.

Phase III: Choose health priorities and target groups. Program objectives and goals are established using data from Phase II.

Phase IV: Choose and conduct interventions. Health interventions are designed and implemented.

Phase V: Evaluate PATCH process and interventions. Programs and the PATCH process are evaluated.

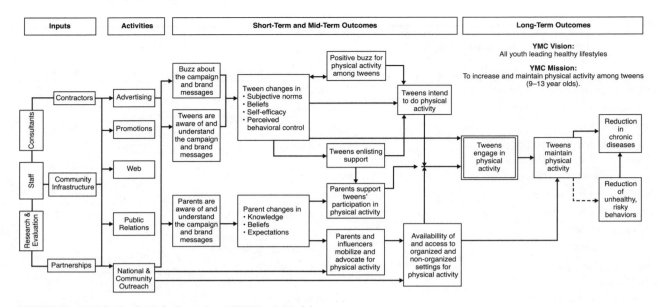

FIGURE 19–1 CDC's Youth Media Campaign, VERB™ Logic Model

Source: Centers for Disease Control and Prevention, *CDC Youth Media Campaign, VERB™ Logic Model.* Available at http://www.cdc.gov/youthcampaign/research/PDF/LogicModel.pdf. Accessed February 24, 2010.

Project models are often placed into one of two categories: ecological models and consumer based models. An *ecological model* strives to explain health-related behaviors and environments, and to design and evaluate the interventions needed to influence both the behaviors and the living conditions that influence them and their consequences. *Consumer based models* are based on consumer input and designed with consumers in mind.

Ecological Models

PRECEDE-PROCEED

PRECEDE-PROCEED is a nine-phase planning model (**Figure 19–2**). Gold, Green, and Kreuter's[6] overarching principle in this model is that most lasting health behavior change is voluntary in nature and must include input from the individual. This principle is reflected in a methodical planning process, which empowers individuals with understanding, motivation, skills, and active engagement in community affairs to improve their quality of life. The model begins with the end or final consequence and works back to the causes. PRECEDE, an acronym for Predisposing, Reinforcing, and Enabling Constructs in Educational/Environmental Diagnosis and Evaluation, is the diagnostic and needs assessment phase. The PROCEED element of this model refers to the developmental stage of planning and begins the implementation and evaluation process. Its acronym is Policy, Regulatory, and Organizational Constructs in Educational and Environmental Development.

MATCH

The Multilevel Approach to Community Health (MATCH) planning model was developed in the late 1980s by Simons-Morton and colleagues.[7] The planning model includes five phases: goal selection, intervention planning, program development, implementation, and evaluation. This model emphasizes that intervention approaches can and should be aimed at a variety of objectives and individuals.

> Examples of MATCH planning models are online:
>
> http://clinicaltrials.gov/show/NCT00385866
> http://www.healthierus.gov/steps/summit/prevportfolio/programs/cancer.htm

Consumer-Based Model

CDCynergy

CDCynergy was developed in 1998 by the CDC's Office of Communication.[8] Its original intent was that it would be used by health education professionals working at the CDC. Because the planning approach generated interest from other public health professionals, in 2001 the CDC in conjunction with the Society for Public Health Education made CDCynergy available for use by others.[9] The program is provided via use of a CD-ROM. A program planner could begin by using CDCynergy's Basic Edition, which includes the planning model, a wealth of reference resources and materials, and a guide to planning and evaluating a health communication project. There are also CD-ROM editions focused on the topics of cardiovascular, micronutrients, diabetes, tobacco prevention and control, American Indian/Alaskan Native Diabetes, Emergency Risk Communication (ERC), social marketing, and sexually transmitted disease

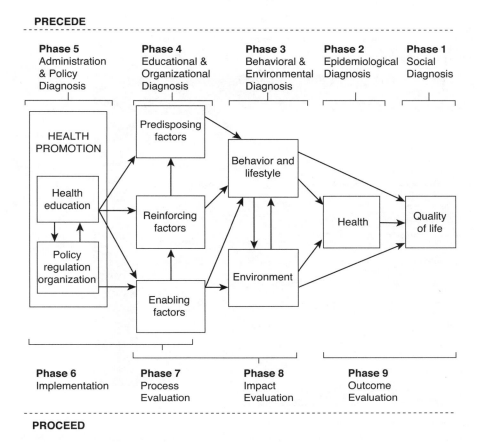

PRECEDE

FIGURE 19–2 PRECEDE-PROCEED Planning Model
Source: Gold RS, Green LW, Kreuter MW. *EMPOWER: Enabling Methods of Planning and Organizing Within Everyone's Reach.* Sudbury, MA: Jones & Bartlett Publishers, 1998.

(STD) prevention. **Figure 19–3** provides an illustration of the content that a program planner can access using the CD-Cynergy model system.

Other Planning Models

The 10-Step Planning Model

The 10-Step Planning Model was developed by Thomas C. Timmreck in his book entitled *Planning, Program Development, and Evaluation.*[3] This chapter provides a brief overview of the 10-step model, but you will find detailed suggestions and guidance by reading Timmreck's entire text.

Step 1 focuses on the development of the mission statement or the information that details the overall direction and purpose of the organization. A strong mission statement can be written by considering five elements: purpose, function, structure, legitimacy, and tangibility.

Step 2 encompasses the completion of an organization and community assessment. In this step, the organization must collect and evaluate data regarding internal and external factors, resources, regulations, and policies that might

affect the feasibility and success of the program being considered for development.

Steps 3 and 6 focus on the development of program goals and objectives. Step 3 establishes the goals and objectives for needs assessment and feasibility studies, and Step 6 focuses on the project goal and objective development. *Goals* are defined as a quantified statement of a desired future state or condition; they are generally long-term and have no deadline associated with them. *Objectives* are any statement of short-term, measurable, specific activity having a specific time limit or timeline for completion. To attain objectives, you must develop a plan of action. Action steps lead to objective accomplishments, which in turn lead to goal attainment. Precision and focus in writing high-quality goals and objectives can make the difference between a program that succeeds and one that fails.

Step 4 deals with the completion of a community needs assessment. The needs assessment must focus on collecting data from an established target population. Important decisions to be made when conducting Step 4 include what data to collect, what tool to use to collect the data, and how

FIGURE 19–3 CDCynergy Model

Source: Centers for Disease Control and Prevention, *Health Marketing*. Available at http://www.cdc.gov/healthmarketing/cdcynergy/. Accessed February 24, 2010.

the data will be analyzed. Revisit Chapter 3 to refresh your memory about needs assessments.

Once the data are collected and analyzed, Step 5 focuses on methods to assist in setting priorities. There are multiple factors in the community that influence prioritization decisions, such as people, politics, and finances. A public health nutritionist can use a variety of decision-making tools and techniques to assist in making sound prioritization decisions.

Step 7 helps determine the activities and procedures that need to be performed in order to implement the programs. Factors to be considered are the actions that must take place and the order in which they should occur. Pilot projects to test certain actions may be warranted prior to large-scale implementation. Managerial elements, such as financial and marketing strategies, need to be considered and planned. Once activities are established in this step, timelines are assigned to each item in Step 8.

Steps 9 and 10 deal with implementation and evaluation, respectively. These planning elements will be discussed in detail later in the chapter.

The P Process Model

The second planning model is Johns Hopkins University Center for Communication Program's P Process.[10] The P Process provides a framework for the development of strategic health communication programs. The process was developed in 1982 and was used to help design effective communication projects for behavior change. The P Process can be used when developing:

- Project and program design
- Workshops and classes
- Brochures, reports, manuals, posters, presentations, and publications

The five steps in the P Process are described in further detail in the following sections.

Step 1: Analysis Two types of analysis should be considered: situation and audience/communication. *Situation analysis* refers to determining the severity and causes of problems, identifying factors inhibiting or facilitating desired changes, developing a problem statement, and carrying out formation research that takes the learners' needs and priorities into consideration. *Audience/communication analysis* focuses on conducting a participation analysis to identify partners, audiences, and field workers for the project, carrying out a social and behavioral analysis at the community and individual level, and assessing communication and training needs.

Step 2: Strategic Design   Step 2 deals with developing a strategic design for the project. Elements of this step include establishing clear objectives, developing program approaches, determining marketing channels, and creating implementation and evaluation plans.

Step 3: Development and Testing   The development and testing phase is where the actual program or project is developed. It is then revised as needed before full implementation. This step should not only consider the technical and scientific accuracy of the products, but also must include an element of creativity in order to better reach and engage the participants.

Step 4: Implementation and Monitoring   Implementation and monitoring deals with taking the product and disseminating it throughout the target population's community. This phase may incorporate some training or development of personnel delivering the program. The program must be monitored and changes made as necessary to assure a high-quality product.

Step 5: Evaluation and Replanning   The final step in the P Process is the evaluation and replanning phase. During this step, outcomes are measured and future needs are assessed. Programs are redesigned and revised as needed based on data collected during this phase. Outcomes during this phase may warrant that the project begin again at Step 1, the analysis phase.

The Health Communication Process

The Health Communication Process is a planning model developed by the U.S. Department of Health & Human Services, the National Institutes for Health (NIH), and the National Cancer Institute (NCI).[11] This model was first designed in 1985, and for almost 25 years an ongoing evaluation of the communication programs has confirmed the value of using specific communication strategies to promote health and prevent disease.

The Health Communication Process has four stages. Upon completion of each stage, the planners can expect to accomplish the goals shown in **Table 19–2**.

A copy of *Making Health Communication Programs Work* can be found on the Internet at http://cancer.gov/pinkbook/ or by calling NCI's Cancer Information Service.

Mobilizing for Action Through Planning & Partnerships

The Mobilizing for Action Through Planning & Partnership (MAPP) planning model was developed by the National Association of County and City Health Officials (NACCHO), in collaboration with the CDC.[12]

TABLE 19–2	**Health Communication Process Stages**

Stage

1. Planning and strategy development
2. Developing and pretesting concepts, messages, and materials
3. Implementing the program
4. Assessing effectiveness and making refinements

What Will Be Accomplished?

- Identify how the organization can use communication effectively to address a health problem.
- Identify intended audiences.
- Use consumer research to create a communication strategy and objectives.
- Draft communication plans, including activities, partnerships, and baseline survey for outcome evaluation.
- Develop relevant, meaningful messages.
- Plan activities and draft materials.
- Pretest the messages and materials with intended audience members.
- Begin program implementation, maintaining promotion, distribution, and other activities through all channels.
- Conduct process evaluation via tracking intended audience exposure and reaction to the program. Determine whether adjustments are needed.
- Periodically review all program elements and make revisions as needed.
- Assess your health communication program.
- Identify refinements that would increase the effectiveness of future programs.

MAPP purpose is to assist communities in developing frameworks to improve public health by helping them to prioritize their public health issues, identify the resources needed to address them, and to implement strategies to fit each community's unique needs.

The MAPP process consists of six phases:

Phase 1: Organize for success and partnership development

Phase 2: Visioning

Phase 3: Assessment phase including identifying community themes and strengths, a local public health system assessment, a community health status assessment, and a forces of change assessment

Phase 4: Identification of strategic issues

Phase 5: Formulate goals and strategies

Phase 6: Action cycle, which includes planning, implementing and evaluating the community's strategic plan

NACCHO provides a variety of tools to help communities in using and implementing programs using the MAPP model. Program managers can access training, a handbook, a field guide, and brochure, to assist them in using the MAPP approach to tackling the public health issues of their organization or community.

Healthy Plan-IT

The Healthy Plan-IT Model is a tool that is used by the CDC's Sustainable Management Development Program.[13] The planning tool kit uses a data-based decision-making process for planning and managing public health programs. This model focuses on preventing and controlling diseases, disabilities and premature mortality through quality management of planning, organizing, monitoring, and evaluating the use of time, personnel, and money.

The model is designed in three modules.

Module 1: Problems and Priorities   Health priorities are rated through the Basic Priority Rating System (BPRS), and which priorities make the most sense to address are determined by using the PEARL assessment system. PEARL is an acronym for propriety, economics, acceptability, resources, and legality.

Module 2: Finding Solutions   Module 2 teaches the steps involved in problem solving: identifying determinants and contributing factors to the selected health issue, setting objectives, designing an intervention strategy, and developing a work plan based on a work breakdown structure (WBS).

Module 3: Evaluation and Budget   Module 3 provides tools for monitoring and evaluating progress toward achieving the set objectives, creating budgets, and using the budget as a management tool.

MAP-IT

The Department of Health and Human Services has a program implementation guide called Healthy People in Healthy Communities, which is focused on helping communities to implement *Healthy People 2020* initiatives. The program management model used for this program is called MAP-IT.[14] (MAP-IT is available at www.healthypeople.gov/publications/HealthyCommunities2001/Chapter_2.htm.)

The MAP-IT technique is a strategy that can be applied by communities to help them to "map out" the changes they want to see in their community.

> Further information about MAPP is at http://www.naccho.org/topics/infrastructure/mapp/framework/index.cfm

MAP-IT's acronym is:

Mobilize individuals and organizations that care about the health of your community into a coalition.

Assess the areas of greatest need in your community, as well as the resources and other strengths that you can tap into to address those areas.

Plan your approach: start with a vision of where you want to be as a community; then add strategies and action steps to help you achieve that vision.

Implement your plan using concrete action steps that can be monitored and will make a difference.

Track your progress over time.

By using the MAP-IT approach, a planning team can devise a structured, step-by-step plan focused on a particular community's specific needs and goals.

■ PROGRAM IMPLEMENTATION

Program implementation can be defined as the process of putting a project, service, or program into full effect. It is the management of the execution of the project. Program implementation is a critical part of the planning process and requires the creation of an implementation action plan.

Eight factors to consider when developing an implementation plan are:

1. *Why:* The effect of the objectives to be achieved
2. *What:* The activities required to achieve the objectives
3. *Who:* The individuals responsible for each activity
4. *When:* A chronological sequence of activities and timing in relation to project implementation activities or organization events
5. *How:* The materials, supplies, technology, devices, methods, media approaches, flow of activities, or techniques to be used. Also, consideration regarding consents, medical clearances, and program safety should be addressed as appropriate.
6. *Where:* Which activities will take place at what locations in the community—at the health promotion site, facility, office, clinic, and center
7. *Cost:* An estimate of expenses for materials, personnel, facilities, and time
8. *Feedback:* When and how to tell if the activities are happening as they should be and if adjustments are needed; use timelines

With all of these elements to consider, a written implementation plan is essential. An easy method to apply when writing an implementation process is to create action plans or timetables. If a dietitian is managing a project, she/he can take elements from the eight implementation factors listed above and create a detailed timetable. Use of a timetable helps to assure that all necessary elements are included and that deadlines are established so that implementation goals may be met in a timely fashion.

There are several types of timetables or action planning formats that can be used by program managers. Some examples of such tools include Task Development Time Lines, Gantt charts, and PERT charts.

Task Development Time Lines and Gantt charts are very similar approaches. They are both a table format, which indicates the timeline in the columns, and the tasks to be completed in the rows. A sample of the Gantt chart can be found in **Figure 19–4**.

The PERT acronym is program evaluation and review technique. There are three elements in a PERT chart. A program manager begins the process of creating it by listing all activities involved in implementation of the program. To create the PERT diagram, each activity would be placed in a circle. Lines are then used to indicate the sequence of events for each task. Solid lines indicate activities that begin with one task and end with another task. Dotted lines are used to show events that are dependent on one another but for which no work is involved. **Figure 19–5** shows an example of a PERT chart.

■ DETERMINING TEAM MEMBERSHIP

An important component of any planning project is working effectively through joint efforts. Working together as a team has many benefits, such as providing the group with a variety of viewpoints and backgrounds, pooling resources to get work accomplished, satisfying personal and professional needs of the team members, and gaining community support for your initiative. Development of team membership procedures, however, often is not easy or without cause for concern. Difficult situations can arise when coordinating teams; these can be managing a large group with slow progress on action plans or decision making; difficulty in obtaining volunteer membership due to busy or conflicting schedules; and conflicts of interest of membership, particularly for those working in for-profit venues.

The *Making Health Communication Programs Work* textbook[11] provides several tools to assist planning groups to

Example: The Gantt chart below shows part of one team's test implementation. Notice the sheer volume of information you can easily absorb simply by looking at this chart. Consider its value as a tracking tool once implementation is under way.

Schedule		Week Number:								
Task	**Assigned to**	**1**	**2**	**3**	**4**	**5**	**6**	**7**	**8**	**9**
Submit draft for review	Team Leader	▓								
Review draft	Review Comm.		▓	▓						
Submit comments	Review Comm.			▓						
Revise manual based upon feedback	Team				▓	▓	▓			
Create camera-ready materials	Team Leader							▓		
Print 100 copies of manual	Print Shop								▓	
Circulate 100 copies to employees	Team Leader									▓

FIGURE 19–4 Gantt Chart

Source: Centers for Disease Control and Prevention. Available at http://www.cdc.gov. Accessed February 25, 2010.

Example: The PERT chart below is mapping out the critical path for printing and distributing a new form.

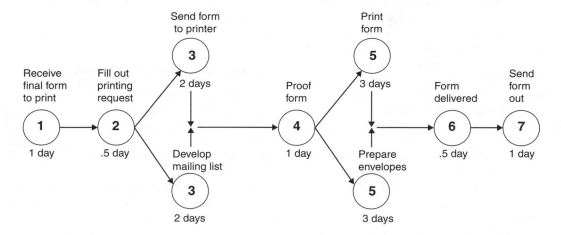

FIGURE 19–5 PERT Chart

Source: Centers for Disease Control and Prevention. Available at http://www.cdc.gov. Accessed February 25, 2010.

establish their membership. A partnership planning worksheet is supplied that asks questions regarding potential partners, partners' roles and tasks, benefits to partners when they participate on the team, as well as many other considerations. This guide also provides an excellent re-

source entitled "Steps for Involving Partners in the Program" (**Table 19–3**).

Sociologist and community planner Xavier de Souza Briggs, currently on leave from the Massachusetts Institute of Technology to serve in the White House in the Depart-

---

TABLE 19–3	**Steps for Involving Partners in the Program**

1. Choose organizations, agencies, or individuals (e.g., physicians) that can bring the resources, expertise, or credibility your program needs.

2. Consider which roles partners might play to best support the program.

3. Involve representatives of the organizations you want to work with as early as appropriate in program planning.

4. Give partners the program rationale, strategies, and messages (in ready-to-use form). Remember that strategic planning, creative messages, and quality production are the most difficult aspects of a communication program to develop and may be the most valuable product you can offer to a community organization.

5. Give partners advance notice so that they can build their part of the program into their schedule, and negotiate what will be expected of them.

6. Allow partners to personalize and adapt program materials to fit their circumstances and give them a feeling of ownership, but don't let them stray from the strategy.

7. Ask partners what they need to implement their part of the program. Beyond the question of funding, consider other

assistance, training, information, or tools that would enable them to function successfully.

8. Provide partners with new local/regional/national contacts or linkages that they will perceive as valuable for their ongoing activities.

9. Give partners an appropriate amount of work. Give them a series of small, tangible, short-term responsibilities as well as a feedback/tracking mechanism.

10. Gently remind partners that they are responsible for their activities; help them complete tasks but do not complete tasks for them.

11. Assess progress through the feedback/tracking mechanism and help make adjustments to respond to the organization's needs and to keep the program on track.

12. Provide moral support by frequently saying "thank you" and by providing other rewards (e.g., letter or certificate of appreciation).

13. Give partners a final report of what was accomplished and meet to discuss follow-up activities and resources they might find useful. Make sure that they feel they are a part of the program's success.

14. Share one final tremendous "Thank you for a job well done."

Source: U.S. Department of Health and Human Services, National Institutes of Health, National Cancer Institute, *Pink Book—Making Health Communication Programs Work.* Available at http://www.cancer.gov/pinkbook. Accessed February 25, 2010.

ment of Housing and Urban Development, promoted an original approach to looking at planning participation in 2003.[15] He suggested that when making project participation decisions, groups often focus on the how-to elements relative to participation tactics and techniques.[15]

Once the project team has been assembled, it can be important to establish guidelines as to how the group will work together. One approach to the development of such a structure is called Terms of Reference (TOR). A TOL template can assist a project manager in communicating effectively and establishing "buy in" with all team members and stakeholders. Information that can be addressed in a project TOR includes the project vision and objectives, a list of the key project deliverables and/or outcomes, a list of the team member and stakeholders along with information of their key roles and responsibilities, and an organizational structure by which the program will operate.

■ HEALTH PROGRAM EVALUATION

Benefits of Evaluation

Evaluation of health programs is essential in order to assure that objectives are being met. Health programs aim to result in efficient, effective, and quality outcomes, and the goal of an evaluation process is to prove that these aims are being realized. Evaluations focus on proving that programs are cost-effective, that managerial practices are accountable, and that the programs are contributing to improvements in the community's health.

Types of Evaluations

Several types of evaluation can be conducted, and definitions for some of them are provided here. A *formative evaluation* assesses whether a problem is occurring in a program, the extent of the problem, and if corrective action is necessary. *Summative evaluation* focuses on program impact and program effectiveness. *Program impact* assesses if interventions are producing desired outcomes, and *program effectiveness* determines if outcomes could be achieved at a lower cost, and deals specifically with cost-benefit and cost-effectiveness analysis. *Process evaluation* assesses the effectiveness of administrative activities and program implementation. It may be helpful to visualize the interrelationships that exist between the program outcomes, types of evaluations, and evaluation objectives.

Impact outcomes look at outcomes correlated with resources and cost. The PRECEDE model presented earlier in this chapter includes an element of impact outcome. This model also includes evaluation elements through the use of intermediate objectives applied to each phase of the model. Program intervention models look at the impact of outcomes. An example of such a model is based on the acronym RASOGO, an acronym for:

R – Resources lead to activities.

A – Activities lead to sub-objectives.

S – Sub-objectives lead to objectives.

O – Objectives lead to goals.

G – Goals produce outcomes.

O – Outcomes.

Evaluation as a Three-Act Play

In his book, *The Practice of Health Program Evaluation*, David Grembowksi[16] describes program evaluation as a three-act play. In the second act of his model, Grembowski discusses program impact and cost-effectiveness evaluation in great detail. Several designs can be used to measure the impact of programs, each having its own strengths and weaknesses. Designs can be pre-experimental, experimental, or quasi-experimental. The design that is chosen to measure program impact should be feasible; fit well with logistical, political, budgetary, and other constraints of the program; and be able to produce reliable results.

Cost-Effectiveness Analysis

There are three types of cost-effectiveness analysis (CEA) that can be conducted for a program:

- *Cost-benefit analysis:* A method of economic evaluation where all benefits and costs of a program are measured in dollars. Programs have value when their benefits are equal to or exceed their costs, or the ratio of $benefits/$costs is equal to or greater than 1.0, or when the benefit/cost ratio of Program A is equal to or greater than 1.0 and exceeds the benefit/cost ratio of Program B.
- *Cost-minimization analysis:* A type of CEA where Program A and Program B have identical benefit outcomes, and the goal of the analysis is to determine which program has the lower cost.
- *Cost-utility analysis:* A type of CEA in which the outcomes of Program A and Program B are weighted by their value, or quality, and measured with a common metric, such as "quality-adjusted life years." The goal of the analysis is to determine which program produces the most quality-adjusted life years at lower cost.

The 10 basic steps to conducting a CEA are:

1. Define the problem and objectives.
2. Identify alternatives.
3. Describe production relationships, or the CEA's conceptual model.
4. Define the perspective of the CEA.
5. Identify, measure, and value costs.
6. Identify and measure effectiveness.
7. Discount future costs and effectiveness.
8. Perform a sensitivity analysis.

9. Address equity issues.
10. Use CEA in decision making.

A CEA can be an intense and complicated evaluation endeavor. If a planning team has minimal experience with this concept, they may find it necessary to partner with individuals with skill and experience in conducting CEA evaluation processes.

CDC's Evaluation Process

The CDC's program evaluation process (**Figure 19–6**) is laid out in a wheel shape. This can help an organization to summarize and organize the essential elements of program evaluation, provide a common frame of reference for conducting evaluations, clarify the steps in program evaluation, review the standards of effective program evaluation, and address misconceptions about the purposes and methods of the program evaluation. A summary of the CDC evaluation model's steps follows:

Steps in Evaluation Practice

1. Engage stakeholders: Those involved, those affected, primary intended users
2. Describe the program: Need, expected effects, activities, resources, stage, context, logic model
3. Focus the evaluation design: Purpose, users, uses, questions, methods, agreements
4. Gather credible evidence: Indicators, sources, quality, quantity, and logistics
5. Justify conclusions: Standards, analysis/synthesis, interpretation, judgment, recommendations

6. Ensure use and share lessons learned: Design, preparation, feedback, follow-up, and dissemination

Standards of Effective Evaluation

1. Utility: Serve the information needs of intended users.
2. Feasibility: Be realistic, prudent, diplomatic, and frugal.
3. Propriety: Behave legally, ethically, and with due regard for the welfare of those involved and those affected.
4. Accuracy: Reveal and convey technically accurate information.

The Health Communication Planning Guide's Outcome Evaluation Process

The *Health Communication Planning Guide* does provide an outcome evaluation process component. Results of the evaluation should be used to help identify areas of the program that should be changed, deleted, or augmented. The outcome evaluation process has nine steps, as follows:

1. Determine what information the evaluation must provide.
2. Define the data to collect.
3. Decide on data collection methods.
4. Develop and pretest data collection instruments.
5. Collect data.
6. Process data.
7. Analyze data to answer the evaluation questions.
8. Write an evaluation report.
9. Disseminate the evaluation report.

FIGURE 19–6 CDC Evaluation Wheel

Source: Centers for Disease Control, *Framework for Program Evaluation in Public Health.* Available at http://www.cdc.gov/epo/mmwr/preview/mmwrhtml/rr4811a1. htm. Accessed February 25, 2010.

TABLE 19–4	Types of Program Designs[1]
Design Type	**Subtypes**
Pre-experimental	One-group posttest-only design
	One-group pretest-posttest design
	Posttest-only comparison group design
Experimental	Pretest-posttest control group design
	Posttest-only control group design
Quasi-experimental	Single time series design
	Multiple time series design
	Repeated treatment design
	Pretest-posttest nonequivalent comparison group design
	Recurrent institutional cycle design
	Regression discontinuity design

[1]Refer to statistical resources for detailed explanations of these designs.

To summarize, evaluation is an essential element in the planning process. When developing plans, groups need to consider what types of evaluation they wish to conduct. Most evaluation plans will include several elements and will deal with analysis of both the outcome and the effectiveness of programs. Several models and references are available for teams when they are developing plans for evaluation components of programs.

■ CONCLUSION

Proper planning, implementation, and evaluation of programs are important managerial functions for the public health nutritionist. A great deal of information is available for reference and support when taking on this critical community health program function. Several models are available for both planning and evaluation. The decision of which prototype to use will depend on the nature of the planning task and the team assembled to complete the work. Spending time planning before approaching an endeavor will be rewarded by a resulting product or program that positively impacts the community's health, thus contributing to professional success for the public health nutritionist and the planning team.

Issues for Discussion

1. Is planning an important skill for a public health nutritionist to possess and justify spending time doing? Justify your answer.

2. A public health nutritionist can potentially be involved in three types of planning. What types of work situations may cause a public health nutritionist to apply skills in strategic planning? Long-term planning? Operational planning?

3. You are working in a public health department and are assigned to implement a weight management program for the community.
   a. Choose a planning model presented in this chapter and discuss how to apply the model to the assigned project.
   b. Create an implementation plan for your weight management program using either a task development timeline, Gantt chart, or PERT diagram.

4. Discuss how a project manager could make decisions regarding what team members and stakeholders to include in a public health project.

5. You are continuing work on your community weight management program. Discuss what types of data and evaluation methods you would use in order to evaluate the program.

References

1. McKenzie JF, Neiger BL, Thackeray R. *Planning, Implementing, & Evaluating Health Promotion Programs: A Primer.* 5th ed. San Francisco, CA: Pearson; 2009.

2. Centers for Disease Control and Prevention (CDC), National Vital Statistics System. *Mortality data.* (2006). Available at http://www.cdc.gov/nchs/deaths.htm. Accessed May 14, 2010.

3. Timmreck TC. *Planning, Program Development, and Evaluation: A Handbook for Health Promotion, Aging, and Health Services,* 2nd ed. Sudbury, MA: Jones and Bartlett; 2003.

4. U.S. Department of Health and Human Services. *Healthy People 2020: The Road Ahead.* (2010). Available at http://www.healthypeople.gov/hp2020/. Accessed June 7, 2010.

5. Campbell C. *Health Education Planning Models—A Review of the Literature, Part II.* Mississippi State, MS: Mississippi Cooperative Extension Service; 1995.

6. Gold RS, Green LW, Kreuter MW. *EMPOWER: Enabling Methods of Planning and Organizing Within Everyone's Reach.* Sudbury, MA: Jones and Bartlett; 1998.

7. Simons-Morton DG, Simons-Morton BG, Guy S, Bunker JF. Influencing personal and environmental conditions for community health: a multilevel intervention model. *Fam Community Health.* 1988;11:25–35.

8. Centers for Disease Control and Prevention (CDC). *Framework for Program Evaluation in Public Health. MMWR Morb Mortal Wkly Rep.* 1999;48(R11):1–40. Available at http://www.cdc.gov/mmwr/preview/mmwrhtml/rr4811a1.htm. Accessed May 12, 2010.

9. CDCynergy. Centers for Disease Control and Prevention, Health Marketing. (2006). Available at http://www.cdc.gov/healthmarketing/cdcynergy/. Accessed May 14, 2010.

10. Center for Communication Programs, Johns Hopkins Bloomberg School of Public Health. *The P Process. Steps in Strategic Communication.* Available at http://www.jhuccp.org/training/scope/Pprocess_070215.htm. Accessed May 14, 2010.

11. National Cancer Institute. *Pink Book—Making Health Communication Programs Work.* Available at http://www.cancer.gov/pinkbook/page1. Accessed May 14, 2010.

12. Mobilizing for Action through Planning and Partnerships (MAPP). National Association of County and City Health Officials. (2009). Available at http://www.naccho.org/topics/infrastructure/mapp/. Accessed May 14, 2010.

13. Centers for Disease Control and Prevention (CDC). *Global Health, 2010.* Available at http://www.cdc.gov/globalhealth/. Accessed June 10, 2010.

14. U.S. Department of Health and Human Services (DHHS), Office of Disease Prevention and Health Promotion. September 1997. *Development Objectives for Healthy People 2010.* Available at http://www.healthypeople.gov/default.htm. Accessed May 14, 2010.

15. Briggs XS. *The Art and Science of Community Problem-Solving Project.* Cambridge, MA: Harvard University; 2003.

16. Grembowski D. *The Practice of Health Program Evaluation.* Thousand Oaks, CA: Sage; 2001.

CHAPTER

20

Managing Data

Elizabeth Barden, PhD

READER OBJECTIVES   After studying this chapter and reflecting on the contents, you should be able to:

1. List the purposes for which data are needed by nutrition professionals.
2. Identify how to triangulate data from different sources to gain a more complete picture of a community's health needs, constituents, and resources.
3. Recognize sources of useful data.
4. List the steps in developing a new data collection, analysis, and reporting system.

■ INTRODUCTION

All nutrition professionals need to have a basic competence with the acquisition, analysis, and interpretation of diverse types of data from various sources. Mastering the skills necessary for dealing with data is essential for any nutrition professional who wants to be able to rely on his or her own interpretation of available data, and not on the analysis of coworkers or the published opinions of others. This set of skills is particularly important in the current economic climate, where divergent agendas in combination with shrinking resources at times lead to contradictory interpretations of the same data, or at least to differing outlooks on the relative importance of competing priorities.

Learning to manage regularly released statistical summary reports and other available data sources, including primary data (also known as *raw data*), can be a tremendous advantage for any professional looking to plan relevant, meaningful, and effective nutrition programs. In addition, nutrition professionals today are not just producers and users of data, but also are consumers of data. Not only do nutritionists generate and utilize data themselves in the course of designing, managing, and evaluating their own programs, but they also stay current in their field and operate in a professional team setting by appraising the work of others. Competence with data management, analysis, and interpretation allows nutritionists to evaluate the positions others put forth, assess the quality of recommendations they receive, and evaluate the reasonableness of published research findings and public health reports.

Data can be defined broadly as information, especially information organized for analysis and decision making.[1] *Data* include, but are not confined to, statistics, which is the branch of mathematics dealing with the collection, analysis, interpretation, and presentation of numerical data.[2] Objective, statistical data (e.g., a community's leading cause of death, the percentage change in the prevalence of teen pregnancy, or per capita healthcare costs for obesity-related illness) certainly are useful for quantifying and comparing the size of need, degree of achievement toward meeting goals, and costs in relation to accomplishment. However, additional types of data, including subjective information (e.g., a community's perceived needs) are important in accurately characterizing a population and its health service requirements. The definition of what constitutes relevant data to a public health nutrition professional has expanded as the availability of information on all facets of life has become easily accessible. For instance, census data about the presence of a telephone in the household at first glance may not appear to be relevant nutrition data. However, it is a pertinent factor to know for a nutritionist who is planning a telephone survey in a given neighborhood, where he or

The valuable input of Jan Kallio, Stephanie Lambou, and Rachel Colchamiro on an earlier draft of this manuscript is greatly appreciated.

she needs to obtain a representative sample of residents, or for a nutritionist who is planning services that include follow-up telephone counseling.

Data are used in many different contexts within nutrition practice. There are at least four dimensions from which data management for nutrition practice can be considered: 1) using data to plan work (program planning and needs assessment); 2) using data to assist managerial oversight and to demonstrate the effectiveness of work (program evaluation); 3) using data to monitor a population (nutrition surveillance), define health objectives and associated benchmarks (e.g., *Healthy People 2010 and 2020*), and monitor progress towards meeting those objectives; and 4) collecting and managing new data, and/or accessing existing data sources, to address identified information deficits. This chapter addresses each of these dimensions to give an overview of some of the major issues and processes involved in managing data in a public health nutrition context.

■ DATA IN PROGRAM PLANNING AND NEEDS ASSESSMENT

An effective, successful nutrition program is achieved by following a conscientious planning process that justifies its need, inventories available resources and identifies service gaps, identifies relevant goals and objectives, defines tasks and activities to accomplish those goals, and explains how results will be evaluated and disseminated.[3] Data are used during every phase of the program planning process to achieve the following outcomes:

- Identify the need for new services or initiatives
- Recognize the need for changes in service delivery
- Prioritize competing health problems
- Identify the most appropriate at-risk target population
- Define goals and objectives
- Make decisions about allocating limited resources
- Define program performance expectations
- Justify a program's budget
- Develop proposals to secure additional funding when necessary

Needs assessment is the portion of the planning process during which a community and its particular health needs are defined. Overall, the needs assessment phase of the program planning process aims to understand the nutrition requirements of the community, prioritize their identified needs, and target resources accordingly. Chapter 3 discusses the topic of needs assessment in detail.

Identifying a specific population with specific health and nutritional status challenges and identifying gaps in existing service delivery is accomplished through close examination of both quantitative and qualitative data. A quantitative assessment includes examination of demographic, socioeco-

nomic, health status, nutritional status, and risk indicators. Data for this assessment come from a review of both regularly published public health reports and scientific research literature that are relevant to the health problem and/or the community. Qualitative methods, such as key informant interviews, focus groups, and informal conversations, derive information from health professionals, community leaders, and community members at-large regarding the community's perceived needs and demands for nutrition-related services. The more subjective information obtained from these sources is necessary to balance the more objective, statistics-driven information that comes from the quantitative assessment; both provide important pieces to the big picture. The needs assessment methodology also includes the compilation of an inventory of existing health and nutrition resources in the community and any major duplication or gaps in available services, as well as service delivery and resource utilization data. A final piece is an assessment by the program planner of the host organization's (usually his or her employer's) mission and willingness to support a proposed nutrition program, both financially and institutionally.

Typically, objective quantitative data are used in nutrition program planning to address four questions:

1. What are the health issues facing a community (problem)?
2. Where are the problems (place)?
3. Who is at risk (person)?
4. When: are problems are increasing or declining over time (time period)?

Problem

Planning often begins with an examination of which health and nutrition issues affect a community. An inventory of the leading causes of morbidity and mortality, the prevalence of chronic and infectious diseases, and the leading causes of hospitalization can give a broad overview of the health concerns of the community. These types of data typically are found in regularly published public health reports, such as state or national vital statistics reports and surveillance system reports. As an example of these types of data, **Table 20–1** presents the leading causes of death among U.S. women in 2006. From the table, it is clear that deaths from heart disease and cancer are far more common than deaths from diabetes or kidney disease, for example.

Place

Place describes geographic units, such as the nation, state, county, clinic, region, or neighborhood. Examination of data by place helps to ascertain the geographic extent of the health problem. Maps are an effective way to visually represent differences in health status data by geographical area. For example, **Figure 20–1** effectively illustrates both the increase in proportion of American adults who are obese in 2007 compared to 2002 (demonstrated by BMI ≥ 30) as well as regional differences in the prevalence of obesity across the United States, with the central and southern states having a greater prevalence of obesity than those in the west. Additionally, maps are useful for illustrating disparities in health status among communities that may be segregated in large part on the basis of certain socioeconomic characteristics, such as ethnicity or income. Use of maps to depict the geographical distribution of health problems and suspected factors in the causal pathway can be very effective in attracting the attention of key stakeholders.[4] Maps that include health, social, economic, and other asset data are relatively easy to construct now that geographical mapping technology is widely available.

Person

An accurate characterization of *person* is necessary because different groups within a larger population have different health problems and different service requirements. Person may be described in many different ways. The words *population* and *community* are sometimes used interchangeably. Most often, though, population refers to all of the inhabitants of a given region (e.g., the U.S. population, or the population of the state of California). Community, on the other hand, is usually a subset of a larger population that is defined on the basis of geographic boundaries, political boundaries, or demographic characteristics.[5] Another way that communities are defined for planning purposes is on the basis of place of residence, occupation, or other shared personal characteristics; membership in a particular insti-

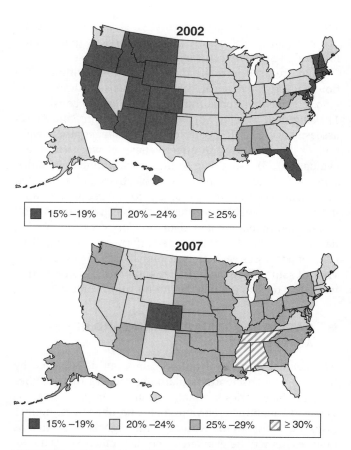

FIGURE 20–1 Obesity Map, 2002 Compared to 2007: BMI > 30
Source: Centers for Disease Control and Prevention, *Overweight and Obesity*. Available at http://www.cdc.gov/obesity/data/trends.html. Accessed February 25, 2010.

tutional setting; or the clientele of a service-delivery organization. **Table 20–2** presents some examples of different ways a community unit may be conceptualized. For instance, a demographically defined community may be described on the basis of age (e.g., preschoolers or senior citizens), gender, ethnicity, income bracket, occupation, or neighborhood (e.g., residents of Center City, Philadelphia, or San Francisco's Chinatown). More commonly, some combination of factors is used to further aggregate individuals by characteristics that may be associated with some known risk,[6] such as defining a community of teenage mothers who have not graduated from high school and who live in a particular state, or a community of housebound elderly Asian American immigrants living in Chicago. A clear, specific definition of the community early in the planning process facilitates data collection and program design.

Time Period

It is important to use data to identify changes in health problems over time. This is relevant to establishing whether existing problems have receded or intensified as well as identifying emerging health problems or an increase in

TABLE 20–1	Leading Causes of Death, Females—United States, 2006	
All Females, All Ages		**Percent[1]**
1. Heart Disease		25.8
2. Cancer		22.0
3. Stroke		6.7
4. Chronic lower respiratory diseases		5.3
5. Alzheimer's disease		4.2
6. Unintentional injuries		3.5
7. Diabetes		3.0
8. Influenza and pneumonia		2.5
9. Kidney disease		1.9
10. Septicemia		1.5

[1]Percent of total deaths due to the cause indicated.

Source: Centers for Disease Control and Prevention, *Women's Health*. Available at www.cdc.gov/women/lcod.htm. Accessed May 17, 2010.

TABLE 20–2	Different Ways of Defining the Community	
Basis of Community	**Examples**
Geographical (may also be a political unit)	town, city, or state county housing complex school district village or neighborhood zip code area
Setting-based	elementary school community group corporate workplace hospital university church YMCA
Occupational or personal characteristics	physicians, nurses, or dentists immigrants ballet dancers vegans marathon runners
Service delivery-based	patients in a private medical practice patients in a community health center VNA clients Meals-on-wheels clients WIC participants

disease prevalence among affected groups who were not previously recognized as being at risk. This often is accomplished through the use of trend charts. *Trends* are annual rates reported over a period of time, usually in terms of years. Interpretation of trends involves examination of similarities and differences among various parameters. For instance, an investigator may initially examine the pattern of change over time to see whether a problem is increasing or decreasing. More refined analyses may include comparison of one time period to another, a comparison of time series trends in different geographic areas or among different populations, or a comparison of trends among high-risk groups relative to the general population. Often, trend charts concisely present several aspects of data that allow for multiple interpretations. For example, **Figure 20–2** demonstrates little change during the 1980s in the incidence of diagnosed diabetes across all age groups, followed by an increase in incidence across all age groups during the 1990s. However, during the 2000s, the rate of increase in incidence seemed to have slowed in the two older age groups, but continued to increase among those in the 18- to 44-year-old category. The inclusion of additional years of data going forward is necessary to confirm what appears to be a promising trend among persons over 45 years old as well as the discouraging upward trend among younger adults.

■ ANALYSIS OF QUANTITATIVE DATA

It is the analysis of the relationship between the parameters of problem, place, person, and time that allows the

FIGURE 20–2 Incidence of Diagnosed Diabetes per 1,000 Population Age 18–79 Years, by Age, United States, 1980–2007
Source: Centers for Disease Control and Prevention, *Data and Trends*. Available at http://www.cdc.gov/diabetes/statistics/incidence/fig3.htm. Accessed February 25, 2010.

program planner to draw conclusions about which priority issue should be addressed within which community. Different data elements should be used in combination to more fully characterize the big picture, and to help narrow down a target audience for intervention. In Table 20–1, data on the leading cause of death among U.S. women was presented as an example of how important health issues can be identified. That information by itself is not enough for program planning, however, unless the program planner is going to tackle one of the top leading causes of death with the entire U.S. female population as the target community! Almost always, the scope of such a project would not be feasible; more commonly, programs are implemented on a much smaller scale. Therefore, it is necessary to narrow the focus. **Table 20–3** includes the same data ranking leading causes of death among U.S. women as Table 20–1 in its second column ("All Races"); however, it also includes the data disaggregated by race/ethnicity. This means that the top 10 causes of death are also listed separately for groups of women on the basis of race/ethnicity. A comparison of how the leading causes of death are ranked within each racial/ethnic group, as opposed to the rank of leading causes of death for all U.S. women, illustrates that there are discrepancies. For example, the percentage of deaths due to Alzheimer's disease among Asian/Pacific Islander women is less than half that of U.S. women overall. Additionally, diabetes is a greater contributor to deaths among women of color than among white women, which might influence a nutritionist interested in diabetes to target a program more specifically for those women than for the population of women in general.

Similarly, an examination of the same cause of death data yields a different picture when the data are disaggregated on the basis of age (**Table 20–4**). As Table 20–1 demonstrated,

TABLE 20–3	Leading Causes of Death by Race/Ethnicity, All Females—United States, 2006*					
Rank	**All Races**	**White**	**Black**	**American Indian/ Alaska Native**	**Asian/ Pacific Islander**	**Hispanic**
1	Heart disease 25.8%	Heart disease 26.0%	Heart disease 25.5%	Cancer 19.2%	Cancer 27.2%	Heart disease 22.8%
2	Cancer 22.0%	Cancer 22.0%	Cancer 21.6%	Heart disease 18.8%	Heart disease 22.7%	Cancer 21.7%
3	Stroke 6.7%	Stroke 6.7%	Stroke 6.8%	Unintentional injuries 8.1%	Stroke 9.3%	Stroke 6.4%
4	Chronic lower respiratory diseases 5.3%	Chronic lower respiratory diseases 5.8%	Diabetes 5.0%	Diabetes 7.0%	Unintentional injuries 3.8%	Diabetes 5.4%
5	Alzheimer's disease 4.2%	Alzheimer's disease 4.5%	Kidney disease 3.2%	Stroke 4.9%	Diabetes 3.8%	Unintentional injuries 5.0%
6	Unintentional injuries 3.5%	Unintentional injuries 3.5%	Unintentional injuries 3.1%	Chronic lower respiratory diseases 4.3%	Influenza & pneumonia 3.0%	Chronic lower respiratory diseases 2.7%
7	Diabetes 3.0%	Diabetes 2.7%	Chronic lower respiratory diseases 2.5%	Chronic liver disease 4.2%	Chronic lower respiratory diseases 2.4%	Alzheimer's disease 2.7%
8	Influenza & pneumonia 2.5%	Influenza & pneumonia 2.6%	Septicemia 2.4%	Kidney disease 2.4%	Alzheimer's disease 2.2%	Influenza & pneumonia 2.6%
9	Kidney disease 1.9%	Kidney disease 1.7%	Alzheimer's disease 2.3%	Influenza & pneumonia 2.0%	Kidney disease 2.0%	Kidney disease 2.2%
10	Septicemia 1.5%	Septicemia 1.4%	Influenza & pneumonia 2.0%	Septicemia 1.7%	Hypertension 1.6%	Perinatal conditions 2.1%

*Percentages represent total deaths in the age group due to the cause indicated. Numbers in parentheses indicate tied rankings. The white, black, American Indian/ Alaska Native, and Asian/Pacific Islander race groups include persons of Hispanic and non-Hispanic origin may be of any race. Some terms have shortened from those used in the National Vital Statistics Report. See the next page for a listing of the shortened terms in the table and their full unabridged equivalents used in the report. To learn more, visit *Mortality Tables* http://www.cdc.gov/nchs/nvss/mortality_tables.htm (HHS, CDC, NCHS).

Source: Centers for Disease Control and Prevention, *Women's Health.* Available at http://www.cdc.gov/women/lcod/. Accessed February 25, 2010.

TABLE 20-4   Leading Causes of Death by Age Group, All Females—United States, 2006

Rank	1–4	5–9	10–14	15–19	20–24	25–34	35–44	45–54	55–64	65+	65–74	75–84	85+	All Ages
1	Unintentional injuries 32.7%	Unintentional injuries 36.0%	Unintentional injuries 33.4%	Unintentional injuries 51.3%	Unintentional injuries 40.7%	Unintentional injuries 27.3%	Cancer 25.7%	Cancer 35.8%	Cancer 41.0%	Heart disease 28.7%	Cancer 36.1%	Heart disease 25.9%	Heart disease 33.9%	Heart disease 25.8%
2	Birth defects 13.0%	Cancer 17.0%	Cancer 14.9%	Homicide 7.9%	Homicide 8.5%	Cancer 14.8%	Unintentional injuries 16.5%	Heart disease 15.3%	Heart disease 18.1%	Cancer 19.3%	Heart disease 20.6%	Cancer 23.1%	Cancer 10.2%	Cancer 22.0%
3	Cancer 8.1%	Birth defects 7.8%	Homicide 5.4%	Suicide 7.7%	Cancer 7.6%	Heart disease 7.9%	Heart disease 12.0%	Unintentional injuries 8.4%	Chronic lower respiratory diseases 5.3%	Stroke 7.6%	Chronic lower respiratory diseases 8.2%	Stroke 7.5%	Stroke 8.5%	Stroke 6.7%
4	Homicide 7.6%	Homicide 6.0%	Heart disease 5.4%	Cancer 6.8%	Suicide 7.4%	Suicide 7.3%	Suicide 4.9%	Stroke 4.1%	Diabetes 4.2%	Chronic lower respiratory diseases 5.8%	Stroke 5.2%	Chronic lower respiratory diseases 7.1%	Alzheimer's disease 7.4%	Chronic lower respiratory diseases 5.3%
5	Heart disease 3.4%	Heart disease 3.5%	Birth defects 5.3%	Heart disease 3.2%	Heart disease 4.8%	Homicide 5.8%	HIV disease 3.8%	Chronic liver disease 3.1%	Stroke 4.1%	Alzheimer's disease 5.2%	Diabetes 4.2%	Alzheimer's disease 4.3%	Chronic lower respiratory diseases 4.0%	Alzheimer's disease 4.2%
6	Influenza & pneumonia 3.0%	Influenza & pneumonia 1.9%	Suicide 4.9%	Birth defects 2.3%	Pregnancy complications 2.9%	HIV disease 3.5%	Stroke 3.4%	Diabetes 3.1%	Unintentional injuries 3.2%	Diabetes 2.9%	Kidney disease 2.1%	Diabetes 3.4%	Influenza & pneumonia 3.6%	Unintentional injuries 3.5%
7	Septicemia 2.2%	Stroke (7) 1.6% Chronic lower respiratory diseases (7) 1.6%	Benign neoplasms 1.6%	Stroke (7) 1.0% Influenza & pneumonia (7) 1.0%	Birth defects 1.9%	Pregnancy complications 2.5%	Chronic liver disease 2.9%	Chronic lower respiratory diseases 2.8%	Chronic liver disease 1.9%	Influenza & pneumonia 2.9%	Unintentional injuries 1.9%	Influenza & pneumonia 2.5%	Diabetes 2.1%	Diabetes 3.0%
8	Benign neoplasms 1.7%		Stroke 1.5%	HIV disease 1.0%	HIV disease 1.4%	Diabetes 2.3%	Diabetes 2.6%	Suicide 2.6%	Kidney disease 1.7%	Kidney disease 2.0%	Septicemia 1.8%	Kidney disease 2.1%	Kidney disease 2.0%	Influenza & pneumonia 2.5%
9	Stroke (9) 1.3% Perinatal conditions (9)	Septicemia 1.3%	Chronic lower respiratory diseases 1.3%	Pregnancy complications 0.9%	Stroke 1.2%	Stroke 1.9%	Homicide 2.4%	HIV disease 1.6%	Septicemia 1.7%	Unintentional injuries 1.9%	Influenza & pneumonia 1.6%	Unintentional injuries 1.9%	Unintentional injuries 1.9%	Kidney disease 1.9%
10	1.3%	Benign neoplasms 1.2%	Septicemia 1.3%	Benign neoplasms 0.8%	Diabetes 1.0%	Birth defects 1.4%	Chronic lower respiratory diseases 1.4%	Septicemia 1.5%	Influenza & pneumonia 1.1%	Septicemia 1.5%	Alzheimer's disease 1.2%	Septicemia 1.7%	Hypertension 1.6%	Septicemia 1.5%

Source: Centers for Disease Control and Prevention, *Women's Health*. Available at http://www.cdc.gov/women/lcod/. Accessed June 22, 2010.

the leading cause of death for U.S. women of all ages is heart disease. However, among women younger than 35 years, the leading cause of death is unintentional injury; among women 35 to 64 years, the leading cause of death is cancer. One potential conclusion for a nutritionist working with preschool children and their parents is that a program aimed to educate kids about a diet that promotes cardiovascular health would be valuable to them with respect to both their current and future health. This nutritionist, however, would need to recognize that an outcome evaluation of the program's effectiveness in reducing deaths from heart disease could not commence for more than 60 years!

Several cautions apply when working with published data. (Jacob provides an excellent overview of errors and remedies associated with using published data for research purposes.[7]) First, before making any comparisons, pay close attention to factors such as the time period represented by the data, the definition of the population (e.g., do the data represent the total U.S. population, only women, or just persons of a specific ethnicity and age, etc.?), how data indicators are defined (e.g., does low birth weight [LBW] refer to all births $< 2,500$ grams, or just to births between 1,500 and 2,500 grams, with very LBW presented as a separate indicator for $< 1,500$-gram births?), and the original data source. High-quality data reports always include this information, and other caveats or definitions are often presented as footnotes. One indicator that is particularly fraught with difficulty is race/ethnicity categories, which are defined in various ways by different data systems. To make valid comparisons, planners must ascertain that the populations being compared are analogous, or at least they must recognize and disclose cases where comparisons are made on the basis of data that differ in some important aspects. This last situation occurs when limited data are available, and inexact comparisons are made knowingly and explicitly to get a preliminary, overall sense of whether discrepancies exist.

It is important to bear in mind that percentages can be deceiving with respect to magnitude; for instance, a mortal event that affects only 1.5% of the population initially may not give the impression of being a big problem, yet when the population is composed of 1 million people, that small percentage actually reflects 15,000 deaths. Program planners must keep the denominators from which the percentages are computed in mind when making decisions about priorities. Additionally, advanced statistical techniques may be necessary to account for the instability of rates and proportions caused by small denominators (associated with small populations and/or small geographic areas) so that appropriate conclusions may be drawn.[4]

It is also important not to look at data in isolation, but to consider relationships between different indicators. For example, when considering the proportion of LBW births, a planner should also consider the total birth rate. A community with five births per year may have a LBW prevalence of 20%, if just one baby is born at less than 2,500 grams. In contrast, a neighboring community with 500 births per year would have a LBW prevalence of only 5% even if 25 babies were born at less than 2,500 grams, and a similar prevalence of 20% in this second community would represent 100 LBW births! In this example, the second community has a bigger LBW problem despite have a smaller percentage of LBW births than the first community, because of the greater birth rate. This example illustrates that a planner cannot just rely on the largest percentage or the biggest numbers to determine the community with the greatest need.

Prioritizing Health Needs

The process of using a range of methods and integrating multiple sources of data to gain a more complete picture of relevant health issues, potential solutions, and effective program evaluation is known as *triangulation*.[8] This technique improves the validity of assessments by reducing biases inherent in the reliance on any single data source or approach.[9] The analysis of health data that is used to derive a list of priority issues for a given community, in order to select a focus of intervention, is based on many sources of information. It is a subjective process to rank the issues based on data collected from the quantitative health assessment, the literature review, and the qualitative sources such as key informant interviews and focus groups. The process also is tempered by the constraints of staff, money, time, community acceptability, and political feasibility; it is because of these factors that resources need to be identified early in the planning process, so that realistic and achievable priorities can be established. For example, a publicly funded community health center, with one nutritionist and a limited budget, would likely prioritize local health issues for its program planning differently than would a well-endowed private charitable trust, with a charter to focus exclusively on perinatal health. Analysis of published statistics is important, but it is equally important to recognize how things work in the real world. What makes sense theoretically (based on how things look on paper) needs to be balanced with how things work in practice.

For this reason, when planning a public health nutrition program, it is essential to consider other sources of information than just the results of demographic, socioeconomic, and health risk assessment analyses. It is crucial to speak with key informants to learn their perspectives on where critical needs lie, and on what types of programming might be acceptable to, and be effective with, the chosen target audience. Key informants usually include a combination of the following: subject area experts, such as local providers (e.g., physicians, nurses, WIC nutritionists, nutrition extension service staff); academics; voluntary health association and professional association spokespeople (e.g., the American Dietetic Association, the March of Dimes, the American Academy of Pediatrics); community leaders (e.g., elected officials, clergy, venerated elders, school officials); and the constituents themselves, in order to learn what their values and health expectations are. It is important to directly hear the voice of the intended target audience, as their perceived needs and interests may or may not converge with the prioritized needs identified during the quantitative health assessment analysis. To ensure a receptive audience, information regarding acceptability, appropriateness, and usefulness of planned interventions is a must. Sometimes a community will accept a health program for which there is little community demand (but a quantitatively demonstrated need) when it dovetails with something that is highly desired. For instance, WIC nutrition educators in California discovered during their planning process that the greatest perceived need among their intended target audience, non-English-speaking WIC participants, was learning English, not receiving nutrition and health education. They designed a creative program that established an English-as-a-second-language (ESL) program, using nutrition concepts as the subject matter. In that way, the target audience received a highly desired product, and the nutritionists were able to convey their education messages simultaneously.[10]

To enhance decision making when prioritizing health needs, objective and subjective data provide the explicit informational criteria upon which the decisions are based. Objective data often are presented using descriptive statistics, such as frequency, mean (a measure of central tendency), and variance and standard deviation (measures of dispersion). These basic statistics can be used to communicate information simply and can be readily computed.[4]

Sample criteria for decision making include the number of persons affected, disease severity, the magnitude of the effects of the problem on quality of life, public perception of the seriousness or changeability of a problem, available resources (including funding, personnel, and redundancy), the political feasibility of intervention, legal mandates, community acceptability, and indicators of organizational support. Criteria should be clearly stated, understood, and agreed upon by those involved in the decision-making process. Assurances should be made that each alternative will be assessed consistently. Various priority rating systems are available that make the prioritization process more systematic, such as the Basic Priority Rating System and the Propriety, Economics, Acceptability, Resources, and Legality (PEARL) System. These approaches assign scores to different factors that are then used in numerical calculations to compute a final priority rating.[4]

Development of grant applications to secure funds for current or future programming is achieved through a similar examination of data and consideration of priorities and interventions as the process just described. A successful grant proposal (or project proposal) demonstrates health disparities among a particular target audience that are amenable to change through the proposed intervention, so that funders are convinced of the need for action as well as the likelihood that the proposed intervention can meet its stated goals.

■ DATA IN PROGRAM MANAGEMENT AND EVALUATION

Evaluation is a core function within program management. The primary purposes of evaluation are to guide program managers and staff members in deciding whether to change or continue a program or specific activities within a program, allow program managers to assess the outcomes of the program on clients' health, and demonstrate to funding sources that their money is being used efficiently and effectively. In the context of program evaluation, data may be used for quality assurance; evaluation of specific initiatives; monitoring of statewide or national data for trends; measurement of progress towards meeting goals and objectives; and assessment of the impact of programs on health outcomes, morbidity, and mortality.[11,12]

Once a priority health issue and a target community have been selected, the next phase in the program planning process is the selection of interventions appropriate to the target audience, health problem, and setting; development of appropriate intervention goals and objectives; and development of an evaluation plan. Goals and objectives provide direction for a program's work and the standards by which its performance is evaluated. *Goals* are broad statements of purpose and direction, and need not be quantifiable and time-limited. *Objectives*, on the other hand, are the framework for program implementation, management, and evaluation. Objectives must be quantifiable and time-limited. Guidelines for writing objectives include the following data categories:

- *Action:* What activities will be undertaken, or what specific changes are desired?
- *Target population:* Who is expected to benefit from these activities?
- *Measurement:* What are the measurable criteria for determining success?
- *Timeline:* Over what period of time will objectives be met?

Well-written objectives always contain statements that express a quantified result expected within a stated timeframe. For example, a physical activity promotion program at a local hospital could have the following objective: "By June 2014, 45% (up from 20% in January 2012) of County Hospital employees will engage in light to moderate activity for at least 30 minutes per day." In this sample objective, the action is 30 minutes of engagement in light-to-moderate physical activity; the target population is County Hospital employees; the measurement refers to the percentage of employees who engage in physical activity (expected to be

45%); and this result is expected by June 2014. The statistic of 20% in January 2012 provides the baseline against which change will be measured.

Thoughtful definition of goals and objectives greatly facilitates the development of an evaluation plan, which also is done during the planning stage. Because objectives are measurable statements of what the program intends to achieve, for whom, and by when, *evaluation statements* are complementary in that they state the extent to which change actually occurred within the given time frame, relative to what was expected. In order to evaluate and monitor the process of implementation (especially targeting), data must be collected to illustrate whether the program is being delivered as planned to the intended target group. Data also must be collected to monitor program outcomes using appropriate, measurable indicators, to assess the impact of the program, and to answer whether the gross outcome was acceptable.[13] In the case of the sample objective provided above, in June 2014, data would be collected regarding how many hospital employees engage in light to moderate physical activity for at least 30 minutes per day. The percentage of employees who actually met the physical activity objective would be compared to the expected percentage of 45%; if the percentage was 45% or greater, the program could be considered a success. If the percentage was less than 45%, planners could pursue the analysis of additional information collected during program implementation to investigate areas for program improvement, or decide to discontinue program efforts.

The evaluation process is integrally dependent on quality data that are collected as part of program operations. It is necessary to decide during the planning stage what elements of the program will be evaluated (i.e., how many client visits were scheduled? When were they scheduled? Who did what activities? Were the actual participants members of the expected target audience? At what cost were the activities delivered? What changes occurred among individuals?). This ensures that the appropriate data will be collected during program implementation, provides ongoing management feedback about how the program is being administered, and allows for outcome assessment once the program has ended (or at some regular interval). If evalu-

ation is not considered until after a program has ended, it is unlikely that the required data will be available. For example, consider an eight-week nutrition education lecture series for elderly adults planned at a local community center. Planning to use something as simple as a weekly sign-in sheet would allow the nutritionist to be able to monitor attendance as the course proceeds (which may show whether interest is increasing or decreasing) and demonstrate, at the course's completion, how many persons actually were served. Collecting additional information on the sheet (such as gender or age) would provide additional information about who attended for comparison to the expected target audience's characteristics. If the actual participants differed from the expected target audience (e.g., if the majority of attendees were < 65 years old), the evaluation process would have illustrated that the needs of the intended target audience were not being met by the program as currently designed, even if the number of participants met the number expected.

Data collected through the course of program evaluation also may be used for program advocacy. In this instance, the data are used to highlight the need for services and to promote visibility for specific aspects of services and for the program as a whole. In addition, data regarding the number of clients served and achievements in meeting goals and objectives often are used to positively reflect on a program and justify requests for future funding and other types of support.

■ NUTRITION MONITORING AND SURVEILLANCE

Nutrition monitoring refers to the ongoing description of nutrition conditions in the population, especially among high-risk groups, for the purposes of planning and evaluation.[14] Nutrition monitoring includes ongoing nutrition surveillance systems as well as periodic nutrition surveys. Both are used to monitor trends and patterns among key indicators of nutritional status, with the goals of identifying existing and emerging needs, targeting and developing appropriate nutrition interventions, and determining public policies. *Surveillance* refers to the continuous, systematic collection of data, as well as its timely interpretation regarding the current and changing condition of the population, and the dissemination of those results to those in a position to act on them.[15]

The definition of *population* varies according to the specific aims of a given surveillance system; often, nutrition surveillance activities are designed to document the status of nutritionally vulnerable groups, particularly where data are lacking. Then, the data can be used to assess the unmet needs of these groups (e.g., pregnant women, children, the homeless, or the elderly).

Nutrition monitoring also includes periodic observation and measurement of the general population, commonly using surveys. A *nutrition survey* refers to the examination of a population's dietary behavior and nutrient intake, often at a single point in time. Major historical examples of nutrition monitoring surveys include the three National Health and Nutrition Examination Surveys (NHANES; NHANES I in 1971–1975; NHANES II in 1976–1980; and NHANES III, conducted in two phases between 1988 and 1994), administered through the Department of Health and Human Services (DHHS), National Center for Health Statistics (NCHS). An additional survey, Hispanic HANES was conducted from 1982 to 1984 to gather comprehensive data on Mexican, Cuban, and Puerto Rican Americans. Since 1999, NHANES has become a continuous annual survey program that has a changing focus on various health and nutrition measurements to meet emerging needs. The U.S. Department of Agriculture (USDA) has conducted surveys for more than 70 years to obtain information about food use and food consumption patterns; the surveys include the Nationwide Food Consumption Survey (NFCS; 1977–1978), the Continuing Survey of Food Intakes by Individuals (CSFII; 1994–1996 and 1998), and the Diet and Health Knowledge Survey (DHKS; 1994–1996). As a result of the National Nutrition Monitoring and Related Research Act of 1990's goal to improve coordination of nutrition monitoring across agencies, CSFII and NHANES have been integrated. The result is that the common dietary intake methodology and processing system utilized by CSFII has been incorporated into the sample and data collection capability of NHANES. This integrated NHANES survey currently includes data collection regarding food intake, dietary supplement intake, food program participation, and other diet-related data, as well as demographic, socioeconomic, and health-related questions and physiological measurements, from about 5,000 respondents per year in counties across the United States.[16,17]

Common nutrition-monitoring data elements include nutritional status indicators for pregnant women, infants, children, school-aged children, or elderly adults. These may include food and nutrient consumption data; knowledge, attitude, and behavior assessments; nutrition service uti-

lization, service delivery, and access to care information; and food supply and food access indicators, in order to address issues such as food security and hunger. For instance, key indicators of childhood nutritional status include height, weight, anemia status, birth weight, and breastfeeding history.

Data collected by nutrition surveillance systems are used for many purposes, including:

- To describe, monitor, and document nutritional status, especially for high-risk subgroups
- To provide early warning data and trend data on the extent of malnutrition and nutrition-related health problems
- To support effective programming, planning, evaluation, and policy making
- To enable departments of public health to provide information on nutrition-related problems to legislators and administrators.

In the context of nutrition program planning, various nutrition surveillance elements may be relevant to define target population characteristics or to demonstrate a health need. In addition, program-specific data can be assessed for monitoring progress toward goals, by using surveillance data as a benchmark for comparison.

Two valuable sources of data regarding the health and nutrition status of women and children are the national Pediatric and Pregnancy Nutrition Surveillance Systems. The Centers for Disease Control and Prevention (CDC) began working with five U.S. states in 1973 to develop a system for continuously monitoring the growth and nutritional status of low-income children who participated in federally funded maternal and child health and nutrition programs. By 2008, the Pediatric Nutrition Surveillance System (PedNSS) had expanded to include 43 states, 2 U.S. Territories, the District of Columbia, and 6 Indian Tribal Organizations, representing approximately 8,165,000 children younger than 5 years of age.[18] PedNSS aggregates data on demographic characteristics, birth weight characteristics, indicators of nutritional status, and infant-feeding practices for children from birth to age 18. All data submitted to the national PedNSS originate from the clinical service records of participating programs. PedNSS data are not representative of the total population of U.S. children because participation in the programs that originally collect the data is dependent upon income, nutrition risk criteria, or other eligibility requirements.[19] Nationally, in 2008, approximately 85.3% of PedNSS data records were submitted from the clinical service records of the Special Supplemental Nutrition Program for Women, Infants and Children (WIC), and the majority of the remaining data were submitted from the Early Periodic Screening Diagnosis and Treatment program (EPSDT), the Title V Maternal and Child Health Program, and other programs. WIC provides supplemental nutritious foods and nutrition education and counseling to low- to moderate-income pregnant and postpartum women and children up to 5 years of age who are at nutritional risk.

The Pregnancy Nutrition Surveillance System (PNSS) is a national surveillance system implemented in 1979 by the CDC to identify and reduce pregnancy-related health risks.

PNSS collects nutrition-related data regarding the medical and behavioral risk factors associated with poor pregnancy outcomes, including weight gain during pregnancy, anemia, timing of initiation of prenatal care, alcohol use, and tobacco use before, during, and after pregnancy. Selected data related to the infant include birth outcome, birth weight, and infant feeding behavior. Data are program-based, primarily obtained from WIC and prenatal clinics funded by Maternal and Child Health Program Block Grants. The states and intertribal organizations that participate in PNSS have varied since its inception.

Comparison of data from a smaller community to data from a larger unit, such as a state or the nation, can identify areas where health improvement efforts may be warranted. For example, comparison of state-level PNSS data to national PNSS data is informative regarding the health and nutritional status of low- to moderate-income women and children in that state, relative to individuals in similar economic circumstances across the nation. Such a comparison could assist that state's WIC program in identifying specific risk factors and needs among its participant population; in planning, implementing, and evaluating nutrition interventions; and in developing and implementing quality assurance protocols. At a more local level, data reports that present data by local program and for the state overall could be produced to enhance targeting of services, provide managerial insights, and facilitate individual local program evaluation. Probert[20] provides a sample format for comparing demographic, socioeconomic, and health status indicators from smaller to larger data collection units. A complete series of worksheets that include nutritional status indicators is available online (http://www.movingtothefuture.org). As described earlier, interpretation stems from analysis of similarities and differences between the smaller population of interest and the broader population. Recognize that, at times, data will not be available for every indicator at both levels of the comparison. Additionally, data may need to be obtained from multiple sources (e.g., if the community of interest is not geographically based, U.S. census data for that community will not be available, but perhaps the relevant data would be available from a community source, such as client service records or membership profiles).

Data also may be used for comparison to health performance objectives. In this instance, existing surveillance data are used to provide a baseline for current conditions and to develop target goals for the future, and ongoing surveillance is used for comparison to the target and to assess progress toward meeting those goals. In 2010, the U.S. DHHS published a national agenda, called Healthy People (HP) 2020[21] that outlined a federal disease prevention and health promotion agenda to achieve by the year 2020. HP 2020 contains objectives in multiple health-related areas, including nutritional status. Areas of particular relevance to nutrition include the three major categories: Nutrition and Overweight; Physical Activity and Fitness; and Maternal, Infant, and Child Health. HP 2020 defines a federally determined target and the recommended state-level data source for comparison to the target. These are areas that need to be addressed in the development of future surveillance systems, and they illustrate cases where a program planner may need to collect original data to demonstrate need or progress in meeting objectives.

■ DATA COMPILATION

Data Requirements, Collection, and Management

The recent expansion in data accessibility at the federal, state, and local levels allows nutrition professionals to be more specific in their planning, which increases the likelihood that a true health need will be addressed by nutrition programming and that such efforts will result in a positive change in nutritional status and health for the intended target audience. However, because of the plethora of available data, it is important than ever to carefully plan for data requirements prior to data retrieval and/or initiation of data collection. Failure to do so can result in a nutritionist becoming mired in data that do not contribute to the primary purpose of the data collection, whether it is for a community profile, program evaluation, or grant development. Additionally, a nutritionist could end up wasting time and money collecting redundant data that is already available.

The most important step when working with data is to define existing data elements and to specify information gaps. When a need for additional data is identified, two processes follow: 1) identifying the goal for data collection, and 2) making procedural plans for the data's acquisition, storage, manipulation, and reporting. Before collecting a single data point, a nutrition program planner first must know the answers to the following questions relative to goal identification:

- Why collect original data at all?
- What type of data will be collected (i.e., demographic and socioeconomic, or nutrition knowledge, beliefs, and behaviors)?
- Which indicators can address the type of data desired?
- How will allowable values for each indicator be defined?
- What method will be used to collect the data?
- What information is expected to be learned from data analysis?
- What will be done with the information?
- How will the information acquired help in meeting client and organizational needs?

For instance, prior to designing a new questionnaire, a program planner should know what problem he or she is trying to solve, what new information must be gained to solve it, and who the target population is for the survey. By specifying exactly what one needs to know, the planner can limit the questionnaire to only critical fields and eliminate the collection of potentially interesting but unusable information, thereby reducing the response burden, cost, and processing time. Often, existing monitoring and surveillance systems already may have collected the desired information. If the nutrition program planner does not know what is being searched for, it is necessary to stop and reconsider why a data collection process is being considered in the first place. It is never good practice to collect data on myriad topics and hope that something useful and informative will emerge.

Second, planning for the data collection procedure begins with a thoughtful self-evaluation of the nutrition program planner's personal and organizational capacity so that data are obtained in a format that can be utilized. For instance, a nutritionist or data analyst who is proficient working with large, complex data files and sophisticated data analysis software may be comfortable obtaining large raw data files from a government Web site and extracting the required information. Others who lack those types of skills or who do not have the necessary computer hardware and software (and associated technical support) may be better off working from summary statistics in published reports or from third-party summary data sources.

The next step in procedural planning is to consider the analytic plan. The nutrition program planner must define exactly what he or she hopes to learn prior to data collection to ensure that the appropriate data for the type of analysis desired are obtained. It is an all-too-common scenario that oversights in data collection result in the inability to process data for desired results, which ends in much frustration and a lot of wasted effort on the part of subjects, data collectors, and data analysts. For instance, if a nutritionist is interested in learning more about nutritional status and weight status (in terms of weight-for-age, height-for-age, and BMI-for-age) among school-aged children, the failure to include gender as a data collection field on the form during the data collection stage ultimately will result in the inability to generate meaningful results during the analysis stage, even if each child's age, height, and weight are collected. This is because the growth charts from which BMI-, weight-, and height-for-age are computed are gender-specific. It cannot be emphasized strongly enough that the best results occur when an analysis plan is defined in advance of data collection. This method ensures that all required variables will be identified prior to data collection.

If it is determined that the required data are nonexistent for a given population and a new questionnaire must be implemented, it can be extremely valuable to borrow questions from existing questionnaires. There are at least two advantages to this approach: 1) the data collected locally can be compared to data collected by the original investigators from a larger population (or a population that differs in some other respect, such as income or education); and

2) the existing questionnaire may have been formally validated. The choice of whether to use existing data or to collect new data also is dependent upon the anticipated survey sample size and the method of survey administration (telephone survey, face-to-face interview, mailed survey, etc.).

Final data collection procedural issues to consider include planning for data processing and database management, and deciding when and how results will be presented and disseminated. Although the nutrition program planner may not perform all of these functions, he or she needs to be familiar with them in order to provide managerial oversight.

Bourque and Clark[22] describe an expanded definition of data processing that goes beyond just data coding, data entry, and verification. In their definition, data processing begins with the selection of a data collection strategy and ends with the completion of data transformations. The process they describe includes:

- Developing response categories during the development of the data collection instrument so that categories for pre-coded and open-ended questions are defined prior to data collection
- Collecting the data
- Creating data files that are compatible with statistical packages (i.e., Statistical Analysis Software [SAS] or Statistical Package for the Social Sciences [SPSS])
- Transforming data into analytically meaningful variables
- Documenting in writing all aspects of the system.

This broad definition is extremely useful as it highlights the multistage process of converting verbal or written information into meaningful data that can be analyzed electronically. Developing operational definitions up front is important so that it is clear exactly what each indicator being collected refers to. This is particularly important when comparison to published data (e.g., from a surveillance system or the U.S. Census) is anticipated, so that similar categorical responses are used, when appropriate. Attention to this process will likely increase success as decisions about data content and format will be addressed at the beginning, decreasing the likelihood that acquired data will not be useable. It also will increase data quality and improve reliability and validity.

The decision of how results will be presented (particularly with respect to content) can save a lot of time during data analysis by preventing superfluous data analyses or unnecessary formatting of results that are not intended to be used. For instance, if data will be used only for internal purposes, perhaps output that contains all analyses printed straight from the analytic software will be acceptable. If results are intended for publication, perhaps a more polished document with summary results and interpretation highlighted will be prepared.

Accessing Existing Data Sources

There are many different sources for quantitative community-level and population-based data on a wide variety of topics. Which types of data and which sources will be used is a matter of strategic choice. Some possible sources include, but are not limited to, population data (e.g., U.S. Census or NHANES), program data (e.g., the WIC program or Head Start), trend data, national objectives (e.g., HP 2020), and cost data. Frequently, national surveillance data also are available at the state level, either from the national agency that operates the system or from the state department that submits the data to the national system.

All of the data sources that are available online are too numerous to mention. FedStats (http://www.fedstats.gov/), described on its Web page as "the gateway to statistics from over 100 U.S. Federal agencies," is a good place to start finding pertinent sources. Other sources may be readily located using a Web search engine. Many online data sources offer the options of viewing predefined reports or generating custom tables with data obtained through searches and queries of summary and micro-data files. Web sites should be visited frequently, because many are constantly in the process of adding new or updated material.

There also are a wide variety of state-level sources of data, particularly through state departments of public health. Other available data sources are hosted by private foundations, such as the Kaiser Family Foundation's State Health Facts (http://www.statehealthfacts.org/), a resource that contains state-level data on demographics, health, and health policy, including health coverage, access, financing, and state legislation, or the Annie E. Casey Foundation's KIDS COUNT Data Center (http://datacenter.kidscount.org/), in which data reflecting measures of child well-being are available as profiles, line graphs, national maps, rankings, and raw data for states, cities, counties, and school districts across the United States.

It is important to pay close attention to the data source attribution when using a secondary data source (i.e., data from an agency that is presenting information that its own staff did not collect). For instance, the U.S. Census Bureau is a primary data source because it publishes data collected only by that agency. The KIDS COUNT Data Center, on the other hand, utilizes multiple federal data sources in producing its reports but does not collect its own original data, making it a secondary data source. Failure to note data's point of origin could result in a program planner collecting data from multiple sources that actually are duplicative rather than complimentary. As indicated previously, it is also critical to note the time period represented by the data, as well as operational definitions for all measures and technical terms used.

■ CONCLUSION

A nutrition program plan to address a specific health issue is strengthened by data that demonstrate a community's health and nutritional status (based on demographic, socioeconomic, and health and nutritional status data), the community's perceived needs (gathered through qualitative methods), and any major duplication and/or gaps in available community services. The use of data in the needs assessment process assures that resources and activities are directed toward a defined target audience with a prioritized health need.

Accurate, timely information is absolutely critical for decision makers, who need to understand a problem's scope as well as its causes and consequences prior to taking action (such as whether to revise a program or initiate something new). Such understanding is achieved through the processes of assessment, analysis, and action. Assessment refers to the detection of the existence of a problem. Analysis is the mechanism by which causes and solutions are identified. Action involves the communication of results to those responsible for initiating action to solve the problem. In addition, related information is essential to monitor and evaluate how well (or poorly) their actions have affected the problem.

The utility of nutrition data is far reaching, as it can be used to improve an agency's capacity to assess, analyze, and design resource-relevant actions; improve organizational and public perception and knowledge; increase effective demand for nutrition-relevant information; and ensure adequate resources for action. This is what is meant by "translating data" into public health action.

Issues for Discussion

1. What is the role of data in the justification for an intervention among a given target audience?

2. What skills are required by a nutritionist to demonstrate a facility with data management and interpretation?

3. What resources should be allocated to collecting, analyzing, and reporting data for program planning and evaluation?

4. When utilizing a secondary data source versus collecting original data, what are the benefits and tradeoffs in terms of simplicity, time, comprehensiveness, and flexibility?

References

1. Morris W, ed. *The American Heritage Dictionary of the English Language.* Boston: Houghton Mifflin; 1982.

2. Spicer DA, Kaufman M. Managing data. In: Kaufman M, ed. *Nutrition in Public Health: A Handbook for Developing Programs and Services.* Rockville, MD: Aspen; 1990:312–341.

3. Probert KL, ed. *Moving to the Future: Developing Community-Based Nutrition Services.* Washington, DC: Association of State and Territorial Public Health Nutrition Directors; 1996.

4. Issel LM. *Health Program Planning and Evaluation: A Practical, Systematic Approach for Community Health.* Sudbury, MA: Jones and Bartlett Publishers; 2009.

5. Aspen Reference Group. *Community Health Education and Promotion: A Guide to Program Design and Evaluation.* Gaithersburg, MD: Aspen; 1997.

6. Cole TJ. Sampling, study size, and power. In: Margetts BM, Nelson M, eds. *Design Concepts in Nutritional Epidemiology.* New York: Oxford University Press; 1991:53–78.

7. Jacob H. *Using Published Data: Errors and Remedies.* Newbury Park, CA: Sage; 1984.

8. Owen AL, Splett PL, Owen GM. *Nutrition in the Community: The Art and Science of Delivering Services*, 4th ed. Boston: McGraw Hill; 1999.

9. Winkelman M. *Culture and Health: Applying Medical Anthropology.* San Francisco: Jossey-Bass; 2009.

10. Wurzbach ME, ed. *Community Health Education and Promotion: A Guide to Program Design and Evaluation*, 2nd ed. Gaithersburg, MD: Aspen; 2002.

11. Centers for Disease Control and Prevention (CDC). Guidelines for evaluating surveillance systems. *MMWR Morb Mortal Wkly Rep.* 1988;37(S-5):1–18.

12. Centers for Disease Control and Prevention (CDC). Framework for program evaluation in public health. *MMWR Morb Mortal Wkly Rep.* 48(RR-11):1–40.

13. Mason JB, Habicht JP, Tabatabai H, Valverdi V. Nutritional surveillance for programme management and evaluation. In: Nutritional Surveillance. Geneva: World Health Organization (WHO); 1984;140–175.

14. Briefel RR. Nutrition monitoring in the United States. In: Bowman B, Russell RM, eds. *Present Knowledge in Nutrition*, 8th ed. Washington, DC: International Life Sciences Institute; 2001:617–635.

15. Birkhead GS, Maylahn CM. State and local public health surveillance. In: SM Teutsch, RE Churchill, eds. *Principles and Practice of Public Health Surveillance*, 2nd ed. New York: Oxford University Press; 2000:253–286.

16. Dwyer J, Picciano MF, Raiten DJ; Members of the Steering Committee. Collection of food and dietary supplement intake data: What We Eat in America—NHANES. *J Nutr.* 2003;133:590S–600S.

17. Centers for Disease Control and Prevention (CDC). *National Health and Nutrition Examination Survey.* Available at http://www.cdc.gov/nchs/nhanes.htm. Accessed May 18, 2010.

18. Centers for Disease Control and Prevention (CDC). *Pediatric and Pregnancy Nutrition Surveillance System.* Available at http://www.cdc.gov/pednss/index.htm. Accessed May 18, 2010.

19. Polhamus B, Dalenius K, Thompson D, Scanlon K, Borland E, Smith B, Grummer-Strawn L. *Pediatric Nutrition Surveillance 2002 Report.* Atlanta, GA: U.S. Department of Health and Human Services, Centers for Disease Control and Prevention; 2004.

20. Probert KL. *Moving to the Future: Developing Community-Based Nutrition Services* (workbook & training manual). Washington, DC: Association of State and Territorial Public Health Nutrition Directors; 1997.

21. U.S. Department of Health and Human Services. *Healthy People 2010* (conference edition in 2 vols). Washington, DC: U.S. DHHS: 2000.

22. Bourque LB, Clark VA. *Processing Data: The Survey Example.* Newbury Park, CA: Sage; 1992.

Managing Money

Katherine Cairns, MPH, MBA, RD

READER OBJECTIVES   After studying this chapter and reflecting on the contents, you should be able to:

1. Discuss the nutritionist's responsibilities for managing money.
2. Identify collaborators in the agency budgeting process.
3. Discuss justifications for each budgeted proposal.
4. Describe the major sources for funding public health nutrition services.
5. List and describe major categories for a nutrition program budget.
6. Specify major items in a grant application.
7. Describe major sources of third-party reimbursement for public health nutrition services.

■ INTRODUCTION: FINANCING PUBLIC HEALTH NUTRITION PROGRAMS AND SERVICES

Providing the community with public health nutrition programs that residents need and want requires that the agency allocate dollars to pay personnel salaries, reimburse their travel, buy equipment and supplies, provide for continuing education of nutrition personnel, and purchase other goods needed to deliver services.

The need for accountability and financial transparency are critical for the public health manager. Every nutritionist who manages a program, service, or project must take responsibility for requesting, justifying, and negotiating a budget and controlling expenditures within the funds allocated. Fiscal management means understanding the financing and budgeting process while working closely with the following key people in an organization:

- Department/agency administrator and board members who set the agency's fiscal policy and determine how the agency's budget will be distributed to programs and overhead.
- Finance/fiscal officer or business manager who maintains accounts, controls expenditures, and can provide

advice on the organization's written and unwritten fiscal policies and procedures.
- Other program directors who request and manage budgets for programs that should utilize nutrition services. These directors may be convinced to

collaborate in funding nutrition services through their internal funding sources or by writing grants for external funding.

Tighter federal, state, and local government agency budgets require nutritionists to compete for the money they need if they want to turn plans for comprehensive nutrition services into action. Convincing a governmental unit or foundation to invest money and become a stakeholder in nutrition services requires that the value of each proposal be justified. Business planning and compelling answers to the following questions will prepare a nutrition

Katherine Cairns, MPH, MBA, RD, was an original author from the *First Edition* of Mildred Kaufman's *Nutrition in Public Health* (1990). Portions of this chapter are reprinted with permission from the publisher.

administrator for the competitive public and private funding environment.

- Is there really a community need for the service?
- What are the competing options for the available and new money? The plan, budget, service, product, and their evaluation must stand out from the competition.
- Is there a strong and persuasive reason for funding this option over others?
- What support does the competition have for the same funding?
- Does your agency/team have the skills and track record of innovative service and project completion?
- Can cost-effectiveness data be provided for the type of nutrition service proposed?
- What stakeholder support and contributions are there for the proposal?
- What additional community support and media attention can be generated prior to, during, and following the funding decisions?
- Are there federal, state, or local requirements/mandates for components of the proposed nutrition service?
- What potential does the proposed service have to generate income for the agency?
- Are there federal or foundation grants available to establish and maintain the service into the future?
- Is it feasible to implement and maintain the service after external funding ends?

Competitive proposals for spending new or ongoing money must show evidence of support from individuals and organizations in the community who will benefit from the product or service. They can demonstrate their support by paying fees for services; making in-kind contributions of staff, volunteer time, or space in offices or clinics; writing letters of support; presenting testimony; lobbying proactively; and donating equipment, materials, or cash contributions.

Interdisciplinary teamwork and networking to increase the number of stakeholders in nutrition programs are discussed in other chapters. Financers prefer to fund a service that fits their mission and responds to a demonstrated need that can be met cost effectively. A well-conceived budget for a new service or product details the cost per unit. Services with high start-up costs should show a reasonable cost per unit after the start-up and within the first six months of operation. Fiscal managers will ask these questions:

- Will the proposed service or product have a reasonable cost-to-benefit ratio? Funders compare the costs and outcomes of varying types of service delivery options.
- Will the service be carried out with the most cost-effective intervention? For example, will reducing anemia in 80% of a population group within six months

of diagnosis be less costly if nutrition counseling is provided by a trained and supervised paraprofessional rather than by a nutritionist? Although the outcome may be the same, the costs of different intervention models may vary.

These and additional questions can be used as a checklist in preparing to request the funds needed to initiate the service. Funds for nutrition services may be secured from a variety of sources. The more diversified the funding base, the more stable the program. The more funding sources used to maintain a public health nutrition program, the less dependent the program is on any single source. However, maintaining accountability for too many small funding sources ($< \$10,000$) may be counterproductive.

■ GENERAL REVENUE

State governments generate funds through state income taxes, sales taxes, various types of business taxes, and taxes on such products as alcoholic beverages and cigarettes. Several states use lotteries and lawsuit settlement proceeds as revenue for public services. Local government units have the authority to tax property owners for municipal services, such as police and fire departments, schools, recreation, and public health. Tax levies are set annually based on the services needed, the priorities of policy makers, the demands of the taxpayers, and outside interests.

Some local government and many state public health departments derive a portion of their income from general revenue. Public health agencies generally seek a reasonable share of general revenue as a cornerstone of their base income. Usually, there is keen competition for these funds in a health agency because they offer programs some funding stability. However, when governmental entities face increasing economic pressure, the general revenue funds become less stable. If there is no general revenue in the budget for nutrition services, nutritionists need to discuss this funding source with agency administrators and business managers to prepare their request for the next budget cycle. Nutritionists may need to be persistent and assertive over several years to succeed. Acquiring some funding that is less restrictive to a specific target population provides flexibility to plan more comprehensive, community-responsive programs.

Grants

Federal Grants

A variety of federal funds are used by state, local, and nongovernmental organizations (NGO) to operate food and nutrition programs. Federal agencies that fund major food/nutrition programs and demonstration projects to over 80 million Americans include:

- The Food and Nutrition Service (FNS) of the U.S. Department of Agriculture (USDA) specific grant funds and innovation grants/contracts

- Centers for Medicare and Medicaid Services (CMS) of the U.S. Department of Health and Human Services (DHHS)
- Centers for Disease Control and Prevention (CDC) of the U.S. DHHS
- Specific health block grant funds from the U.S. DHHS

Requests for Proposals (RFPs): Invitations to suppliers to bid on supplying products or services that are difficult to describe for a company, or in this example, a public agency.

Personal contacts within each of the major federal or state agencies are useful to obtain advance notice of Requests for Proposals (RFPs) and special project funding.

State Grants

State departments of health, health and human services, agriculture, and education usually provide some funds for nutrition services. The state funds may support selected statewide and/or local services. In many states, a per capita or preestablished formula is used for allocating state and federal funds to local health agencies. State agencies may have special legislated funding for nutrition programs. State agencies also serve as the conduits for federal funds earmarked for local program implementation. Specific federal project funds that state governmental agencies administer through a grants process include:

- Special Supplemental Food Program for Women, Infants and Children (WIC)
- Other supplemental food programs for targeted groups (Farmer's Market, Senior Food Program, Summer Food Programs, Special Milk Programs, Daycare Programs, School Lunch/Breakfast Programs, Congregate Dining)
- Nutrition education special projects
- Maternal and child health special projects
- Health promotion special projects
- Chronic disease intervention/reduction special projects
- Targeted agricultural marketing special projects

Each state's grant application procedure has special requirements that need to be determined by consulting the local agency administrator, state agency, or regional/central office nutrition consultants.

Local Grants or Contracts

Local human or social service agencies, home health agencies, area agencies on aging, mental health agencies, developmental disabilities councils, school districts, jails, community colleges, and other governmental units frequently need nutrition services or have special initiatives or ongoing projects that require nutrition expertise. When agencies do not employ a full-time nutritionist on their own staff, they will often contract for these services as the most efficient method for getting the short- or long-term services they need. Those local agencies that need part-time nutrition services frequently maintain lists or files of available contractors and their specialties. It is important to cultivate contacts within the local agencies who can advise on their needs, availability of funding, and interest in developing contracts.

Local voluntary health agencies (e.g., American Heart Association, American Diabetes Association, American Cancer Society, Cystic Fibrosis Association, or March of Dimes chapter or affiliate offices) also may need and contract for nutrition services or offer small competitive project grants. For short-term community projects, funds may be obtained from local businesses, banks, civic organizations, or churches.

Foundation Grants

Millions of dollars of private foundation projects are funded annually for foundation-specific priorities. The Internet and the public library are the most valuable resources for identifying these foundation funders. Foundation and grant information centers maintain information on:

- Names and contact persons for local, state, regional, or national foundations
- Information on past funding priorities and projects funded
- Dollar amount of awards for foundation projects
- Criteria and format for submitting funding requests
- Timeline for review of grant requests

Priorities of foundations may change annually. Putting a new twist on an old idea or need thus may be required for the foundation to consider the proposal. Some foundations prefer that proposals be submitted on behalf of a nongovernmental, nonprofit agency. Nutritionists working in a governmental agency who seek a foundation grant might collaborate with a nonprofit agency that will submit the proposal and subcontract the nutrition work to the public health agency.

Fee for Services

A fee-for-service adjusted for each target population is a useful method for recovering program costs. A basic market analysis is required to determine the range of fees appropriate to charge the various target populations. Fees must be based on actual costs, not guesswork. Making a fee-for-service plan more acceptable to clients of a public health service is a second task, after calculating actual costs. In presenting a plan to establish fees to administrators, government officials, the public, and coworkers, three alternatives might be offered:

1. Sliding scale fee-for-service: The fee is based on the client's ability to pay, with the maximum fee being the actual cost of the service; this can be used for all basic public health services.

2. Actual cost fee-for-service: The actual cost of providing a service is calculated and revised annually. It is charged for public health services where there are other private and nonprofit providers of the services within a community. These service charges are not put on a sliding scale because of the potential legal issues of unfair competition by a governmental provider. A public agency will by design have few of these services because of need-based planning.

3. Cost plus fee-for-service: This pricing model permits a nonprofit agency to recover the actual cost of a service in addition to a profit, which is then used to subsidize another service within the agency. These "cash cows" may include innovative services or products

(healthy cooking demonstrations, diet and fitness classes, customized nutrition services for community organizations), or long-standing, fully capitalized services (laboratory tests).

These "price" versus "cost" strategies are dependent on an accurate cost determination and are discussed later in this chapter.

THIRD-PARTY REIMBURSEMENT

Third-party reimbursement income is received by billing insurance carriers, such as governmental healthcare programs (Medicaid, Medicare), workers' compensation, health maintenance organizations (HMOs)/managed care organizations (MCOs), and/or other special health insurance pools (catastrophic health, state-sponsored alternative care pools, organized employer groups). Each health carrier has its own billing procedures that the agency accounting office must determine and continuously keep updated. It is most cost effective for the agency accounting department to select the three or four third-party reimbursement sources that cover the majority of the agency's clients and bill these carriers. Clients not covered by those carriers would be treated as fee-for-service clients and advised to collect reimbursement from their own carrier. Some organizations contract with healthcare reimbursement firms that require an assignment

of benefits from all clients and handle all agency billing for a predetermined fee.

Emerging opportunities for income generation are developing in the area of third-party reimbursement. Nutrition services are increasingly being reimbursed for preventive services, and chronic and acute care interventions. Nutrition and health programs are identifying ways to protect revenue raised from third-party reimbursements to allow a carryover of these funds between fiscal years for program-specific initiatives.

PREPARING BUDGETS AND DETERMINING PROGRAM COSTS

Generating the funds to cover the cost of delivering a nutrition service is an important part of fiscal management. Determining the real cost of a product or service is crucial to setting fees, collecting reimbursements, and writing grants. Preparing a budget for an array of services and then breaking it down into the actual cost of each product/service is the next step.

The budget defines what services can be implemented with the amount of funding available. An annotated budget, as shown in **Table 21–1**, is one way to walk through the process.

> **Annotated budget:** A budget supplied with critical or explanatory notes.

BUDGET SUMMARY

Controlling the budget requires a monthly comparison of projected income to actual expenses and encumbrances (items purchased but not yet paid for). The agency's accounting section should provide a monthly financial summary listing the current status of expenditures compared to the amounts budgeted. **Table 21–2** displays an example of this analysis. The program manager must monitor this carefully so that all budgeted resources are wisely used. The monthly financial summary also enables the manager to determine when the income flow is inadequate compared to projections. Fund transfers between program accounts may be needed to balance the budget.

The monthly budget summary should be used to determine when there is a need to:

- Communicate with staff about the program's financial position
- Trim discretionary costs (supplies, printing, etc.) or increase spending on consumable supplies
- Increase or decrease staffing (overtime/voluntary reduction of hours/layoffs)
- Generate more income (find out why some health carriers are slower to pay or slow down the agency billing process)

TABLE 21–1	The Annotated Program Budget

Income
A diversified income base is critical to a strong nutrition program. Client fees and reimbursements are projected based on past income-generating experience

Allocation		Amount
Grant A		$ XXX
Grant B		$ XXX
Client fees		$ XXX
Program A	$ XXX	
Program B	$ XXX	
Third-party reimbursement		$ XXX
General revenue (tax levy)		$ XXX
State grant/allocation		$ XXX
Total income		**$ XXXX**
(Note: This should equal or exceed total expenses.)		

Expenses

Salaries		$ XXX
Full-time (specify FTEs)	$ XXX	
Part-time (specify FTEs)	$ XXX	
Fringe benefits		$ XXX
Mileage for local travel		$ XXX
Other travel		$ XXX
Phone fees: local, long-distance, cell		$ XXX
Internet and technology allocation		$ XXX
Postage		$ XXX
Film/video reproduction		$ XXX
Printing		$ XXX
Supplies		$ XXX
Office	$ XXX	
Food for demonstrations/clients	$ XXX	
Books, other educational materials		$ XXX
Subscriptions		$ XXX
Software		$ XXX
Space, rental/allocation		$ XXX
Equipment rental/allocation[1]		$ XXX
Copy machines	$ XXX	
Computers	$ XXX	
Telephones	$ XXX	
Video	$ XXX	
Equipment, purchase[2]		$ XXX
Computer/other hardware	$ XXX	
Other office equipment	$ XXX	
Utilities, actual/allocation		$ XXX
Staff training and continuing education		$ XXX
Out-of-town travel	$ XXX	
Lodging	$ XXX	
Registration fees	$ XXX	
Registrations, local	$ XXX	
Memberships	$ XXX	
Other		$ XXX
Indirect costs[3]		$ XXX
Central service charge[4]		$ XXX
Consultant fees[5]		$ XXX
Student stipends[6]		$ XXX
Contingent reserve fund[7]		$ XXX
Total expenses		**$ XXXX**
(Note: Total expenses should be less than total income.)		

[1]Carefully evaluate the rent vs. buy decision on all equipment.
[2]It is important to plan for life-cycle replacement of equipment in each annual budget.
[3]There may be a negotiated administrative overhead charge included as a percentage of each budget for overall agency indirect costs.
[4]Additional overhead may be charged by the county/city/state to cover the costs of attorneys, accountants, executive directors, and central purchasing that provide service but are outside of the nutrition or health department.
[5]Include fees for graphic consultants, contract professional/technical assistance, external evaluation specialists, and auditor fees for federal funds received. Contract physician fees for grants/third-party reimbursement requirements, especially if third-party reimbursement will cover the costs and result in nutrition reimbursement.
[6]Try to build in student stipends for internships if quality supervision can be provided for the students.
[7]A carryover fund for emergencies, reimbursed initiatives.

A computer spreadsheet is a clear, time-saving tool for preparing the budget summary. There are many fine financial software packages available. Most governmental agencies will require their departments to use their purchased financial software.

Determining Costs for Each Service

Determining the costs for each specific service or product requires a slightly different adaptation of the program budget. The program manager must know the approximate utilization of staff and resources directed to each service. Staff time is the largest expense in any service. Time studies or tracking of billable hours are frequently used to assess the amount of staff time each product or service requires. If a time study is not feasible for a variety of reasons (lack of time, staff issues, etc.), a quick, less precise method can be used to approximate the amount of staff time spent in each specific service area. This method is displayed in **Table 21–3**. Note that administrative time is factored into each service category.

The next step is to cost out staff, supplies, equipment, and other resources for each service area (**Table 21–4**), then divide the total cost by the number of clients or client visits (or relative value units, a productivity measuring unit used by some programs) expected to be served during the year. This yields a *cost-per-contact*, or the actual cost to provide each unit of service.

Starting from the program budget, this cost determination analysis takes approximately two hours to calculate for each service. A program manager could devote about two hours per month to identifying the actual costs of one program per month and make needed adjustments in charges. More complicated systems of cost determination exist, especially for federally funded programs. These can be developed with the guidance of the agency's business manager or accountant. Public health programs have been able to increase their operating income after doing this type of analysis. Health screening programs, therapeutic counseling, and group educational programs are examples of programs for which this cost determination would be useful to document actual costs compared to reimbursed costs. The goal is to move reimbursed costs closer to the actual costs of the public health nutrition service.

Divide total cost by number of clients or client visits (or relative value units used by some programs) expected to be served this year. This gives a cost per contact or encounter, which is the actual cost to the program to provide each unit of this service. This can also be analyzed by the actual number of clients served in the most recent reporting period.

Service Productivity Analysis

A second stage of analysis for program managers concerned about the high cost of a given service is a service productivity analysis. A simple analysis of service productivity levels

---

TABLE 21–2	**Monthly Financial Summary**				
	Month		**Year-to-Date (YTD)**		**Previous YTD**
	Actual	**Budgeted**	**Actual YTD Received**	**YTD Budgeted**	**Previous YTD**
Income (List all sources)					
Total Income					
	Actual	**Budgeted**	**Actual YTD**	**YTD Budgeted**	**YTD Last Year**
Expenses (List All Expense Categories)					
Total Expenses					
Variance					

---

involves multiplying the total full-time equivalent (FTEs) allocated to each service by 2,080 (paid hours) or 1,800 (billable hours) for each full-time equivalent position and dividing by the number of clients or contact visits (**Figure 21–1**).

Cost-Effectiveness and Cost-Benefit Analysis of Services

The third and final challenge of fiscal management is to evaluate the service/product once the costs and providers have been identified. Cost-benefit analysis and cost-effectiveness analysis are most commonly utilized for evaluations. A cost-benefit analysis is used in the planning process to decide if a program/service should be undertaken. A cost-effectiveness analysis is undertaken in planning to determine the least costly way to provide the service or program.

Through the application of these analysis tools, the nutritionist can make services generate income and become increasingly self-supporting. There is great risk in taking an

---

TABLE 21–3	**Staff Allocation by Service/Cost Center for Cost Determination**					
Staff	**Total FTE**	**WIC**	**Clinic**	**Home Visit**	**Education Sessions**	**Weight Reduction**
Clerical						
Amy Jones	1.0	0.9	0.0	0.0	0.0	0.1
Jean Brown	0.8	0.1	0.1	0.3	0.2	0.1
Nutrition Assistants						
Tom Smith	1.0	1.0	0.0	0.0	0.0	0.0
Symon White	0.8	0.8	0.0	0.0	0.0	0.0
Pam Johnson	0.7	0.7	0.0	0.0	0.0	0.0
Terry Jones	1.0	0.5	0.0	0.5	0.0	0.0
Nutritionists						
Mary Stokes	0.8	0.8	0.0	0.0	0.0	0.0
Sue Austin	1.0	0.0	0.0	0.2	0.3	0.5
Steve Doe	1.0	0.0	0.0	0.2	0.3	0.5
Tia Vang	1.0	0.2	0.1	0.2	0.4	0.1
Total	**9.1**	**5.0**	**0.2**	**1.4**	**1.2**	**1.3**

Abbreviation: FTE = full-time equivalent.

TABLE 21–4   Cost Determination for a Nutrition Service

Service: Nutrition counseling in-home visits
Date of cost determination: 9-21-20XX

Salaries	$	Comments
Jean Brown, .3 FTE	$ XXX	Full-time equivalent (FTE) by salary
Terry Jones, .5 FTE	XXX	
Sue Austin, .2 FTE	XXX	
Steve Doe, .3 FTE	XXX	
Tia Vang, .4 FTE	XXX	
Fringe benefit allocation	XXX	Based on required allocation
Mileage for home visits	XXX	Allocated or actual use
Telephone	XXX	Allocated on estimated/actual use
Postage	XXX	Allocated on estimated/actual use
Copies	XXX	Allocated on estimated/actual use
Supplies	XXX	Allocated on estimated/actual use
Office rental	XXX	Allocated based on space occupied
Equipment	XXX	Allocated based on use
Training/education	XXX	Allocated
Other	XXX	
Subtotal	XXX	
Indirect cost rate (___%)	XXX	Apply to subtotal
Total cost of service	**$ XXX**	

Divide total cost of service by number of units (or Relative Value Units) to determine the cost per unit or per service.

Service: Nutrition counseling in-home visits

Date of cost determination: 12-21-20XX   650 home visits

1. **How long should it take to provide one unit (visit) of this service?**

   2 hours (includes direct service time, travel time, charting, case conference, and administration)

2. **How long does it take to provide each unit (visit) of this service?**

   Agencies may calculate this based on:
   - 2,080 hours (1.0 FTE paid with vacation/sick days included) *or*
   - 1,800 billable hours (1.0 FTE excluding vacation/sick/holiday hours)

   Total service units: 650 home visits
   2,520 divided by 650 budgeted
   home visits = 3.87 hours per home visit

3. **Explain the difference between the answers to 1 and 2.**

   - 3.87 hours per visit (actual) compared to 2.0 hours per visit (estimate) is significant. Thus, staff take almost twice as long to complete the home visit service as what they estimated during the budget cycle or too many staff are assigned to this activity or case complexity has changed from initial budget or newer, less experienced staff have been assigned to work and it takes them longer to complete service.

   - Suggest that staff re-adjust expectation to 2.0 hours per visit and expect 1,260 home visits this year, or reduce staff to .72 FTEs to provide 650 visits. In order to break even financially for this service, staff productivity must increase or staff must be reassigned/reduced.

   - The budget for home visit service is based on an actual reimbursed cost of $65.00 per home visit. If the number of home visits can be increased from 650 to 1,260 with the existing staff, the program will generate an additional $39,650 this year (1,260 − 650 = 610; 610 additional visits × $65/visit = $39,650). Healthcare payers will not reimburse more than $65.00 per visit this year. Suggest that staff initiate a quality improvement audit of existing clients to document outcomes. Bring results with actual higher costs to health payers to attempt negotiated reimbursement increases for serving high-risk Medicaid/Medicare population in the next year.

FIGURE 21–1 Service Productivity Analysis

innovative service idea, guessing at a charge for the service, providing the service, and later questioning why the staff time commitment is so excessive in relation to the financial return. An analysis of the project, including the documented need, the population to be served, favorable pricing, and realistic income expectations could turn the innovation into a source of income.

■ DEVELOPING SKILLS IN GRANT WRITING

Most nutritionists need to become grant writers so that they can obtain outside income to support innovative services, reach new populations, develop and test interventions, and initiate special projects; any or all of these may then turn into long-term, income-producing services. Some grant writing tips are as follows:

- Maintain a grant idea folder in which to file innovative ideas that would require external funding. These can be ideas with a one-paragraph description as contributed by staff members. The community needs assessment will help produce some ideas for needed community services.
- Foster staff development by conducting an internal seed grant program within the section or agency. Allocate a small amount of money each year to this research and development (R&D) fund.

Project Title (5 to 7 words):

_____

Amount Requested: _____

Total Project Cost: _____

Project Collaborators:

Project Summary:

Statement of specific problem or need:

Target population:

Project Goal:

Measurable Objectives	Methods	Lead Staff	Timeframe	Deliverables/ Evaluation

Budget, including in-kind contributions:

Sustainability opportunities once grant funding has ended:

Opportunities for replication in other geographic locations or with other target populations:

Letters of support to be sought:

FIGURE 21–2 Sample Grant Application Internal Worksheet

- Find several grant writers and reviewers within the agency with whom to brainstorm ideas and advice on writing grant proposals.
- Reduce all grant proposals to one-page worksheets as an initial step. A sample worksheet is shown in **Figure 21–2.**
- Maintain a large network of project collaborators to work with on grant proposals of mutual interest.
- Identify reliable people and organizations that can be counted on to write support letters, even on short notice. Some of these individuals/agencies may prefer that the support letter be written for their signature.
- Plan on writing grants that will generate three to four times the dollar amount from the grant as the program is committing.
- Practice writing concisely. If the idea cannot be conveyed in two double-spaced pages, including needs statement, methods, objectives, budget, and collaborators, grant writing will be too time-consuming.
- Maintain a file of agency information that can be pulled for grant attachments. Items such as Agency Internal Revenue Tax Exemption 501(c)(3) statements, audited budgets, lists of board members, agency descriptions, federal identification numbers

for the agency, and personnel curriculum vitae should be in this file.

- Maintain a file of copies of grants submitted previously.
- Use word processing and spreadsheet software to write the narrative and prepare the budget spreadsheet. This makes it easier to revise the proposal without introducing errors.
- Get on the mailing lists of every agency and foundation that announces related grant/contract RFPs that can be identified.

■ SUMMARY OF GRANT WRITING

Undoubtedly, additions will be made to these grant writing tips and they will be shared with other people. Sharing the work and the glory when a new grant comes to the agency is the mark of a true professional. Researching grant funds and writing proposals takes time. Alas, well-written proposals are not always funded. Even experienced grant writers receive rejections. It takes persistence. If a proposal is rejected, ask for a copy of the grant evaluation sheet and try again, and again.

Issues for Discussion

1. Given the staffing patterns described in Table 21–4 and Figure 21–1, is the nutrition program using the best mix of staff and allocation of staff time to result in the desired outcomes? What additional information would be useful? What productivity-enhancing strategies would be useful for the nutrition staff involved in the home visiting service?

2. Suggest a grant application idea to increase financial resources for the home visiting service. Complete a Grant Application Internal Worksheet (Figure 21–2) for your idea and discuss.

3. How should fees for nutrition services be established, and how should this income be allocated most effectively?

4. Explore the healthcare billing/coding references for your state Medicaid program and identify two potential billing codes for public health nutrition services. Identify the state and federal requirements (documentation, supervision, service provider, eligibility) for use of these billing codes. Medicaid reimbursement rates paid by the state Medicaid agency should be public information. Request the reimbursement rate for the billing codes you identified from different healthcare providers. Discuss your findings.

5. Explore the use of Relative Value Units (RVUs) in other health professions and describe how this could be adapted to dietetic practice.

6. Explore www.grants.gov for a grant opportunity that would involve public health nutrition. Complete a Grant Application Internal Worksheet for this grant possibility.

Suggested Reading

Baker J, Baker RW. *Healthcare Finance: Basic Tools for Non-Financial Managers*, 3rd ed. Boston: Jones & Bartlett; 2010.

Chima C, Pollack H. Nutrition services in managed care—an ADA position paper. *J Am Diet Assoc.* 2002;102:1471–1478.

Conklin MT, Simko MD. Cost-benefit and cost-effectiveness analyses of nutrition programs. *Quality Rev Bull.* 1983;9:166–168.

Dever GEA. *Improving Outcomes in Public Health Practice: Strategies and Methods.* Gaithersburg, MD: Aspen; 1997.

Disbrow D. The costs and benefits of nutrition services: a literature review. *J Am Diet Assoc.* 1989;89(suppl):S4–S63.

Frank HA. *Public Financial Management.* Boca Raton, FL: CRC Press and Taylor & Francis; 2006.

Gapenski L. *Healthcare Finance: An Introduction to Accounting and Financial Management,* 2nd ed. Chicago: Health Administration Press; 2001.

Honore P, Clarke R, Mead D, Menditto S. Creating financial transparency in public health–examining best practices of system partners. *J Public Health Manag Pract.* 2007;13:121–129.

Lighter D, Fair D. *Principles and Methods of Quality Management in Healthcare.* Gaithersburg, MD: Aspen; 2000.

Omachonu V. *Total Quality and Productivity Management in Healthcare Organizations.* Norcross, GA: Institute of Industrial Engineers; 1991.

Schramm WF. WIC prenatal participation and its relationship to newborn Medicaid costs in Missouri: a cost/benefit analysis. *Am J Public Health.* 1985;75:851–857.

Warren C, Reeve J, Duchac J. *Accounting,* 23rd ed. Cincinnati, OH: South-Western College Publishers; 2009.

PART

VII

Mobilizing Personnel

CHAPTER 22

Staffing Public Health Nutrition Programs and Services
CYNTHIA TAFT BAYERL, MS, RD, LDN

CHAPTER 23

Managing Public Health Nutrition Personnel
ESTHER OKEIYI, PhD, RD, LDN

CHAPTER 24

Leveraging Nutrition Education Through the Public Health Team
DEEPA ARORA, PhD

In Part VII, Chapter 22 reviews the core functions of the professionals who make up the public health nutrition team and designate job responsibilities needed to carry out the programs and services. In addition, Chapter 23 educates the reader on effective management skills that enable the public health nutrition profession to perform necessary services, including public health nutrition education, which is discussed in Chapter 24. Education is the final result of all the program planning, scientific data collection and findings, nutrition policy, money appropriation, and safeguarding and distribution of food for the American public.

CHAPTER

22

Staffing Public Health Nutrition Programs and Services

Cynthia Taft Bayerl, MS, RD, LDN

READER OBJECTIVES

After studying this chapter and reflecting on the contents, you should be able to:

1. Discuss changing trends that impact public health nutritionists' job functions.
2. Compare and contrast the job functions of nutrition personnel who work in public health and community settings.
3. Describe the educational requirements for nutritionists who work in public health settings and how those qualifications might be obtained.
4. Discuss how job satisfaction and salary impact staffing.
5. List various work settings for public health nutrition positions.

■ INTRODUCTION

A working knowledge of current and emerging trends in public health is important to appreciate more fully the roles and responsibilities of staffing in public health nutrition programs. Healthcare trends greatly influence the public health nutritionist's scope of practice and thus the roles and functions she or he assumes in the healthcare arena. Recent consumer trends indicate that there is an increased interest in both personal health and health information to be provided by qualified providers, including nutrition personnel.[1,2] This trend may be attributed, in part, to major changes that have occurred in the healthcare environment as well as more media coverage of relevant consumer-focused research findings. These changes have begun to impact how nutrition personnel work to provide more effective public health services. Some of these changes include:

- Socioeconomic and demographic changes, including ethnic diversification within the U.S. population[3]
- Changes in eating habits and food preparation, resulting in more obesity[4]
- New advances in food technology and biochemical and molecular research, which have changed what types of food we eat, how we eat it, and who prepares it

- Adverse economic factors that affect food supply and demand as well as health and nutritional status

To understand and to meet the challenges associated with these emerging trends, public health agencies must hire and train staff with the knowledge and skills to provide effective services beyond the traditional model of direct-care nutrition counselors.[5] In order to understand the role and function of today's public health nutrition personnel, an understanding of the definition, role, and responsibilities of these providers is important.

■ STAFFING TRENDS

Public health nutritionists in community agencies are responsible for nutrition and physical activity programs, which focus on community-wide health promotion and disease prevention. The term *public health nutritionist* is used for the professional who has completed academic course work in biostatistics, epidemiology, environmental studies, health program planning and evaluation, and advanced nutrition. Historically, public health nutritionists are differentiated from the dietitian on the basis of providing community care, rather than direct care, to individual patients/clients.

My thanks to: Carol E. Chan, MS, Combined Didactic Program in Dietetics/Master of Science and Dietetic Internship, Boston University, for her assistance in updating the references for this chapter.

In many agencies, both dietitians and public nutritionists perform similar job functions and can be classified in similar job categories.[6] Public health nutrition services, including those at federal, state, and local levels, are described in detail by Kaufman and colleagues within the Association of State and Territorial Public Health Nutrition Directors (ASTPHND).[7] The landmark publication *Personnel in Public Health Nutrition for the 1990's* provides an excellent basis for defining job titles of professional and paraprofessional staff and their roles, responsibilities, and function within state and local programs.[8] Within the field of public health nutrition, the 2006–2007 survey by the ASTPHND serves as the common definition for most current job descriptions and functions for public health staff.[9]

Current trends, which have shifted the focus of the public health system from an individual to a population-based system, is described best by the Institute of Medicine (IOM) in *The Future of Public Health*[10] and The Future of the *Public's Health in the 21st Century*.[11] The IOM further describes trends in the public health system, detailing the roles and responsibilities of public health personnel, including those within the Maternal and Child Health (MCH) programs, one of the largest employers of nutritionists through the Special Supplemental Nutrition Program for Women, Infants and Children (WIC). IOM definitions are based on a detailed study of public health systems and include strong recommendations on the purpose, function, and mission of public health as a system to assure conditions in which people can be healthy. The IOM used this detailed study to act as a catalyst to inform the public about the improvements in Americans' health, which have prevented countless deaths and improved the quality of life. These improvements, in many instances, are due to the successes of public health systems. The IOM also used its study to address a concern that the nation has lost sight of its public health goals and has allowed the public health system to fall into disrepair. The study has been used to communicate a sense of urgency about the need to maintain current preventative efforts to sustain the capability of existing public health programs and to meet future public health needs. The IOM recommends that public health staff will need to focus on the following three core functions in order to transition from the current client-focused system to a population-based approach:

1. Community assessment: The IOM recommends that every public health agency collect, assemble, analyze, and document information on the health of the community on a regular and systematic basis. Community assessment includes ongoing data collection and dissemination of statistics on the community's health status and needs. Systemized studies would result from these assessments, and would include population health trends and controlled epidemiological studies of community health problems. Nutrition assessment and the study of the nutrition profile of the population will provide the basis for developing new, population-focused nutrition programs. As the IOM has specified, the state public health agency bears the responsibility for leadership in the development and implementation of nutrition assessment at the state level. At both the state and local community levels, staff responsibilities for the assessment function would include monitoring and surveillance of nutritional status and population needs, as well as resource identification and collection and interpretation of data. Identifying community needs using multiple data sources, forecasting trends, ensuring a safe supply of food and water, and evaluating outcomes are important components to an effective state-of-the-art public health nutrition program. In order to successfully accomplish community nutrition assessment, personnel must have the skills necessary to evaluate how interrelated systems such as health, education, human services, food supply, and

Epidemiological studies: Research that is derived from data compiled from a population. Some different types of epidemiologic studies include:

- **Correlational studies:** Comparison of the frequency of events between two populations, which do not have to be at a specific time.
- **Cross-sectional studies:** Comparison of the frequency of events between two populations at the same specific time.
- **Cohort or incidence studies:** A population is followed over time to assess data incidences.
- **Case-control studies:** Subjects with specified characteristics are followed and compared to other subjects who don't have those characteristics.
- **Controlled trials:** Usually the study of subjects, using randomized selection and a double-blind method (both researcher and test subject are not privy to study group assignment), to evaluate a hypothesis.

Review nutritional studies in Chapter 1 and 2.

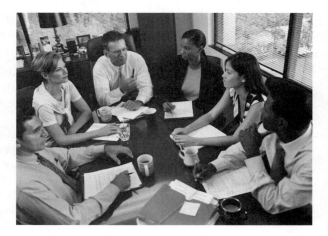

financial and insurance systems are interconnected as well as how these systems are interdependent. Interactions among these arenas and between nutrition and the public health system as a whole will need to be assessed.

2. Policy development: The IOM advocates the use of scientific knowledge in decision making (see Chapter 2). Public health agencies should lead in the development of public health policies that take a strategic approach to public health and use a democratic process (see Chapters 7 and 8). For example, policies and programs that address the highest perceived needs of the community will need to include nutrition and health policy. Policy development also includes:
   - Setting priorities
   - Development, implementation, and evaluation of community plans
   - Assumption of leadership, where overall goals include nutrition programs

3. Public health assurance: The IOM places the public health agency in the leadership role to assure the community that the services necessary to achieve agreed-upon goals will be provided. Policy can be implemented by encouraging actions by other entities (in both the private and public sector) through regulation and/or by direct-care service. The public health agency would invite key policy makers and the general public to collaborate in determining community-wide health policies, which would govern every member of that community including those who are unable to afford it. Public policy assurance also includes a wide scope of functions, which are described by Probert.[12] In her book, *Moving to the Future*, the author indicates that the following public health policy functions should exist:
   - Implementation of effective nutrition strategies
   - Access to services and quality in the implementation of public health and community nutrition plans
   - Ensuring safety, access, and adequacy of the food supply to promote and maintain the health of the population
   - Responding to food and nutrition crises
   - Support for monitoring and surveillance systems
   - Provision of population-based and culturally competent nutrition education
   - Provision of nutrition services to high-risk, underserved, and culturally diverse populations
   - Nutrition counseling to persons with health conditions related to poor nutritional status (e.g., diabetes, cardiovascular disease, hypertension)
   - Planning for emergency preparedness
   - Marketing
   - Providing nutrition information to the public

- Encouraging public and private sector collaborations
- Mobilizing nutrition resources
- Setting standards for various levels of nutrition staff, including maintaining accountability to the community through setting goals and measuring progress towards those goals

For nutrition personnel to carry out these core functions, they will need to be supported by strong administrative and managerial leadership, which is essential to provide a successful transition from direct-care services to those that include all three of these core functions.

CORE FUNCTIONS IN NUTRITION SERVICE SYSTEMS

Generally, the state public health agency is recognized as the lead agency to develop and implement systems that will assess, monitor, and evaluate the nutritional status of the entire state.[10] Personnel, at both the state and local levels, need to have the necessary skills to participate in the planning, implementation, and evaluation of nutrition service systems. Qualified personnel will enable the community to identify and procure funding and resources from local, state, and federal agencies to provide services that focus on nutrition and physical activity. Community public health programs include services to low-income populations [e.g., school breakfast and lunch programs, SNAP (food stamps), and WIC] as well as services targeted to promote the health of the general public.[5]

In 2006–2007, the ASTPHND surveyed public health personnel and reported that more than 66.6% of the public health nutrition workforce indicated that their primary area of practice was in direct client services or the assurance core function. Approximately 10.5% indicated that management/administration of these programs was their primary area of focus; 10.5% reported focusing on assessment; and 5.9% indicated public policy including population interventions (e.g., community organization, advocacy and policy development) as their primary area of focus. About 90% (88.6%) of the public health nutrition workforce works in the WIC program. WIC remains the largest public health nutrition program in the United States.[7-9]

CORE PUBLIC HEALTH FUNCTIONS INTERRELATED WITH ESSENTIAL PUBLIC HEALTH FUNCTIONS

Core public health functions and essential public health functions are interrelated. Creation of public health programs, which are based on both core and essential public health functions, are important in providing comprehensive, standard community-based programs. In work funded by the Department of Health and Human Services (DHHS), entitled *Public Health in America* (**Figure 22–1**), the essential functions and interrelationship of the core public health functions are described.[13] This information is supported by research in community settings, which is based on science as well as the practice of public health.

Historically, the work of public health nutritionists has been studied by and supported through collaborations with colleagues in academia. The collaboration has been essential to understanding the issues from both the research perspective and in practice. The lessons learned have been used to effectively teach emerging and seasoned nutritionists public health solutions to nutrition issues. For example, Haughton, Story, and Keir[5] propose using the IOM studies on public health systems, including core functions, to develop curriculum and continuing education. This includes providing distance and on-campus education to prepare the workforce with the knowledge and skills necessary to understand and practice core public health functions.[5,6]

Integration of core and essential public health services moved the health of the nation closer to the objectives outlined in Healthy People (HP) 2010 and 2020, which are highlighted in Figure 22–1. According to the 2008 Progress Review of HP 2010, of 37 objectives and sub-objectives defined in the original HP 2010 text aimed at improving public health agencies' infrastructure, 12 have met or are successfully moving toward their targets, while 7 are showing no progress or are moving away from their targets. The remaining objectives lack sufficient data to evaluate progress.[14]

Further success of meeting HP 2020 objectives will continue to depend in part on how healthcare professionals, including nutritionists, integrate the core functions and essential health functions into their portfolio of skills.

ESSENTIAL PUBLIC HEALTH SERVICES

Nutrition services and the recruitment and hiring of effective personnel to staff these nutrition services depend on a thorough understanding of the relationship between core public health functions and subsequent public health programming. Probert, in *Moving to the Future*,[12] described the following essential public health services:

- Monitor health status to identify community health problems.
- Diagnose and investigate health problems and health hazards in the community.
- Inform, educate, and empower people about health issues.
- Mobilize community partnerships to identify and solve health problems.
- Develop policies and plans that support individual and community health efforts.
- Enforce laws and regulations that protect health and ensure safety.
- Link people to needed personal health services and assure the provision of health care when otherwise unavailable.
- Assure a competent public health and personal health-care workforce.
- Evaluate effectiveness, accessibility, and quality of personal and population-based health services.
- Research for new insights and innovative solutions to health problems.

If public health programs are to provide both core and essential functions, then staffing will need to reflect training, expertise, and time spent in delivery of both of these services. This recommendation supports thinking that the functions of nutrition personnel have not undergone the recommended systematic changes as outlined by the IOM.[7,8]

NUTRITIONISTS' ROLE IN CORE FUNCTIONS AND ESSENTIAL PUBLIC HEALTH SERVICES

Current thinking indicates that the core functions and essential public health functions can be addressed at the federal, state, and local levels. Probert[12] described the importance of nutrition services as part of a comprehensive public health system in addressing the mission of public health, as outlined by the IOM. Current trends reflect the importance and need for nutrition personnel at all levels to be aware of the essential public health services, as they are the foundation for their scope of practice. The essentials and core functions

FIGURE 22–1 Healthy People 2020 Core Functions

Source: U.S. Department of Health and Human Services. *Healthy People.* Available at http://www.healthypeople.gov/. Accessed February 25, 2010.

are the drivers of change from the traditional model of assurance to the inclusion of assessment and public policy in current public health models.

According to Probert, essential public health nutrition services are[12]:

- Assessing the nutritional status of specific populations or geographic areas
- Identifying target populations that may be at nutritional risk
- Initiating and participating in nutrition data collection
- Providing leadership in the development of and planning for health and nutrition policies
- Recommending and providing specific training and programs to meet identified nutrition needs
- Raising awareness among key policy makers about the potential impact of nutrition and food regulations and budget decisions on the health of the community
- Acting as an advocate for target populations on food and nutrition issues
- Planning for nutrition services in conjunction with other health services, based on information obtained from an adequate and ongoing database focused on health outcomes
- Identifying and/or assisting in development of accurate, up-to-date nutrition education materials
- Ensuring the availability of quality nutrition services to target populations, including nutrition screening, assessment, education, counseling, referral for food assistance, and follow-up
- Participating in nutrition research and demonstration and evaluation projects
- Providing expert nutrition consultation to the community
- Providing community health promotion and disease prevention activities that are population based
- Providing quality assurance guidelines for personnel dealing with food and nutrition issues
- Facilitating coordination with other providers of health and nutrition services within the community
- Evaluating the impact of the health status of populations who receive public health nutrition services

■ HEALTHY PEOPLE 2010 AND LEADING HEALTH INDICATORS WITH CONTINUATION INTO HEALTHY PEOPLE 2020

The HP 2010 objectives were developed by the U.S. DHHS and released in 2000.[15] HP 2010 was a set of health objectives for the nation to achieve over the first decade of the new century. Many different people, states, communities, professional organizations, and others used these objectives to help develop programs to improve health care. The report contained approximately 400 goals, of which 66 were directly related to nutrition, with 21 specifically related to improving the nutritional status and eating habits of Americans. HP 2010 built on initiatives pursued over the prior two decades. The 1998 Surgeon General's report, *Healthy People*,[16] along with Healthy People 2000: National Health Promotion and Disease Prevention Objectives,[17] established national health objectives and served as the basis for the development of state and community plans. Like its predecessors, the HP 2010 and 2020 objectives supported the broad goals of the Surgeon General's report by increasing the quality and years of healthy life and eliminating health disparities among different segments of the population. Healthy indicators, one way to categorize the health objectives, were used for the first time in the HP 2010 and will be continued to be used 2020.

> Read about Healthy People 2010 and 2020 at http://www.healthypeople.gov.

Several of the leading health indicators are relevant to the field of nutrition/dietetics. These include overweight and obesity, physical activity, and access to health care. These health indicators are focal areas for many public health providers, including nutritionists. In order to effectively work with clients, these providers require a variety of skills.[18] The effectiveness of nutrition personnel working within their communities helps determine the success of the community in meeting the targeted public health outcomes.[18]

Work groups prepared the Healthy People 2020 document. Details are on the Internet. Public participation was critical in shaping Healthy People 2020, its purpose, goals, organization, and action plans. DHHS sought input from communities and stakeholders through public meetings across the country and public comment periods. As a national initiative, Healthy People's success depends on a coordinated commitment to improve the health of the nation. Subscribe to the Healthy People listserv for the latest information on Healthy People 2020 and to receive e-mail notices of related news, events, publications, and more! To become an active supporter of Healthy People, join the Healthy People Consortium.

Healthy People 2020 was released in two phases. The framework (the vision, mission, goals, focus areas, and criteria for selecting and prioritizing objectives) was released in 2010. Its objectives were released along with guidance for achieving the new decade's targets. For more information as it is released go to (http://www.healthypeople.gov/hp2020/).

■ EMERGING TRENDS THAT IMPACT STAFFING

The Bureau of Labor Statistics (BLS)[1] and the American Dietetic Association (ADA)[19] have reported trend data, which include projections on the impact of the economy and other factors on staffing. The BLS publishes information biennially in the *Occupational Outlook Handbook* (OOH).

Read about the Bureau of Labor Statistics' *Occupational Outlook Handbook*[1] at http://www.bls.gov/oco/home.htm.

The *Handbook* utilizes employment and census data to predict the growth in employment for specific occupations, including nutrition services. However, it does not differentiate between the commonly used terms *registered dietitian*, *dietitian*, and *nutritionist*. This lack of differentiation among the job descriptions makes it difficult to clearly identify which types of nutrition personnel or specific staffing will benefit from the projection statistics. The 2008–2009 OOH reported that dietitians and nutritionists held 57,000 jobs in 2006. Jobs were held in the following areas[1]:

Hospitals

Nursing care facilities

Outpatient care centers

Offices of physicians and other health practitioners

Correctional facilities

Health Departments

Other public health–related areas

Food service establishments on contract to facilities such as colleges and universities, airlines, correctional facilities, and company cafeterias

Public and private educational services

Community care facilities for the elderly (including assisted-living facilities)

Individual and family services

Home health care services

The U.S. Department of Veterans Affairs

Self-employment as consultants to facilities or individuals

The BLS OOH[1] reported employment to increase by 9% during the period 2006–2016, which is a comparable job growth rate to all occupations. Dietitians and nutritionists with specialized training, advanced degrees, or certifications beyond the particular state's minimum requirement for employment will experience the best job prospects.[1]

In their ADA study, Kornblum[19] utilized the BLS data to report the projected number of jobs for various nutrition positions and services into the year 2005, and in which sectors of the job market they would occur. This report indicated that the demand for dietetics professionals will increase as the demand for food service expertise and nutrition counseling increases in a variety of settings, including hospitals, nursing homes, schools, prisons, community health programs, and health clubs.[20] The following areas of public health interest have generated the increase:

- The public's interest in nutrition and the emphasis on health education and prudent lifestyles will add to the present demand for credentialed and highly skilled nutrition personnel to provide the service.
- As life expectancy increases and the elderly are more commonly living to 100 + , community-based settings such as nursing homes will need the services of skilled nutrition providers to assist the geriatric population with emerging health- and nutrition-related issues.
- Contract food services, as found in residential care facilities and other social service agencies, will require qualified nutrition personnel to oversee compliance as well as provide therapeutic programs to residents.

Within these sectors, the greatest growth in the number of nutrition personnel needed is projected to be in physicians' offices (54%), offices of other health practitioners (63%), personal services such as Diet Workshop (60%), childcare services (64%), home health care (91%), and residential care (129%). Third-party reimbursement and the aging of the population are projected to play a role in demand. Industries projected to have a lower growth rate for nutrition personnel include hospitals (7%), education (16%), and government (0.5%).[19]

In 2005, Payne-Palacio and Canter identified several societal changes that will affect the field of dietetics in the coming future[21]:

- Aging population and cultural diversity. As the baby boomer generation ages, more dietetics professionals will be needed to work with the elderly. The increasing ethnic diversity in the country will require not only a greater need for culturally competent dietetics professionals, but also more ethnic diversity within the profession as well.
- Changing lifestyles and changing workplace. The public is perpetually concerned with efficiency in all aspects of life, including diet and nutrition. Dietetics professionals will be increasingly needed to help individuals and institutions meet health and wellness goals as efficiently as possible. Furthermore, with more families with both parents spending more time in the workplace than at home, as well as with children spending more time in school, there will be an increased need for dietetics professionals in school foodservice, and in foodservice industries to provide healthy options while depending on prepared and packaged foods.

Technology plays a major role in societal change. With integrative technology becoming increasingly prominent in society, dietetics professionals will need to be comfortable with computers, telecommuting tools and resources, and stay updated with new technological advances in various food and agriculture, nutrition, pharmacologic, and health-related fields. The continuous expansion of the Internet will require an increased presence on the Web. With the overwhelming amount of information available on the Internet, there is an immense need for dietetics professionals to effectively educate the public using evidence-based research and to sort out the facts from the fiction.[21]

- Eating away from home: Snacks and "grab-and-go" food items are increasingly popular as the public spends less time away from home. Dietetics professionals therefore are needed in foodservice industries and establishments that serve this growing population.
- Nutraceuticals and government policies: Qualified dietetics professionals must be skilled and knowledgeable about functional and designed foods, known as nutraceuticals, to guide consumers about the growing number of products widely available in grocery and health stores.
- Obesity and diabetes: As obesity and diabetes continue to be top public health concerns, and with medical nutrition therapy being the best tool to combat these and other health problems, dietetics professionals need to continuously work toward including medical nutrition therapy (MNT) in Medicare and other insurance programs.

A new publication by the ADA, *Achieving Excellence: Clinical Staffing for Today and Tomorrow*,[22] outlines parameters for clinical nutrition staffing for registered dietitians and dietetic technicians in both inpatient and outpatient settings. Biesemeier acknowledges various challenges, including that there is no universally accepted method for staffing, and that budget constraints are the lead factor negatively impacting staffing ratios. This is further hindered by the fact that the service model is being used, rather than focusing on desired patient outcomes or benchmarking reports.

A wide range of nutrition care procedures are used by practitioners and facilities to meet various standards, including those of the Joint Commission on Accreditation of Healthcare Organizations (JCAHO), as discussed in Chapter 15. JCAHO standards, which in the past were mainly used by hospitals or by dietitians in clinical settings, are now used by many community-based healthcare facilities. The ADA reports' authors propose the use of staffing in any setting to correlate with desired patient outcomes.[22] A variety of strategies, based on the performance improvement model, should be used to monitor clinical indicators and outcomes. A performance-based model measures performance indicators using measurable characteristics of products, such as processes, services, and systems used to track and improve performance. One of the tools with the model is called a "dashboard," which consists of the indicator, the actual performance, a performance benchmark, an indicator value, a data source, a benchmark source, trends, and comments. Information is collected and reported on a quarterly basis. Biesemeier discussed a system of nutrition care based on evidence-based practice using a host of tools, including data and validated measures and procedures, on which to base performance and management.[22]

Other Tools to Assess Nutrition Services and Staffing

Tools such as *Moving to the Future: Developing Community-Based Nutrition Services*[13] and the *Bright Futures* series, which includes publications on nutrition[23], oral health[24], and physical activity[25], have been developed for healthcare providers and nutritionists to expand their skills. These and other tools provide effective communication vehicles to help deliver clear, focused messages to motivate healthy behavior changes to meet the goals established within the HP 2010 objectives.

Read about the Joint Commission on Accreditation of Healthcare Organizations (JCAHO) at http://www.jcaho.org.

■ AMERICAN DIETETIC ASSOCIATION'S DEFINITION OF NUTRITION PERSONNEL

The ADA is the nation's largest organization of food and nutrition professionals, with over 70,000 members.[26] Approximately 75% of the ADA's members are registered dietitians (RDs), and 4% of its members are registered dietetic technicians (DTRs). Other members include clinical and community dietetics professionals, consultants, food service managers, educators, researchers, and students. ADA members represent a range of practice areas and interests including: public health; sports nutrition; medical nutrition therapy; diet counseling; cholesterol reduction; diabetes; heart and kidney disease; vegetarianism; food service management in business, hospitals, restaurants, long-term care facilities, and education systems; education of other healthcare professionals; and scientific research. The following are ADA definitions of qualified personnel[27]:

- Registered dietitian (RD): The RD must pass a national examination administered by the Commission on Dietetic Registration and complete continuing professional educational requirements to maintain registration. Some RDs hold additional certifications in specialized areas of practice, such as pediatric or renal nutrition, nutrition support, and diabetes education. Most RDs work at hospitals and medical centers, in private practice, or at other healthcare facilities. Many work in community and public health settings, academia, and research. A growing number work with the food and nutrition industry and business, journalism, sports nutrition, corporate wellness programs, and in other nontraditional settings. Nearly half of all ADA members hold advanced academic degrees.
- Dietetic technician, registered (DTR): A food and nutrition practitioner, often working in conjunction with a registered dietitian, who has met the minimum

academic and professional requirements to qualify for the credential "DTR." In addition to DTR credentialing, some states have regulatory laws for registered dietetic technicians. Like RDs, DTRs must complete professional educational requirements to maintain their registration. DTRs work in hospices, home healthcare programs, food service operations, and government and community programs such as Meals on Wheels. DTRs must complete at least a two-year associate's degree in an approved dietetics technology program from an accredited U.S. college or university and additionally must have supervised practice experience in community programs, healthcare, and food service facilities. DTRs must pass a nationwide examination and continuing education courses throughout their careers.

- Public health nutritionist: This title is reserved for positions that require dietetic registration status and a graduate-level science degree, which includes environmental sciences, health program planning, management, and evaluation. The term is usually used for an individual with a master's degree in public health nutrition.
- Community nutritionist/dietitian: An individual with a baccalaureate degree who is a registered dietitian or registration-eligible dietitian.
- Community nutrition educator: An individual with a baccalaureate degree with a minimum of 15 hours of course work in nutrition from a regionally accredited college or university.

It is important to understand the academic preparation guidelines so that nutritionists/dietitians can more fully understand a host of factors including various job functions, skills, employee performance, job expectations, recruitment and retention issues, and job satisfaction.

Academic Preparation of the Nutrition Staff

Academic preparation of the nutrition staff can vary significantly depending upon the job function. Information from the 2006–2007 ASTPHND workforce survey[9] indicates that more than half of public health staff had at least a bachelor's degree with a focus on nutrition or dietetics. Among the WIC workforce, 48.9% had a bachelor's degree in nutrition or dietetics, whereas 57.6% from the non-WIC workforce had a similar degree.[6] In contrast to 1999–2000 survey results, fewer WIC personnel had bachelor's degrees (4.2%) than their non-WIC counterparts (4.9%), although both statistics are higher in 2006–2007 than in 1999–2000 (2.3% for WIC personnel and 1.8% for non-WIC personnel). The non-WIC workforce had a higher percentage of advanced degrees (21.4%), such as a master's degree in nutrition/dietetics, versus 17.5% with a master's degree in public health.[6] For information on which nutrition/dietetic

programs have been approved by the American Dietetic Association, refer to the ADA Web site,[24] which also lists additional references to public health programs having a nutrition program.

In addition to definitions of job classifications, the ADA has established a definition of nutrition services for Medicare-eligible clients, which is referred to as medical nutrition therapy (MNT).[28] MNT

> Find the ADA Web site at http://www.eatright.org/public/7782_13280.cfm for current nutrition/dietetics programs.

includes nutritional diagnostic, therapeutic, and counseling services provided by a registered dietitian and can effectively treat and manage disease conditions. MNT can:

- Reduce or eliminate the need for prescription drug use
- Help reduce complications in patients with disease
- Improve patients' overall health and quality of life

The academic preparation for registered dietitians and other nutrition personnel who work in public health/community settings must include MNT training as a part of direct-care services to individuals.[28]

The ADA's *Future Practice and Education Task Force Report* was focused on entry-level practitioners and various employment trends of the future. The Task Force made the following recommendations[29]:

Education and Supervised Practice for Entry-Level DTR

- The Promotion of the DTR within the ADA membership and its organized units as a valuable member of the dietetics team.
- Increased promotion of dietetic technician programs to community colleges, and the further development of articulation agreements between Dietetic Technician Programs and Didactic Programs in Dietetics (DPD) or Coordinated Programs (CP) to foster the career ladder.
- The creation of opportunities for DPD students/graduates to obtain quality dietetics practice experience for eligibility to sit for the Registration Examination for Dietetic Technicians after completion of the DPD and baccalaureate degree.

Future Education and Supervised Practice for Entry-Level RD

- The faculty of dietetics education programs to continue to implement a variety of innovative quality education models with the support of Commission on Accreditation for Dietetics Education (CADE), and the continued implementation of an array of experiential routes that satisfy entry-to-practice requirements.
- Pathways for entry into the profession be developed for individuals who have earned master's or doctoral

degrees in food and nutrition or related fields from U.S. regionally accredited colleges and universities or the equivalent. Initial priority should be for implementation for the doctoral prepared individuals, and these individuals must successfully complete the academic and experiential competencies for eligibility for registration exam (one aspect for the preparation must be through a CADE-accredited program).

Future Specialty Practice   ADA to continue to recognize specialty practice areas in dietetics and provide support for additional appropriate education and credentialing opportunities.

Future Advanced Practice   ADA to define and recognize advanced practice. Advanced practitioners will be supported with educational programming and the appropriate credentials.

Implementation and Resource Allocation   Adequate resources to be allocated by the ADA board of directors to support the planning and implementation of a Future Practice and Education Summit involving both Dietetic Practice Groups and all types of dietetics education programs.

The establishment of a two-prong grant program to promote the integration of practice and education by supporting educators to obtain updated practice experience and practitioners to increase their exposure to academic settings.

Enhancement of the efficiency and effectiveness of academic and experiential education through development of practice simulations and utilization of other appropriate educational technologies; development of educational opportunities for dietetic educators to obtain updated practice exposure, and for practitioners to enhance skills in developing and evaluating practice experiences of students; and continuing education to assist dietetic education program directors in managing programs effectively.

■ OPPORTUNITIES IN GOVERNMENT EMPLOYMENT

Federal Government

The largest employer of public health nutrition personnel, the federal government, funds many nutrition programs through state and local community agencies. The United States Department of Agriculture (USDA) is one branch of the federal government that administers primary food assistance programs, which include the (SNAP) Food Stamp Program, the National School Lunch Program, and WIC. In the fiscal year 2008, these three programs, along with the School Breakfast Program and the Child and Adult Care Food Program, accounted for the majority (95%) of the $60.7 billion spent on USDA food assistance.[30] In addition, the USDA funds other public health nutrition programs

and the staffing of food assistance programs, including the Cooperative Extension and the Center for Nutrition Policy and Promotion, which coordinates government efforts to review and publish the Dietary Guidelines for Americans (in coordination with the Department of Health and Human Services).[31] Local agencies also contribute to the funding of public health nutritionist staffing, but the amount varies from state to state.[32]

The federal government is the largest single funding source of nutrition programs as well as departments of education, public health, and public assistance, with some states providing additional staffing funds. Nearly 69% of public health personnel work for state or local government health agencies.

The WIC program is the major employer of public health nutrition staff. This program alone funds 79.3% of the full-time-equivalent public health nutritionists.[33] The results of the 2006–2007 ASTPHND survey indicated that 88.6% of respondents worked in WIC, as compared to 85.4% in 1994 and 90.4% in 1999–2000.[6,9] The WIC program provides nutritious foods, nutrition education, and healthcare referrals to meet the special nutrition needs of low-income pregnant, postpartum, and breast-feeding women, and their infants and children up to five years of age, who are at nutritional risk.[34] Because WIC is the largest employer of public health nutritionists in the country, it is important to understand the goals and current challenges of the program[33] as well as the personnel issues such as recruitment and retention.[35] Information on the roles of personnel and the WIC service standards are outlined in the WIC Nutrition Services Standards.[36]

> Read more about the WIC program at http://www.fns.usda.gov/wic/.

Administrative Staff

Personnel in Public Health Nutrition for the 1990's[8] identified three professional job classifications with management and budgetary responsibility: the public health nutrition director, assistant public health nutrition director, and public health nutrition supervisor. In the 2006 ASTPHND survey, the degree to which the job descriptions matched the public health nutrition workforce was quite high. Ninety-one percent of the workforce were public health nutrition directors, 71.1% were assistant directors, and 76.7% were public health nutrition supervisors. In addition to supervising personnel, 62% of directors responded that they had responsibility for the agency's entire nutrition budget, while 32.4% of directors and 46.4% of assistant directors had responsibility for a more limited budget.[9] Other issues that nutrition personnel need to consider when developing and implementing effective nutrition service systems and hiring qualified providers include the following:

- Number of providers versus the number of clients
- Cultural and ethnic diversity of services and staffing
- Training needs
- Effective use of resources
- Salary
- Job satisfaction
- Reimbursement by third-party payers for nutrition services

Staffing Ratios

Personnel in Public Health Nutrition for the 1990's proposed a mathematical formula to estimate the ratio of nutrition personnel to clients.[8] Haughton, Story, and Keir[5] proposed a recommended staffing ratio of 1 public health nutritionist to 50,000 people. They estimated the number of public health nutritionists from the 1990 census data for all states and territories to be approximately 4,379, which was an 83% increase from the those levels identified in prior ASTPHND surveys.[5] More recent articles describing the roles and responsibilities of the nutrition workforce hypothesized a shift to population-based services, and subsequently to add the two core functions of public policy and community assessment. It is difficult to estimate whether these calculations remain pertinent. No other study to date has been identified that provides information on staffing ratios in public health settings.

Diversity

One of the two major goals of HP 2010 and 2020 is to eliminate ethnic and class disparities in the workforce. The development of a culturally competent health service workforce is one strategy that will help accomplish this goal. HP objective 1-8 specifically addresses the goal of increased representation of ethnic minorities in the health professions.[16] Greenwald and Davis[35] surveyed newly credentialed RDs, DTRs, and education program directors to better understand why males and minorities were underrepresented in the field of nutrition. RDs and DTRs primarily attributed the underrepresentation of minorities to the limited visibility of the field; they attributed the underrepresentation of men to the traditional association of the field of nutrition to women, an association typically characterized by low salaries. Educators, in contrast, attributed the minority underrepresentation to a disadvantage in education, particularly in science. Proposed solutions included flexible time lines for completion of programs, outreach to elementary and lower-division college students, tutoring, mentoring, encouragement by program faculty, scholarships, and the creation of professional networks to identify potential new minority entrants into the field.

In the ASTPHND survey, professionals and paraprofessionals were asked to rank their top-10 training needs when communicating with their clients; responses included dealing with low-literacy populations (60.9%) and cultural competency (43.7% for the WIC workforce, and 64.5% for the non-WIC workforce).[9] Although low literacy and cultural competency were not ranked high under communication needs, nutritionists did not identify the need to improve their own skills in this area. However, the lack of diversity in the public health nutrition workforce was evidenced in several parameters within other areas of survey results. Over 95% of the ASTPHN survey respondents were female. Ethnic diversity was greater among the WIC workforce as compared to non-WIC staff: Latino/Hispanic Americans made up 20.9% of the WIC workforce versus 9.1% of the non-WIC workforce; African Americans were 11.6% versus 6.5%, and Asian Americans were 5.5% versus 4.3%. Although the diversity of the WIC workforce was more representative of the population than the non-WIC workforce, it was not considered representative of the WIC participants themselves, which is an important component if culturally and linguistically diverse nutrition services are to be effective.[36] Ninety percent of the ASTPHND respondents reported English as their primary language (non-WIC 93.3% vs. WIC 88.5%), which does not demonstrate linguistic diversity.[4]

New initiatives, such as the American Public Health Association's (APHA) initiative, have been established to help public health nutritionists increase the diversity of the workforce. To assist current and emerging nutrition programs, two organizations have developed initiatives to address diversity issues. The ADA has developed a model to help practitioners develop multicultural competencies as well as learn to identify how the profession can more effectively work with diversity issues of practitioners and clients.[36,37] The APHA's initiative targets undergraduates to enhance educational opportunities in public health nutrition.[38]

Staff Training Needs

Nutrition personnel who responded to the 2006–2007 ASTPHND survey[9] identified the following practice areas where they could use more training for their current work:

- Breastfeeding
- Prenatal nutrition
- Infant and preschool age nutrition
- Childhood nutrition
- Nutrition counseling, behavior change, and client education

A list of ADA's nutrition and dietetics training programs are on the Internet at: http://www.eatright.org/students/education/accreditedprograms.aspx

The focus on maternal and child health areas for training was surprising because a large number of respondents who work in public health nutrition programs work in the WIC program. Haughton and George[9] hypothesized that if official health agencies were to shift to performing public health core functions, as recommended by the IOM, they would need to obtain the knowledge and skills necessary to practice assessment and evaluation in order to be more knowledgeable to meet the nutrition objectives. The ASTPHND report proposed that continuing education interventions should be offered by professional organizations (i.e., ASTPHND, ADA, and APHA). Distance and on-campus educational opportunities should be offered through approved public health nutrition programs so that more staff will have access to educational opportunities to enhance their skills. As an adjunct to existing funding, nutrition personnel will need to advocate for new funding streams to provide training in areas focused on public health core functions. These include cultural diversity and linguistic competency training, so public health staff can communicate more effectively with their clients and more fully understand the needs of their community.

Staff Resources

Many resources and tools are available to expand the skill level of nutritionists working in public health or community settings. Multiple Web sites from federal and state agencies, such as the CDC and USDA, provide tool kits and best practices. In addition, resources such as the ADA's *Guidelines for Community Nutrition Supervised Experiences*[39] were developed for various levels of personnel (e.g., registered dietitians, associate-level diet technicians, and bachelor's degree nutritionists) to help expand their skills. The tool was developed to assist those who lack the training or supervised experiences in community nutrition and who work in nutrition positions that are based on the traditional client-focused model (assurance) but need to transition to a practice that will be more population/systems focused (public policy and assessment). The knowledge and skills of nutrition personnel need to be consistent with the mission of public health, which is to assure conditions in which people are healthy. Cutting-edge tools and training as well as mentoring programs are needed to guide emerging practitioners and mid-career change candidates who want to enhance their skills and be prepared for the future. Using newer computer-based online tools such as virtual classroom, tele-seminars and Webinars, and self-study courses hopefully encourages both emerging and seasoned personnel to take advantage of continuing education experiences to enhance their knowledge and skills. Announcing these educational opportunities using communication vehicles such as YouTube, Facebook, Twitter, and Photo voice are ways to market educational opportunities.

Comparative studies of online and other learning avenues are still in progress, but will be important to consider in the quality and depth of knowledge and skills. These alternative learning methods may be particularly helpful for those practitioners within public health and community settings where income is more limited than in private sector employment. The ADA has several resources through The Center for Professional learning that offer accredited courses online. By encouraging and supporting public health personnel who may have financial, time, and other challenges to traditional avenues of education to learn online and by other means, a wider diversity of language and culture can be brought to the practice of dietetics.[40]

Other resources/tools to enhance staff knowledge and skills include the position papers of professional associations such as the ADA, the American Academy of Pediatrics, and the National Association of WIC Directors. Position papers can be used to support public policies, which guide the best practice strategies of nutritionists.

Position papers are derived from the latest available research and focus on such issues as promotion of breast feeding, child and adolescent nutrition programs, food technology and safety, effectiveness of medical nutrition therapy, and elderly nutrition. In addition to including relevant data in a practice area, they discuss implications on practice and staffing of nutrition programs. For example, one study, "The Role of Dietetics Professionals in Health Promotion and Disease Prevention"[37] supported the hypothesis that diet plays an important role in health promotion and disease prevention. Hampl, Anderson, and Mullis proposed that nutrition personnel should be trained in primary prevention in addition to the more traditional role in clinical settings (secondary and tertiary prevention), which focuses more on a disease management model. ADA position statements are available at its Web site.[38]

Position papers also can be used with policy makers and community leaders to provide evidence that healthy eating habits, coupled with other healthy lifestyle behaviors, have the potential to reduce the risk of chronic disease. Nutritionists and dietitians can use the information as part of the public policy core functions used to shape safe and supportive environments, build community coalitions, and redirect health services to include health promotion as a primary approach to delivering high-quality health care. Professional organizations are good resources of evidence-based research. Examples are the ADA's Evidence Analysis Library and Nutrition Care Process and Quality Assurance tools and practice based protocols; various ADA specialty certifications (pediatrics and sports medicine; the Pediatric and Adolescent Weight Management course; ADA Leadership Institute; CPE toolkit) that help practitioners at various points in the educational process to use the most current research and guidelines to best meet their individual needs and prepares them to provide quality patient care.

Job Satisfaction

Studies of public health personnel in the Virginia[41] and North Carolina[42] WIC programs found that associations exist between employee job satisfaction and consumer satisfaction. These associations translate to improved program participation rates. WIC benefits—namely food vouchers and nutrition education—were found to be insufficient incentives for the participants to continue to return on a regular basis to the program. The burden of other considerations, such as transportation to the clinic, wait time to obtain an appointment, and/or food vouchers, were deterrents to program participation. A negative correlation among low pay, low visibility, and limited resources was associated with giving a poor image of the nutrition profession, which was shown to lead to some job dissatisfaction. Negative effects identified by participants in public health nutrition programs (e.g., long wait, language and transportation barriers, limited culturally diverse food options, limited cost of food package) were also thought to be inversely tied to the job dissatisfaction felt by many nutrition personnel working directly with these clients, making job retention a challenge.[6,41]

Reimbursement Impacts Staffing

Changes in the healthcare system, including fee-for-service and other methods such as prepaid capitated and managed care, have had profound effects on the number and types of jobs available to dietetics professionals, the settings in which they work, and their roles and responsibilities. Although health promotion and prevention activities that include screenings and health education should be a top priority for healthcare providers and organizations, the value of these activities still is under debate. Many managed care organizations offer preventative services (e.g., health education workshops, discounts at fitness centers) for their enrolled populations. Population-based prevention activities (i.e., changes in the community environment to promote health) have not been considered the responsibility of private healthcare organizations. Studies by the ADA on the cost effectiveness of MNT are in progress and are expected to support the hypothesis that prevention and control of chronic illness would save healthcare costs. A finding consistent with this theory would both support and justify third-party payers providing nutrition services as part of subscribers' healthcare benefits, as it would be a cost-effective way for both the insurer and the client to save precious healthcare dollars.[42]

■ CONCLUSIONS

Staffing public health programs with qualified people to meet the challenges of the rapidly changing environment and emerging research is an exciting opportunity for public health nutritionists. Trend data support the concept that nutrition positions are increasing at the same rate as other healthcare provider jobs. These same studies also demonstrate that consumers have an increased awareness of and interest in nutrition and health. The expanding cultural and ethnic diversity of the U.S. population offers opportunities to advocate for nutrition services for populations who are interested in good healthcare as part of the American dream. The types of job settings are expanding, thanks to

heightened interest in nutrition and the aging and diversification of the population. While this is occurring, the public health system is transitioning from a traditional model of direct care services (assurance) to one that focuses on population-based health promotion and disease prevention that includes public policy and assessment of core functions.

To meet these new challenges, low-cost, accessible, and flexible training opportunities need to be available so that public health staff can expand their skills while working to support themselves and their families. Training opportunities coupled with competitive salaries will enhance recruitment and retention of qualified personnel.

Nutrition services, including MNT, offer exciting new opportunities to qualified nutrition care providers, which include registered dietitians, nutritionists, registered dietetic technicians, and other nutrition personnel, both professional and paraprofessional. Reducing challenges to securing third-party reimbursement for MNT, as part of public health intervention to prevent such conditions as obesity, will go a long way to expand the horizons beyond disease-based intervention.

Additional research is needed to measure outcomes of nutrition intervention as they relate to decreasing chronic illness. Securing government funding for research in combination with additional research monies from industry is critical to support best practices and intervention protocols. These studies are necessary to demonstrate the cost effectiveness and efficacy of nutrition services, which also includes the cost associated with staffing.

Staffing public health nutrition programs is a continuing challenge. The ever-changing healthcare landscape, diversity issues, and the rising cost of doing business in the United States continue to challenge the already burdened healthcare system. Despite rapidly rising healthcare costs, consumers continue to demonstrate an increased interest in nutrition. Americans want quick access to information and qualified professionals. Simultaneously, nutritionists are interested in achieving gains in several areas, including:

- Increased recognition by consumers and the profession
- Training opportunities to enhance their skills
- Equitable income

To improve job satisfaction, employers must provide a wide range of educational opportunities for public health nutritionists. Continuing flexible educational opportunities is a step in the right direction towards improving job satisfaction. Distance and Web-based learning programs offer flexibility for employers to continue to support the continuing education needs of our profession.

The impending retirement of long-time WIC staff will affect the number of qualified personnel ready and able to assume a seamless transition to management of WIC programs. In order to prepare for the shortage of nutrition personnel, the profession has developed outreach programs to potential nutrition students from diverse cultural and linguistic populations, and is actively addressing the issues of income parity, job satisfaction, and continuing education.

Issues for Discussion

1. Shortage of personnel: The traditional model of public health nutrition services is one-to-one and group counseling. Discuss two ways that nutrition assessment and public policy could enhance the role of nutritionists and improve nutrition services on the local, state, and federal levels, and use of new technology to educate clients (e.g., phone, chat room) as well as practioners (e.g., virtual classroom, Webinar, and teleconferences).

2. Funding: The federal government has historically funded public health nutrition services. With increased constraints on federal budgets, discuss two or more potential ways that nutritionists can use their new skills in assessment and public policy to advocate for an increased level of nutrition services budgets.

3. Job satisfaction: Discuss how the publics' participation and satisfaction with public health nutrition services impacts staff recruitment and retention both positively and negatively.

4. Aging of providers: How do you propose to recruit and retain new staff to meet the challenge of the upcoming waves of retirement of public health nutritionists?

5. Training opportunities: In the present healthcare system, it is difficult for public health nutritionists who work full time to enhance and expand their skills when most higher education programs are full time, costly, and held during work hours. What types of low cost, free, or scholarship opportunities and programs and or resources or tools would you suggest to academic institutions and other interested partners so that ethnically and culturally diverse nutrition staff can move up the career ladder and provide much-needed services to a culturally diverse U.S. population?

6. Job functions of nutrition staff: Compare and contrast the various major job functions of nutrition personnel who work in public health and community settings, and how they already intersect or could intersect to provide seamless services for consumers.

7. Recruitment and retention of staff: Encouraging people to enter and stay in public health positions is problematic due to dissatisfaction with low salary and benefits. What are some ideas you could suggest that might help retain and recruit nutrition personnel?

References

1. U.S. Department of Labor. *Occupational Outlook Handbook*, 2008–2009 ed. Available at http://www.bls.gov/oco/. Accessed May 10, 2009.
2. *United States Census 2000*. U.S. Census Bureau. Available at http://www.census.gov/main/www/cen2000.html. Accessed May 20, 2009.
3. The Institute for the Future. *Health and Healthcare in 2010*. San Francisco: Jossey-Bass; 2000.
4. Jarratt J, Mahaffie JM. Trends affecting the dietetics profession and the American Dietetic Association. *J Am Diet Assoc*. 2002;102:1821.
5. Haughton B, Story M, Keir B. Profile of public health personnel: challenges for population/system-focused roles and state-level monitoring. *J Am Diet Assoc*. 1998;98:664–670.
6. McCall M. *Survey of Public Health Nutrition Workforce: 1999–2000*. Washington, DC: USDA, FNS; January 2003.
7. Kaufman M. *Nutrition in Public Health: A Handbook for Developing Programs and Services*. Rockville, MD: Aspen; 1990.
8. Dodds JM, Kaufman M. *Personnel in Public Health Nutrition for the 1990's*. Washington, DC: The Public Health Foundation; 1991.
9. Haughton B, George A. *Survey of the Public Health Nutrition Workforce: 2006–2007*. Available at http://www.fns.usda.gov/wic/resources/workforcesurveyreport.htm. Accessed May 10, 2009.
10. Institute of Medicine (IOM), Committee for the Study of the Future of Public Health, Division of Health Care Services. *The Future of Public Health*. Washington, DC: National Academy Press; 1988.
11. Institute of Medicine, Committee on Assuring the Health of the Public in the 21st Century. *The Future of the Public's Health in the 21st Century*. Washington, DC: National Academy Press; 2002.
12. Probert KL. *Moving to the Future: Developing Community-Based Nutrition Services*. Washington, DC: Association of State and Territorial Public Health Nutrition Directors; 2003:87–88.
13. U.S. Department of Health and Human Services. *Public Health in America*. Available at http://www.Health.gov/phfunctions/public.htm. Accessed April 26, 2009.
14. U.S. Department of Health and Human Services, Public Health Service. *Progress Review: Public Health Infrastructure*. April 16, 2008. Available at http://www.healthypeople.gov/data/2010prog/focus23/. Accessed June 28, 2010.
15. U.S. Department of Health and Human Services. *Healthy People 2010: Understanding and Improving Health*, 2nd ed. Washington, DC: U.S. Government Printing Office; November 2000. Available at http://www.health.gov/healthypeople. Accessed June 28, 2010.
16. Public Health Service, Office of the Surgeon General of the United States, Department of Health and Human Services, Nutrition Policy Board. *The Surgeon General's Report on Nutrition and Health 1998*. Publication No. 88-50210. Available at http://profiles.nlm.nih.gov/NN/B/C/Q/G/.
17. U.S. Department of Health and Human Services. *Healthy People 2000: National Health Promotion and Disease Prevention Objectives*. DHHS Publication No. 91-50212. Washington, DC: U.S. Government Printing Office; 1991.
18. U.S. Department of Health and Human Services. *What Are the Leading Health Indicators?* Available at http://www.health.gov/healthypeople/LHI/lhiwhat.htm. Accessed April 26, 2009.
19. Kornblum TH. Professional demands for dietitians and nutritionists in the year 2005. *J Am Diet Assoc*. 1994;94:212–222.
20. Bryk JA, Kornblum T. Report on the 1999 membership database of the American Dietetic Association. *J Am Diet Assoc*. 2001;101:947–953.

21. Payne-Palacio J, Canter DD. *The Profession of Dietetics: A Team Approach*, 3rd ed. Philadelphia: Lippincott Williams & Wilkins; 2005:192–194.

22. Biesemeier C. *Achieving Excellence: Clinical Staffing for Today and Tomorrow.* Chicago, IL: American Dietetic Association; 2004.

23. Story M, Holt K, Sofka D, eds. *Bright Futures in Practice: Nutrition*, 2nd ed. Arlington, VA: National Center for Education in Maternal and Child Health; 2002. Available at http://www.brightfutures.org/nutrition/resources.html. Accessed April 26, 2009.

24. Casamassimo P, ed. *Bright Futures in Practice: Oral Health.* Arlington, VA: National Center for Education in Maternal and Child Health; 1996. Available at http://www.brightfutures.org/oralhealth/pdf/index.html. Accessed April 26, 2009.

25. Holt K, Sofka D, eds. *Bright Futures in Practice: Physical Activity.* Arlington, VA: National Center for Education in Maternal and Child Health; 2001. Available at http://www.brightfutures.org/physicalactivity. Accessed April 26, 2009.

26. The American Dietetic Association. Qualifications of a Registered Dietitian. Available at http://www.eatright.org/HealthProfessionals/content.aspx?id = 6857. Accessed April 26, 2009.

27. The American Dietetic Association. *Accredited or Approved Education Plans.* Available at http://eatright.org/public/7782_13280.cfm. Accessed April 26, 2009.

28. American Dietetic Association. *Evidence Mounts on the Effectiveness of Medical Nutrition Therapy.* Available at http://www.eatright.org/Public/GovernmentAffairs/98_evidence2000.cfm. Accessed April 26, 2009.

29. American Dietetic Association. *Final Report of the Phase 2 Future Practice and Education Task Force.* Available at http://www.cdrnet.org/pdfs/Final%20Task%20Force%20Report%20July%2015%2008%20FINAL.pdf. Accessed June 14, 2009.

30. Oliveira V. *U.S. Department of Agriculture. The Food Assistance Landscape FY 2008 Annual Report.* Available at http://www.ers.usda.gov/Publications/EIB6-6/EIB6-6.pdf. Accessed May 10, 2009.

31. U.S. Department of Agriculture. Revitalizing Quality Nutrition Services in WIC. Available at http://www.fns.usda.gov/wic/CONTENT/RNQS/RNQS.htm. Accessed April 4, 2009.

32. U.S. Department of Agriculture, Food and Nutrition Services. Survey of public health nutritionists workforce. Alexandria, VA: USDA; 2007. Available at http://www.fns.usda.gov/WIC/resources/SurveyofthePublicHealthNutritionWorkforce2006-07.pdf. Accessed June 9, 2010.

33. U.S. Department of Agriculture, Food and Nutrition Service. *WIC Nutrition Service Standards.* Available at http://www.fns.usda.gov/wic/. Accessed April 4, 2009.

34. Harris-Davis E, Haughton B. Model for multicultural nutrition counseling competencies. *J Am Diet Assoc.* 2000;100:1178–1185.

35. Greenwald HP, Davis RA. Minority recruitment and retention in dietetics: issues and interventions. *J Am Diet Assoc.* 2000;100:961–966.

36. Food and nutrition section exposes students to public health careers. *The Nation's Health.* 2002; XXXII.

37. Hampl J, Anderson J, Mullis R. The role of dietetics professionals in health promotion and diseases prevention. *J Am Diet Assoc.* 2002;102:1680–1688.

38. American Dietetic Association. ADA Position and Practice Papers. Available at http://www.eatright.org/positions/. Accessed June 28, 2010.

39. Mixon H, Dodds J, Haughton B. *Guidelines for Community Nutrition Supervised Experiences*, 2nd ed. Public Health/Community Nutrition Practice Group, American Dietetic Association; 2003. Available at http://www.phcnpg.org. Accessed February 2009.

40. Wallner S, Kendall P, Hillers V, Bradshaw E, Medeiros LC. Online continuing education courses enhance nutrition and health professionals' knowledge of food safety issues of high-risk populations. *J Am Diet Assoc.* 2007;107:1333–1338.

41. Chance KG, Green CG. The effect of employee job satisfaction on program participation rates in the Virginia WIC program. *J Public Health Manage Pract.* 2001;7:10–20.

42. Olecko WA, Blacconiere MJ. Job satisfaction in public health: a comparative analysis of five occupational groups. *J Roy Soc Health.* 1995;115:386–390.

Suggested Reading

Association of State and Territorial Public Health Nutrition Directors (ASTPHND). *Guidelines for Comprehensive Programs to Promote Healthy Eating and Physical Activity.* Nutrition and Physical Activity Work Group. Available at http://www.fns.usda.gov/oane/menu/nuteducation.htm.

Association of State and Territorial Public Health Nutrition Directors (ASTPHND). *Strategies for Success: Curriculum Guide*, 2nd ed. Association of Graduate Programs in Public Health Nutrition, Inc.; 2002. Available at http://nutrition.Utk.edu/resources/StrategiesForSuccess.pdf. Accessed April 26, 2009.

Hatner-Eaton C. Public health departments and the quality movement: a natural partnership. *Clin Perform Qual Health Care.* 1995;3:35–40.

Hess AMN, Haughton B. Continuing education needs for public health nutritionists. *J Am Diet Assoc.* 1996;96:716–718.

Johnson DB, Easton DL, Wahl PW, Gleason C. Public health nutrition practice in the United States. *J Am Diet Assoc.* 2001;101:529–534.

Owen, AL, Splett PL, Owen GM. *Nutrition in the Community: The Art and Science of Delivering Services*, 4th ed. Boston, MA: WCB/McGraw-Hill; 1999.

Starbaugh C, ed. *Call to Action. Better Nutrition for Mothers, Children, and Families.* Washington, DC: National Center for Education in Maternal and Child Health; 1990.

Tuttle CR, Derrick B, Tagtow A. A new vision for health promotion and nutrition education. *Am J Health Promot.* 2003;18:186–191.

U.S. Department of Health and Human Services, Public Health Service. *The Public Health Workforce: An Agenda for the 21st Century.* Washington, DC: APHA; 2000.

Wellness Councils of America. Steps to a healthier U.S.: joining forces: health promotion takes the hill. *Absolute Advantage.* 2004;3(6). Available at http://www.eatright.org.

CHAPTER

23

Managing Public Health Nutrition Personnel

Esther Okeiyi, PhD, RD, LDN

READER OBJECTIVES

After studying this chapter and reflecting on the contents, you should be able to:

1. List at least 10 responsibilities of a public health nutrition director or manager.
2. Describe the five major management functions involved in managing nutrition personnel in the nutrition division of public health.
3. Explain the "six M's" of management.
4. Explain at least three activities performed under each of the five major functions of a director.
5. Differentiate between strategic planning and operational planning as well as between a job description and a job specification.
6. Describe the relationships among the following: job analysis, job description, and job specification.
7. Distinguish between the characteristics of a manager and the characteristics of a leader.
8. Discuss the characteristics of a good performance appraisal.
9. List the advantages of a performance appraisal.
10. Compare the goals and objectives, job descriptions, and mission statements of the nutritional division of the two types of public health divisions represented in this chapter.
11. Compare the job description for the directors of the two nutrition divisions discussed in this chapter.
12. Develop a mission statement for the two types of public health nutrition divisions discussed in this chapter.
13. Define the following terms: planning, organizing, delegating, controlling, and Behavioral Anchored Rating Scale.

■ INTRODUCTION

Today's public health nutrition managers recognize the need for a clear understanding and effective application of management principles in day-to-day operations. However, sometimes they may feel overwhelmed by the various terms applied in the field of scientific management. Public health nutrition directors or managers therefore need to become familiar with these terms and principles, because no unit in the public health department will provide a greater opportunity for applying these management skills. Mackenzie,[1] building

on the works of Fayol, illustrated the elements, continuous and sequential functions, and activities of managers.

Mackenzie[1] indicated that the elements that today's managers are faced with are ideas, things, and people. These are considered the main components of an organization. The manager's task related to ideas thus is to think conceptually about issues or matters that need to be resolved. The tasks relating to things are to administer or manage the details of the director's affairs. The task relating to people is to exercise leadership and influence people so that they accomplish desired goals.

■ ROLE OF A PUBLIC HEALTH NUTRITION DIRECTOR/MANAGER

A public health manager, also referred to as a *director of nutrition services*, wears many hats as a leader in his or her department. The responsibilities of a public health manager or director may include, but are not limited to:

- Providing leadership in all areas of a nutrition division of a public health department
- Recruiting, orienting, and training nutritionists in the nutrition division
- Supervising nutritionists and their work
- Motivating employees, conducting performance appraisals, and disciplining employees when necessary
- Maintaining good communication between the nutritionists and staff, and between the director and employees
- Handling concerns and grievances
- Planning, implementing, and evaluating program and service outcomes
- Organizing the nutrition division
- Planning the budget and controlling costs
- Interacting and working with other divisions in the public health department
- Representing the health department as an expert in the area of nutrition within and outside the public health department
- Ensuring *esprit de corps* among the nutritionists
- Generating income by soliciting grants and writing grant proposals for funding programs and employee positions in the division
- Networking and partnering with the community
- Keeping abreast of laws, changes in the community, community needs, and health needs

The major role of a public health nutrition director or manager can be divided into five areas: planning, staffing, organizing, leading, and controlling. The director utilizes available resources to accomplish the organizational goals. There are six main resources available to the director, which are known as the "six M's" of management: manpower, market, machine, method, material, and money. *Manpower* represents the employees. *Market* represents the clients and the community that the nutrition division serves. *Machines* include the equipment used in producing services, such as assessment tools, computers, and storage cabinets. *Materials* represent the supplies, software, training and promotional materials needed to run programs. *Methods* represent the processes, policies, procedures, and guidelines stipulated by the division, government, and funding agencies. *Money* represents the financial aspect of the operation. The following sections take a closer look at the major roles of the nutrition director in a health department.

Planning

Planning is the establishment of a mission statement, goals, and objectives, and the determination of strategies to accomplish the goals and objectives. A mission statement is the first step in planning; it represents the philosophy or purpose that drives an organization. The division's *mission statement* must be derived from the overall mission of the public health department and pro-

vides an overall direction for the organization. Although *goals* are stated in general terms, *objectives* are specific and must be stated in measurable terms related to actions or activities. The following are examples of short-range objectives and goals pertaining to personnel:

GOALS:
1. The nutrition division will reduce the employee turnover rate annually.
2. To make employees successful.

OBJECTIVES:
1. The nutrition division will reduce the employee turnover rate from 50% to 25% by the end of 2011.
2. The number of employees indicating satisfaction with their productivity will increase by 25% the first year and 50% the second and third years.
3. All employees will participate in at least two professional conferences annually.

The three types of planning are the strategic plan, the intermediate plan, and the operational plan. The *strategic plan* involves making decisions about the future, forecasting for the future, and making decisions based on the environment and the current and anticipated available resources. A strategic plan serves for 3 to 15 years and should be reviewed regularly. Managers at the top of the organizational structure develop the strategic plan. In strategic planning, strengths and weaknesses of the organization or the unit are analyzed. The strategic plan document serves as a foundation for an intermediate plan, which covers a one- to three-year period. Middle level managers or supervisors may develop an *intermediate plan*. It is through the intermediate plan that policies are developed. Finally, the *operational plan* describes a day-to-day action plan. It dictates the plan for a period of one year or less.

There are three major levels of managers, each of whom is responsible for a different level of planning. Top managers function at the policy-making level of the organization. They are responsible for broad, comprehensive planning involving strategic planning and long-range goals. Middle-level managers are responsible for developing policies; first-line managers, at the technical or operational level, are responsible for developing procedures and methods.

The level of managers involved in developing any plan may be based on the size of the organization/unit and the levels of management in that unit. It is clear from the organizational chart in **Figure 23-1** and job descriptions in **Figure 23-2** that a director and a supervisory staff nutritionist in different nutrition divisions in the public health department may perform different responsibilities, based on the division's size, levels of management, and how that particular organization is structured. For example, a director of nutrition delegates most of the first-line and middle management functions to her team leaders. These team leaders plan, orient, train, and provide direct supervision to their area employees. The nutrition manager or director works with other division managers internally, planning and coordinating efforts relating to the public health department, and representing the division by providing expertise in matters relating to nutrition. An example of a public health department issue that can affect all divisions is bioterrorism. The nutrition director may contribute ideas regarding how the nutrition division may handle such matters in terms of managing food sanitation and safety. Externally, the manager or director represents the public health department, negotiating for community partnerships, contracts, funding, and projects. In addition, the manager implements nutrition programs and works with other stakeholders, such as government agencies and community key players.

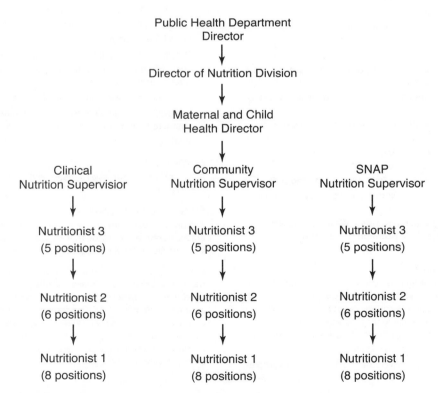

FIGURE 23-1 Example of an Organizational Chart from a Public Health Department Nutrition Division

NUTRITIONIST Manager

DEFINITION

Under direction, develops, administers, and maintains administrative and program aspects of the Women, Infant and Children (WIC) Food Nutrition Program; consults with other public health programs and special projects on nutrition matters; supervises subordinate staff and performs other duties as required.

CLASS CHARACTERISTICS

Functions with minimum direction to provide direct supervision and evaluation of subordinate nutritionists and support personnel in the operation of the WIC program. Administrative direction is received from the Community Health & Prevention Service Manager. The class is distinguished from Nutritionist and Senior Nutritionist in the comprehensiveness and scope of responsibility for program planning, staff supervision, orientation and in-service education, and assistance in formulation, implementation, and evaluation of policies and procedures, and budget preparation.

DUTIES

- Plans, organizes, and directs the operations of the WIC in accordance with State and Federal Regulations.
- Organizes, coordinates, assigns, directs and evaluates the work of WIC program personnel.
- Prepares schedules and plans staffing needs for all WIC Clinics.
- Inventories and secures food vouchers.
- Provides nutrition assessment and counseling for enrollment and recertification clinics.
- Coordinates nutrition services between WIC and Marin Maternity Services to assure consistency and quality of service.
- Coordinates all outreach efforts.
- Prepares yearly WIC budget for submission as part of the Department budget.
- Monitors participant enrollment changes.
- Oversees breast feeding promotion component of WIC program including supervision of paid peer counselors.
- Participates in workshops and conferences aimed at promoting better nutrition.
- Reviews and adjusts monthly financial reports submitted to the State.
- Prepares and/or reviews and signs Monthly Transaction Reports of food vouchers issued and exchanged.
- Investigates vendor complaints from participants and staff.
- Reviews and edits yearly WIC Nutrition Education Plan prepared for the State.
- Works collaboratively with the Nutrition Wellness Program and participates in the Marin Nutrition & Physical Activity Collaboration and Nutrition Task Force.

EMPLOYMENT STANDARDS

Any combination of education and experience that would provide the knowledge and skills listed below. Typically, equivalent to a Bachelor's degree in Food and Nutrition, Dietetics, Nutritional Sciences or closely related field, and three years of experience in public health nutrition which includes lead work experience in the operation of a public health nutrition program.

A Master's degree in Public Health Nutrition which includes studies in community and perinatal nutrition may substitute for one year of the experience.

Knowledge of:

- Human nutrition and its relationship to health and disease.
- Investigative and research methods as applied to public health nutrition.
- Content, organizational structure and goals of a public health nutrition program.
- Social, cultural and economic problems of individuals and families as they apply to public health nutrition.
- The field of nutrition as it relates to public health practices.
- Appropriate educational principles and methods as applied to public health nutrition practices.
- Safe food handling practices.
- Principles of consulting.
- Principles and techniques of supervision.
- Principles and techniques of budgeting.

Ability to:

- Organize, coordinate and direct a Public Health Nutrition program.
- Provide direct nutrition services.
- Analyze and evaluate nutrition data and services.
- Prepare acceptable materials for use by communication media.
- Provide technical assistance on nutrition and food service management.
- Explain the nutrition aspects of the public health program.
- Present ideas clearly and concisely, both orally and in writing.
- Plan, implement and organize work effectively.
- Work independently.
- Suggest policy implementation and changes.
- Train others in the principles of nutrition and their application in public health programs.
- Train, supervise and evaluate subordinate staff.
- Establish and maintain effective working relationships with those contacted during the performance of duties.
- Work in a standard office environment.

CERTIFICATE

A current registration as a Dietitian by the American Dietetic Association.

PHYSICAL CHARACTERISTICS

The physical demands and working conditions described here are representative of those that must be met by an employee to successfully perform the essential functions of this job.

Work is performed in an office or clinic setting and may require travel to alternative off site work locations and meetings. Hand-eye coordination is necessary to operate computers and various pieces of office equipment. While performing the duties of this job, the employee is occasionally required to stand or sit; walk; use hands to operate equipment, tools, and/or controls and to reach with hands and arms. The employee is occasionally required to stoop, kneel, crouch, talk and hear.

continues

FIGURE 23-2 Sample Job Descriptions for a Nutrition Manager and a Nutritionist 1 Positions

Nutritionist 1 - WIC

Description of Work

Performs entry-level professional work in providing WIC services; plans and coordinates the operation of assigned WIC clinics including supervision of Nutrition Assistants; and performs related duties as assigned.

Works under the technical, general, and/or administrative supervision of a unit or division manager.

Exercises technical supervision over lower-level support, technical, or professional staff.

Typical Duties Performed

- The listed examples may not include all the duties performed by all positions in this class.
- Supervises the daily activities of Nutrition Assistants and other WIC staff including assigning, training and conducting performance evaluations.
- Oversees operation of WIC nutrition clinics by providing guidance and direction to clinic staff on day-to-day clinic operation.
- Participates with other staff in planning for and developing unit or program policies, procedures and activities.
- Develops and writes grants as needed.
- Conducts state-mandated chart audits and observations of Nutrition Assistants.
- Performs clinical services as required.
- Maintains records and reports.
- Organizes and carries out designated specialized WIC program services.
- Adheres to a regular work schedule as assigned.

Competencies

- Considerable knowledge of the theories, principles, and practices of community nutrition and nutrition education.

- Considerable knowledge of nutrition counseling techniques and nutrition education.
- Considerable knowledge of the WIC program, its policies, procedures, rules and regulations.
- Considerable knowledge of the principles of maternal and child nutrition.
- Working knowledge of the technology, principles, and processes of normal and therapeutic nutrition, food science, public health nutrition and food programs.
- Working knowledge of community nutrition needs and resources.
- Considerable ability to provide normal and therapeutic nutrition screening, assessment, counseling, and referral services.
- Considerable ability to plan, organize, and coordinate activities.
- Considerable ability to communicate effectively, both orally and in writing.
- Considerable ability to interact effectively with a wide variety of people.
- Working ability to assign, train, and supervise the work of others.
- Working ability to provide leadership, training, and development of paraprofessional staff, student interns, and volunteers.
- Working ability to lift and weigh children, load and transport nutrition equipment to clinics or off-site locations.

Requirements

Bachelor's degree in dietetics, food and nutrition, or a related field and must be a registered dietitian with the American Dietetic Association or eligible to take the Dietetic Registration examination. (No substitution for education.) Must have a valid driver's license or equivalent out-of-state driver's license with no suspensions for driving related offenses or revocations within two years prior to the date of appointment.

FIGURE 23–2 *(Continued)*

A good plan is vital to a successful organization. It determines how well and smoothly an operation performs. In the long run, a good plan prevents many problems for both the director and the division as a whole. Planning increases effectiveness and efficiency. Effectiveness refers to an operation's ability to accomplish its goals and objectives. Efficiency refers to an operation's ability to achieve maximum results with minimum input. It is important that employees are involved in the planning. It keeps everyone knowledgeable of what is going on in the unit. In addition, employees are more likely to buy into the plan if they are part of the planning team.

Staffing and Employee Evaluation

Directors are responsible for hiring the right people for the positions in their divisions. Once employees are hired, they are introduced to the job and organization during a formal orientation program, and subsequently are given an organized training period in preparation for their job. The orientation process may take three to five days. The amount

and length of training are dependent upon each employee's previous training and experience. Over time, the employees are evaluated periodically, typically after the first 90 days on the job and annually by the manager to inform them of how well they are doing. This is referred to as a *performance appraisal*. A performance appraisal is a formal method of providing constructive feedback to an employee regarding how well or poorly the employee is performing his or her job. The objectives are to positively influence, motivate, strengthen, and enhance the employee's work performance. The performance appraisals must be job-related.

Performance appraisals have many advantages, including:

- Aiding employees in defining future goals and providing an objective set of criteria to measure job performance
- Providing a basis for modifying poor work habits
- Providing a means of gathering employees' suggestions for improving performance, methods, and morale

- Demonstrating a source of documentation in the event of litigation
- Providing a basis on which to determine promotions and wage increases
- Providing a means to seek an alternative to termination
- Helping to pinpoint personal weaknesses and how to improve them

Overall, a performance appraisal is an effective motivational tool. The appraisal should not be used as a punishment or as an opportunity for vindictiveness. Also, it must not be a one-way process, but should be a mutual discussion between an employee and the manager. For the evaluation to be effective, the employee must be informed about the process prior to starting work and a week or two before the actual evaluation. A performance appraisal must be conducted in a private environment.

Employees are entitled to be informed about how they are progressing in regards to their jobs. Every employee is also entitled to be informed about the criteria being used for their evaluation. These criteria can be covered during orientation, training, or in-house meetings. Opportunities should be given to the employees to ask questions about information that is not clear to them. Although there are many evaluation tools available, the Behavioral Anchored Rating Scale (BARS), as documented by Payne-Palacio and Theis,[2] is generally considered the best and most effective tool for employees' performance appraisals. This tool identifies specific behaviors for each performance level in each task and job category and provides a scale with which to rate employees. The Management by Objectives (MBO) system is another performance evaluation tool managers can use. With this tool, both the manager and the employee agree on performance objectives, and the employee is evaluated on how well the objectives are accomplished.

Discipline is used when all other measures have failed to bring the employee up to standard regarding desired work performance. Any disciplinary action against an employee should be legally defensible. It may be advisable to double check with the legal office of the department before taking disciplinary action. Disciplinary actions should be immediate, consistent, and impersonally based, and the evaluation criteria must be known in advance. The work rules must be clear, fair, and reasonable, and they must be reviewed regularly.

A manager must be alert to signs of grievances in employees, whether verbal or nonverbal, and should have a plan to deal with these. Some of the signs may include indifference toward the job or toward other employees, excessive tardiness and absences, decline in quality of work, and excessive complaints. The first line of action by a manager may be to have a face-to-face, private discussion with the employee. The manager may point out changes observed and concern for the employee's progress. Discussion of the problem may lead to brainstorming strategies between the employee and the manager for solving the problem. If the problem persists, documentation and a Grievance Action Form may be completed and serve as a warning to the employee. A Grievance Action Form is a form for written record of a grievance and action taken. Grievance proceedings usually follow three to four steps after discussion: verbal warning, written warning, second written warning, and final warning, followed by termination, if the employee has been ruled against.

Organizing

In order for the goals and objectives of a nutrition division to be accomplished, the manager must organize the resources in an orderly fashion. Organizing is the act of carefully grouping the organization's resources and activities, including human resources, by type of tasks performed. The organizing process establishes relationships among all functions of management. How the public health nutrition division is organized is based on its mission, goals and objectives, and areas of nutrition services provided to the community. For example, whereas some nutrition divisions of public health departments focus on providing nutrition services to women, infants, and children through the WIC program, others focus on preventing and reducing disabilities among individuals or groups, such as the elderly, children, and home-bound individuals. Convalescents and the poor in the community, both of whom are at nutritional risk, also can be provided nutrition-related services. The nutrition division may serve those who come to a clinic for another health reasons, but are identified as candidates at high nutritional risk. In each case, the service areas of a public health nutrition division will be easily discernable on the unit's organizational chart. Figure 23–1 is a typical example of an organizational chart for a public health nutrition division.

The following steps are used in developing an organizational structure:

1. Define organizational goals and objectives.
2. Analyze and classify work to be done.
3. Describe in detail the work or activity in terms of the employees.
4. Determine and specify relationships of the jobs to each other and to management.
5. Organize the employees by tasks and activities and show their relationship to each other and to management.
6. Clearly delineate staff and line positions. Line positions are in the direct chain of command that are responsible for the achievement of organizational goals.[3] Staff positions, in contrast, provide expertise, advice, and support for the line positions. Examples of staff positions are the advisory board, consultants, and secretaries. In an organizational chart, line positions are shown with solid unbroken lines, whereas staff

positions are shown with broken lines or dotted lines. The lines depict lines of communication and control. Scalar principle indicates that a clear and unbroken line of authority flow from the bottom position to the top position in the organization.

7. Organizational charts should be reviewed and updated periodically as positions change. Proper organization of employees requires that managers be assigned a number of employees that they are capable of managing. This is known as *span of control*. According to the principle of unity of command, under no circumstance should an employee report to more than one supervisor or manager.

The tools for structuring an organization include job descriptions, job specifications, job breakdowns or analyses, and job design. A *job description* is an organized list of duties, skills, and responsibilities required in a specific position. A *job specification* is a written statement of minimum standards that must be met by an applicant for a particular job. It covers duties involved in the job, working conditions specific to the job, and personal qualifications required to carry out the responsibilities successfully. A *job analysis or breakdown* is written documentation of a study conducted on all aspects of a specific job. It provides information used in developing job descriptions. Figure 23–2 shows examples of job descriptions for a managerial position and one nutritionist position in two different types of public health nutrition divisions with different missions. A *job design*, developed from job analysis, is concerned with structuring jobs to improve organization efficiency and employee satisfaction. Jobs are divided into manageable units based on employees' expertise.

Leading

Leadership and management are not the same, although the words are sometimes used interchangeably.[4,5] Characteristics of managers and leaders are outlined in the book entitled, *Executive Leadership*, by Tamel and Reynolds.[5] *Leadership* is the activity of influencing other people's behavior toward the achievement of desired objects. It involves influencing others without coercion to achieve the organization's goals and objectives. Simply stated, it is getting people to do what you want them to because they want to do it. There are many different types of leadership styles (see **Figure 23–3**). *Management*, on the other hand, is the function of running an organization by effectively integrating and coordinating resources in order to achieve desired objectives. Managing a nutrition division should be combined with leadership qualities and activities. A director leads the human resources in an organization while managing the nonhuman resources used in operating the division.

Leaders share decision making, information, authority, reward, trust, drive, motivation, and vision with their employees. They work well with employees and demonstrate respect, concern, and empathy. They honor differences in employees. The leader takes risks for the benefit of a work group. On the other hand, a good manager may effectively plan, organize, and control finances and productivity, but have less success in dealing with employees.[6]

A common characteristic of a leader is *native intelligence*. This means he or she has the ability to acquire and retain knowledge, and respond quickly and productively to a new situation. Leaders have drive, which they need in order to achieve and feel successful. They have integrity and self-confidence, and are experts in what they do. George and Jones[7] summarized the traits that correlate strongly with leadership. Leadership skills are partly innate and partly learned.[8] Leaders have strong personal mastery that impels them to struggle for change in an organization. They seek out risks, dislike mundane tasks, are concerned about people, and strive to achieve personal goals. They derive power from personal relationships and relate with people in intuitive ways. They question established procedures and create new concepts. They are concerned with results.[5(p.59)] There is a high correlation between leadership and the ability to relate, influence, motivate, coordinate, delegate, and communicate.[9]

Leading and Influencing

In leading, the manager and subordinate's relationship is critical. McGregor's[10] X and Y Theories of leadership are based on the fact that a leader's attitudes toward employees influence their job performances. The Contingency Theory of leadership promotes the idea that the type of leadership provided should be contingent on the type of employees and the situation in which the organization exists.[10,11] Drucker[12,13] noted that directors can obtain peak performance from their employees if they set high standards and stick to them, put the right people in the right position, keep them informed about their performance, and allow them to be an active part of the process.

Democratic—This style is also called participative, because it encourages employee participation in decision making. The manager checks with the employees before making a decision and can act as a coach or problem solver for the group.

Autocratic—A leadership style that does not encourage employee input. The manager makes all decisions. Employees are expected to obey management decisions without asking any questions.

Laissez-faire—A leadership style also known as the "hands-off" style. The manager provides little or no direction and gives employees as much freedom as possible. All authority or power is given to the employees, and they must determine goals, make decisions, and resolve problems on their own.

FIGURE 23–3 Different Leadership Styles

McGregor's X and Y Theories: Different ways in which managers view employees. There are two theories: Theory X and Theory Y.

Theory X: Managers believe that workers are motivated by only one thing: money. They are selfish, lazy, and hate work. The manager believes that workers need to be closely controlled and directed.

Theory Y: Managers believe that workers are motivated by many different factors apart from money. They enjoy their work. The manager believes that employees will **happily take on responsibility and make decisions for the business**.

Contingency Theory: The belief that performance is a result of interaction between two factors: leadership style and situational favorableness.

Maslow's Theory: The theory of a hierarchy of human needs. The needs of an individual exist in a logical order (physiological, safety, belonging, esteem, and self-actualization); the basic root needs must be satisfied first.

Herzberg's Theory: A theory regarding motivation; also called the two-factor theory. Work characteristics causing dissatisfaction (i.e., work conditions, pay, and interpersonal relationships) are quite different from those causing satisfaction (i.e., achievement, recognition, and opportunity for growth).

McClelland's Theory: An individual's motivation and effectiveness in certain job functions are influenced by three needs: achievement, affiliation, and power.

Motivating

Another aspect of leading is creating an environment in which subordinates can be motivated and excited to perform their job well. A leader must understand the concepts of human motivation. To accomplish the goals and objectives of the division, the people who produce the products and services need to be well led and motivated. Interaction between a leader and his or her subordinates will result in the leader being able to elicit what motivates the employees. There is no one method to create conditions that will motivate employees. Maslow,[14] Herzberg,[15] McClelland,[16] and Vroom[17] all developed theories on how employees are motivated in a work environment. An experienced leader may employ Abraham Maslow's Hierarchy of Needs Theory[14] by first determining the point of motivation need for each subordinate. Herzberg's two-factor theory,[15] which is similar to Maslow's needs theory, identified two major factors—job satisfiers and job dissatisfiers—that can motivate or dissatisfy employees, respectively. Job satisfiers are motivators that include achievement, recognition, responsibility, advancement, the work itself, and potential for growth. The job dissatisfiers are known as maintenance or hygiene factors that must be present for job satisfaction to occur. They include pay, supervision, job security, working conditions, organizational policies, and interpersonal relationships on the job. McClelland's Motivation Theory[16] supported Maslow's theory and emphasized that employees are usually at different levels of need, which can be high or low.

An employee will respond positively to motivation if the degree of need is high. Vroom's Expectancy Theory[17] stipulates that employees will be motivated if they can link the job performance to the expected reward. For example, if they expect a better reward for better performance, then they will be motivated to perform. Motivators can range from a simple pat on the back, affirming work well done, to public recognition of the employee in a meeting, publishing an employee's accomplishments, offering incentives, or rewarding an employee by delegating managerial tasks.

Coordinating

A director must coordinate all aspects of the various parts of employees' work so that they flow smoothly. The public health nutrition division director can accomplish this through departmentalization or specialization by functions, clients, geographic areas, number of persons, or time. Some tasks may be delegated to free the director's time to do other tasks. Delegating is essential in distributing workloads. It enriches and enlarges employees' jobs and contributes to employees' improved job knowledge, job motivation, professional development, and job accomplishment. When job responsibilities are delegated, authority must accompany them. The manager must guide the employee to understand the limits of the authority, and what decisions and actions can be made without consultation. Delegating, developing, and motivating employees are all acts of leading.

Vroom's Theory: Assumes that behavior results from conscious choices among alternatives whose purpose is to maximize pleasure and minimize pain. The key elements to this theory are referred to as expectancy, instrumentality, and valence.

Communicating

Effective leadership depends on the ability of the leader to communicate with his or her subordinates. Communication includes being able to transmit ideas and goals, receive messages from internal environments, listen, network, interact with others, and manage both formal and informal organizations. A true leader must resist the temptation of showing favoritism among employees.

The director represents both the employees and management. The employees look up to the director as representative of management. The director, therefore, must be able to 1) interpret the mission, goals, objectives, and policies of the organization to the employees in a way that garners their cooperation and confidence; 2) motivate and guide the employees with their job; 3) assist in employees' professional development; 4) listen to and empathize with employees as needed; 5) provide training to both individuals and groups; and 6) evaluate employees and implement discipline when needed.

Leading and directing are synonymous. Directing requires continuous decision making, conveying these decisions to subordinates, and ensuring appropriate actions. Also, it requires coordinating and directing the work of employees to accomplish organizational goals. The director as a leader organizes and fits the right employees to jobs based on their abilities, assists in the orientation and training of employees, listens to and handles grievances, solves problems, and makes decisions in a timely and logical manner. She or he schedules and conducts employee meetings regularly. As a leader, she or he must keep abreast of the legal ramifications regarding public health nutrition. There is no one best style of leadership; rather, style must be adapted to fit the situation. Leaders can use different styles of leadership—democratic or participative, laissez-faire, or autocratic—depending on the employees they lead. The leader must accept leading responsibilities as well as earning the employees' trust. The quality and the amount of supervision may determine the success or failure of the organization in accomplishing its goals and its ability to attract government funds to stay afloat.

Managers of today's employees must understand that good communication is essential in managing cultural, ethnic, and racial diversity. As the ethnic composition of the workforce continues to become increasingly more diverse, good communication will become essential. A good leader must understand and accept ethnic pluralism. Ethnic pluralism is the coexistence of ethnic and racial groups. For example, it is okay to be both Cuban and American. Individuals do not have to shun or deny their Cuban ethnicity to be Americans or vice versa because they have dual ethnic identities and are bicultural.[18] The leader must correct misconceptions, misunderstandings, biases, and stereotyping within and outside the unit. It is the leader's responsibility to help employees to understand and respect their own and each other's culture as well as work better with each other. Knowledge of ethnicity is fundamental to being an effective multicultural manager.

Conflicts between employees and between employees and management do occur from time to time. A leader must not ignore conflicts that exist in the work environment or allow them to linger for a long period of time because they affect team morale, efforts, and productivity. The leader must facilitate conflict resolutions by attempting to influence behavior change among the individuals involved.

Controlling

Controlling is a mechanism to ensure that resources, quality of services, and client satisfaction are regulated appropriately and adequately. It also involves regulating the activities of employees in the division to ensure that they meet the established standards and goals. Control functions require the director to determine which activities need control, such as establishing and communicating standards to employees, measuring performance, and correcting devia-

tions. This means staffing positions with the right qualified employees, developing and retaining them, and ensuring quality in programs and services provided to the clients. It also means making sure that clients indicate satisfaction with services provided, and ensuring that funding partners are satisfied with how their funds are managed. All of these are control functions. Additionally, managing the budget, costs, and information is considered a control function. The ability to reallocate personnel or realign the budget when facing financial constraints and still accomplishing objectives is control.

Studies by Snead, Burnell, and Anderson[19] and Rogers, Leonberg, and Broadhurst[20] revealed that control management is a major aspect of a manager's responsibility in nutrition and dietetics. Budgeting includes both planning and controlling functions. Managers must be able to prepare and report financial analyses, control program costs, generate income, detect irregularities in client services or cost overruns, and handle complex projects and programs. The American Dietetic Association (ADA) role delineation study of 1998[21] agreed that managers or directors in public health are responsible for preparing financial analyses and financial reports, controlling program costs, monitoring program financial performance, documenting program operations, and making decisions regarding capital expenditure. The nutrition division usually undergoes periodic review or audits of its accounts. Directors must be able to manage and report the status of the thousands of dollars entrusted into their care.

The public health nutrition director therefore must have basic knowledge of accounting, preparing a budget, interpreting financial documents, and preparing financial reports for all income and expenses generated in the unit. It is important that as the director, he or she must know how to write for grants, develop the budget for grants, justify the reasons for requesting the amount being sought, and manage programs. Usually, the amount funded is dependent on how well the justification is written.

Managers and directors must regularly and continuously monitor productivity of their employees. Quality control, quality assurance, continuous quality improvement, and total quality management are all related concepts and can serve as tools for accomplishing this managerial function. *Quality control* is defined as determining if the products or services being provided meet the minimum standards of acceptability. *Quality assurance* is defined as a process of identifying "problem areas" within a unit and taking action to correct them. The results are monitored over time to see if the problems have been resolved and remain resolved. Quality assurance monitoring may necessitate a development of policies and procedures in patient (client) care protocols, thereby ensuring consistency from practitioner to practitioner. For example, a typical problem may be timeliness in screening to identify high-risk patients. Another example may be inconsistent methods for determining desirable body weight. Quality assurance must be ongoing, using a method such as *continuous quality improvement (CQI)*, which helps identify areas that can be strengthened, and working to make those areas better. When all the departments or areas of the organization are studied to determine problem areas and work to correct them, it is called *total quality management (TQM)*.

For a nutrition unit in a public health department, quality assurance is a most applicable tool. Some county health departments use weekly and monthly meetings as a quality assurance strategy. The team leaders of each focus area meet weekly with their employees and discuss the week's events and challenges. Team leaders, in turn, meet with the director weekly to apprise her of their work productivity, issues, and challenges from their individual areas. During the monthly meeting of the division, each of the focus area team leaders give a progress report presentation to all employees. Controlling, therefore, provides a process of making sure that established objectives and plans are being accomplished.

While public health nutrition directors or managers aim at being successful at what they do (i.e., being able to plan, staff, organize, lead, and control as well as being able to utilize available resources to accomplish the organizational goals), public health directors must continuously strive to improve themselves through professional development. They must keep abreast with what is currently happening in the profession. Status quo is never an option for successful directors in a dynamic environment. These managers or directors must continually assess the competitive environment, assess their strengths, and areas for improvements, build organizational skills, and managerial (people and process) skills. As noted by Drucker,[12,13] directors need to develop themselves while they develop their employees. An important skill essential for a successful leadership is being personally organized amidst myriad roles and activities that that must be performed on a daily basis. This is called *self-organization*. *Time management* is essential to a self-management style that leads to success. Developing a timeline in planning what needs to be accomplished, requires effective time management. For example, time spent organizing electronic data files, folders, and information is time saved in the long run. Directors must learn to say "no" to new projects not originally included in their management plan except they are very sure of the availability of time and resources to accomplish the additional projects. In the planning stages, directors or managers should not overwhelm themselves with too many objectives that cannot be accomplished. Also, delegation is a way of managing time while developing the employee. For in the end, it is best to manage limited resources such as "time."

■ CONCLUSIONS

This chapter discussed how employees in a nutrition division of a public health department are managed. The manager or director must combine management and leadership skills in managing the resources (the six M's of management) in his or her unit. The five main functions in directing the activities of the employees work in tandem to accomplish the goals and objectives of the nutrition division. The director or the manager must use strategies for the success of the organization by continually assessing the competitive environment, recognizing the strengths and areas for improvement in the organization, building organizational skills, building the staff skills, as well as the process.

Issues for Discussion

1. Why is it important to have job descriptions? How is having appropriate job descriptions a win-win for both the employee and the manager?

2. Discuss some problems you have experienced at your workplace. How could these have been avoided if a good manager was in place? What disciplinary actions should have occurred?

3. List and discuss the five top time wasters for a public health manager or a director?

References

1. Mackenzie A. The management process in 3-D. A diagram showing the activities, functions and basic elements of the executive's job. *J Nurs Adm.* 1979;11:30–33.

2. Payne-Palacio J, Theis M. *Introduction to Foodservice*, 11th ed. Upper Saddle River, NJ: Prentice Hall; 2009.

3. Griffin RW. *Management*, 2nd ed. Upper Saddle River, NJ: Prentice Hall; 1999.

4. Bittle LR, Newstrom JW. *What Every Supervisor Should Know*, 6th ed. New York: McGraw-Hill; 1990:189–190.

5. Tamel ME, Reynolds H. *Executive Leadership*. Englewood Cliffs, NJ: Prentice Hall; 1981:59.

6. Hudson N. *Management Practice in Dietetics*. United States: Cengage Learning; 2005.

7. George JM, Jones GR. *Organizational Behavior*, 3rd ed. Upper Saddle River, NJ: Prentice Hall; 2002.

8. Boyle MA, Holben DH. *Community Nutrition in Action: An Entrepreneurial Approach*. Belmont, CA: Wadsworth, Thompson Learning; 2010.

9. Hudson N. *Management Practice in Dietetics*. Belmont, CA: Wadsworth, Thompson Learning; 2006:53–87.

10. McGregor D. *The Human Side of Enterprise*. New York: McGraw Hill; 1985.

11. Fielder FE, Garcia JE. *New Approaches to Effective Leadership*. New York: John Wiley & Sons; 1987.

12. Drucker PF. *Profession of Management.* Boston, MA: Harvard Business Print; 2003.

13. Drucker, PF. *Management Responsibilities, Practices.* Burlington, MA: Butterworth Heinemann Publishers; 1999.

14. Maslow AH. A theory of human motivation. *Psychology Rev.* 1943;50:370–396.

15. Herzberg F. *Work and Nature of Man.* Cleveland, OH: World; 1966.

16. McClelland DC. *The Achievement Society.* New York: Free Press; 1985.

17. Vroom VH. *Work and Motivation.* San Francisco: Jossey Bass; 1994.

18. Tanke ML. *Human Resources Management for Hospitality.* Albany, NY: Delmar; 1990.

19. Snead J, Burnell EC, Anderson M. Development of financial management competencies for entry level dietitian. *J Am Diet Assoc.* 1992;92:1223–1229.

20. Rogers D, Leonberg BL, Broadhurst CB. Commission on dietetic registration, dietetics practice audit. *J Am Diet Assoc.* 2002;102:270–292.

21. American Dietetic Association. The American Dietetic Association standards of professional practice for dietetics professionals. *J Am Diet Assoc.* 1998;98:83–87.

CHAPTER 24

Leveraging Nutrition Education Through the Public Health Team

DEEPA ARORA, PhD

READER OBJECTIVES

After studying this chapter and reflecting on the contents, you should be able to:

1. Discuss how a nutritionally balanced diet can prevent the onset and development of several diet-related, preventable, chronic diseases.

2. Explain why education is an important tool for modifying diet-related behavior.

3. Describe how nutrition education campaigns provide a low-cost method for encouraging and sustaining healthy food habits.

4. Discuss the challenges nutrition educators routinely face, including noncompliance with their recommendations and providing services that are culturally and linguistically sensitive.

5. Clarify why nutrition education is best provided by a team of qualified public health professionals.

6. Explain why continuing education programs and in-service programs are vital for sharing recent developments in the field of nutrition with all members of the nutrition education team.

7. Explain why the members of the nutrition education team must adhere to the principles of effective teamwork and group development in order to establish an effective nutrition education program.

■ INTRODUCTION

Lifestyle choices, such as nutrition, smoking, drinking, physical activity, and psychological stress, have the greatest impact on health and longevity. Innumerable studies in the literature show the detrimental effect of poor dietary habits on health and on the development of disease.[1] Dietary factors have been shown to be linked to 4 of the 10 leading causes of death: coronary heart disease, stroke, some types of cancer, and type 2 diabetes.[1] It has been shown, for example, that obesity and/or being overweight significantly increases the risk of developing diabetes, heart disease, stroke, and hypertension.[1] According to the report titled, *Statistics Related to Overweight and Obesity*, released in 2010, obesity and overweight affect approximately $2/3$ of the adults in the United States and are linked to medical problems that cost the U.S. economy billions.[2] Early intervention to encourage weight loss before an individual becomes overweight or obese thus may be the desired course of action. Public health personnel can encourage changes in dietary choices to help reduce the incidence of preventive disorders in those populations most susceptible to them.

Read about *The Surgeon General's Call to Action to Prevent and Decrease Overweight and Obesity* at http://www.surgeongeneral.gov/topics/obesity/calltoaction/CalltoAction.pdf.

Many studies have effectively shown that changes in people's dietary patterns can reduce the incidence of chronic diseases such as heart disease and cancer. In the past 35 years, deaths due to heart disease have declined by 45%, although it is still the leading cause of death in the United States.[3] This reduction is attributed to a decrease in the intake of animal fat and cholesterol as well as a decline in smoking. In 2001, the U.S. Department of Health and Human Services released the findings from the Diabetes Prevention Program.[4] This program was a major clinical trial that compared the effects of dietary modifications and exercise with the effects of an anti-diabetes drug in combating the development of type 2 diabetes in individuals with an impaired glucose tolerance test and who were at risk for developing the disease. The results were dramatic in that the risk of developing type 2 diabetes decreased by 58% in participants who exercised and followed the suggested diet, as compared to 31% in those who took the anti-diabetes drug. Introducing dietary modifications to meet the Dietary Guidelines for Americans thus can significantly impact the health of an individual and society.

> More about the 2010 Dietary Guidelines for Americans can be found at http://www.nal.usda.gov/fnic/dga/.

◼ MODIFYING NUTRITION-RELATED BEHAVIOR

As discussed in previous chapters, the U.S. Public Health Service, along with public and private organizations, developed a set of public health objectives called Healthy People (HP). The goals of the HP initiative include helping individuals of all ages increase life expectancy and improve their quality of life.[1] These goals are to be met through a variety of approaches that aim to improve the nutritional status of the population by improving access to comprehensive, high-quality healthcare services; increasing the availability and effectiveness of educational and community-based health promotion programs designed to prevent disease and improve health and quality of life; and improving core competencies in health providers' training.

> The Healthy People Initiative is at http://www.healthypeople.gov.

Health-related behaviors show a strong correlation with education. People who are better educated make healthier choices and show better health-related behaviors. Public health practitioners can use the medium of education to promote healthy behaviors and healthy lifestyles. A big challenge for public health professionals is to develop educational programs and initiatives for nutrition education and health promotion in communities that are characterized by a lower socioeconomic status and low levels of education.

◼ DEFINITION OF NUTRITION EDUCATION

Nutrition education is a process of learning that influences the knowledge, beliefs, attitudes, and behavior of an individual or a community and allows them to make more intelligent decisions regarding dietary choices in order to improve health and reduce the risk of developing chronic diet-related disorders, such as obesity, diabetes, heart disease, hypertension, and osteoporosis. A group of public health professionals can provide nutrition education by studying nutrition-related health problems and then planning, developing, organizing, and implementing educational programs to address some of the frequently occurring health concerns.

◼ IMPACT OF NUTRITION EDUCATION

Education can impact the behavior of families and communities in a very strong and powerful manner. Individuals gain knowledge of the world and their surroundings, helping them build certain skills and capabilities that, in turn, boost their self-confidence and self-esteem.[5] As the family and the community develop, there is an improvement in health and health resources, reduced exposure to environmental health hazards, gains in socioeconomic status, and, thus, additional purchasing power for buying health care and medical care. Along this road to development, public health professionals can play a very important role in improving the nutritional status of communities by imparting nutrition education with a message of "managed lives/healthy lives." Nutrition education can be provided in hospitals, health agencies, schools, churches, workplaces, and recreational facilities. Public health professionals have a diverse array of venues where they can reach their target populations. Target populations can include individuals, families, organization leaders, community leaders, and influential people who could make a greater impact on the community to facilitate voluntary actions conducive to a nutritionally balanced and healthy diet.

How Effective Are Nutrition Education Campaigns?

Millions of dollars are spent on marketing and advertising for high-profit foods, including those rich in refined carbohydrates and fats. Regrettably, not enough money is available for nutrition education campaigns that promote healthy food choices. In contrast, the advertising budget for junk foods could be as high as $100 to $500 million.[6] In a recent report, the Kaiser Family Foundation stated that the media contributes significantly towards childhood obesity by airing advertisements worth billions of dollars showing candy, cereal, and fast food.[7] This has contributed significantly to the increased incidence of overweight children aged 6 to 11 years, which has risen from 6.5% in 1976–1980 to 17% in 2003–2006.[8] There lies an ever-widening gap between the funds available for advertising for fast foods and those available for promoting healthy food choices. A suggestion was made to generate funds for public health campaigns[6] by imposing a small tax on fast foods and junk foods. This could generate significant revenue, which could be added to the pool of funds available for nutrition education to promote healthy food choices. The question remains, however, as to whether advertising and marketing strategies can lead to an improvement in the dietary choices made by individuals. Reger and colleagues[9] studied the impact of different health promotion strategies, such as paid advertising, public relations, and community education, on inducing people to switch from consuming high-fat milk to consuming low-fat milk. They reported that these low-cost measures did result in a change in the type of milk consumed and that these changes were sustained. In a study reported from Finland, an educational campaign to reduce heart disease incidence in affected communities was highly effective in improving dietary habits, reducing the risk factors for heart disease, and lowering the incidence of disease and death.[6] Because the funds for nutrition education campaigns are limited, it is essential to design and implement low-cost programs that use multiple strategies, have a simple and clear message, involve the family, and are repeated over a long time period. Such programs will be effective in encouraging and sustaining improved dietary habits in communities.

Challenges Faced by Nutrition Educators

By providing nutrition education programs to communities at risk of developing nutrition-linked chronic diseases, nutrition educators hope to provide information, skills, and reinforcements in order to encourage people to introduce modifications into their dietary patterns to protect or improve their health. It is easy to impart knowledge related to nutrition to the target population, but difficult to actually introduce changes in the dietary pattern because those changes are not inherently rewarding or satisfying.[5]

Providing nutrition education thus involves not just dispensing knowledge and information, but also supplying ways and means to change attitudes and behavior. The challenge is for people to retain and follow the recommended changes in dietary practices. Noncompliance can result from a number of factors, including 1) communication is ineffective; 2) the client is not paying attention; and 3) the message is misinterpreted.[10] The whole concept of nutrition education therefore needs to be viewed differently. It is just not enough to design programs and deliver information to the public in a one-time interaction.[11] To bring about any significant change in the lifestyle of individuals or communities and impact health in a positive manner, the process of imparting knowledge and encouraging changes has to be continued over a period of time. The approach has to be slow, but consistent. Nutrition educators must understand that most individuals know what they need to do in order

to remain healthy, but strongly resist making any modifications in their daily habits. Individuals and communities thus have to be motivated to change; the individual must be taught that he or she is responsible for his or her own health decisions and is in full control over his or her own well-being, particularly as it relates to food and nutrition.

It is much more challenging to introduce behavioral changes through educational programs that depend entirely on mass media and have little interpersonal contact. While designing programs that target nutrition education, public health professionals must realize the value of one-on-one communication with individuals. Developing a good relationship and maintaining close contact with the target population is an integral component of a successful nutrition education program.

To produce a strong desire to change and an intense motivation to incorporate changes into their dietary patterns, people need more than just knowledge transfer, information availability, and attitude change. Skills and adequate resources must be available to support the motivated individual. Social support and rewards for the behavioral change are necessary if the changes are to be incorporated and sustained over time. Public health professionals must therefore train individuals, families, employers, community leaders, and influential people in the community to provide support for recommended changes in their dietary habits.

A major barrier faced by nutrition educators is the lack of linguistically and culturally appropriate services.[12] There is a dearth of translated materials in different languages for audiences who are not adequately proficient in English. Such individuals have trouble understanding even basic information related to nutrition, health, and healthcare services. This problem is further compounded by the fact that the number of bilingual providers and trained interpreters is limited. The public health team must be cognizant of this issue and have appropriate training procedures prepared for communities that are Hispanic American, Asian American, or non-English speaking. In order to convey the message of sound nutrition and help audiences imbibe the principles of nutrition in health and in different disease states, public health personnel thus must bridge the language gap. Another challenge along similar lines is that dietary habits are culturally sensitive. Health promotion programs that emphasize nutrition will have to be designed specifically, or be "custom-made," for the target communities, keeping in mind their dietary food habits, regional food choices and selection, food preferences, and cultural limitations. Any recommendation that is not culturally appropriate will not be easily acceptable to the public. In a policy adopted in 2001, the American Public Health Association advocated that federal agencies use resources that are culturally sensitive and linguistically relevant, along with translators.[13] The association also encouraged healthcare providers to collaborate with federal agencies to provide culturally and linguistically appropriate services.

See the American Public Health Association's Web site at http://www.apha.org.

It is also imperative that public health professionals consider gender differences in designing nutrition education programs. Women in several societies have a tendency to take a back seat in their own healthcare decisions and neglect their own health. The resources available at home are used to take care of the health requirements of other family members at the expense of their own health. Clearly, improvements in health via nutrition education have to be targeted towards all family members. Women must be encouraged to view themselves as important members of their family and the community, with a great responsibility towards themselves, their family, and the community. They must recognize that they are a powerful tool to bring about change in society, including societal values and thinking.

The public health team also must recognize the need to remove cultural barriers that impede the progress of healthy change in communities. Along with outreach programs for health promotion and nutrition education, additional programs must address the problem of cultural and social barriers to change.

It is also important to keep in mind that if nutrition education and health promotion programs are to be successful, they should be imparted not only at the level of the individual, but also at the level of the community. Public health professionals in community health centers and community-based organizations can reach communities that are otherwise disenfranchised. They can target their programs towards specific populations so the message can be delivered more effectively, and be better retained and implemented. Community-based organizations are important because many of them arise out of personal experiences and thus better understand the pulse of the community.[12]

Who Should Provide Nutrition Education?

To prevent the spread of nutrition misinformation, consumers must have access to trained/qualified nutrition professionals and other health and allied health professionals who have received sound training in nutrition. The providers of nutrition information must be registered or licensed nutritionists who have fulfilled the requirements and standards established by state and national regulations. It has been noted, however, that to improve the acceptance and inclusion of suggested dietary modifications, as well as compliance, the desired dietary patterns must be emphasized repeatedly. A client/patient must meet with several health professionals during his or her care, so it is important that every member of a person's medical care team be well-trained and well-versed in the principles of nutrition. Repeated emphasis on improving dietary habits and remaining healthy will have a greater impact than counseling by a single individual. If the message of managed lives/healthy lives is to be delivered, it thus must entail a combined strong effort by a group of individuals (the nutrition education team) who can shape public health efforts to promote health in communities. It is the responsibility of the public health nutrition education team to spread the message of nutrition, particularly in communities where the risk for developing preventable chronic disorders like diabetes and heart disease are high.

■ THE NUTRITION EDUCATION TEAM

Many professionals in public health disciplines are involved in providing total care to the individual. Some of these can be important members of the nutrition education team, which can include public health nutritionists/dietitians, dietetic technicians, physicians, nurses, pharmacists, social workers, psychologists, health educators, medical educators, and physical and occupational therapists, among others.[14,15] Each of these professionals can contribute his or her expertise towards the nutritional care of the community as a whole or to an individual client. Activities that these professionals can provide at a healthcare facility include assessing the nutritional status of the patient and prescribing an appropriate diet, indicating possible food-drug interactions, planning modified diets and menus, supervising food services, assisting the patient with meal selection, helping those unable to feed themselves, recording data on food allergies and acceptance, providing nutrition counseling, and making arrangements for financial assistance and home services. The following sections discuss the responsibilities of each member of the nutrition education team.[14,15]

Nutritionists/Dietitians and Dietetic Technicians

Nutritionists/dietitians and dietetic technicians play a very important role in providing comprehensive nutrition care to the client. They are an integral part of the professional staff working in hospitals, health clinics, well-baby clinics, nursing homes, schools, and daycare centers. In hospitals, health clinics, and nursing homes, dietitians assess the nutritional status of patients, provide dietary counseling, prescribe diets, plan menus, and supervise food services. In addition, dietetic technicians assist patients in menu selection, and record daily dietary intake and data on food acceptance. In schools and daycare centers, nutritionists are responsible for planning nutritionally balanced meals for children, providing a variety of foods that meet the Dietary Reference Intakes for different nutrients.

In hospitals and medical settings, nutritionists also must be actively involved in client case discussions and exchange information with the physicians and the nursing staff on the patient's dietary intake. While providing nutrition care to the patient, they must actively educate the patient about the nutrition modifications necessary for controlling his or her medical disorder and preventing any further deterioration. This close interaction with the other members of the team allows for reinforcement of the information delivered to the patient, fills in any gaps in information, and prevents any contradictory message from reaching the patient. To reinforce the message of nutrition education, it is therefore imperative that nutritionists, physicians, nurses, and other professionals involved in the care of the patient collaborate closely in the screening, diagnosis, treatment, and follow-up. Each professional should be cognizant of the important role played by others, respect their professional qualifications, and leave room for all to contribute to the nutrition care of the patient.

As a member of the public health team, another responsibility of the nutritionist is to provide updated nutrition information to the other members of the team. Recent developments related to nutrition in children or adults that focus on normal or therapeutic nutrition, as well as recently published articles from refereed scientific publications or journals, should be shared with the other members of the nutrition education team. This ensures that all of the public health professionals are on top of new developments in the field of nutrition and can provide appropriate education to their clients. Nutritionists can invite the other members of the team to some of their nutrition counseling sessions to observe their interactions with the client and learn some effective approaches for conveying dietary information. Special sessions could be arranged by the nutritionist to reinforce the principles of nutrition in a state of health or disease for the other members of the patient care team. This also strengthens the ability of other team members to provide nutrition education to clients in the absence of the nutritionist.

In addition to group sessions, nutritionists can consult on individual cases with the other members of the nutrition education public health team. The responsible physician, nurse, pharmacist, and nutritionist can have a conference to discuss the medical records of the client, family history, the medical treatment prescribed, and the nutrition approaches involved in caring for the patient. The team also can discuss

the most effective strategies that can be employed for the dietary care of the patient. The progress made by the client should be evaluated on a regular basis to ensure compliance with the dietary recommendations.

Physicians

Medical doctors obtain anthropometric, clinical, biochemical, and general dietary intake data from their patients to diagnose disease and assess the health and nutritional status of the patient. Following the diagnosis, they recommend the type and course of treatment in order to control the disease and prevent further health deterioration. As part of treatment as well as disease prevention and health promotion, physicians suggest the appropriate diet for the patient. In the case of patients with disease conditions that need extensive dietary modifications, most physicians will provide a referral to a qualified nutritionist for detailed assessment, planning, and patient counseling concerning the preparation of the diet. It is very important at this stage that the physician maintain a positive and encouraging attitude toward the dietary modifications recommended. They should be able to convince their patients as to why the dietary change is essential and how it will help treat the disease and prevent any further damage to their health. This positive attitude is developed only if physicians themselves are convinced of the importance of sound nutrition; this can be achieved only through proper training in their medical curricula. Physicians who fail to emphasize the importance of nutrition at this stage and do not encourage changes in dietary habits deter the patient from following any diet-related advice provided by another member of the nutrition team.

Nurses and Nursing Assistants

Nurses interact with the patient frequently and assist the patient in menu selection, help those unable to feed themselves, record data on food intake and acceptance, and counsel patients on health and nutrition promotion. Nurses also can educate their patients using standard educational materials available in health clinics and hospitals. They can provide overall dietary guidance for different diet-related disorders and refer the patient to the nutritionist for more detailed and specific information on the dietary modifications recommended. They can motivate and reinforce the dietary recommendations to their patients for an extended period of time and thus serve as very valuable sources of nutrition education.

It is very important that the members of the nutrition team interact with each other to discuss the progress made by the patient in following the suggested dietary recommendations. Frequent dialogue with a patient allows nurses to know more personal information about the patient than the other members of the team. In particular, nurses that pay home visits recognize the physical, emotional, and financial limitations of the patient. Sharing their experiences with the other members of the team can also pave the way for making additional suggestions and changes in the prescribed diet to better fit the environmental, social, physical, and financial circumstances of the patient.

Pharmacists

In some scenarios, the role of the pharmacist is to provide information to the patient on possible interactions between different drugs and food. Additionally, pharmacists form an integral part of the medical team that will screen and treat the patient. Close interaction among the pharmacist, physician, nutritionist, nurse, and patient thus allows the pharmacist to explain any food-drug interactions to the patient and prevent complications.

Social Workers

Social workers help those patients who are in need of placement services. They are able to assess the physical, emotional, financial, and social stresses encountered by the patient that would prevent him or her from following the recommended medical and dietary advice. Social workers provide guidance and suggestions to patients to allow them to face challenges and find workable solutions, and help prepare them to follow the recommended medical and dietary advice. Because they interact with the patient on a more personal level, social workers can serve as an important vehicle for the delivery of nutrition information, help the family with meal budgeting and meal planning, and be an active contributor to the process of nutrition education.

Psychologists

The role of the psychologist is to counsel clients on their mental health condition and suggest treatment. They study the emotional, financial, and social constraints faced by the patient in following the desired treatment, help the patient to deal with emotional stresses, and strengthen him or her psychologically to accept and follow the recommendations. Psychologists provide emotional security and support to patients in need, enabling their patients to think clearly and make the right eating and drinking choices.

Physical and Occupational Therapists

Physical and occupational therapists interact closely and for an extended period of time with clients in need of therapy. Patients who have difficulty eating or swallowing need help from these therapists to overcome their handicap to function more efficiently. Therapists must work closely with the nutritionist to decide which foods will be appropriate for the patient as well as provide the desired nutrition. Subsequently, they interact with the family and the client to train them as to appropriate feeding procedures and regimen. During each session, these therapists could prove invaluable in transferring nutrition-related information to the client. Patients usually receive therapy over a period of time, which may extend into weeks or even months in some cases, so adequately trained physical/occupational therapists could serve as a vehicle for slow dispersal of knowledge to the patient. Because nutrition education is an ongoing endeavor, these professionals can play an invaluable role as a member of the nutrition education team.

Dentists and Dental Hygienists

Promoting oral hygiene and preventing the development of cavities and tooth-related disorders is the function of the dentist. Dentists and dental hygienists, in their interaction with the client, discourage the use of high-sugar food items and encourage the use of nutritive foods. In other words, these professionals also contribute significantly to improving the nutritional status of their clients.

Health/Medical Educators

In public health departments, health clinics, and hospitals, health/medical educators play a very important role as members of the nutrition education team. Being education specialists, they design, implement, and assess educational activities that involve all the other professionals of the public health nutrition team. They can develop and revise the curriculum, select appropriate methods and materials, and also train the staff effectively. Health educators must be able to develop good relationships with the public so that they can identify the needs and problems of the community and then develop programs to address these concerns. The health educator can also market educational campaigns to the target audience.

Veterinarians

The American Public Health Association recognized the need for veterinarians in public health services, in every health department and health clinic.[13] They recommended that schools of public health and applied public health programs provide facilities for continuing education and recruitment outreach to veterinarians. Veterinarians play an important role in promoting food safety, especially pathogen control, and in the surveillance of food-borne diseases.[13]

The Public

Public health should not be limited to only experts who advise the public on what to do and what not to do. There are not enough public health educators available to interact with the public. The onus of improving the diet and health of communities also lies on the public itself. More active participation is required of the public.[16] Each individual must recognize his or her own responsibility towards maintaining good health. Each individual must consider his or her own actions to understand what needs to be changed to improve nutritional status and maintain good health.

It would be ideal if each trained professional could associate with a community-based organization long enough to train some of their members. The responsibility thereafter could be taken up by these members to train others in the organization. The organization could then expand its educational activities to other organizations. A chain reaction would follow whereby one individual would educate another until the whole community was informed. "Each one, educate one." Such could be the motto of all community organizations to achieve good nutrition and health for all.

Are These Professionals Adequately Trained in the Discipline of Nutrition?

Clearly, if the members of the nutrition education team have a responsibility to provide advice that impacts dietary choices, they must have adequate training in the discipline of nutrition. Registered dietitians are trained nutritionists with national accreditation; licensed or certified dietitians are also qualified nutritionists with state accreditation; and some professionals have academic degrees in nutrition from an accredited institution.[17] These individuals possess, in addition to satisfactory training in the principles of nutrition, membership in relevant professional societies, such as the American Dietetic Association, American Society for Clinical Nutrition, Society for Nutrition Education, and Institute of Food Technologists, to keep them informed of recent advances in the field of food and nutrition. In order to maintain their professional status, registered dietitians must take a certain number of continuing education credit hours every five years to update their skills and knowledge. The American Dietetic Association holds registered dietitians to high standards to assure they are reliable and trustworthy sources of nutrition information.[17]

American Dietetic Association: http://www.eatright.org.

American Society for Nutrition: http://www.nutrition.org

Society for Nutrition Education: http://sne.org

Institute of Food Technologists: http://www.ift.org

In 1985, the Committee on Nutrition in Medical Education, a branch of the Food and Nutrition Board of the National Research Council, identified the lack of adequate training for medical students in the United States and recommended that nutrition be added to the curriculum as a required course.[18] The National Nutritional Monitoring and Related Research Act was passed in 1990 to ensure that medical students and practicing physicians in the United States have adequate training in the field of nutrition and how it relates to human health. Despite efforts to improve training for medical students and physicians in the discipline of nutrition, however, the curriculum offered at many U.S. medical schools still does not adequately concentrate on this discipline. This is reflected in clinical practice, where physicians provide very limited nutrition education during patient care. Physicians routinely fail to underscore the importance of diet in the treatment of nutrition-related diseases like diabetes, heart disease, obesity, osteoporosis, and anemia, among others. In 2004, it was reported that annually 400,000 deaths in the United States were linked to poor diet and nutrition.[19]

For the treatment of major public health disorders such as obesity, diabetes, and atherosclerosis, pharmaceutical and technological approaches are preferred over nutritional interventions. The Nutrition Academic Award program[20] was developed in 1997 by the National Heart, Lung and Blood Institute to improve nutrition-related knowledge and skills among medical school students, residents, fellows, faculty, and practicing physicians. This initiative is intended to improve the application of nutrition principles in patient care and clinical practice. It should reinforce the existing efforts to improve the qualifications and training of physicians in the science of nutrition. In addition to training medical students, some recipients of the Nutrition Academic Award provide training to students of other health professional schools, such as dental programs, dietetic programs, nursing schools, pharmacy schools, physician assistant programs, public health programs, exercise physiology programs, physical education programs, and health ecology programs.

◼ EDUCATION PROGRAMS

Continuing Education Programs

Accrediting agencies provide continuing education programs for health professionals, including physicians, nurses, pharmacists, and nutritionists, to provide an avenue to the most updated and recent information about innovative clinical intervention strategies, clinical trials, and medical success stories. Such continuing education programs can be planned for all health professionals, regardless of whether they work in private practice, healthcare facilities, community health centers, public health departments/agencies, or educational institutions.[15] Medical and health professional schools also can plan these continuing education programs for health professionals, because they provide both knowledge and practical training tips for successful clinical practice.

In-Service Education Programs

In-service education programs can be planned in hospitals and public health agencies for their public health personnel. A committee of medical educators, physicians, nurses, nutritionists, pharmacists, social workers, and psychologists can plan the program in order to address the most common medical concerns.[15] This would be a good platform for sharing recent developments in the scientific literature, exchanging ideas, asking questions, and sharing critical thinking. Any challenges and concerns can be addressed, and constructive suggestions can be made. Such educational programs could also provide an avenue for reinforcing the existing information related to suggested dietary practices in a state of health or disease. The team can discuss the existing nutrition care for different medical conditions, any new modifications to be introduced, any existing drawbacks, and new suggestions for overcoming some of them. The dietitian can demonstrate the planning of modified diets to the group so they can share these ideas with their clients.

As with any educational program, program assessment should form an integral part of the educational effort. Participants should evaluate the program to see if learning occurred. Any suggestions for improvement should be taken into consideration while planning the next in-service education program. The nutrition department in healthcare facilities and public health nutritionists can provide a monthly newsletter highlighting new findings for the benefit of the other members of the public health team. Collectively, all these measures may ensure that the nutrition knowledge of healthcare professionals meets the professional standards set by accrediting agencies.

NATIONAL INITIATIVES TO PROMOTE NUTRITION EDUCATION

Team Nutrition Initiative

The Food and Nutrition Service of the U.S. Department of Agriculture developed the Team Nutrition Initiative in order to improve the nutritional quality of meals served to schoolchildren and to encourage foods that reflect the dietary guidelines and are low in fat and sodium.[21] As part of its activities, Team Nutrition has developed messages and educational materials linked to nutrition that can be used in schools throughout the country. Team Nutrition provides training to food service professionals in schools to help them prepare and serve meals that meet both the nutrition requirements of children and appear appetizing. This initiative also provides nutrition education for parents as well as children to help them make healthy food choices and improve their health. For additional support of this activity, Team Nutrition involves school administrators and community leaders who can reinforce the message effectively. Team Nutrition spreads its message using different communication strategies, such as food service interventions, activities in the classroom, school-wide events, promoting healthy actions at home, programs in the community, media events, and media coverage. The effectiveness of Team Nutrition depends on successful partnerships among federal, state, and local agencies. The Team Nutrition initiative shows that school administrators, teachers, community leaders, and

See the Team Nutrition Initiative at http://www.fns.usda.gov/tn/.

agencies at the local, state, and federal levels can all play a very important role in spreading the message of nutrition education to families and communities.

Action for Healthy Kids

As discussed in previous chapters, the U.S. Department of Agriculture, the U.S. Department of Education, and the Centers for Disease Control and Prevention have partnered with other organizations to establish Action for Healthy Kids.[22] The main objective of Action for Healthy Kids is to improve the health of schoolchildren by encouraging the consumption of nutritionally balanced meals and promoting physical activity. Schoolchildren are faced with serious diet-related health problems, and this organization, which works at the local level, can make a significant impact by disseminating nutrition information to address these concerns.

TEAMWORK

Strategies for Developing an Effective Public Health Team

A team consists of a group of individuals working together to achieve a shared goal.[15] In an ideal team, members function synergistically, leading to increased efficiency and productivity. The emphasis is seldom placed on individual team members; rather, the team as a total entity is always paramount. To achieve the shared goal, team members are involved in activities that are interdependent instead of independent. With different individuals contributing their skills and knowledge to the team, each member of the team learns about the important role and position of different professional contributors on the team. They learn to respect each other's expertise and also appreciate how all the disciplines come together to address a common goal. In the public health arena, teamwork is crucial because the efforts of the physician, nutritionists/dietitians, dietetic technicians, nurses, pharmacists, social workers, psychologists, health educators, medical educators, and physical and occupational therapists contribute tremendously towards improving the health and nutritional status of the individual, family, or community. As discussed earlier, such integrated efforts are necessary to address the physical, emotional, social, economic, cultural, and personal issues linked to the individual, family, or community. Not only can these professionals address the problem from different perspectives, but they also can reinforce the message of health and nutrition education to bridge the gap between knowledge and practice. Teamwork thus can prove to be an economical way of addressing the health and nutrition needs of an individual, family, or community.

Teams can serve a patient group or a population, and their membership is fluid depending on the needs of the people served. Team functions can include planning, program delivery, and case discussions and conferences. A nutrition education team can assess the needs of its client population, identify areas that need emphasis, design and develop programs to address those needs, and set up conferences for clients with complex and chronic problems. Subgroups may form within a team to provide special services. In a team, leadership roles are clearly defined and assigned.

Strategies and Characteristics of a Properly Functioning and Effective Team

For a team to function in the most productive and efficient manner, its members have to be focused on the objectives, share leadership roles, and be accountable for their actions. Some defining features of a successful team are the following[23]:

- *Zero in on the objectives:* Any team should, at the onset, be aware of the goals to be achieved. Each member of the team should be very clear about the goals and objectives of the project. Additionally, the team members should be in agreement regarding the specific outcomes and parameters to be used to assess whether the goals have been adequately reached.
- *Accentuate a participatory style:* In a team as diverse as a public health team, different ideas are bound to arise because members originate from different disciplines. Members must be encouraged to listen and acknowledge alternate points of view in order to obtain a view of the "big picture."[23] As team members begin to respect each other, recognize each other's contributions, and trust each other, they can address the health issue more appropriately. While some members look at the broader picture, others look at small details; while some address the physical aspect, others deal with emotional issues; while others stress the economic aspect, some will focus on social influences. This is perhaps one of the best ways of finding solutions together.
- *Increase the sense of belonging and connectedness:* The work of any team is considerably enhanced if the members have a strong sense of connection with other team members and with the objectives of the team. All members of the team should have a sense of belonging and a strong desire to meet the defined goals and objectives.
- *Organize the team:* The specific responsibilities for the team should be mutually agreed upon by all team members. Because a public health team is inherently multifaceted, as are the problems it intends to address, clear leadership roles should be defined for different team activities.[23] Team members should be identified by discipline, knowledge, skills, specialization, experience, and interests.
- *Promote team responsibility:* Given the interdependent nature of any team, members of the team must

be encouraged to take responsibility for completing individual duties in a timely manner.[23] When necessary, team members also should assist one another to collectively achieve the objectives of the team.
- *Encourage equal influence:* The team must be built on the premise that the viewpoints and contributions of all members are of equal value, and therefore all members must be willing to yield influence on all issues facing the team. Each member of the team must recognize and respect the contributions made by the other members of the team. Members must pay close attention to the suggestions made by others and then collectively arrive at one decision.
- *Establish a timeline for the work to be done and commit to allotting time to do the work:* After the activities necessary to achieve the desired goals and objectives are planned and explained to all the members of the team, every member must then assume responsibility for the activities and make the necessary time commitment to work towards them.
- *Define measurable outcomes and work products:* As per the commitment of each team member, at the end of the time period designated for the activity, tangible work products should be visible. Each person on the team must show his or her contribution towards attaining the planned goals and objectives of the team. The resources available to the team must be shared equally by all the members; there should be no competition or turf guarding. Team members come from different disciplines, so there should be complete understanding between all the members about the role and responsibilities of each member. Cooperation with each other along with administrative support will allow the team to function efficiently and effectively.
- *Discuss and resolve all problems together:* As each member of the team undertakes activities to move in the planned direction, some problems and challenges may arise. For smooth resolution of all such problems, the team members must communicate on a regular basis to discuss and formulate solutions. All challenges thus must be faced by the team collectively and solutions finalized with mutual consent.

Team Leader

All teams must be led by a team leader. This individual must have the skills of a manager to lead the team smoothly in the planned direction. The leader is selected from the team itself not just for professional expertise, but also for possessing management skills to keep the team cohesive. The team leader must understand very clearly the mission of the team and communicate this mission to all members. It is the responsibility of the team leader to charge the team and orient all the members with the goals and objectives of the team. The leader must be involved in the selection of the team members and be able to delineate the roles and responsibilities of each one.[15] After setting the direction of the team, the leader must follow up the progress of the team on a regular basis, encourage cooperation and collaboration among the team members, and peacefully resolve any conflicts that may occur. The team leader must have the skills to deal with differences of opinion and power struggles within the team.[23] The leader plans for regular team meetings to monitor progress, share any achievements, discuss concerns and challenges, and encourage exchange of ideas and suggestions. The leader encourages participation by all team members to facilitate close interaction among all members of the team and promote an atmosphere of openness and trust. The leader must guide the discussion during each meeting to promote effective decision making, and also ensure that the focus remains on the topic under consideration.[24] To develop a productive team, selection of an efficient and effective leader is very important. To function as an effective leader, an understanding of the process of group development is of paramount importance.

Group Development

A group can face different issues as it matures, including interpersonal relationships, group behavior, and leadership. To address issues of interest, groups can be organized on a temporary or permanent basis.[24] Groups can be small or large, formal or informal, and with membership that may remain constant over a period of time or undergo frequent changes. A group must develop a sense of cohesiveness so that even group members who originate from different backgrounds view the interests of the group over the interests of the individual. Some strategies for successful group development are highlighted in **Table 24–1**.

Stages of Group Development

Table 24–2 highlights the feelings and behavior of group members as they progress through the different stages of group development. These stages are discussed further in the following sections.

Stage 1: Forming

Group members get to know each other in Stage 1, which is called *forming*. They form impressions about the different members of the group and recognize similarities and differences. An atmosphere that is informal, not intimidating, and encourages conversation is a good start for the first stage of group development.[25–27] The group leader is looked to for orientation, guidance, and direction.[15] The reason for the existence of the group—the group's charge—is indicated clearly by the leader to the members of the group.[24,26,27] Members become acquainted with the goals and objectives of the team—in short, the mission of the team. They discuss the activities to be undertaken to accomplish the goals and objectives, and the ground rules are well established and understood.[26,27] Any controversial issues are avoided during the discussion. No one wants to get into conflicts; every member wants to feel a part of the group and has the desire to belong and be accepted by the group.

Stage 2: Storming

In the next stage, called *storming*, group members plan and organize the activities for the task. At this point, conflicts may arise between the members and also between the members and their leader.[24,26,27] Controversies arise over leadership, structure of the group, the power of each member, and who is in charge. The responsibility of each member, the rules and regulations, the rewards associated with performance, and the criteria for evaluation are constant

TABLE 24–1	Strategies for Successful Group Development
Strategy	**Activity/Advantage/Outcome**
Shared leadership	Responsibility for group facilitation should be given to all group members. Several leadership roles are necessary; they need not be performed by one person.
Clearly stated goals	Group members must reach a consensus on the group's goals and objectives; the group's mission should be periodically reexamined and amended, if necessary.
Ground rules established	Acceptance of rules and procedures adds to the cohesiveness of the group.
Acceptance of conflicts	Group members must recognize that conflicts and disagreements are inevitable. All decisions cannot be unanimous; groups should work hard to reach a consensus.
Members are effective listeners	Group members should listen to alternate points of view to improve the quality of decision making; all members should be encouraged to participate to make the group a successful "learning team."
Group meetings are constructive	Although group decisions should not be rushed or forced, discussions should not continue indefinitely. All group sessions should be wrapped up meaningfully.

TABLE 24–2	**Stages of Group Development: Member Feelings and Behaviors**	
Stage	**Member Feelings**	**Member Behavior**
Forming	Apprehension; excitement; desire to belong	Form impressions about other group members; try to understand the goals and objectives of the group; try to define activities; avoid conflicts and disagreements.
Storming	Resistance; resentment; jealousy	Arguments over group structure, leadership, ground rules, and responsibilities; competition between the team members.
Norming	Acceptance; respect; trust; sense of belonging	Work together towards the goal; group more creative and cohesive; resources pooled together for maximum efficiency.
Performing	Ease; comfort; acceptance; encouragement; unity; confidence; interdependence	Team is highly productive; members respect the contributions of all others on the team; team is focused and united in problem solving.
Adjourning (Deforming, Mourning)	Relief; pride; happiness	Members discuss the group's achievements and future projects and collaborations.

issues of debate. There is an underlying competition between the team members as all tend to evaluate each other, and this generates hostilities.[15,25-27] Some members tend to dominate over others and try to gain influence and support, whereas others remain completely silent. Subgroups may form as a result of this internal conflict and may even challenge the leader of the group.[15] No problem solving occurs at this stage.

Stage 3: Norming

In Stage 3, called *norming*, group members begin to respect each other and support each other.[15] This makes the group more cohesive and close-knit. Group members begin to acknowledge and accept the knowledge, skills, and expertise of different professionals in the group.[26,27] As the group members begin to know and trust each other, they change their preconceived ideas or notions about each other and work together to resolve group issues.[25-27] The group becomes more cohesive and productive. Members develop a sense of belonging to the group and begin to exchange ideas and thoughts. This stage is, therefore, characterized by high creativity.

Stage 4: Performing

Stage 4 is referred to as *performing*. In this stage, the team is most productive. All team members are fully cognizant and fully accepting of the contributions and roles of the other members of the team.[15] Team members are at ease with each other in problem solving and working towards the planned objectives.[26,27] They can work comfortably as

a group, as a subgroup, or individually. Initiatives and suggestions made by different members are accepted by all others; members encourage feedback from each other.[15] Members are highly focused on task functions and obtaining the desired goals and objectives. The group is united in its efforts; group morale and confidence are very high.[25-27]

At this stage, the performance and the productivity of the group peak. The pitfalls that might have troubled the group until this stage are avoided, and the group forges ahead with a renewed sense of accomplishment. And accomplish the group does, with self-assurance. Group members concentrate on finding optimal solutions to problems at hand. Interdependence among the group members reaches an all-time high, with no need to seek validation from the other members. Because the members identify very strongly with each other at this stage, group loyalty reaches a new crest. Further, members refuse to let themselves be pigeonholed into specific categories and roles, and regularly switch gears from being independent members to being members of a subgroup to being a complete unit. The "means" at this stage is hard work, and the "end" is greater productivity.

Stage 5: Adjourning

This stage is also referred to as "deforming" or "mourning." Rather than viewing this stage as an extension of the above four stages, one can look at this stage as an adjunct. Clearly, this stage is not critical to the overall functioning of the team. Rather, the focus is solely on the emotions of the people who had made up the team until now.[26,27] In this stage, after the group has accomplished its task, it is effectively disbanded. The group members could reiterate their support of the steps they have taken together to achieve results. They also could discuss whether they would consider working together again. Members highlight individual and collective accomplishments and make decisions regarding future collaborative efforts. They may also feel opposing emotions at this stage: on one hand, some pain of farewell could be felt; on the other hand, there could be considerable relief that the project is finally over.[26,27]

Although five stages have been identified in the process of group development, not all groups will pass through them. Some groups may not be successful in overcoming the challenges associated with the earlier stages and never get past them. Groups that are able to negotiate all the stages eventually prove to be the most productive and efficient.

■ CONCLUSION

In this chapter you learned that the significance of nutrition in preventing the onset of disease and controlling the progression of chronic diseases cannot be underestimated. However, the benefits associated with a healthy diet can be achieved only if the public is aware of the principles of nutrition in a state of health and in a state of disease. It is the responsibility of public health professionals like nutritionists, physicians, nurses, pharmacists, social workers, psychologists, and others to make conscious efforts individually and collectively to provide nutrition education for the benefit of the community.

Issues for Discussion

1. What criteria can be used to assess the impact and effectiveness of a nutrition education program?

2. What strategies can be adopted to emphasize the importance of nutrition to professionals in the health and allied-health disciplines involved in providing complete care to the patient?

3. What level of training in the field of nutrition is considered to be "adequate" for medical school students?

4. What measures can be taken to reduce the challenges faced by nutrition educators?

5. Is nutrition education the responsibility of nutritionists alone? Defend your answer.

6. How can the effectiveness of in-service education programs be enhanced?

References

1. U.S. Department of Health and Human Services. *Healthy People 2020: Understanding and Improving Health*, 2nd ed. Washington, DC: U.S. Government Printing Office; November 2010.

2. U.S. Department of Health and Human Services.. *Statistics Related to Overweight and Obesity*. Available at http://www.win.niddk.nih.gov/statistics/index.htm#econ. Accessed June 10, 2010.

3. Ernst ND, Sempos CT, Briefel RR, Clark MD. Consistency between U.S. dietary fat intakes and fetal serum cholesterol concentrations. *Am J Clin Nutr*. 1997;66(suppl):965S–972S.

4. National Institute of Diabetes and Digestive and Kidney Diseases, National Institutes of Health. *Diabetes Prevention Program*, NIH publication No. 09-5099, Oct 2008. Available at http://diabetes.niddk.nih.gov/dm/pubs/preventionprogram. Accessed June 29, 2010.

5. Green LW, Potvin L. Education, health promotion, and social, and lifestyle determinants of health and disease. In: Detels R, McEwen J, Beaglehole R, Tanaka H, eds. *Oxford Textbook of Public Health. The Scope of Public Health*, 4th ed. Vol 1. New York: Oxford University Press Inc.; 2002:113–130.

6. Nestle M, Dixon LB. Do education campaigns induce communities to change their diets and improve health? In: Nestle M, Dixon LB, eds. *Taking Sides. Clashing Views on Controversial Issues in Food and Nutrition*. Guilford, CT: McGraw-Hill/Dushkin; 2004:174–175.

7. The Henry J. Kaiser Family Foundation. *The Role of Media in Childhood Obesity. Program for the Study of Entertainment Media and Health*. Publication Number 7030; February 2004. Available at http://www.kff.org. Accessed June 7, 2010.

8. Childhood Obesity and the Impact of Food Marketing to Children. CDC Congressional Testimony. September 23, 2008. Available at http://www.cdc.gov/washington/testimony/2008/t20080923.htm. Accessed June 29, 2010.

9. Reger B, Wootan MG, Booth-Butterfield S. A comparison of different approaches to promote community-wide dietary change. *Am J Prev Med*. 2000;18:271–275.

10. Tones K. Health promotion, health education, and the public health. In: Detels R, McEwen J, Beaglehole R, Tanaka H, eds. *Oxford Textbook of Public Health. The Methods of Public Health*, 4th ed., Vol 2. New York: Oxford University Press Inc.; 2002:829–831.

11. Breckon DJ, Harvey JR, Lancaster RB. Current perspectives of practice and professional preparation. In: *Community Health Education—Settings, Roles and Skills for the 21st Century*. Gaithersburg, MD: Aspen Publication, 1998.

12. Ro M. Moving forward: addressing the health of Asian American and Pacific Islander women. *Am J Public Health*. 2002;92:516–519.

13. American Public Health Association. Policy statements adopted by the governing council of the American Public Health Association, October 24, 2001. *Am J Pub Health*. 2002;92:468.

14. Weigley ES, Mueller DH, Robinson CH. Food, nutrition and health. In: *Robinson's Basic Nutrition and Diet Therapy*, 8th ed. Upper Saddle River, NJ: Merrill Prentice Hall; 1997:4–5.

15. Joyner G, Kaufman M. Leveraging nutrition education through the public health team. In: Kaufman M, ed. *Nutrition in Public Health*. Gaithersburg, MD: Aspen Publications; 1990:420–436.

16. Avery B. Who does the work of public health? *Am J Public Health*. 2002;92:570–575.

17. Leeds MJ. Good nutrition for a healthy life. In: Leeds MJ, ed. *Nutrition for Healthy Living*. Boston, MA: WCB McGraw-Hill; 1998:13–15.

18. Pearson TA, Stone EJ, et al. Translation of nutritional sciences into medical education: the Nutrition Academic Award Program. *Am J Clin Nutr*. 2001;74:164–170.

19. Mokdad AH, Marks JS, Stroup DF, Gerberding JL. Actual causes of death in the United States. *JAMA*. 2004;291:1238–1245.

20. *About the Nutrition Academic Award (NAA) Program*. Available at http://www.nhlbi.nih.gov/funding/training/naa/about.htm. Accessed June 29, 2010.

21. Food and Nutrition Information Center, U.S. Department of Agriculture, Agricultural Research Service. *Team Nutrition*. Available at http://www.fns.usda.gov/tn/. Accessed June 29, 2009.

22. U.S. Government Accounting Office. *School Lunch Program: Efforts Needed to Improve Nutrition and Encourage Healthy Eating*. GAO-03-506; May 2003. Available at http://searching.gao.gov/index.html. Accessed June 7, 2010.

23. Management Sciences for Health and the United Nations Children's Fund. Strategies for Developing an Effective Team. Available at http://erc.msh.org/quality/building.cfm. Accessed May 2, 2009.

24. Breckon DJ, Harvey JR, Lancaster RB. Working with groups in leadership roles. In: Breckon DJ, Harvey JR, Lancaster RB. *Community Health Education—Settings, Roles and Skills for the 21st Century*, 4th ed. Gaithersburg, MD: Aspen Publications; 1998:245–251.

25. Manion J, Lorimer W, Leander WJ. Building new teams: a discipline. In: *Team-Based Health Care Organizations: Blueprint for Success*. Gaithersburg, MD: Aspen Publications; 1996: 55–84.

26. Tuckman B. Developmental sequence in small groups. *Psychological Bull.* 1965:63;384–399.

27. Tuckman B, Jensen M. Stages of small group development. *Group and Organizational Studies*. 1977:2;419–427.

PART

VIII

Surviving in a Competitive World

CHAPTER 25

Networking for Nutrition

PATTI S. LANDERS, PhD, RD/LD

CHAPTER 26

Marketing Nutrition Programs and Services

NANCIE HERBOLD, EdD, RD
PAUL N. TAYLOR, PhD

CHAPTER 27

Earning Administrative Support

JEANNETTE BEASLEY, PhD, MPH, RD

CHAPTER 28

Striving for Excellence and Envisioning the Future

MARCIA THOMAS, MS, MPH, RD
PAMELLA DARBY, MS, MPH, RD

Many factors are important to any program: networking, marketing, earning internal administrative support, striving for excellence, and envisioning the future. For a program to be successful, these elements must be present, although they continue to be some of public health nutrition's most daunting challenges. In order for programs to work and meet the needs of those targeted to receive help, networking and marketing must be planned carefully. Chapters 25 and 26 give the reader an insight into these important tools to reach the public. Chapter 27 stresses the need for us to also market our nutrition programs within the organization of public health to assure survival. Finally, Chapter 28 reminds us all that public health nutrition is a dynamic process that changes constantly. As professionals, we must be able to anticipate needs and provide for them if we are to serve our communities successfully.

CHAPTER 25

Networking for Nutrition

Patti S. Landers, PhD, RD/LD

Call it a clan, call it a network, call it a tribe, call it a family. Whatever you call it, whoever you are, you need one.[1]

READER OBJECTIVES

After studying this chapter and reflecting on the contents, you should be able to:

1. Define common terms related to networking.
2. Discuss the difference between networks, alliances, and coalitions.
3. Give examples of nutrition issues that might be addressed by networks or coalitions.
4. List the benefits of networking for nutrition.
5. Identify characteristics of a successful nutrition coalition.
6. Describe the responsibilities of a lead agency and steering committee in maintaining a nutrition coalition.
7. Develop your own professional networking plan.

INTRODUCTION

Think of your network of contacts as a professional family. Networks are important both personally and professionally. The purpose of this chapter is to explore how relationships ranging from a network to coalition building are constructed and nourished. These interactions can benefit you personally. In addition, they are vital to promoting nutrition and making better health available to the individuals and families that we seek to reach and serve. Later in the chapter, you will find tips about how to improve your own networking skills.

NETWORKS, ALLIANCES, COALITIONS, AND CONSORTIUMS

Nutrition experts interact with one another at varying levels of organization. There are many terms used to describe these groups. They are often called networks, alliances, associations, coalitions, consortiums, leagues, or federations. Here we discuss a few of these terms that are representative of them all.

In the most informal sense, a *network* is a group of people who form relationships to share ideas, information, and resources. *Alliances* are often semi-official and loosely organized. In alliances, instead of people acting as individuals, the members tend to be made up of representatives from different organizations with similar goals. *Coalitions* are the most structured type of group, and are more formal in nature. Built for a specific purpose, coalitions are often formed to address a particular problem or need in the community. *Consortiums* are similar; they are large groups of organizations, formed to undertake enterprises beyond the resources of any one member.

Networks

We all have links of communication that connect us to other people. For example, most nutrition professionals attend district, state, or national meetings as a means of keeping up with new information and maintaining continuing education requirements. Telephone conference calls and Internet listservs also provide valuable contacts. These types of informal networks can be an excellent way of finding out about employment opportunities and gathering data to be used in program planning and evaluation.

An Internet nutrition Web site can be used as a community for nutrition students and dietitians. There may be a message board where students exchange information about class work, explore different academic programs, and discuss internships. A career center part of the Web site may provide information about writing resumes and examples of which questions to expect at a job interview. It can even tell prospective employees how to negotiate for a better salary. Employers may pay to place listings on the site. Job seekers may sometimes post their resumes for free and view a list of open positions and their locations. A speaker's network may be available, where an organization needing a speaker can view people's credentials. Or, members can enroll in a referral network, if it exists, where others wanting nutrition services can find contact information.[2]

At a higher level, nutrition networking efforts can be encouraged or even mandated by funding agencies. The Food and Nutrition Service (FNS) of the United States Department of Agriculture (USDA) provides matching funds for states and communities to provide education to those who receive Supplemental Nutrition Assistance Program (SNAP) benefits (formerly known as Food Stamps). The goal is to increase the likelihood that all SNAP recipients will make healthy food choices and engage in active lifestyles consistent with the Dietary Guidelines for Americans and MyPyramid. Because of the tremendous growth in expenditures for SNAP Education (SNAP-Ed), from $661,000 in 1992 to over $343 million in 2008,[3] networking has become very important and is being mandated by the USDA to avoid duplication of services.

The following provides an example of how the USDA promotes networking: If a Cooperative Extension Service or community agency writes a SNAP-Ed plan that includes breast-feeding education, the group must document that it is collaborating with WIC (the Special Supplemental Nutrition Program for Women, Infants and Children). Why? Both SNAP and WIC are USDA programs and many women participate in both. USDA wants to be sure that the information each woman receives is consistent. Because the WIC program has primary responsibility for breast-feeding education, it takes the lead.[4]

> **Cooperative Extension Service:** A research-based program that provides outreach services and education to consumers.

Alliances

According to the *Merriam-Webster Dictionary*, "An alliance is the state of being allied: a bond or connection between families, states, parties, or individuals."[5]

Alliances and consortia may be sponsored by professional organizations. For example, The National Nutrition Alliance is an arm of the American College of Nutrition. It was established to bring industry, academia, and nutrition practice together for the purpose of improving human health through better nutrition. Through this organization, industry scientists can interact with academicians.[6]

Local groups also form alliances to meet a community need. The Metropolitan Area Neighborhood Nutrition Alliance (MANNA) is a group of over 1,000 volunteers and a small paid staff who provide over 60,000 home-delivered, medically appropriate meals per month to people with life-threatening illnesses.[7]

Consortia and Coalitions

As defined by the *Merriam-Webster Dictionary*, "A consortium is a group formed to undertake an enterprise beyond the resources of any one member, while a coalition is defined as a temporary alliance of distinct parties, persons, or states for joint action."[5] Coalition building is considered a formal process where public and private agencies, communities, businesses, and volunteers unite as partners to combine resources and work together toward a common goal.

An example of a consortium at the national level is the U.S. Department of Health and Human Services' Healthy People. Since 1979, the initiative has promoted partnerships designed to enable diverse groups to work together to improve health. There are partners from all sectors. Federal agencies serve as coordinators. All state and territorial health departments and a multitude of national membership organizations, including the American Dietetic Association, the American Public Health Association, and the Institute of Food Technologists, belong to the Healthy People Consortium.[8] The plan is updated every 10 years as the U.S. Department of Health and Human Services (DHHS) leverages scientific insights and lessons learned from the past decade, along with new knowledge of current data, trends, and innovations. Healthy People 2020 will reflect assessments of major risks to health and wellness, changing public health priorities, and emerging issues related to our nation's health preparedness and prevention.

By engaging in networks, alliances, coalitions, and consortia, nutritionists can design interventions and services that are more likely to meet community needs and priorities. In order to effectively network, the nutritionist must have community-leader contacts, so it is important to dedicate time to community and professional service. At the heart of an effective network are successful relationships that lead to productive partnerships. Some benefits of networking include:

- Expanding understanding about an issue
- Generating innovative approaches
- Overcoming political, cultural, and bureaucratic barriers

- Reducing duplication of effort
- Bringing together complementary resources
- Sharing risks and limiting liability

■ COLLABORATING WITH OTHERS FOR NUTRITION NETWORKS

When forming a nutrition network, alliance, or coalition, the first step is to bring individuals together to explore an issue and clearly identify their purpose or define a problem. It is vital to come to a consensus about purpose and problem. Where do you find people and organizations that will become good partners? *Moving to the Future: Developing Community-Based Nutrition Services* (Workbook & Training Manual),[9] provides potential sectors that may include organizations and businesses that deal with food and nutrition issues.

After you have assembled a group of potential partners, one of the most important features of this stage is relationship building. Each person must feel that she or he has had an opportunity to give a perspective and that others in the group have heard them. This may take several meetings and a significant amount of time.

After a problem or general purpose has been identified, it is helpful if each member of the group tells how his or her organization is related to the problem. As illustrated in **Figure 25–1**, you may want to use a RACK analysis to inventory partners. This acronym stands for *Resources, Access, Constraints,* and *Knowledge.*

Consider the example problem of hunger in a community. The following RACK analysis gives examples of resources, access, constraints, and knowledge that can be provided by members of a community nutrition network. These represent inputs that community agencies make toward the problem or purpose of the network or coalition.

Resources

A primary resource would be food or funds to buy food. Which agencies would you want to enlist who could help with this resource? Examples would include emergency food assistance pantries, a regional food bank, area food markets and food processors, and the local agencies responsible for administering the Food Stamp program and other food distribution programs such as WIC.

Other resources, such as space, furniture, telephones, office equipment, and supplies, would also be needed. The next issue is: Who could provide personnel to take applications from hungry people and send them to the right agencies? This may be solved in the "access" category.

Access

Who has access to people who do not have enough food? Partners who can help in this area may include schools, places of worship, healthcare facilities, childcare centers, and social service agencies. Even if we know who needs the food, however, constraints may prevent distribution.

Constraints

Most partners in a network will have constraints of one kind or another. For example, a regional food bank may have plenty of food but be unable to distribute it directly to hungry people. Local food pantries can perform that role. Other constraints may be cultural or political barriers to service. For example, a community agency may be able to provide office space and telephones, but have no funds to hire personnel who speak languages other than English.

Knowledge

A university may have expertise in research and how to evaluate a program but lack access to data for analyses. Social service or cooperative extension agencies may employ nutritionists or paraprofessionals who are trained as nutrition education aides to provide instruction about dietary quality, food safety, and food resource management; however, they may not be able to teach hungry people who are not enrolled in their programs.

Any coalition should engage in frequent evaluation. New problems may be identified and a RACK analysis may prove helpful in identifying which new partner agencies or business the coalition should seek to involve.

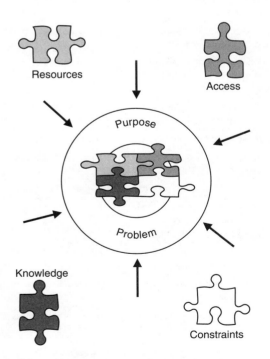

FIGURE 25–1 Elements of a RACK (Resources, Access, Constraints, and Knowledge) Analysis
Source: Developed by Patti Landers, PhD, RD/LD.

■ DEVELOPING A COMMUNITY-BASED NUTRITION NETWORK

In *Moving to the Future: Developing Community-Based Nutrition Services* (Workbook & Training Manual),[9] Karen Probert defines a coalition as a structured arrangement for cooperation and collaboration between otherwise unrelated groups or organizations. Each group retains its identity, but all agree to work together toward a common, mutually agreed upon goal. In the handbook, Probert lists seven items that need to be in place for a coalition to succeed[9]:

1. Staff support
2. Focal point of coordination
3. Specified system of communication
4. Actively involved community leaders
5. Strong relationships between private and public sector groups
6. Communication networks within the community
7. A constituency for public health that can advocate for resources and for the attention of elected officials

Probert also provides job descriptions and lists ways for members to participate. These tools may aid in building a successful coalition. The book is available online, and for a small copyright fee the forms can be customized for use by other organizations.[9]

Community Tool Box: Available at http://ctb.ku.edu.

The Community Tool Box[10] provides over 6,000 Internet pages of practical skill-building information on over 250 different topics, including how to build partnerships and coalitions. In his book *Quick Tips: Principles for Coalition Success*,[10] Tom Wolff of AHEC/Community Partners states that a shared mission and goal is vital to a successful coalition. Members must be able to set aside their own self-interest in favor of what will benefit the target audience. Wolff also emphasizes that the coalition membership must be diverse, and should include representatives from business, government, and the clergy as well as members of neighborhood groups, young people, and the disenfranchised.

When forming a nutrition coalition, it is essential to identify a lead agency. This organization should be willing and able to commit personnel and financial resources as well as have some experience in coalition building. If an agency, rather than an individual, is committed to lead the group, the project will continue even if a personnel vacancy occurs and the individual who was serving as contact person leaves.

Because coalitions are formal and structured, it is important that members write a mission statement, goals, and objectives. Bylaws should be put in place, too. Most coali-

tions have a steering committee. This subgroup also may be called the executive or coordinating committee. Typically, the steering committee includes the coalition chairperson and a representative from the lead agency. The chair or facilitator is often, but not always, from the lead agency and conducts coalition meetings.[11] Some groups prefer to rotate the position. Although someone must chair the group, leadership should be shared as much as possible, and everyone should feel they have input into decisions through a clear, democratic process. To aid in good communication, the coalition should have regular meetings. The chair or secretary should send out minutes to all members.

Successful coalitions have clear short-term and long-term goals. The members plan often, focus efforts, and measure results. They engage in ongoing evaluation at all stages of their work. The coalition should have an annual meeting that includes all of the members. The chair or steering committee should publish and distribute a yearly report. **Table 25–1** lists examples of potential issues and partners who might come together in a nutrition coalition.

TABLE 25–1	**Food and Nutrition Potential Partners**
Organization or Agency	**Web Site**
U.S. Department of Health and Human Services (DHHS)	http://www.aids.gov
Centers for Disease Control and Prevention	http://www.cdc.gov
Federal Interagency Forum on Child and Family Statistics	http://www.Childstats.gov
National Consumer Protection (A group of 17 federal and private agencies)	http://consumer.gov/ncpw/
U.S. Department of Health and Human Services (DHHS)	http://www.dhhs.gov
Food and Drug Administration	http://www.fda.gov
President's Council on Physical Fitness and Sports (DHHS)	http://www.fitness.gov
Federal Food Safety Information	http://www.FoodSafety.gov
Grants.gov (A group of 7 federal agencies sponsor this online grant search and application site)	http://www.grants.gov
Office of Disease Prevention and Health Promotion (DHHS)	http://www.health.gov
U.S. Department of Health and Human Services (DHHS)	http://www.healthfinder.gov
Executive Office of the President and DHHS	http://www.healthierus.gov

Source: USDA, *Nutrition.gov.* Available at http://riley.nal.usda.gov/nal_display/index.php?info_center=11&tax_level=1&tax_subject=384. Accessed February 25, 2010.

■ PROFESSIONAL NETWORKING

Professional organizations provide a support and networking system for public health nutritionists. The American Dietetic Association (ADA) is the nation's largest organization of food and nutrition professionals and serves the public by promoting optimal nutrition, health, and well-being.[12] The ADA has state, district, and student affiliate groups that provide for excellent peer networking through meetings and the annual Food & Nutrition Conference & Expo. ADA members also can choose to participate in the Nationwide Nutrition Network. At the ADA Web site (http://www.eatright.org), consumers, doctors and other healthcare professionals, restaurant owners and managers, and food manufacturers and distributors can enter a zip code to find local dietetics professionals for individual consultations, program development, workshops and seminars, and special projects. ADA holds an annual Public Policy Workshop in Washington, D.C., where dietitians network and focus on how they can become involved with members of Congress to impact legislative issues key to the profession and the nutritional health of Americans. ADA dietetic practice groups (DPGs) also provide opportunities for networking with others. Of particular interest to public health nutritionists are the following DPGs: Public Health/Community Nutrition, School Nutrition Services, Hunger and Environmental Nutrition, Nutrition Education for the Public, Gerontological Nutritionists, Nutrition Educators of Health Professionals, Pediatric Nutrition, Weight Management, and Women's Health and Reproductive Nutrition.

The American Public Health Association (APHA) is the oldest and largest organization of public health professionals in the world. APHA has been influencing policies and setting priorities in public health for over 125 years. Throughout its history it has been in the forefront of numerous efforts to prevent disease and promote health.[13] The APHA Food and Nutrition section contributes to long-range planning in food, nutrition, and health policy, which may affect the nutritional well-being of the public. Priorities of the section include promotion of public health nutrition policy, elimination of racial and ethnic health disparities, education and training for public health workers, and increasing and strengthening membership. An advantage of membership in APHA is the opportunity to interact not only with nutrition professionals, but also with the wider public health community, including physicians, nurses, and health educators.

The Society for Nutrition Education (SNE) is an international organization of nutrition education professionals who are dedicated to promoting healthful, sustainable food choices and who share a vision of healthy people in healthy communities.[14] Members conduct research in education, behavior, and communication; develop and disseminate innovative nutrition education strategies; and communicate information on food, nutrition, and health issues to students, professionals, policy makers, and the public. SNE members share ideas and resources through the *Journal of Nutrition Education and Behavior*, a newsletter, an annual conference, and a members-only e-mail listserv. Divisions offer networking opportunities for members with similar interests and expertise.[14] Groups of special interest may include the Public Health Nutrition and the Social Marketing Networks divisions.

Networking Tips

Developing a strong network requires planning and deliberate action. First, list your personal and professional goals and the contacts you need to make in order to achieve them. The book entitled, The *WetFeet Insider Guide to Networking*[15] suggests that your existing and potential contacts are comprised of your inner circle, your expanded network, and the network you never knew you had. People who know you well are in your inner circle; these are your family, friends, and current and former colleagues. Your expanded network includes acquaintances with whom you've had brief contact, other members of professional groups, or e-mail correspondents. The network you never knew you had includes "friends, relatives, and colleagues, relatives, and colleagues or friends."[15]

Here are some tips that will help you develop your personal network:

- Cultivate a wide circle of friends and acquaintances in many different venues.
- Stock a good supply of business cards and carry them with you at all times. Every time you meet someone you believe might be a good contact, take out one of your cards. Write a personal note on the back before you give it to them. This will let the person know about your interests and make them more likely to keep up with your contact information. They will usually offer you one of their business cards in return. Immediately write a reminder to yourself on the back. Just a phrase like "childhood obesity poster in Atlanta" will help you to remember them. Then, when you contact that person later, they will be impressed that you know who they are and what they did.
- Have a date book or personal digital assistant (PDA), and keep it handy and current.
- Keep an updated resume template on file at all times. You will want to customize it for each specific situation. For example, your resume needs different emphasis areas depending on the type of position you are seeking. If applying for a job as a clinical dietitian, you would highlight education and work in hospital settings. If you are looking for a position in a nonprofit agency, you would stress your training and experience in collaborating with other people. Listing volunteer

activities that show your community involvement would be important. Demonstrating skill with grant writing would be especially impressive.

- Be a member of one or more professional organizations. Always attend local and state meetings. Volunteer to be on committees and help at events. Always do a good job, even with small tasks. Your skills will become known and soon you will be asked to take a leadership role.
- Attend a national conference, at least every other year. If possible, travel with someone in the organization whom you do not know well. Getting out of town and having block time to network is very important.
- Immediately follow up on contacts you make with a card, brief phone call, or e-mail message.
- Prepare in advance for follow-up meetings.
- Work to improve social skills. Good social skills are essential to networking. At meetings or parties, be outgoing, even if it is not natural for you. Do not stand in a corner by yourself. Go up to others who look lonely and strike up a conversation, or join a group and introduce yourself. Do not forget your business cards. Keep them handy even at social events. If social occasions are painful, investigate a public speaking group like Toastmasters where you can improve communication skills.
- Be sincere. Help others and they will help you.
- Always remember to say thank you.

■ CONCLUSIONS

It is important to be professionally competent in what you know; however, who you know may be just as vital to accomplishing your objectives in promoting better health and nutrition.

Networking includes relationships built at both personal and professional levels. These associations may range from informal interactions with individuals and groups of people for information, ideas, and resources, to semi-official alliances, and then on to structured coalitions that were purposefully organized to address a particular nutrition problem or need in the community.

When building a coalition, it is important that membership be diverse and representative. You may want to use a RACK analysis to categorize resources, access, constraints, and knowledge of potential coalition member organizations. Write a mission statement, goals, objectives, and bylaws. Choose a steering committee and chair to interact with both coalition members and the lead agency that has committed personnel and financial resources to the coalition.

Networking, allying yourself with others, and coalition building will allow you to maximize resources, increase access to target audiences, minimize or overcome constraints, and use knowledge to benefit yourself and others. Use the tips listed near the end of the chapter to help you develop a strong personal system of contacts.

Issues for Discussion

1. How do the benefits of networking justify your investment of time and effort?

2. How can professional networking relationships benefit you personally?

3. Where do you want to go in your professional career? How can networking help you to achieve that goal?

References

1. Howard J. *Families*. New York, NY: Simon and Schuster; 1978.
2. Job Ventures, LLC. *My Nutrition Jobs*. Available at http://www.nutritionjobs.com. Accessed June 2, 2009.
3. U.S. Department of Agriculture. Approved Federal Funds for Supplemental Nutrition Assistance Education by Fiscal Year. Available at http://www.nal.usda.gov/snap/Approved%20FederalFundsSNAP-EdFY2004-2010.pdf. Accessed June 2, 2010.
4. U.S. Department of Agriculture. *Supplemental Nutrition Assistance Program Education SNAP-Ed Plan Guidance*. Available at http://snap.nal.usda.gov. Accessed June 2, 2009.
5. *Merriam-Webster Online Dictionary*. Available at http://www.m-w.com. Accessed June 2, 2009.
6. American College of Nutrition. *National Nutrition Alliance*. Available at http://www.americancollegeofnutrition.org/Default.aspx?tabid=103. Accessed June 5, 2010.
7. The Stephen Korman Nutrition Center. *Metropolitan Area Neighborhood Nutrition Alliance (MANNA)*. Available at http://www.mannapa.org. Accessed June 5, 2010.
8. U.S. Department of Health and Human Services. *Healthy People 2010*. Available at http://www.healthypeople.gov. Accessed June 5, 2010.
9. Probert K. *Moving to the Future: Developing Community-Based Nutrition Services*. Johnstown, PA: Association of State and Territorial Public Health Nutrition Directors, 1997. Available at http://www.movingtothefuture.org. Accessed June 5, 2010.
10. Wolff T. Community Tool Box. *QuickTips: Principles for Coalition Success*. University of Kansas. Available at http://ctb.ku.edu/en/tablecontents/sub_section_main_1168.htm. Accessed June 5, 2010.
11. Cohen L, Baer N, Satterwhite P. *Developing Effective Coalitions: An Eight-Step Guide*. Available at http://www.nblca.org/capacitybooks/Developing_Effective_Coalitions%5B1%5D.pdf. Accessed June 5, 2010.
12. American Dietetic Association. *Welcome. American Dietetic Association*. Available at http://www.eatright.org. Accessed June 5, 2010.
13. American Public Health Association. *About APHA*. Available at http://www.apha.org. Accessed June 5, 2010.
14. Society for Nutrition Education. *Identity Statement*. Society for Nutrition Education. Available at http://www.sne.org. Accessed June 5, 2010.
15. WetFeet. *Networking Works!* San Francisco: WetFeet Inc.; 2004. Available at http://shop.wetfeet.com/Browse/Career-Management/Networking-Works!.aspx. Accessed June 5, 2010.

Marketing Nutrition Programs and Services

NANCIE HERBOLD, EdD, RD
PAUL N. TAYLOR, PhD

READER OBJECTIVES   After studying this chapter and reflecting on the contents, you will be able to:

1. Compare and contrast simple marketing, business marketing, and social marketing.
2. List and define the four Ps of marketing and some additional Ps of social marketing.
3. Discuss types of market research and how they can be used in preparing a plan for a public health nutrition program.
4. Compare and contrast the ethics of business marketing and social marketing.

■ INTRODUCTION

The opening years of the 21st century clearly indicate that nutritionists must understand the nuances of marketing and how its concepts are used, not only to promote public health through nutrition, but also to counter messages that may not be in the best interests of the public health. Whereas you would be hard pressed to find MyPyramid explained in a television or newspaper advertisement, it is easy to find examples of marketing for weight-loss supplements, meal replacements, and "low-carb" foods. Relatively recently, healthcare professionals and organizations realized the value of marketing to reach desired objectives. As an important member of the healthcare team, the nutritionist must understand the power and value of marketing as a tool, and use marketing concepts to inform and educate the public as part of an effective nutrition program.

How, then, does the nutritionist define marketing? The National Public Health Leadership Institute provides this comprehensive definition:

> "Marketing" can denote a continuum of efforts and activities ranging from simple "marketing" to the more complex "media advocacy"; each form of marketing involves a relationship and two-way interaction between the marketer and those to whom the marketing is being directed. Simple "marketing" involves targeted communication of information based on audience research. "Social marketing" aims to create attitudinal and/or behavioral change in a target audience by emphasizing relevant benefits to that audience. "Branding" strives to define and establish a positive image or impression for a product via a linked association with a visual or auditory cue that will, when re-experienced, stimulate a quick, almost hard-wired short-cut reminder of the positive value of the product. "Media advocacy" is a strategy designed to bring about a political action and/or policy change through the reframing of issues in mass media.[1]

In this chapter we focus on simple marketing and social marketing, although other forms of marketing will be mentioned. We also distinguish between traditional or business marketing and social marketing.

■ BUSINESS MARKETING VERSUS SOCIAL MARKETING

A practical definition of business marketing is given by Pride and Ferrell[2]: "The process of creating, distributing, promoting, and pricing goods, services, and ideas to facilitate satisfying exchange relationships with customers in a dynamic environment." In business marketing, therefore, an exchange of goods or services occurs between a buyer and a seller such that both buyer and seller are satisfied. The dynamic environment in which these exchanges occur consists of uncontrollable forces (consumers, competition, the economy, politics, government, the media, and technology) that affect the marketing mix. Because the marketing environment is dynamic, the most successful marketers continuously evaluate their marketing plans and change them as necessary to ensure that their product is available at the right time, in the right place, and at an acceptable price.

Social marketing, when introduced in 1971, was defined as:

> ...the design, implementation, and control of programs calculated to influence the acceptability of social ideas and involving considerations of product planning, pricing, communication, distribution, and marketing research.[3]

More recently, Andreasen[4] described social marketing as:

> ...the application of commercial marketing technologies to the analysis, planning, execution, and evaluation of programs designed to influence the voluntary behavior of target audiences in order to improve their personal welfare and that of their society.

These definitions describe the activities of nutritionists, public health agencies, and other government and private agencies (e.g., the Centers for Disease Control and Prevention [CDC], the Robert Wood Johnson Foundation) who desire to change food choices and eating behaviors among their constituents. Whereas business marketing focuses on maximizing organizations' profits by fulfilling customers' needs and desires, social marketing focuses on benefiting the target audience and the general society by influencing social behaviors.[5]

Andreasen proposes six benchmarks to identify approaches that could be legitimately called social marketing[6]:

1. Interventions are designed and evaluated using behavior change as a benchmark.
2. For all projects, formative research is conducted to understand the target market, intervention elements are pre-tested before being implemented, and interventions are monitored as they are introduced.
3. Resources are used to maximum efficiency and effectiveness by carefully segmenting target audiences.
4. Influence strategies are designed to create attractive, motivational exchanges with target audiences.
5. All four Ps of the traditional marketing mix are considered in developing strategy: create attractive benefit packages (products); minimize costs (price); make the exchange convenient and easy (place); and communicate powerful messages through media appropriate to the target audiences (promotion).
6. The program strategy anticipates and accounts for the competition likely to be faced by the desired behavior.

In the more than 30 years since the advent of social marketing, two separate lines of thought have emerged regarding its definition. A nutritionist implementing a program to inform the public about the role of *trans*-fatty acids in the prevention of heart disease thus is following the premise of Kotler and Roberto, that social marketing programs are "aimed at increasing the acceptability of a social idea or practice in one or more groups of target adopters."[7] In contrast, the 5-A-Day campaign, a joint venture between the National Cancer Institute (NCI) and the Produce for a Better Health Foundation that encourages the public to eat five servings of fruits and vegetables per day, is following the premise of Andreasen that the ultimate objective should be behavior change in the target population.[6,8]

Whatever definition of social marketing one wishes to adopt (and there are others besides those mentioned[9]), the use of social marketing to develop a nutrition program plan requires commitment from top-level management, adequate funding and personnel, marketing skills, and vision.

As with any nutrition program, the foundation is thorough research, beginning with defining the problem. Once data have been collected and analyzed, recommendations can be made to form the outline of the program and to delineate the marketing plan.

■ MARKETING RESEARCH

Marketing research is necessary to plan, develop, and implement a successful social marketing program for an organization. Market research begins with defining the problem and gathering data to understand all aspects, a process that is similar to a nutrition assessment. Data will consist of both objective and subjective information. Marketing research provides information on the knowledge, beliefs, attitudes, wants, and practices of the targeted population necessary to develop strategies for behavioral change.[10] The better the problem is understood, the greater the likelihood of developing a successful plan.

Secondary Data

Secondary data are information collected by other groups and agencies. Health indicators collected by the federal government, such as the National Health and Nutrition Examination Survey (NHANES) data, are one example of secondary data. State Departments of Public Health collect state health statistics, such as infant mortality rate, teen pregnancy rate, and chronic disease incidence and prevalence, which are all are examples of secondary data. There are many helpful Web sites for data collection (**Table 26–1**). Private polling data collected by organizations such as AC Nielsen and the Roper Center also may be helpful.

Secondary data collected within an organization are referred to as *internal data*. The number of patients who visit the nutrition cardiac program, the costs of the services, and

TABLE 26–1	Helpful Web Sites
Web Site	**Sponsoring Organization**
http://www.eatright.org	American Dietetic Association
http://www.apha.org	American Public Health Association
http://www.diabetes.org	American Diabetes Association
http://www.americanheart.org	American Heart Association
http://www.marketingpower.com	American Marketing Association
http://www.social-marketing.org	Social Marketing Institute
http://www.restaurant.org	National Restaurant Association
http://www.fao.org	Food and Agriculture Organization of the United Nations
http://www.ift.org	Institute of Food Technologists
http://www.who.org	World Health Organization
http://www.cdc.gov	Centers for Disease Control and Prevention
http://socialmarketing-nutrition.ucdavis.edu	Center for Advanced Studies in Nutrition and Social Marketing
http://www.cdc.gov/mmwr/	Morbidity and Mortality Weekly Report
http://www.cdc.gov/nchs/	National Center for Health Statistics
http://www.census.gov	National Census Bureau
http://www.phli.org	National Public Health Leadership Institute
http://www.fda.gov	Food and Drug Administration
http://www.fedstats.gov	Fedstats
http://www.hhs.gov	U.S. Department of Health and Human Services
http://www.usda.gov	U.S. Department of Agriculture
http://www.healthstats.gov	Healthstats
http://www.ropercenter.uconn.edu	Roper Center for Public Opinion Research

A review of the professional literature is an important part of collecting information. This review can provide clarity on the problem and uncover successful and unsuccessful approaches to the same or a similar problem. A literature review also can lead to helpful Web sites. For example, Project LEAN (Leaders Encouraging Activity and Nutrition) and Team Nutrition both address the issue of healthy eating and physical activity in schoolchildren. These groups' Web sites provide background information and examples of activities used in these programs.[11,12] The literature will discuss details of programs and provide authors' names and affiliations, making it easy to contact someone for additional information. The review of the literature can also uncover food, nutrition, and health trends (e.g., consumer use of fortified foods,[13] attention to body image prompting adherence to low-fat diets,[14] and increased fish consumption to aid heart disease prevention[15]).

Data also can be gathered from trade association research. The National Restaurant Association (NRA) collects information on food eaten away from home and the latest trends on new foods, diners' preferences, and spending patterns. Nearly 70% of consumers believe that takeout meals make the lives of families with children easier, while 80% believe that restaurant dining is a better use of leisure time than cooking at home, according to information retrieved from the NRA Web site.[16] American Demographics and Brandweek are other sources of information on consumer trends and buying practices.[17] *Brandweek*, for instance, reports that women were targeted with an advertising campaign for a new cereal fortified with nutrients and vitamins (Harmony™) that described the product as a "support system for women."[18]

After gathering the secondary data, the nutritionist should assess what is lacking. Once gaps in the collected secondary data are identified, primary data collection should begin.

■ PRIMARY DATA

Primary data are types of information collected from focus groups, observations, mail or telephone surveys, interviews, and the like. Primary data help to focus the problem and define targeted audiences. For example, after interviewing mothers with young children, it was uncovered that fresh fruit was not being offered to children at home. While the parents did not lack knowledge about the health benefits of fruits and vegetables, it was found that the local supermarket had closed recently. Parents were now shopping at a local convenience store where only a limited variety of

popular days and times for services are all considered *internal secondary data*. In contrast, the data collected by an outside entity are regarded as *external secondary data*. It is important to gather as much secondary data as possible to save time, effort, and money.

fresh produce was available and was more expensive than what had been available at the supermarket.

Collecting primary data can provide insight on the attitudes, beliefs, and consequent nutrition and health behaviors of a population. For example, if a cultural group (e.g., Chinese American, Indian American, or Latin American) believes in the humoral theory of health—where illnesses are classified as either "hot" or "cold" and remedies and food are classified into the same two categories—a "hot" illness needs to be treated with a "cold" remedy to bring the body into balance.[19] A person ill with a common cold might not be willing to consume orange juice because orange juice is classified as a "cold" food by humoral theory health practitioners.[20]

Qualitative and Quantitative Data

Primary information includes qualitative and quantitative data. *Qualitative data* are usually obtained from small samples of the targeted group. Here, interviewers frequently use open-ended questions in focus-group formats or in-depth interviews with key informants to obtain knowledge about the problem. *Key informants* are individuals who are knowledgeable about the targeted population and can provide insight and history on the specific problem. Because of the small sample size, the results cannot be generalized to the larger target population. *Stakeholders* should be interviewed also. These are individuals who are interested in addressing the problem, such as the community health educator, the school nurse, or the area Director on Aging.

Formative evaluation uses qualitative data to help understand attitudes, beliefs, and perceptions. Formative evaluation is undertaken during the development of a social marketing program. It includes pre-testing of ideas and materials, allowing for revisions prior to implementing the full program.[21]

Quantitative data are objective indices from a selected sample where results are expressed in numerical terms. As an example of quantitative data, Yussman and colleagues reported "17% of adolescents and children reported using herbal remedies."[22] Both qualitative and quantitative data are used in the planning of social marketing strategies.

■ MARKET SEGMENTATION

Market segmenting is used to target a social marketing strategy to a particular group. Rather than apply the "average" approach where mean age, income, and education are used to produce an "average American,"[23(p.13)] market segmenting more narrowly focuses groups (e.g., Latina American women, adolescents, urban dwellers).

Market segmentation is based on:

- *Demographics:* Age, race, sex, income, education
- *Geographics:* Country, state, urban/rural, climate

- *Psychographics:* Attitudes, values, beliefs, personality traits
- *Behavior:* Benefits wanted, usage

To best tailor your marketing strategy, it is important to identify the market segment. Subgroups within populations may be further segmented; for instance, African Americans might be subcategorized into men with hypertension and men without hypertension. Individuals with diabetes might be subcategorized into low-literacy individuals with diabetes and high-literacy individuals with diabetes.

It is important in social marketing to consider the multicultural nature and beliefs of our society and the media habits of the various ethnic groups.[23(p.113)] Even when a marketing campaign is targeted to Asian Americans, you may want to subdivide this market even further. For example, is the population you want to reach Chinese American or Vietnamese American? Both groups share many cultural values, but there are differences as well. Most Asian cultures are rooted in Confucianism, where deferring to the father/husband and holding elders in high esteem is part of the Confucian practice.[23(p.263),24] The extent to which these behaviors and cultural norms are practiced, however, may be influenced by how long the group has lived in the United States, income level, and education.

The ¡Salud! Campaign targeted Latino American children and their caregivers to increase knowledge of folic acid's effect on neural tube defects. The campaign was culturally sensitive and included public service announcements (PSAs) in both Spanish and English. Latina celebrities were used in advertisements on billboards, buses, and bus stop shelters, and in magazines and newspapers. Seventy-seven percent of those surveyed responded that they were aware of the ¡Salud! campaign. The number of individuals who knew about the positive association between folic acid and the decrease in neural tube detects, although small, increased by 10%.[25]

Age can be a factor also when segmenting a market. Different generations have different identifying characteristics (**Table 26–2**). For example, adults over the age of 45 have contributed to an increase in alcohol consumption at dinner because of their exposure to the message that alcohol may decrease heart disease.[26] Children are another segmented market, one with great influence on purchasing decisions. For example, The Institute of Medicine reports "strong evidence that television advertising influence the food and beverage preferences of children ages to 2–11 years."[27] By using market segmenting, a customized plan and strategy can be developed that increases the likelihood of yielding greater success.

■ THE SOCIAL MARKETING MIX

In traditional business marketing, the specific combination of marketing elements used to achieve objectives and

TABLE 26–2	Characteristics to Consider When Planning a Social Marketing Campaign for Different Generations

Veteran Generation (born before 1945)

- Fastest growing group of Internet users is over age 55.
- Military/war background; influential voters.
- Like gadgets; are patient; conservative; range from fixed income to substantial investments.
- Respect teachers because of rank; polite; use proper grammar.
- Dislike off-color humor or language.
- Like to interact with people, not machines.
- Don't like to be put on the spot.

Baby Boomers (born 1946–1965)

- Were socialized to do work; workaholics; married later, had children later.
- Think work is recreation; are very competitive.
- Have high levels of expectations; optimistic; idealistic; interested in social causes.
- Value education; treat them as though they are young.
- Have a lot of information but little hands-on experience.
- Know how to share.
- Are obsessive about themselves; "me" generation.

Generation X (born 1966–1976)

- Environmentally conscious.
- Humor is critical for communication; loud music; fast moving images.
- Want the truth directly; cynical.
- Invented casual clothes at work.
- Technology is very important; use minimal written material.
- Demand more visual variety on the page.
- Do not read for pleasure; give short bits of information.

Generation Y (born 1977–1994)

- Have a lack of future expectation; most multicultural generation in United States thus far.
- Computers and the Internet are natural to them; media savvy.
- Will live in smaller families with single parents; 75% have working moms.
- Family values are very important; have much in common with their grandparents.
- Use hands-on, interactive creativity and games.
- There are more of them than there are baby boomers.
- Want to make money and have less stress in life.

Sources: Compiled from: Marconi J. *Future Marketing*. Lincolnwood, IL: NTC Business Books, 2001; Stetter L. *Learning with Style*. Boston, MA: Pottruck Technology Resource Center, Simmons College, May 22, 2003; and Tharp M. *Marketing and Consumer Identity in Multicultural America*. Thousand Oaks, CA: Sage Publications, 2001.

satisfy the target market is known as the marketing mix. Those variables over which an organization has control include the four Ps of marketing: product, place, price, and promotion.[28] Social marketing plans also use the four Ps, and some authors espouse additional Ps for social marketing, such as partnership, policy, politics, positioning, publics, and purse strings.[29–31] These additional Ps, with the possible exception of Positioning, usually pertain to the uncontrollable variables of the marketing environment. Alcalay and Bell[31] regard *positioning* as "a psychological construct that involves the location of the product relative to other products and activities with which it competes." As such, the nutrition program manager must position the product to maximize benefits and minimize costs. For instance, breast-feeding could be repositioned as a way for a family to establish a special relationship with their child from birth, as was done in the National WIC (Special Supplemental Nutrition Program for Women, Infants, and Children) Breast-feeding Promotion Project (described further later in this chapter).[32]

Product

In traditional business marketing, the product is either tangible (a good) or intangible (a service or an idea). Public health nutrition products are usually intangible (e.g., distributing weight-control counseling, consulting on developing food service menus). Tangible public health nutrition products might include such things as humanitarian rations distributed to populations in disaster-stricken areas or surplus dry milk powder distributed to low-income populations. In stark contrast to business marketing, the social marketing product may be offered or provided to the customer without considering whether the customer wants or needs the product. For example, a patient diagnosed with diabetes or cardiovascular disease may be automatically referred for nutrition counseling whether or not the service is wanted. To overcome reluctance or outright denial of service benefits, the product must be carefully designed, implemented, and followed up to maximize the probability of the patient's acceptance of a need for the service and eventual beneficial behavior change.

Nutrition Program Product Design

Designing a nutrition program product that will have maximum potential for success requires careful planning. Some factors to consider include:

- Naming the product (establishing a brand)
- Product packaging
- Differentiating the product from its competitors
- Considering product lifetime

Read more about the Social Marketing Institute at http://www.social-marketing.org.

● Continually revising to adapt to a changing market environment

As an example, consider the National WIC Breast-feeding Promotion Project described by the Social Marketing Institute.[32] Started in 1989, the breast-feeding project failed to effect significant behavioral changes in the WIC population. When the product—breast-feeding as a medical health decision—was redefined to emphasize the loving bond the mother would share with her child, breast-feeding rates in the target population rose significantly both in-hospital and at six months postpartum.

In packaging the product, planners considered that focusing on the emotional benefits of breast-feeding would be more appealing to the target audience than focusing solely on the health benefits of breast feeding. They differentiated the product from its competitor (formula feeding) by positioning the product in the target audience's view in a specific and appealing way (familiar bonding from birth), and also by defining and understanding all aspects of the competition's product, including the competing product's related components of price, place, and promotion.

When developing a nutrition product, include long-range planning to ascertain the probable lifetime of the product. Remember that the marketing environment is dynamic and that today's ideal product may be obsolete in the future due to changes in, for example, technology or public policy. Just as the successful business marketer looks beyond the product being designed to forecast future needs and demands of the consumer, so too does the successful social marketer include strategic planning as part of product development. The National WIC Breast-Feeding Promotion Project was succeeded at the U.S. Department of Agriculture (USDA) by the Fathers Supporting Breast-Feeding Project,[33] targeting African-American fathers to positively influence a mother's decision to breast-feed. This change was made as a result of strategic planning coupled with National WIC Breast-Feeding Promotion Project evaluation results.

Pre-Testing the Nutrition Program Product

Pre-testing the product, using a sample of the target market, will provide useful information on the appropriateness of the product's design. The National WIC Breast-Feeding Promotion Project was pre-tested in 10 states from 1996 to 2000.[32] The only state with pre-testing data at this writing is Iowa, which showed an increase in awareness of the breast-feeding messages targeted in the campaign and more positive attitudes on breast feeding.[34]

Place

Place denotes the location where tangible goods are offered and also includes the product's distribution system, that is, the channels through which the product is offered to the target market (including storage, transport, sales, and delivery). For intangible products, place may denote the location where a service is offered, including the channels through which the target market will be reached (e.g., clinics, hospitals, daycare centers, congregate meal sites, shopping malls, agricultural fairs, in-home demonstrations). When considering place, remember to ensure that the product will be accessible to the target market and that product delivery is of high quality.

When place was considered for the National WIC Breast-Feeding Promotion Project, the partners focused on identifying the locations where mothers and their friends and relatives would seek infant care information: homes, hospitals, and birthing centers. Additional partnerships were formed to develop the distribution channels; hospital environments were made more supportive of breast-feeding mothers; and other breast-feeding promotion organizations and professional associations were called upon to endorse and disseminate the program.[32]

Price

Price is perhaps the most critical component of the marketing mix for both traditional business and social marketing, because price is the component most evident to the consumer in the target market. In business marketing, *price* is often a competitive tool and can assist a business to develop product image.[35] In most cases, business marketers establish a product's price so that the business will profit and the consumer will be happy with the value received. Social marketers, however, are not usually interested in generating a profit. (Remember that the ultimate objective in social marketing is to effect a behavioral change that will benefit the individual, the community, or the society.) In social marketing situations where money is involved as part of the exchange between parties, program managers may want to recover all or a portion of their costs for goods or services. They must then develop a pricing strategy that will not negatively affect participation in the program. Options range from full-cost recovery through sliding-scale fees to "suggested donations." A public fundraising campaign aimed outside the target market might also be employed. A balance must be sought. For example, too low a price may diminish the consumer's perception of product quality, whereas too high a price might be unaffordable for some consumers. A free product not only might diminish perception of product quality but also might diminish the consumer's sense of self-esteem.[36]

In social marketing, the price component is often not monetary; rather, it may be based on such intangibles as time, effort, disapproval, or embarrassment. If these costs are thought to outweigh the benefits, then the consumer will perceive the product's value to be low and will be less likely to "buy" it.[36]

The pricing strategy for the National WIC Breast-Feeding Promotion Project aimed to minimize or eliminate the barriers (perceived costs) to breast feeding for new and prospective mothers. Women who doubted their breast-feeding ability, those who perceived breast feeding to be embarrassing, and those for whom breast feeding conflicted with active lifestyles and relationships were targeted. For each group of women, public education materials and a counseling program were developed so that healthcare providers could assist them in identifying and working through the misperceptions.[32]

Promotion

Promotion is the means to introduce the product to the targeted audience. Promotion involves communicating a message through a variety of media to create awareness and promote action. The Fruits & Veggies–More Matters™ campaign (which replaced the 5-A-Day campaign), for example, is a promotion to encourage the public to eat a variety of fruits and vegetables every day. The campaign is a partnership between the Centers for Disease Control and Prevention (CDC), the Department of Health and Human Services, and the National Cancer Institute (NCI). The promotion features an interactive calculator for obtaining individual fruit and vegetable consumption recommendations.[37]

Advertising

Advertising is an important part of a promotional campaign. Advertising can take many different forms, from print to television. Advertising is expensive; therefore, choosing the correct medium is important. Reach and frequency are important to consider when selecting the advertising medium. *Reach* refers to the number of people exposed to a message during a given period of time (how many people the message will "reach"). *Frequency* is the number of times an individual will be exposed to the message.[21] Paying for expensive advertising that does not reach the targeted audience, is a costly mistake. Sometimes, lower-level ad campaigns, such as flyers, are more effective than television advertising. Flyers can saturate a particular neighborhood on bulletin boards, as health fair handouts, on car windshields (check local ordinances), or packed with groceries at a local supermarket. Advertising of any kind needs to be more than a one-time event.

The targeted population must be reminded of the action to take, and reinforcement is needed for behavior change to occur. Advertising, as part of a social marketing campaign, may promote social/nutritional services such as School Breakfast or health promotion measures like increase whole grains. **Table 26–3** outlines a social marketing campaign to increase physical activity and healthful eating.[38] The Small Step campaign uses a combination of publicity, public relations, and advertising techniques to maximize the potential for exposure and success.

Advertising must be accurate, its message must be clear and consistent, and the main points must be repeated. The message must be relevant to the target population. For example, children are interested in food that tastes good and is "fun," whereas adults are interested in nutritional value.[39] The advertisement should also stress the action to be taken. The National Diabetes Education Program, for example, in a radio public service announcement (PSA) tells listeners to serve more fruits and vegetables, lean cuts of meat, and high fiber foods (**Figures 26–1** and **26–2**).

An advertisement can be amusing or frightening, provide a testimonial, or use a celebrity spokesperson. Whatever tone the advertisement takes must be acceptable to the targeted population. PSAs are advertisements for a social action or cause. Television and radio stations set aside free airtime for PSAs to meet Federal Communications Commission requirements. Most PSAs are aired during non-prime-time hours, however, which limits their reach.[40]

Web Sites

The younger generation grew up with many technologies, including the World Wide Web, cell phones, iPods, and Internet social media and platforms such as Facebook and MySpace blogs, and tweets (message-based updates of 140 characters).[41] Savvy marketers use these tools to advertise their products cost-effectively.[42] Health professionals must tap these same resources when launching social marketing campaigns.

How do you get consumers to use Internet Web sites? Web sites can be referenced in your print advertisements or your radio and television PSAs. Consumers should be given the site's Uniform Resource Locator (URL) address, so that they can log on to it for more information. If a consumer has not seen your promotional materials but uses the Internet to find information, the nutritionist or health organization needs to make sure that the site is included in the major search engines' referencing systems. Also, the location where a Web site link appears in a search engine's results is important. Is it the first site listed or the fiftieth? How many times a Web site is visited ("hits") is valuable information and should be tallied using readily available automatic counters.

We suggest the following steps for Internet marketing:

1. Acquire a domain name.
2. Build a Web site.
3. Put the Web site on a server.
4. Promote the site.
5. Update the site frequently.[43]

TABLE 26–3	United States Department of Health and Human Services: SmallStep Adult, Teen, and Kids Healthy Lifestyles and Disease Prevention Campaign		
Strategy	**Adults/Teens**	**Kids**	**Education Professionals (Grades 2–4)**
Message to Each Audience	Take a small step to get healthy. Core ideas: -Get the facts -Eat better -Get active -Learn more -Small step ideas -Success stories	Find out cool stuff about food and what it can do for you!	Small steps overtime make a big difference in performance.
Delivery Formats to Launch Campaign	Use humor to inspire: -TV PSA -Radio PSA -Magazine ads -Internet ad banners -Print and out of home ads	Interactive information: -Internet games -Small Step Challenge -Web activities with Shrek -TV PSAs with NFL players	Classroom activities: -Lesson plans -Activities for classroom - Posters
Public Relations Activities	TV/Radio PSAs Web interactive activities: -Newsletters' signups -e-mail content to others -Activity tracker -Internet ad banners	Interactive activities: -Internet games -Challenges -Healthy food ideas -TV PSAs with NFL players	-TV and Radio PSAs -Web site links -Posters
Advertising Activities	- TV spot (network and cable) - Print ad - Radio spot - Internet ad banners - Outdoor activities	-TV spot (network and cable) - Print ad - Radio spot -Internet ad banners	-TV spot (network and cable) -Print ad -Internet ad banners - Radio spot - Outdoor venues

Source: U. S. Department of Health and Human Services & The Advertising Council. Healthy Lifestyles and Disease Prevention Media Campaign. *Take A Small Step To Get Healthy.* (March 2004) Available at http://www.smallstep.gov.

Compiled by Margaret Schade, 2009.

Personal Selling

Personal selling is another tool used in promotional campaigns. *Personal selling* is achieved through one-to-one counseling, group meetings, roundtable discussions, classes, presentations, telephone conversations, and electronic mail (e-mail). Characteristics of positive personal selling include the following:

- Initiating positive contacts, not negative situations
- Being reliable, not unavailable
- Making recommendations, not demands
- Using candid, not accommodative language
- Using "we" problem-solving, not "I want" language
- Using easily understood terms or local jargon, not long, scientific explanations
- Showing respect and concern, not disdain, hostility, or indifference
- Being courteous, not abrupt
- Being attentive, not interruptive[42]

Public Relations

Public relations is a means to gather free publicity for your product, business, service, or idea. Public relations is a valuable component of a social marketing campaign. Although publicity is free, time and materials are not. It is important to develop publicity objectives for guidance to advance your social marketing agenda. Examples of public relations that can garner publicity include:

- Health fairs
- Athletic events (walkathons, road races, golf tournaments)
- Cook-offs, cooking demonstrations, and taste testings
- Fruit and vegetable gardening competitions
- Weight loss and physical activity competitions
- Nutrition poster design contests
- Eating clubs

Any of these activities can be sponsored with other like-minded organizations, such as the American Heart As-

---

Healthy Celebrations (:60 PSA)

American Indians, here's an important message from the [organization]. As American Indians, we gather for many ceremonies and celebrations. There's nothing harder for family members and friends with diabetes than making healthy food choices at a big feast. Let them know you're on their side. Offer a variety of low-fat, high-fiber foods. That means lots of fruits and vegetables. Cut the fat by serving lean cuts of beef and mutton, fish, and poultry without the skin. Use vegetable oil instead of lard in your cooking. And serve more high-fiber foods, like corn, beans, squash, and whole grain breads. Make your next gathering a celebration of healthy eating for everyone. Make it a time to help your loved ones control their diabetes for life. Call [**organization**] at [**phone number**] to learn more.

FIGURE 26–1 National Diabetes Education Program Indian Campaign: Healthy Celebrations Live-Read Radio Script.
Source: U.S. Department of Health and Human Services, *National Diabetes Education Program*. Available at http://ndep.nih.gov. Accessed February 25, 2010.

Healthy Family Reunion (:30 PSA)

There's nothing harder for a person with diabetes than making healthy food choices at a big family reunion. Let your family members with diabetes know you're on their side. Serve a variety of low-fat, high-fiber foods. That means lots of fruits and vegetables . . . lean meats, fish, and chicken . . . whole grain breads, peas, and beans. Help your family members control their diabetes for life. Call [**organization**] at [**phone number**] to learn more.

FIGURE 26–2 National Diabetes Education Program African-American Campaign: Healthy Reunion Live-Read Script.
Source: U.S. Department of Health and Human Services, *National Diabetes Education Program*. Available at http://ndep.nih.gov. Accessed February 25, 2010.

sociation, the President's Council on Physical Fitness, or the Fruit and Vegetable Grower's Association. An example of a joint public relations activity was the "Milk Run," a 10K road race sponsored by the Massachusetts Dietetic Association in collaboration with the Milk Promotion Board. Activities associated with the event include:

- A carbohydrate-loading dinner available to all race registrants
- A series of nutrition talks
- Booths with nutrition information open to the public the day of the race

By holding the Milk Run a week prior to the Boston Marathon, some world-class athletes were in the city and ran the Milk Run as a warm-up for the marathon. Because elite runners participated in this road race, there was more media coverage of the event than might otherwise have occurred. Press releases, PSAs, and media interviews were a few of the publicity activities that the Dietetic Association's public relations committee provided during the months leading up to the race.

Other means to achieve publicity objectives include:

- Public speaking at community events, schools, and senior centers
- Writing nutrition columns for local newspapers
- Providing short nutrition messages for local radio stations
- Acting as a nutrition resource expert for the media on late-breaking nutrition news

Because this publicity is free, you have limited control over where, when, and how the information will be used. Few professional writers will send you copy of an interview for your approval before publication, although nutritionists have occasionally reviewed copy of an interview for accuracy. A nutrition television spot may end up being cut during editing, so your PSA may be aired at 2 AM. For successful publicity when working with the media, you must be prepared to:

- Develop a fact sheet on your issues
- Have photographs and other props available for media interviews
- Provide anecdotal information that personalizes your message
- Develop case histories of interesting people who achieved positive health outcomes

Send query letters and press releases, or call local newspapers, television stations, and radio stations to promote your nutrition topic. Discuss why this topic is of interest to audiences. Do not be discouraged if inroads are not made immediately; be persistent. If a reporter or writer needs a quote from a nutrition professional, your name may come to mind. If you receive a call from a media person, be prompt in returning the call; the caller usually has a deadline to meet. If a reporter knows you are prompt with your reply and that you have interesting information, you are more likely to be called again. This starts the building of a media relationship.

Public relations is not only publicity, but also includes providing the following:

- Comfortable and user-friendly environments to obtain nutrition services
- Locations that are accessible
- Operating times that are convenient for customers
- Helpful personnel
- Education materials that are clear and easy to read

All of these qualities can generate goodwill from the customer and positive "word of mouth" publicity to their family and friends.

■ EVALUATION

Important components of any social marketing effort are evaluation and estimating success. Evaluation is an ongoing process and should not be left until the entire project is complete. Evaluation should start with the inception of the idea and the problem to study. The following questions are important to consider at the beginning of the evaluation process:

- How do we define the problem?
- What are our goals and objectives?
- Who is the market we want to reach?
- What information do we have about the problem and the target market?
- What is our message?
- What communication media will we use?
- Will they be cost effective?
- What is the timing?
- How will we measure our goals and objectives?
- How will we evaluate the program?[44]

Three types of evaluation should be considered when assessing your social marketing campaign: formative evaluation, process evaluation, and outcome evaluation.

Formative Evaluation

Formative evaluation begins during the development of the social marketing program. Formative evaluation helps to define the problem and to refine possible interventions. It includes pre-testing of ideas, procedures, and materials, and using focus groups, surveys, and interviews.[21] For example, you may ask, "Did the target market understand the PSA message?" "Was the print material at a readability level appropriate to the audience?" "Was the action requested of the target market realistic?" This type of information allows revisions to be made before the full program is implemented.

Process Evaluation

Process evaluation assesses the implementation of the social marketing program. Did the plan proceed as outlined? Did the PSA air during the appropriate month? Were print materials delivered in adequate quantities to the correct locations? Are activities occurring according to schedule? Did the program reach the target market?[21] Process evaluation uses continuous quality improvement (CQI) to monitor progress. CQI is a tool based on the premise that there is always room for improvement.[45] Customers are asked how satisfied they are with the services, materials, venues, and costs associated with a program. CQI has been used in health care, including nutrition services, since the 1990s.[45-49]

Outcome Evaluation

Outcome evaluation (sometimes referred to as summative evaluation) determines whether the goals and objectives of the social marketing campaign are met.[21] It is important that the goals and objectives are well defined at the inception of the social marketing process, otherwise it is difficult to measure the success of meeting them. Goals and objectives should be specific in order for them to be evaluated effectively. An example of an objective that can be measured is: "Twenty percent of the target audience/market will increase fruit and vegetable consumption by 1 serving within 3 months of initiating the campaign."

■ MARKETING ETHICS

The opening years of the 21st century were marked by several major business scandals in the United States and other countries.[50-53] In this climate, it is important to revisit the topic of business ethics, in general, and of marketing ethics, in particular.

Whether engaging in business or social marketing, the marketer must begin with a strong code of personal ethics. With a good sense of the moral principles and values that govern individual and group behavior within a society, one can reliably choose the right and just action when faced with a moral dilemma. Ethics courses may be found in colleges and universities, and ethics may be incorporated into the curriculum in elementary and high schools. The elementary school curriculum is not consistent across the country, however, and there is debate about the best approach for teaching ethics (AKA "building character"[54]) as well as over where and when ethics can be taught. Many believe that codes of personal ethics are already formed by the time a person enters college,[55] and there is evidence that geographic and cultural variables affect the process.[56,57] Others hold that ethics can be taught at the college level.[58,59] It is evident that the process of ethical development is multifactorial and that some elements of truth may be found in each of the disparate views.

Kerin and colleagues[60] hold that in marketing, ethics are concerned with personal morals and values in juxtaposition with organizational, legal, and societal morals and values. Situations present themselves in an ethical, legal matrix in which technically legal actions could be viewed as unethical, or in which ethical actions may not be seen as legal. In such an environment, the nutritionist must learn to think and plan like a marketer, under the guidance of personal ethics informed by sociocultural, business/industry, and corporate ethical guidelines.

Traditional business ethics in the last century were largely guided by the principle of *caveat emptor*. By the 1990s, consumer interests had overtaken those of business, ushering in an era of "consumer sovereignty."[61] Although exceptions exist, today most traditional business marketing ethics are guided by the principle that the customer's wants and needs are paramount, and profit-generating activities are aimed at customer satisfaction. Social marketers, too, are focused on the customer, but with the ultimate aim of improving their personal welfare and that of their society.[4]

The social marketer thus faces ethical challenges that are not seen in traditional business marketing, challenges that are only now being identified and studied.[62] As the dimensions of marketing ethics in both traditional business and social marketing contexts are explored and debated, the nutritionist, drawing on a strong personal code of ethics, would do well to follow the guidelines of the American Dietetic Association's Code of Ethics.[63]

In closing this overview of marketing ethics, we must point out that many of the ethical dilemmas that a public health nutritionist is likely to face will arise from cultural differences between the nutritionist and the client or the population being served. The United States is a multicultural land with minority ethnic populations from most parts of the world. When serving those whose ethnic backgrounds differ from your own, make an effort to understand the societal culture and norms that govern them, as well as those that underlie the prevailing U.S. societal culture and norms. When entering into partnerships with multinational or global organizations, be sure to consider the often-great differences in marketing ethics of the cultures represented.[64–69]

Caveat emptor: The principle in commerce that the buyer alone is responsible for assessing the quality of a purchase before buying.

Consumer sovereignty: Alludes to the power consumers have in directing market economies because goods and services are produced and exchanged mostly to satisfy consumer desires.

Issues for Discussion

1. How can a nutritionist promote healthful eating practices to people who are convinced that a currently popular diet plan is appropriate for everyone?

2. What opportunities exist for a public health agency to form partnerships to address the need for people to consume water for optimum health while conserving water for protection of the resource?

3. How can and should a nutritionist approach promoting healthful eating practices for children in partnerships with multinational fast food and toy companies?

References

1. National Public Health Leadership Institute. CB #8165, Chapel Hill, NC. February 11, 2002.
2. Pride WM, Ferrell OC. *Marketing: Concepts and Strategies*, 12th ed. Boston: Houghton Mifflin Co.; 2003:4.
3. Kotler P, Zaltman G. Social marketing: an approach to planned social change. *J Marketing.* 1971;35:5.
4. Andreasen AR. *Marketing Social Change: Changing Behavior to Promote Health, Social Development, and the Environment.* San Francisco: Jossey-Bass; 1995:7.
5. Andreasen AR, Kotler P. *Strategic Marketing for Nonprofit Organizations*, 6th ed. Englewood Cliffs, NJ: Prentice-Hall; 2003:15.
6. Andreasen AR. Marketing social marketing in the social change marketplace. *Journal of Public Policy & Marketing.* 2002;21:3.
7. Kotler P, Roberto E. *Social Marketing.* New York: The Free Press; 1989:24.
8. Andreasen AR. Social marketing: definition and domain. *Journal of Public Policy & Marketing.* 1994;13:108.
9. Maibach EW. Explicating social marketing: what is it, and what isn't it? *Social Marketing Quarterly.* 2002;8:7.
10. Kotler P, Roberto E. *Social Marketing: Strategies for Changing Public Behavior.* New York: The Free Press; 1989:290.
11. Public Health Institute. *California Project LEAN, Leaders Encouraging Activity and Nutrition.* Available at http://www.californiaprojectlean.org. Accessed June 5, 2010.
12. U.S. Department of Agriculture, Food & Nutrition Service. *TEAM Nutrition.* Available at http://www.fns.usda.gov/tn. Accessed July 1, 2009.
13. Sloan AE. Functional food trends. *Food Technol.* 2008;62(4):24.
14. Gruber AJ, Pope Jr. HJ, Lalonde JK, Hudson JI. Why do young women diet? The roles of body fat, body perception, and body ideal. *J Clin Psychiatry.* 2001;62:609.
15. Kris-Etherton PM, Harris WS, Appel LJ. American Heart Association Nutrition Committee: fish consumption, fish oil, omega-3 fatty acids, and cardiovascular disease. *Circulation.* 2002;106:2747.
16. Hensley, S, Donohue, M. "Restaurant Industry Expected to Post Modest Sales Growth in 2009 as it Copes with the Weakest Economy in Decades. National Restaurant Association." December 19, 2008. Available at http://www.restaurant.org. Accessed July 1, 2009.
17. Marconi J. *Future Marketing.* Chicago: American Marketing Association, NTC Business Books; 2001:46.
18. Reyes S. Shopping list: quick, classic, cool for kids. *Brandweek.* June 17, 2002;43:S52.
19. Bogumil C. Humoral theory in cultural food beliefs. June 10, 2002. Available at http://food.oregonstate.edu/ref/culture/humoral.html. Accessed July 1, 2009.
20. Cai J. *Eating Your Way to Health. Dietotherapy in Traditional Chinese Medicine*, 2nd ed. Beijing: Foreign Languages Press; 1996:181.
21. U.S. Department of Health and Human Services. *Making Health Communication Programs Work: A Planner's Guide.* NIH Publication No. 92–1493. Washington, DC: National Cancer Institute; 2004.
22. Yussman SM, Auinger P, Weitzman M, Ryan SA. Complementary and alternative medicine use in children and adolescents. *J Adolesc Health* 2002;30:105.
23. Tharp MC. *Marketing and Consumer Identity in Multicultural America.* Thousand Oaks, CA: Sage Publications; 2001.
24. Wong AM. *Target: The U.S. Asian Market.* Palos Verdes, CA: Pacific Heritage; 1997:69.
25. Perez-Escamilla R, Himmelgreen D, et al. Marketing nutrition among urban Latinos: the !Salud! campaign. *J Am Diet Assoc.* 2000;100:698.
26. Whitaker L. A tasty business. *Psychology Today.* 1999;32:52.
27. Institute of Medicine. *Food Marketing to Children and Youth. Threat or Opportunity.* Washington, DC: National Academic Press; 2006:8.
28. Mulin, R. Cummins, J. *Sales Promotion: How to Create, Implement, and Integrate Campaigns that Really Work*, 4th ed. London, UK: Kogan Page Publishers; 2008:23,24.

29. Weinreich NK. *Hands-On Social Marketing: A Step-by-Step Guide.* Thousand Oaks, CA: Sage Publications; 1999:5.

30. Mississippi Urban Research Center, Jackson State University, Southern Prevention Intervention Center. What is social marketing? Social marketing tools promote health issues. *Adinkra Newsletter.* Fall 2001:2. Available at http://www.apinonline.org/Pubs/Newsletters/Adinkra.SPIC-Fall2001_Issue2.pdf. Accessed June 8, 2009.

31. Alcalay R, Bell RA. *Promoting Nutrition and Physical Activity through Social Marketing: Current Practices and Recommendations.* Davis, CA: Center for Advanced Studies in Nutrition and Social Marketing, University of California; 2000:3.

32. Social Marketing Institute. *Success Stories: National WIC Breast-feeding Promotion Project.* Available at http://www.social-marketing.org/success/cs-nationalwic.html. Accessed July 1, 2009.

33. U.S. Department of Agriculture, Food & Nutrition Service. *Fathers Supporting Breast-feeding.* Available at http://www.fns.usda.gov/wic/Fathers/SupportingBreastfeeding.HTM. Accessed July 1, 2009.

34. Szcodronski H, Dobson B, Losch ME, Bryant C. *Iowa's Implementation of the WIC National Breast-feeding Promotion Project. Loving Support Makes Breast-feeding Work. Project Report and Summary of Findings.* Des Moines, IA: Iowa Department of Public Health; May 2002:29.

35. Gregoire M. *Foodservice Organizations: A Managerial and Systems Approach,* 7th ed. Upper Saddle River, NJ: Prentice-Hall; 2010:98.

36. Weinreich NK. *What Is Social Marketing?* Weinreich Communications; 2003. Available at http://www.social-marketing.com/whatis.html. Accessed July 1, 2009.

37. Centers for Disease Control and Prevention. *Eat a Variety of Fruits & Vegetables Every Day.* Available at http://www.fruitsandveggiesmatter.gov/index.html. Accessed July 1, 2009.

38. United States Department of Health and Human Services & The Advertising Council. *Healthy Lifestyles and Disease Prevention Media Campaign: Take a Small Step to Get Healthy.* (March 2004). Available at http://www.smallstep.gov. Accessed July 1, 2009.

39. Baltas G. The effects of nutrition information on consumer choice. *J Advertising Res.* 2001 (March–April):57.

40. Cury I. *Directing and Producing for Television: A Format Approach,* 3rd ed. St. Louis, MO: Focal Press; 2006:179.

41. Hawn C. Take two aspirin and tweet me in the morning: how twitter, Facebook, and other social media are reshaping health care. *Health Aff.* 2009;28:2.

42. Conklin MT, Parks SC. Marketing strategies can maximize food and nutrition professionals' effectiveness with children. *Top Clin Nutr.* 2005;20:54–63.

43. Kaufman M. *Nutrition in Public Health.* Rockville, MD: Aspen; 1990:308.

44. McDonald MH, Keegan WJ. *Marketing Plans That Work.* Boston: Butterworth Heinemann Publishers; 1997:113,114.

45. Leebov W, Ersoz C. *The Healthcare Manager's Guide to Continuous Quality Improvement.* Lincoln, NE: iUniverse, Inc., Authors Choice Press; 2003.

46. McLaughlin CP, Kaluzny AD. *Continuous Quality Improvement in Healthcare: Theory, Implementation and Applications,* 3rd ed. Boston: Jones and Bartlett Publishers; 2006.

47. Slepin J. Need for education in quality improvement and evidence-based on practice. *Joint Commission Journal on Quality Improvement* 2002;28:463–474.

48. Behrens RI, Blocker AK. *Continuous Quality Improvement and Nutritional Care Planning: A Manual for Long-Term Care Facilities.* Rockville, MD: Aspen; 1993.

49. Edelstein S. *Managing Food and Nutrition Services: For Culinary, Hospitality and Nutrition Professionals.* Boston: Jones and Bartlett Publishers, 2007:75.

50. Keeping an eye on business. *Economist.* 2004;371:68.

51. Verschoor CC. Unethical workplace is still with us. *Strategic Finance.* 2004;85:15.

52. Tsianiar B, Shannon E. Cooking the books. *Time Magazine.* November 17, 2003;162:55.

53. Colvin G. Scandal outrage, part III. *Fortune Magazine.* October 28, 2002;146:56.

54. Davis M. What's wrong with character education? *American Journal of Education.* 2003;110:32.

55. Carroll AB, Scherer RW. Business ethics in the current environment of fraud and corruption. *Vital Speeches of the Day.* June 15, 2003;69:529.

56. Mayer D. Community, business ethics, and global capitalism. *Am Business Law J.* 2001;38:215.

57. Barker TS, Cobb SL. A survey of ethics and cultural dimensions of MNCs. *Competitiveness Review.* 2000;10:123.

58. Lawson RA. Is classroom cheating related to business students' propensity to cheat in the "real world"? *Journal of Business Ethics.* 2004;49:189.

59. Alsop R. The top business schools (a special report): right and wrong: can business schools teach students to be virtuous? In the wake of all the corporate scandals, they have no choice but to try. *Wall Street Journal.* September 17, 2003; eastern edition:R9.

60. Kerin RA, Berkowitz EN, Hartley SW, Rudelius W. *Marketing,* 7th ed. New York: McGraw Hill; 2003.

61. Smith NC, Lawler III EE, Berndt ER. Marketing strategies for the ethics era. *Sloan Management Review.* 1995;36:85.

62. Brenkert GG. Ethical challenges of social marketing. *Journal of Public Policy & Marketing.* 2002;21:14.

63. American Dietetic Association. Code of ethics for the profession of dietetics. *J Am Diet Assoc.* 1999;99:109.

64. Palazzo B. U.S–American and German business ethics: an intercultural comparison. *Journal of Business Ethics.* 2002; 41:195.

65. Pitta DA, Fung H-G. Ethical issues across cultures: managing the differing perspectives of China and the USA. *Journal of Consumer Marketing.* 1999;16:240.

66. Singhapakdi A, Rawwas MYA. A cross-cultural study of consumer perceptions about marketing ethics. *Journal of Consumer Marketing.* 1999;16:257.

67. Taka I. Business ethics in Japan. *Journal of Business Ethics.* 1997; 16:1499.

68. Izraeli D. Business ethics in the Middle East. *Journal of Business Ethics.* 1997;16:1555.

69. Stajkovic AD, Luthans F. Business ethics across cultures: a social cognitive model. *Journal of World Business.* 1997;32:17.

CHAPTER

27

Earning Administrative Support

Jeannette M. Beasley, PhD, MPH, RD

READER OBJECTIVES

After studying this chapter and reflecting on the contents, you should be able to:

1. Review environmental factors that influence the administration's priorities.
2. Describe components of the strategic plan that help to provide insight into administrative goals and objectives.
3. Delineate elements of the community needs assessment that are important to highlight to administrators.
4. Discuss strategies for increasing the administrators' perceived value of the nutrition division, including partnering with other divisions within the agency, working with the policy board, and developing positive relations with the media.
5. Identify potential funding sources to bolster support for nutrition services.

■ INTRODUCTION

Earning the support of the administration within your agency begins with understanding both external and internal forces influencing agency priorities. By remaining current with the agency's focus, the nutrition division can adapt the nutrition plan to meet the changing needs of the agency and survive in the current healthcare environment.

Another important strategy to increase the relevancy of the nutrition division within your organization is to partner with other divisions sharing common goals. Along with developing positive working relationships internally, involvement with the policy board as well as the local media can increase the exposure and value of the nutrition division in the eyes of both the agency administration and the general public.

In networking with the community, gaps in nutrition-related services may be identified and brought to the attention of the administration. If funding is a barrier to developing a new program, identify potential external funding sources and seek administrative support to apply for grant monies.

■ THE ADMINISTRATION'S PERSPECTIVE

Management and delivery of healthcare services is influenced by economic, political, and social forces. In order to promote nutrition services within your organization, it is critical to analyze the dynamics operating within your agency. By doing so, you will better understand the influences and motivations of the administration. Shortell and Kaluzney (2000) identified several key forces impacting healthcare delivery that have implications for management, and for the nutrition department in particular, including the increased focus on evaluation of programs and services, the integration of information technology, the aging of the population, and changing demographics of the United States that are leading to increased cultural diversity.

Understanding the impact of these trends on the healthcare system is important in ensuring that the nutrition division progresses along with the rest of the agency. In this environment of increased accountability, evaluating both the implementation and the effectiveness of existing nutrition programs and services is now routinely expected. Nutrition departments that integrate information technology into

> Excellent Web-based sources for nutrition information in a large number of diverse languages are available at http://ethnomed.org/ ethnomed/patient_ed/ and http://www.spiral.tufts.edu.

daily practices will be more time and cost efficient. Reaching out to elderly populations by implementing programs to improve food security for community members who do not have convenient access to grocery stores is an example of addressing the aging of the population. Consider ethnic and cultural diversity by providing nutrition education materials in languages that are highly prevalent in your community, and provide culturally sensitive recipes and meal plans. Examples such as these illustrate to the administration that the nutrition division is current with issues critical to improving the community's public health infrastructure.

Healthy People (HP) 2010 objectives (as discussed in other chapters) provide a framework for understanding national priority areas for health promotion and disease prevention. The 467 objectives in 28 focus areas offer guidelines for focusing program planning within healthcare organizations. Reviewing the *HP 2010* objectives listed in the Nutrition and Overweight focus area, along with focus areas related to nutrition including cancer, chronic kidney disease, and diabetes, can provide the nutrition professional with a better understanding of the healthcare needs of the nation, the government's priorities with respect to funding initiatives, and the administrator's perspective. Furthermore, nutrition-related *HP 2010* objectives can be used to build administrative support for initiatives. For example, one of the *HP 2010* objectives is to "increase the proportion of persons aged 2 years and older who consume at least two daily servings of fruit." Based on Continuing Survey of Food Intakes by Individuals (CSFII) data, 28% of the population currently meets the goal; the *HP 2010* target is to increase the percentage of the population consuming two fruits daily to 75%. Presenting this data to the administration provides justification and support for the fruit and vegetable promotion programs within the nutrition division.

Presenting state and local data, if available, will increase the relevancy of the problem for decision makers. For example, state-level statistics estimating fruit and vegetable consumption, derived from Behavioral Risk Factor Surveillance System (BRFSS) data, are available from the Centers for Disease Control and Prevention's (CDC) Web site. These data can also be used to explain to administrators why a social marketing program will be targeted to a specific high-risk group, because average fruit and vegetable intake can be grouped by demographics, including age, level of education, race, and income level.

The HP 2010 Nutrition and Overweight focus area is available at http://www.healthypeople.gov/Document/HTML/Volume2/19Nutrition.htm.

The National Health and Nutrition Examination Survey data are available at http://www.cdc.gov/Nchs/about/major/nhanes/wweia.htm.

The Behavioral Risk Factor Surveillance System (BRFSS) is available at http://www.cdc.gov/brfss/.

The Centers for Disease Control and Prevention's Web site for promoting fruit and vegetable consumption is available at http://www.fruitsandveggiesmatter.gov/.

■ UNDERSTANDING THE AGENCY VISION AND STRATEGIC PLAN

The extent to which each of these environmental factors and *HP 2010* objectives influence the vision, goals, and objectives of individual public health agencies may be better understood by reviewing the organization's planning documents, such as the strategic plan, annual report, and budget. By reviewing the agency's strategic plan, the nutrition professional will better understand the underlying philosophy of the agency as well as the current priorities and perspectives of the administrators. The following are the key components of a strategic plan, along with a description of how they can assist you in identifying areas of interest to the agency administration:

- *Mission statement:* Defines the purpose of the organization, and can often provide a better understanding of the underlying philosophy of the agency.
- *Major objectives:* Highlight the priorities of the organization with realistic, measurable, achievable outcomes.
- *Action plan:* Delineates a method for achieving objectives. This section provides an indication of the agency's approach to finding solutions to current issues of interest.
- *Resources needed:* Includes personnel, funds, equipment, and space required to meet objectives. Identify areas where nutrition-related resources could assist in achieving goals, and bring these to the attention of the administrator.
- *Evaluation system:* Delineates the process for assessing the effectiveness of the plan. A description of the evaluation process can provide insight into ways in which the performance of the administration is measured within the organization.

■ SYNERGIZING WITH THE STRATEGIC PLAN

By reviewing the agency's planning documents in concert with the community needs assessment (discussed in Chapter 3), public health nutritionists can evaluate whether their role in the organization is meeting the needs of the public they are serving and is within the framework of the organization's goals. Using components of the community needs assessment can be an effective tool in garnering support for nutrition services from administrators, funding agencies, and the public alike. The following list describes how elements of the community needs assessment can be used to directly increase administrative support for nutrition programs:

- *Assessment:* Composed of copious amounts of data related to community demographics, the health and nutrition of community members, perceived needs, and community assets; this section can be reframed for presentation to decision makers to highlight the need for nutrition services in the community. If your assessment included focus group data regarding the impact of the WIC program on participants, share a direct quote from a participant about ways the program can be improved along with program numbers to support these suggestions. By providing both testimonials from community members and data to support initiatives, you are showing the administration that your department is in touch with the needs of the community.
- *Priorities, goals, and objectives:* Present concise, realistic, measurable objectives to the administrators in order to show that the nutrition department is organized around common goals that are relevant to community needs.
- *Nutrition plan:* Use the nutrition plan to highlight the steps required to achieve the stated objectives. Emphasize the assets of the nutrition department, and also identify gaps along with proposed solutions for addressing barriers to achieving the objectives.
- *Implementation:* Summarize the implementation process to the extent needed to highlight the efficiency, organization, and teamwork of the nutrition division in working toward common goals.
- *Evaluation:* As discussed in Chapter 19, evaluating activities of the nutrition division is important for documenting program impact as well as identifying areas for continuous quality improvement.

Prior to preparing evaluation results for presentation to the administration, review the agency's annual report for ideas on how to format results. For example, if the report relies heavily on charts and graphs rather than qualitative data, recognize that the administrator is more familiar with reviewing quantitative data within agency documents. In addition to increasing the likelihood the administrator will respond favorably to the activities of the nutrition division, results presented in this manner will be more likely to be included in next year's annual report, thereby increasing exposure of the nutrition division's activities to policy makers and budget reviewers.

■ PARTNERING TO ACHIEVE SHARED GOALS

Forging partnerships between the nutrition division and groups sharing common goals and objectives provides the opportunity to capitalize on the benefits of combining resources and avoiding the duplication of services. Although the administration's expectations of the nutrition division may seem ambitious given the limited staff and budget allocated to the department, a review of the responsibilities of other divisions within the organization may provide insight into opportunities for working together on initiatives with common goals.

Effective teams focus on the shared purpose of the collaboration by developing goals and priorities required to fulfill the need. In doing so, the process is directed towards a shared commitment, and members identify skills and contributions required for the effort. Fostering positive relations with team members further integrates the nutrition division into the framework of the healthcare organization and provides the potential to increase the overall productivity of the agency.

■ RELATIONS WITH THE POLICY BOARD

The Board of Health or Board of Directors, often appointed by elected officials, is responsible for approving policies and programs, appointments of personnel, budgets, and legislative initiatives. Special interests of individual board members may influence policy decisions that directly impact the nutrition department. Representing the nutrition division at board meetings and advocating for nutrition-related programs will increase the likelihood that nutrition services will be viewed as important to improving the public's health, rather than being marginalized as major events shift resources to high priority areas. It therefore is important for representatives from the nutrition department to attend meetings and interact with board members in order to remain current with the priorities of the Board.

For example, an outbreak of foodborne illness in the community resulting in hospitalizations and lost productivity provides an opportunity for nutritionists to educate food service workers regarding proper procedures for prevention of further outbreaks. By reaching out to the community when the relevancy of the issue is high, you increase the likelihood that food safety tips will be translated into behavior change. Furthermore, the education campaign increases exposure of the nutrition department to the community as well as policy makers, and will show the administrator that the nutrition division is responsive to high-priority health issues within the community.

■ COMMUNICATIONS WITH THE MEDIA

Another opportunity for strengthening both administrative and community support for nutrition-related initiatives is to build a good rapport with the local media. There are several ways to build a relationship with the media, including inviting the media to cover events sponsored by the nutrition division, providing copy for nutrition-related topics of interest to the public, and answering questions for nutrition-related news stories. Each of these methods can promote positive public relations between the public and the public health agency.

Before communicating with the media, it is important to contact both the public relations division within your agency and your administrator to be certain you understand the rules and regulations associated with media communications. For example, you may need to obtain approval of press releases from the public relations department prior to dissemination to media outlets.

Preparing and Distributing Press Kits

Press kits are packets of information describing an event or program written in a format conducive to dissemination by media outlets. Press kits can include a press release, pictures, program logos, press passes to the event, an invitation to participate in the program, and/or fact sheets related to program activities and time lines. By announcing programs and events in advance, the publicity could result in increased attendance and lead to a more successful intervention.

To increase the likelihood that your information will be noticed by various local media organizations, including radio, television, and newspaper outlets, ask the public relations department within your agency for strategies that have worked in the past. There may be a particular person at each organization to whom health information press kits should be directed, or a template that facilitates publicizing the event in the format familiar to each specific organization. If your agency doesn't have a public relations department to assist you, contact a colleague who has worked successfully with the organization in the past, or call the organization directly for assistance. More information on marketing your message is in Chapter 26.

Promoting Nutrition Messages Through Media

Nutrition is in the news daily, hitting the headlines with topics ranging from newly released surveillance statistics and epidemiological evidence associating particular foods with risk for cancer to the latest fad diet book extolling the benefits of a particular dietary regimen. The media seeks credible sources to interpret the implications of research

findings on the public's health. Registered dietitians have a responsibility to promote evidence-based recommendations based on sound scientific research, and assisting the media in reporting research findings is another way to provide nutrition education. As an added benefit, the media will credit their source, thereby providing an opportunity to promote the image of the nutrition division within your agency.

One way to establish positive relationships with the media is to offer to write copy for a particular topic area of interest to the media organization. For example, if new research findings are published on the benefits of cruciferous vegetables for reducing cancer risk, you could suggest writing a piece summarizing the evidence and providing tips for preparing cruciferous vegetables for the newspaper's health section. In your correspondence to the editor, outline a few nutrition-related topics you consider to be newsworthy and would be willing to research in order to write an educational piece for the paper. This provides a service to the media, who are often under pressure to meet deadlines, while promoting the image of the nutrition division within your agency as a credible source for health-related information.

Maintain records of newspaper articles, letters to the editor, public service announcements, and any other correspondence the nutrition division has with the media. Estimate the impact of your message by tracking the reach, such as the circulation of the newspaper or the size of the audience for the radio station. If the message was part of a particular nutrition program or service, include this data when writing up the impact evaluation for the project.

Obtaining Financial Support for Nutrition Programs and Initiatives

As the nutrition division reaches out to the community, it is likely that gaps in the public health infrastructure will be identified that are not addressed in the planning documents of the agency. Possible reasons the problem was not addressed in the strategic plan include lack of awareness, no known solutions, or emergence after the development of the strategic plan. In discussing the problem with the administrator, you may both agree that the problem is important and that a workable solution has been proposed, but the administrator does not have the funds to allocate to the proposed program. Discuss the possibility of applying for grants to address the problem. The administrator will likely support proposal writing as a mechanism to increase revenue and appreciate the initiative displayed by the nutrition division. Obtaining funding from a range of sources also increases the stability and capacity of the nutrition division to provide programs and services.

The administrator may direct you to funding sources likely to be interested in reviewing your proposal. Potential funding sources include the government, foundations, corporations, or charges for services rendered. Several Web-based resources are available to identify funding agencies and provide guidance in preparing applications. Given the time-sensitive nature of requests for proposals, searching online funding databases is often more productive than searching through paper-based directories. **Table 27–1** provides a list of available Internet resources for identifying grant opportunities.

TABLE 27–1	Internet Resources for Identifying Grant Opportunities

Organization	Web site
U.S. Department of Health and Human Services	http://www.grants.gov/
Catalog of Federal Domestic Assistance	http://12.46.245.173/cfda/cfda.html
Food and Nutrition Service	http://www.fns.usda.gov/fns/
National Institutes of Health	http://grants.nih.gov/grants/oer.htm
American Dietetic Association	http://www.eatright.org/
Foundation Center	http://fdncenter.org/
Robert Wood Johnson Foundation	http://www.rwjf.org/index.jsp

Issues for Discussion

1. Discuss why getting internal support for nutrition programs is as important as controlling external variables.

2. Describe how internal marketing is different from external marketing.

3. What is the competition that public health nutrition faces, and why should public health nutrition be maintained?

Suggested Reading

Centers for Disease Control and Prevention, National Center for Chronic Disease Prevention and Health Promotion. *Physical Activity*. Available at http://www.cdc.gov/physicalactivity/. Accessed May 10, 2010.

Beasley, J. Earning administrative support. In: Edelstein, S. ed. *Nutrition in Public Health: A Handbook for Developing Programs and Service*, 2nd ed. Sudbury, MA: Jones and Bartlett Publishers; 2006:757–766.

Endsley S. *Innovation in Action: A Practical Guide for Healthcare Teams*. St. Louis, MO: Wiley-Blackwell; 2010.

Liebler JG, McConnell CR. Planning. In: JG Liebler, CR McConnell, ed. *Management Principles for Health Professionals*. Gaithersburg, MD: Aspen; 2007:114–121.

Shortell SM, Kaluzny AD, eds. Organization theory and health services management. In: *Healthcare Management: Organization, Design, and Behavior*, 5th ed. Albany, NY: Delmar Thomson Learning; 2005:8–9.

U.S. Department of Health and Human Services. *Healthy People 2010: Understanding and Improving Health*, 2nd ed. Washington, DC: USDHHS. Available at http://www.healthypeople.gov/Publications/. Accessed June 11, 2010.

U.S. Department of Health and Human Services. *Healthy People 2020: Understanding and Improving Health*, 2nd ed. Washington, DC: USDHHS. Available at http://www.healthypeople.gov/Publications/. Accessed June 11, 2010.

CHAPTER 28

Striving for Excellence and Envisioning the Future

Marcia Thomas, MS, MPH, RD
Pamella Darby, MS, MPH, RD

READER OBJECTIVES

After studying this chapter and reflecting on the contents, you should be able to:

1. Identify the multidisciplinary roles of the public health nutritionist.
2. Describe the ways in which such roles help to advance public health nutrition efforts.
3. Suggest strategies for successful professional development.
4. Describe future challenges and ethical considerations facing public health nutritionists.

■ INTRODUCTION

The public health nutritionist has stepped into a 21st century full of both opportunities and challenges. On the one hand, there are an assortment of innovative technologies at our fingertips, technological advances in medicine, and improved methodologies for implementing and evaluating public health interventions. On the other hand, we live and work in communities struggling with obesity, food insecurity, chronic disease, lack of medical insurance, and health disparities. The current health environment leaves us with no other choice but to challenge ourselves professionally, constantly striving for excellence in the field of public health so that we may meet such challenges and advance our efforts.

The motivation to achieve excellence in our field should stem from an understanding that existing opportunities must be embraced in such a way as to foster collective action toward improving the nutritional status of populations. Such opportunities include utilization of innovative technologies, enhanced modes of communication and education, collaboration, advocacy, professional development, and academic training. Globally, health is on the forefront of political and social agendas, with an ever-increasing awareness and interest in food and nutrition. This chapter seeks to encourage today's nutritionists to confront with confidence the professional demands that arise, prepared to take on the many challenges of our field.

Multidisciplinary Roles of the Public Health Nutritionist

Most of us enter the field of public health nutrition with the goal of educating the public about healthy eating to prevent and manage illness and disease. What we find when we begin our work is that there is so much more than just food involved in teaching people how to eat well.

The Institute of Medicine's 2003 report, *The Future of the Public's Health in the 21st Century*, encourages a broad training and practice of public health "because integrated interdisciplinary teaching is important to the preparation of a well-trained workforce that is capable of addressing today's broad array of public health issues...."[1] To be effective leaders in today's dynamic health environment, public health nutritionists must take on multidisciplinary roles, often wearing different hats at the same time. Success in the field, which translates to public health action, requires that nutritionists be ready to serve as educators, researchers, and advocates throughout the course of their careers.

Nutrition Educator

A hat we all wear is that of nutrition educator, even though efforts occur on many levels and the characteristics of communities and population groups may vary. Needs assessments therefore prove invaluable to community nutrition activities and help to provide a framework for program planning and evaluation. From considering the location of super-

Evidence-based practice: Utilizing nutritional information that is based on scientific studies from reputable sources.

markets to cultural beliefs about food and health, ongoing assessment is necessary to understand how to begin and maintain work within populations and communities.

In a time when such huge health disparities exist, public health nutritionists must take on the role of educating the public about those inequalities and helping to move communities towards healthier behaviors. We know that the public values the role of nutrition in prevention of disease, but making dietary changes has proved difficult.[2] To improve results, nutritionists must be included in the planning, implementation, and evaluation of health promotion and disease prevention programs.[3] Furthermore, nutritionists in public health are in the uniquely qualified position to educate not only the lay public, but also other health professionals, policy makers, the media, and private organizations about evidence-based practice.

Nutrition Researcher

Nutritionists in public health settings should also wear the hat of researcher. Investigation is critical to our understanding of the many nutritional concerns and risk factors facing our communities and vital to the development of effective public health practice and interventions. Through dissemination of research, we can reach a larger audience (via publications, presentations, and media) by sharing findings and recommendations for practice to colleagues, policy makers, and the general public.

Not all nutritionists focus full-time on research or become part of large, multidisciplinary studies, such as working as epidemiologists, in academia, or in research centers. Many are involved in research activities that are intertwined in ongoing work such as program evaluation, assessment of intervention effectiveness, or focus groups to qualitatively assess a population of interest. The information collected from nutritionists working within small, local community programs can be extremely valuable to others working within similar environments and may direct work done within a larger population. Frequently, public health nutritionists collect data but never share their results with others. Program evaluations, small quality assurance projects, and lessons learned from building partnerships should all

be shared with the rest of the field and may be just what is needed to help drive future research. In almost all settings, nutritionists can engage in various levels of research, either independently or collaboratively. Nutritionists are encouraged to collect data, as data directs policy and policy drives action. It is our responsibility as public health nutritionists to ensure that policy favors optimal nutrition for all populations. Evidence-based practice is the cornerstone of all health-related initiatives and, therefore, the successful public health nutritionist should look at research as a means to turn obstacles into opportunities.

The hallmark of public health inquiry is community-based participatory research (CBPR). CBPR emerged in the past few decades to become a focus of public health research. CBPR differs from community research in that partnerships are built among multidisciplinary teams, where members of the community are active partners in all aspects of the research and have equal weight in the research process. Partners bring their own expertise and interest to the group and view the health problem from their own perspective. By looking at health problems from the community level, we can focus on the social, cultural, and physical environment and, hopefully, come closer to creating healthy and sustainable communities.[4]

Nutrition Advocate

A third hat worn by nutritionists is that of advocate. Nutritionists have the responsibility to push their ideas forward. For example, nutritionists advocate for the following:

- Elimination of health disparities
- Equal access to nutrition services for all who need them
- Inclusion of nutrition professionals in multidisciplinary teams
- Improved nutrition reimbursement for services
- Increased funding for nutrition programs and community resources

For nutritionists to be heard, we need to stand up for our services and ensure that nutrition professionals are in the position of providing necessary information to the public.

Education in Public Health and Nutrition

Given the advances in public health and the complexity of our nutrition environment, a formal education in both nutrition and public health prepares professionals to meet the dynamic challenges presented locally and internationally. Increasingly, community nutrition jobs seek candidates who are registered dietitians (RD) and who possess advanced training in public health. This combination ensures that the professional has a rooted knowledge of nutrition science, expertise in clinical assessment and nutrition education, and can combine such principles with socioeconomic determinants to improve nutrition in community settings. Although degrees in both nutrition and public health are not required to work in the field of public health, such credentials will increase one's credibility in the job market and allow for advancement in the field.

Both schools of public health and programs in public health provide the primary professional degree for nutritionists seeking public health training, the Master of Public Health degree (MPH). The MPH degree trains professionals to approach health problems with an ecological framework, wedding biological risk factors with behavioral, social, and environmental determinants. Although they vary by program, areas of specialization are offered and several programs offer a concentration specifically in public health nutrition. In addition to one's area of specialization and fieldwork, there are five core components of a public health degree: biostatistics, epidemiology, health services administration, environmental health, and social and behavioral sciences. In recognition of the ongoing evolution and complexity of such determinants of health, the Institute of Medicine's (IOM) Committee on Educating Public Health Professionals for the 21st Century has recently identified eight additional areas that will benefit the trained public health workforce: informatics, genomics, communication, cultural competence, community-based participatory research, policy and law, global health, and ethics.[5] Many programs have already incorporated these new areas of public health into their existing coursework, and it is likely that in the future all public health programs will be required to include these components in their curriculum. (In addition, several other college degree and university programs have been developed that also share the goals of health promotion and public health.) For those wishing to pursue further advanced training in public health research and leadership, doctoral degrees are available (either PhD or DrPH).

Several systems are in place to monitor and assess the quality of public health educational programs. The Council on Education for Public Health (CEPH) was created in 1974 by the American Public Health Association (APHA) and the Association of Schools of Public Health (ASPH) to accredit schools and programs of public health.[6] CEPH is recognized by the U.S. Department of Education and was established to serve the community by ensuring that graduates of public health programs are adequately prepared to serve as leaders in public health.

In response to an increasing need for adequate education of our future public health workforce, the Council on Linkages between Academia and Public Health Practice (composed of public health leaders in the community and academia) developed Core Competencies for Public Health Professionals in 2001.[7] The skill set provides specific competencies in the following eight areas:

1. Analytical assessment
2. Policy development/program planning
3. Communication
4. Cultural competency
5. Community dimensions of practice
6. Basic public health sciences
7. Financial planning and management
8. Leadership and systems thinking

The skill sets are further divided by professional level—front line, senior level, and supervisory/management staff—and have been acknowledged by the Centers for Disease Control and Prevention (CDC) and the APHA. In addition, the Association of Graduate Programs in Public Health Nutrition, Inc. (AGPPHN) developed the *Strategies for Success: Curriculum Guide* to provide a recommended framework for the content of graduate-level public health nutrition programs.[8] Like the *Core Competencies for Public Health Professionals*, the *Curriculum Guide* provides a skill set, but is specific to public health nutrition curriculum, including:

- Knowledge and skills
- Food and nutrition sciences
- Research and evaluation
- Communication and culture
- Management and leadership
- Public health fieldwork

■ IMPORTANCE OF PROFESSIONAL DEVELOPMENT

Throughout this book, we have discussed the various roles of the nutritionist and the impact that public health efforts can have on improving the health of communities. To ensure that those efforts have a positive and lasting impact, adequate and ongoing training of the public health workforce is essential.[9,10] Advances in research, epidemiology, and technologies have increased our awareness of the prevalence and burden of diseases and associated risk factors. At the same time, progress in intervention and evaluation methodologies, social marketing, and health promotion have allowed us to move forward in effecting positive change within our communities. A combination of public health training and ongoing professional development will equip the nutrition workforce with the tools needed to take an active role in such complex efforts.

Keeping Abreast of Current Knowledge

As with all health professionals, it is imperative that nutritionists working in public health stay abreast of current events, advancements in nutrition knowledge, and ongoing public health activities in order to serve the community effectively. Although nutrition and public health education provides the necessary foundation upon which to build a successful career, the nutritionist is held accountable for maintaining and enhancing professional practice. This involves ongoing continuing education and participation in professional development. For example, the Commission on Dietetic Registration (CDR) requires that all dietitians report continuing professional development activities to maintain registration status. Through individualized self-assessment, dietitians identify ongoing strategies to ensure professional competence. Although there is no parallel monitoring system for MPH credentials, the Continuing Education Program of the APHA was established to "maintain and enhance professional knowledge, to increase technical proficiencies, and to enable members to promote and protect environmental and community health."[11]

Strategies for ongoing professional development include the following.

Membership in Professional Organizations

Membership in professional organizations such as the ADA and the APHA provides public health professionals with numerous opportunities for professional development through:

- Continuing education activities
- Professional committees
- Discussion groups
- Professional meetings
- Scholarly publications
- Professional resources and networks

The ADA supports numerous professional interest groups (dietetic practice groups or DPGs), which allow nutrition professionals to be active in specific areas of nutrition. Several DPGs of the ADA may be of particular interest to public health professionals, including Hunger and Environmental Nutrition, Nutrition Education for the Public, Public Health/Community Nutrition, and School Nutrition Services. APHA members can choose from 25 discipline-based sections and 7 special primary interest groups (SPIGs), including the APHA's Food and Nutrition Section. In addition to national organizations, there are numerous state and local professional societies, including affiliates of both the ADA and the APHA. Through professional memberships, nutritionists not only stay informed of current events in the field, but also build lasting professional and social networks.

> View the variety of available DPGs at http://www.eatright.org.

Listservs

Listservs are an efficient and convenient way of keeping up with the latest news and activities surrounding nutrition and public health. They provide information on the latest media news, journal articles, policy actions, and upcoming events in public health. Many international, national, and local agencies allow both professionals and the general public to join distribution lists. Examples of listservs of interest include:

- Agency for Healthcare Research and Quality: http://www.ahrq.gov/
- The American Dietetic Association: For members only, http://www.eatright.org/
- The Centers for Disease Control and Prevention: Includes the Morbidity and Mortality Weekly Report and National Health and Nutrition Examination Survey, http://www.cdc.gov/subscribe.html
- International Food Policy Research Institute: http://www.ifpri.org
- National Institutes of Health: http://list.nih.gov
- U.S. Department of Health and Human Services: http://www.usda.gov
- U.S. Food and Drug Administration: http://www.fda.gov
- World Health Organization Weekly Epidemiological Record: http://www.who.int/wer/en/
- World Health News, Harvard School of Public Health: http://www.worldhealthnews.harvard.edu

Obviously, these are just a few examples. To avoid being overwhelmed with e-mails, listserv memberships should be individually prioritized to those that are most useful. Also, many listservs permit members to customize e-mails, allowing you to choose the number and/or content of notifications received.

Conferences, Lectures, and Workshops

Conferences, lectures, and workshops are another way to stay abreast of the latest news and research in the field; gain insight into new, innovative public health interventions and activities; network and build valuable resources; and share best practices among colleagues. In addition to annual meetings of larger organizations, nutritionists should take advantage of the many workshops, meetings, and lectures that take place on a variety of public health topics throughout the year. Listservs, journals, and Web sites (both the ADA[12] and the APHA[13] provide a calendar of events on their Web sites) serve as excellent resources for upcoming public health events.

Journals and Public Health Publications

Peer-reviewed articles and other public health publications provide a rich source of knowledge on the latest research, insights, and lessons learned in practice. To engage in interdisciplinary dialogue, nutritionists should embrace a wide variety of topics and be aware of the various perspectives shaping public health systems in the current social, medical, and political environment. Furthermore, by keeping up with recent publications, the nutritionist can help to separate fact from fiction when nutrition information reaches the general public.

Academic Courses and/or Programs

Public health is an evolving discipline with ever-emerging methodologies and practices. When possible, the public health nutritionist should consider strengthening his or her current state of knowledge with additional coursework in public health or nutrition programs. For example, you might enhance your current job performance through additional training in language and culture, computer and Internet technologies, communications and media, or research and statistical methodologies. If you do not have formal training in public health as mentioned previously, you should strongly consider advanced training through graduate or certificate public health programs. Formal education in public health prepares the nutrition workforce to meet the challenges of complex health issues facing communities, adds credibility and marketability to professional pursuits, and provides the skills necessary to advance to leadership roles in agencies or organizations.

Maintaining Political Awareness

Much of public health action is influenced by politics, so it is critical that nutritionists stay abreast of current events and the political environment. Although some nutritionists may be directly involved in the political scene through advocacy and grassroots efforts, all nutritionists are affected in some way by political agendas, perhaps through funding, changes in school policies, insurance reimbursement, or community resources. Many professional organizations provide resources through Web sites and listservs that keep members informed of political action and policy development. Newspapers and political publications should be included in the list of resources for all public health nutritionists.

Utilizing Technology

Technological improvements have made the 21st century an exciting time to practice public health. In addition to new advancements in science and medicine, the public health workforce is witnessing innovations in surveillance, communication, and geographic information systems (GIS). As they become mainstream, utilization of such technologies will be important for all public health professionals in order to fully participate in professional activities. Based on the IOM report on preparing the public health workforce, it is likely that more and more educational programs in public health will require such instruction as part of their curriculum. In the meantime, most colleges and universities as well as government public health agencies provide opportunities for training in computer programs, GIS, statistics, surveillance, and Web design.

Collaborations

One of the most significant strategies for professional advancement is through partnerships and collaboration. Collaboration allows for a synergistic approach to public health issues, pulling together the skills and resources of multiple parties to improve the health of populations, which is the ultimate goal of public health professionals. Through professional and community partnerships, nutritionists can augment individual resources, ideas, and political momentum to accomplish a greater good than by acting alone. Such collaborations lead to creative, comprehensive, practical, and transformative thinking.[14] In addition, partnering with the community helps to foster trust and empowerment, thereby allowing for the implementation of community-based interventions that improve health outcomes. As the health of communities improves, especially when the community members themselves actively participate in the process, trust between the health professional and the community is likely to be further strengthened. The cycle thus continues, leading to the potential formation of additional collaborations.

To encourage sustainable action, partnerships should exist beyond the professional circle to welcome community participation. Depending on the desired outcome and goal, nutritionists should seek collaborations with community leaders and community-based organizations, school administrators, universities, government officials and policy makers, parent groups, and private organizations and businesses. The more people on the same team, the easier it will be to build trust, and the more consistent the messages to the public.

■ FUTURE CHALLENGES IN PUBLIC HEALTH NUTRITION

Continuing Issues for Discussion

As we move into the future and find an older, more inactive population, higher rates of chronic disease, and enormous health disparities, nutritionists must serve as authorities on nutrition issues and be ready to jump into the solution of the health problems facing our world today. As we forge ahead with scientific and technological advances in health improvement, ethical issues emerge in many aspects of public health practice. As we decide on a research objective or a treatment/prevention protocol, we must think about the moral values and implications involved in the decisions. We should know the issues, the differing opinions, and where we, and the community, stand on these ethical questions.

According to the University of Pittsburgh's Center for Bioethics and Health Law[15]:

Technology has changed the very boundaries and possibilities of life. Scientific discoveries have blurred the traditional distinctions among birth, life and death as well as given us a vast array of new treatments to combat pain and suffering.

For example, as we move forward with genomics, what will that mean for nutritional science? Will we no longer need to change our behaviors to prevent disease? Will parents want to test their unborn babies for unwanted chronic diseases?

Many current-day issues, not quite as obvious as the aforementioned questions, provide examples of ethical dilemmas that we face on a regular basis:

1. Who should provide nutrition education to the public: nutrition professionals, the media, government, physician groups, or private industry? What is the responsibility of government in ensuring appropriate nutrition care for the public?
2. Given the increasing rates of childhood obesity, what are the implications for children of food advertising on television? Should the food industry have a role in the prevention of childhood obesity?
3. Despite the rise in obesity, there are still a large number of food-insecure households. Who is responsible for ensuring that all Americans have access to enough food?
4. Given technological advances, should genetically modified foods be sold in the marketplace? If so, does the public have the right to know if their food is genetically altered?
5. As we face a new era where the public health workforce is increasingly involved in bioterrorism preparedness, how are public health nutritionists being trained to ensure the safety of our food and water supply?
6. What role does the government play in regulating our food choices? Does the government have an obligation to step in and, if so, how far?
7. In an aging society with rising healthcare costs, are the elderly being forced to choose between adequate nutrition and health care? How are public health nutritionists working as advocates for our seniors?

Public health nutrition is a dynamic and exciting field. Its issues challenge us daily and allow us to grow and develop in ways we may not have imagined when we selected this career path as students. Public health allows us to deal with complex issues, technology, an ever-changing environment, and ethical issues, all of which present new opportunities. In order to meet the demands of the field, we need to be prepared for the associated challenges. Our work places us in a unique position where we are able to inform on food and nutrition policy, advocate for nutrition services, serve as media spokespeople, and help create healthier communities. The rigorous training and life experiences should enable us to survive and thrive in this dynamic field.

References

1. Institute of Medicine. *The Future of the Public's Health in the 21st Century*. Washington, DC: The National Academy Press; 2003:366.
2. O'Sullivan Maillet J, Borra ST, Niedert K, et al. Dietetics in 2017: what does the future hold? *J Am Diet Assoc*. 2002;102:1404–1406.
3. American Dietetic Association. Position of the American Dietetic Association: the role of dietetics professionals in health promotion and disease prevention. *J Am Diet Assoc*. 2002;102:1680–1687.
4. Israel BA, Schulz AJ, Parker EA, Becker AB. Review of community-based research: assessing partnership approaches to improve public health. *Annu Rev Public Health*. 1998;19:173–202.
5. Gebbie E, Rosenstock L, Hernandez LM, eds. *Who Will Keep the Public Healthy? Educating Public Health Professionals for the 21st Century*. Washington, DC: The National Academy Press; 2003.
6. Council on Education for Public Health (CEPH). *About CEPH*. Available at http://www.ceph.org/i4a/pages/index.cfm?pageid=3274. Accessed June 5, 2010.
7. Public Health Foundation, Council on Linkages. *Core Competencies for Public Health Professionals*. Available at http://www.phf.org/link/corecompetencies.htm. Accessed June 5, 2010.
8. Association of Graduate Programs in Public Health Nutrition, Inc. *Strategies for Success: Curriculum Guide*, 2nd ed. Available at http://nutrition.utk.edu/resources/StrategiesForSuccess.pdf. Accessed June 5, 2010.
9. U.S. Department of Health and Human Services. *The Public Health Workforce: An Agenda for the 21st Century*. Available at http://www.health.gov/phfunctions/pubhlth.pdf. Accessed June 5, 2010.
10. Centers for Disease Control and Prevention. *Task Force Report on Public Health Workforce Development*. Available at www.health.gov/phfunctions/pubhlth.pdf. Accessed May 18, 2010.
11. American Public Health Association. *Continuing Education Program Mission Statement*. Available at http://www.apha.org/programs/education/. Accessed June 5, 2010.
12. American Dietetic Association. *Calendar of Events*. Available at http://www.eatright.org. Accessed June 5, 2010.
13. American Public Health Association. *Calendar of Events*. Available at http://www.apha.org/meetings/. Accessed May 11, 2009.
14. Lasker RD, Weiss ES, Miller R. Partnership synergy: a practical framework for studying and strengthening the collaborative advantage. *Millbank Q*. 2001;79:179–205.
15. University of Pittsburgh's Center for Bioethics and Health Law. *Overview*. Available at http://www.pitt.edu/~bioethic/overview.htm. Accessed June 5, 2010.

Helpful Nutrition Web Sites

Aim for a Healthy Weight
  Patient and public education materials from the
  National Heart, Lung, and Blood Institute.
  http://www.nhlbi.nih.gov/health/public/heart/
  obesity/lose_wt/

Centers for Disease Control and Prevention (CDC)
Health Topics: Nutrition
  Fact sheets on various nutrition topics, from the
  Centers for Disease Control and Prevention.
  http://www.cdc.gov/nutrition/index.html

CDC's Nutrition and Physical Activity Program
  Addresses the role of nutrition and physical activity
  in health promotion and the prevention and control
  of chronic diseases.
  http://www.cdc.gov/nccdphp/dnpao

Center for Science in the Public Interest
  Health and nutrition information.
  http://www.cspinet.org

Consumer Nutrition and Health Information
  Nutrition and health information from the Food
  and Drug Administration.
  http://www.cfsan.fda.gov/ ~ dms/lab-cons.html

Dietary Guidelines for Americans
  Recommended Dietary Guidelines from the U.S.
  Department of Health and Human Services and the
  U.S. Department of Agriculture.
  http://www.health.gov/dietaryguidelines

Food and Nutrition Information Center (FNIC)
  Located at the National Agricultural Library,
  collects and disseminates information about food
  and human nutrition.
  http://www.nal.usda.gov/fnic

Health Information: Weight Loss and Control
  The National Institute of Diabetes and Digestive
  and Kidney Diseases of the National Institutes of
  Health provides information on obesity, weight
  control, physical activity, and nutrition.
  http://www.niddk.nih.gov/health/nutrit/
  nutrit.htm

Healthfinder: Obesity
  Links to a variety of sites on obesity.
  http://www.healthfinder.gov/scripts/
  SearchContext.asp?topic = 592

MEDLINEplus
  Nutrition
  http://www.nlm.nih.gov/medlineplus/nutrition.html
  Obesity
  http://www.nlm.nih.gov/medlineplus/obesity.html
  Weight Loss and Dieting
  http://www.nlm.nih.gov/medlineplus/ency/article/
  001940.htm

Nutrition.gov
  A guide to nutrition and health information on
  federal government websites.
  http://www.nutrition.gov

Obesity Education Initiative Web Site
  Information for health professionals and the public,
  from the National Heart, Lung, and Blood Institute.
  http://www.nhlbi.nih.gov/health/public/heart/
  obesity/lose_wt

Overweight and Obesity
  Information on trends and health consequences of
  obesity, from the Centers for Disease Control and
  Prevention (CDC).
  http://www.cdc.gov/nccdphp/dnpa/obesity/
  index.htm

The American Dietetic Association
  An organization of food and nutrition professionals,
  ADA's mission is to promote optimal nutrition and
  well-being for all people.
  http://www.eatright.org

Weight Loss and Nutrition Myths
  Corrections to common myths about dieting and
  nutrition.
  http://www.niddk.nih.gov/health/nutrit/pubs/
  myths/index.htm

Public Health Nutrition List
  Preventive and primary nutrition services and
  public health nutrition core functions.
  Message: subscribe PHNUTR-L your-name.
  subscribe to: http://listproc@u.washington.edu

APPENDIX

B

State Health Department Web Sites

TABLE B-1 — State Health Department Web Sites

State	Web site	State	Web site
Alabama	http://www.adph.org	Missouri	http://www.health.state.mo.us
Alaska	http://www.hss.state.ak.us/dph	Montana	http://www.dphhs.state.mt.us
Arizona	http://www.hs.state.az.us	Nebraska	http://www.hhs.state.ne.us
Arkansas	http://www.healthyarkansas.com	Nevada	http://www.hr.state.nv.us
California	http://www.dhs.cahwnet.gov	New Hampshire	http://www.dhhs.state.nh.us
Colorado	http://www.cdphe.state.co.us/cdphehom.asp	New Jersey	http://www.state.nj.us/health
Connecticut	http://www.state.ct.us/dph	New Mexico	http://www.health.state.nm.us
Delaware	http://www.state.de.us/dhss/dph/index.htm	New York	http://www.health.state.ny.us
District of Columbia	http://dchealth.dc.gov/index.asp	North Carolina	http://www.state.nc.us/DHR
		North Dakota	http://www.health.state.nd.us
Florida	http://www.doh.state.fl.us	Ohio	http://www.odh.state.oh.us
Georgia	http://www.ph.dhr.state.ga.us	Oklahoma	http://www.health.state.ok.us
Hawaii	http://www.state.hi.us/health	Oregon	http://www.ohd.hr.state.or.us
Idaho	http://www2.state.id.us/dhw	Pennsylvania	http://www.health.state.pa.us
Illinois	http://www.idph.state.il.us	Rhode Island	http://www.health.state.ri.us
Indiana	http://www.state.in.us/isdh	South Carolina	http://www.scdhec.net
Iowa	http://www.idph.state.ia.us/default.asp	South Dakota	http://www.state.sd.us/doh/index.htm
Kansas	http://www.ink.org/public/kdhe	Tennessee	http://www.state.tn.us/health
Kentucky	http://chs.ky.gov/publichealth	Texas	http://www.tdh.state.tx.us
Louisiana	http://www.dhh.state.la.us	Utah	http://hlunix.hl.state.ut.us
Maine	http://www.state.me.us/dhs/boh/index.htm	Vermont	http://www.healthyvermonters.info
Maryland	http://www.dhmh.state.md.us	Virginia	http://www.vdh.state.va.us
Massachusetts	http://www.state.ma.us/dph/dphhome.htm	Washington	http://www.doh.wa.gov
Michigan	http://www.michigan.gov/mdch	West Virginia	http://www.wvdhhr.org
Minnesota	http://www.health.state.mn.us	Wisconsin	http://www.dhfs.state.wi.us
Mississippi	http://www.msdh.state.ms.us	Wyoming	http://wdhfs.state.wy.us/wdh

APPENDIX C

Learning Activities

CAROL E. O'NEIL, PHD, MPH, LDN, RD

THERESA A. NICKLAS, DRPH

■ LEARNING ACTIVITIES

1. Learn more about the science behind the U.S. *Dietary Guidelines for Americans* and how to teach the guidelines to the public through the online course at: http://www.health.gov/DietaryGuidelines/. Then work with your instructor to develop a lesson plan to deliver (and evaluate) to a community group, such as a school. This is called *service-learning*. To find out more about service-learning, go to The National Service-Learning Clearinghouse: http://www.service learning.org or to your university's service-learning office. If you work with children, check out this Web site for ideas for nutrition and kids: http://www.nal. usda.gov/fnic/etext/000100.html.

2. It is easy for nutrition students and health professionals to understand the food label and to monitor changes. It's not so easy for most consumers to understand the nuances, and it's not so easy for students or entry-level practitioners to explain it. To be sure you understand the nutrition label and everything it has to offer, go to http://www.cfsan.fda.gov/~dms/foodlab.html; then design, execute, and evaluate a lesson to another community group. You also could work with a local high school to teach the food label, or help them learn how to teach it to a younger group. At http://ific.org/ publications/other/tnfl.cfm, a food label education program for high school students is available from the International Food Information Council.

3. What else could you do? Work with your instructor to write up this experience for publication! For example, *The American Biology Teacher* is a nationally recognized journal that provides specific how-to suggestions for the classroom and laboratory, field activities, interdisciplinary programs, and articles on recent advances in biology and life science. You, your group, and your teacher could write about this project for publication. Your paper might be part of the science base that is used to set nutrition policy.

4. Much of Chapter 2 was devoted to discussing nutrition policy: how it is developed and how it is changed. In a presentation, choose a policy to explain to a group—your classmates or community stakeholders— and discuss how this policy has changed or can be changed to reflect current science and consumer issues.

5. Discuss the importance of the food label as a health education tool. Explain how scientific evidence is used to support each health claim that can be used on a food label and why it is so difficult to have health claims added to labels for given foods. Could (should) this process be shortened? For validated claims, think about how you would integrate specific foods into a client's diet or into consumer health messages.

6. Read and evaluate the article by Dr. Marlene Most (*J Amer Diet Assoc* 2003;103:729–735) on controlled feeding studies. She provides information on the knowledge and skills that dietetics professionals must have to do these studies, including suggestions for working with study participants. Discuss how you would work with clients that you would be counseling.

7. DASH and DASH sodium were landmark studies on how behavioral change can improve hypertension and, subsequently, health. Explain the science behind the DASH diet, what other potential beneficial effects this blood pressure–lowering diet can have, and how you can bring the DASH diet home to your clients.

8. Many agencies promulgate similar recommendations. Prepare a table or chart looking at the similarities and differences in the recommendations of the American Heart Association, the National Cancer Institute, The National Cholesterol Education Program, Healthy People 2020, and the *2010 Dietary Guidelines*. Explain how some of the differences are tailored to each agency's specific target audience.

Index

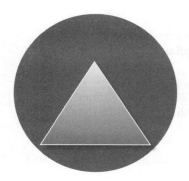

Photo Credits

Chapter 22
Page 342 © BananaStock/Alamy Images

Chapter 23
Page 356 © Endostock/Dreamstime.com;
page 357 © Photodisc

Chapter 24
Page 367 © PhotoCreate/ShutterStock, Inc.;
page 370 © Photodisc

Chapter 25
Page 382 © Photodisc

Chapter 26
Page 389 © Jack Kunnen/Dreamstime.com;
page 393 © Andresr/ShutterStock, Inc.

Chapter 27
Page 401 (right) © Dmitriy Shironosov/ShutterStock, Inc.;
page 402 © Damian Palus/ShutterStock, Inc.

Chapter 28
Page 405 © Monkey Business Images/ShutterStock, Inc.;
page 408 © Photodisc